Workbook for

Radiographic Image Analysis

Fourth Edition

Kathy McQuillen Martensen, MA, RT(R)
Instructional Service Specialist, Radiologic Technology Education
University of Iowa Hospitals and Clinics
Iowa City, Iowa

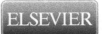

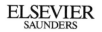

ELSEVIER
SAUNDERS

3251 Riverport Lane
St. Louis, Missouri 63043

WORKBOOK FOR RADIOGRAPHIC IMAGE ANALYSIS,
FOURTH EDITION

ISBN: 978-0-323-28071-6

Copyright © 2015, 2011, 2006, 1996 by Saunders, an imprint of Elsevier Inc. All rights reserved.

All rights reserved. No part of this publication may be reproduced or transmitted in any form or by any means, electronic or mechanical, including photocopying, recording, or any information storage and retrieval system, without permission in writing from the publisher. Details on how to seek permission, further information about the Publisher's permissions policies and our arrangements with organizations such as the Copyright Clearance Center and the Copyright Licensing Agency, can be found at our website: www.elsevier.com/permissions.

This book and the individual contributions contained in it are protected under copyright by the Publisher (other than as may be noted herein).

Notices

Knowledge and best practice in this field are constantly changing. As new research and experience broaden our understanding, changes in research methods, professional practices, or medical treatment may become necessary.

Practitioners and researchers must always rely on their own experience and knowledge in evaluating and using any information, methods, compounds, or experiments described herein. In using such information or methods they should be mindful of their own safety and the safety of others, including parties for whom they have a professional responsibility.

With respect to any drug or pharmaceutical products identified, readers are advised to check the most current information provided (i) on procedures featured or (ii) by the manufacturer of each product to be administered, to verify the recommended dose or formula, the method and duration of administration, and contraindications. It is the responsibility of practitioners, relying on their own experience and knowledge of their patients, to make diagnoses, to determine dosages and the best treatment for each individual patient, and to take all appropriate safety precautions.

To the fullest extent of the law, neither the Publisher nor the authors, contributors, or editors, assume any liability for any injury and/or damage to persons or property as a matter of products liability, negligence or otherwise, or from any use or operation of any methods, products, instructions, or ideas contained in the material herein.

Transferred to Digital Printing 2018

Content Strategist: Sonya Seigafuse
Content Development Manager: Laurie Gower
Content Development Specialist: Charlene Ketchum
Publishing Services Manager: Hemamalini Rajendrababu
Project Manager: Manchu Mohan/Kiruthiga Kasthuriswamy
Cover designer: Gopalakrishnan Venkatram

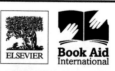

Working together
to grow libraries in
developing countries

www.elsevier.com • www.bookaid.org

Preface

This workbook has been designed to provide students with a means of testing their understanding of the information covered in the *Radiographic Image Analysis* textbook. It follows the same format as the textbook with the first two chapters focusing on the image analysis guidelines, and technical and digital imaging concepts that are considered when all procedures are evaluated for quality. The workbook includes questions and images to evaluate for each of the image analysis guidelines, and technical and digital concepts presented in the first two chapters of *Radiographic Image Analysis*. The remaining chapters guide the student through the image-analysis procedural process of each body structure in a systematic fashion. The chapters can be followed as written, or the student may skip from chapter to chapter or procedure to procedure.

For these chapters, the workbook provides the following features for each procedure presented:

- Study questions that focus on how the patient should be positioned to obtain an accurately positioned projection and what guidelines should be present when proper positioning is obtained. Also, some questions concentrate on improperly positioned projections. The student is asked to state how the patient, CR, or IR was mispositioned to obtain such a projection.
- Poorly positioned projections that separately focus on each topic and procedure. The images are different from those found in the textbook and sometimes present multiple positioning problems. Nonroutine scenarios are also presented.
- Answer keys to the study questions at the end of the workbook.

STUDENT GUIDELINES

Prerequisite: It is suggested that a course in anatomy and basic medical terminology be taken before studying radiographic procedures and analysis. For best understanding, it is effective to study the radiographic procedure in conjunction with the analysis.

Guideline 1: Read the learning objectives provided in the *Radiographic Image Analysis* textbook for the chapter being studied. These objectives outline key issues within the chapter and identify the knowledge you should understand after the chapter has been studied.

Guideline 2: Read the corresponding chapter in *Radiographic Image Analysis* and attend the procedure and analysis courses that focus on the subject matter.

Guideline 3: Fill in as many of the study question blanks as you can without referring to the textbook or the workbook answer key. Any blanks that you were unable to complete indicate the areas that require further study. If you left any questions unanswered or if you were uncertain of the correct answers, restudy the information covered in those questions.

Guideline 4: Check your study question answers with the answers provided at the end of the workbook. Restudy the information covered in any questions you answered incorrectly.

Guideline 5: Consult with your instructor about taking a final examination.

Copyright © 2015, 2011, 2006, 1996 by Saunders, an imprint of Elsevier Inc. All rights reserved.

Reviewers

Laura Aaron, PhD, RT(R)(M)(QM), FASRT
Director & Professor School of Allied Health
Northwestern State University of Louisiana
Shreveport, LA

Becky Farmer, MSRS, RT(R)(M)
Associate Professor of Allied Health and
Radiologic Science
Northwestern State University
Shreveport, LA

Copyright © 2015, 2011, 2006, 1996 by Saunders, an imprint of Elsevier Inc. All rights reserved.

Contents

Copyright © 2015, 2011, 2006, 1996 by Saunders, an imprint of Elsevier Inc. All rights reserved.

1 Guidelines for Image Analysis

1. An optimal radiographic image demonstrates what desired features?

   A. _____

   B. _____

   C. _____

   D. _____

   E. _____

   F. _____

   G. _____

Using the Key Terms listed at the beginning of Chapter 1 in the *Radiographic Image Analysis* textbook, complete the following.

2. Use the lateral chest drawing in Figure 1-1 to complete the following statements.

   Figure 1-1

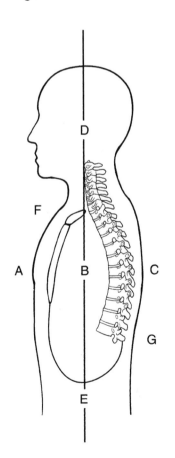

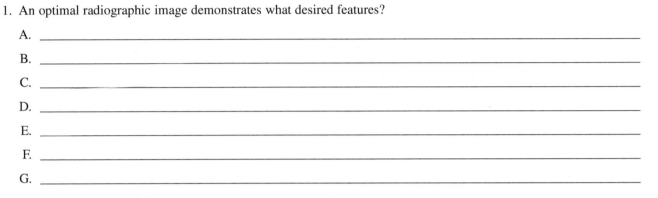

A. Letter B is situated on the _____ plane.

B. Letter A is placed _____ to letter B.

C. Letter C is placed _____ to letter B.

D. Letter D is placed _____ to letter B.

E. Letter E is placed _____ to letter B.

F. Letter F is placed _____ to letter B.

G. Letter G is placed _____ to letter B.

Copyright © 2015, 2011, 2006, 1996 by Saunders, an imprint of Elsevier Inc. All rights reserved.

3. The inferior scapular angle moves toward the front and outer edge of the body when the humerus is abducted. What combination of the positioning terms is used to describe this movement? _____

4. When the humerus is brought from an abducted position to the patient's side, the inferior scapular angle moves toward the patient's back and closer to the midsagittal plane. What combination of the positioning terms is used to describe this movement? _____

5. What combination of the positioning terms is used to describe the portion of the scapula that is positioned closest to the patient's front and head? _____

6. If the IR was placed against the lateral aspect of the patient's leg and the CR was centered to the medial aspect, what projection of the leg was taken? _____

7. Use the abdominal drawing in Figure 1-2 to complete the following statements.

Figure 1-2

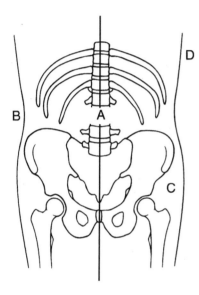

A. Letter A is situated on the _____ plane.

B. Letter B is placed _____ to letter A.

C. Letter A is placed _____ to letter B.

D. Letter C is placed _____ to letter A.

E. Letter D is placed _____ to letter A.

8. Use the drawing of the knee in Figure 1-3 to complete the following statements.

Figure 1-3

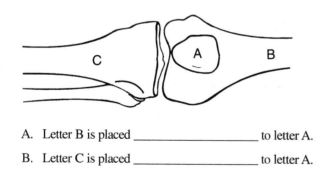

A. Letter B is placed _____ to letter A.

B. Letter C is placed _____ to letter A.

Chapter **1** **Guidelines for Image Analysis**　　　　Copyright © 2015, 2011, 2006, 1996 by Saunders, an imprint of Elsevier Inc. All rights reserved.

9. State the distances indicated in Figure 1-4.

Figure 1-4

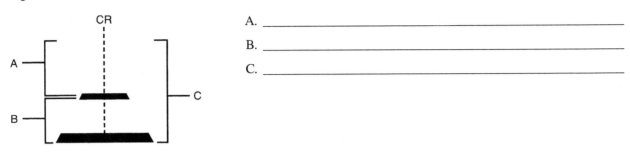

A. _____

B. _____

C. _____

10. Use the following (1 to 6) to define how radiographic projections of the listed body parts are accurately displayed on the monitor.
    1. Displayed as if the patient were standing upright
    2. Displayed as if hanging from the fingertips
    3. Displayed as if hanging from the shoulders
    4. Displayed as if hanging from the toes
    5. Displayed as if hanging from the hip
    6. Displayed as if hanging from the anterior surface

    A. _____ Chest

    B. _____ Wrist

    C. _____ Lumbar vertebrae

    D. _____ Humerus

    E. _____ Toes

    F. _____ Oblique foot

    G. _____ Lateral foot

    H. _____ Ankle

    I. _____ Lower leg

    J. _____ AP hip

    K. _____ Axiolateral shoulder

    L. _____ Cervical vertebrae

    M. _____ Abdomen

11. Evaluate the following projections for displaying accuracy.

    Figure 1-5

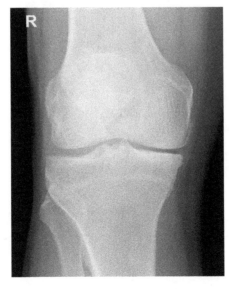

    A. AP knee (Figure 1-5): _____

    _____

Copyright © 2015, 2011, 2006, 1996 by Saunders, an imprint of Elsevier Inc. All rights reserved.   Chapter **1** **Guidelines for Image Analysis**

Figure 1-6

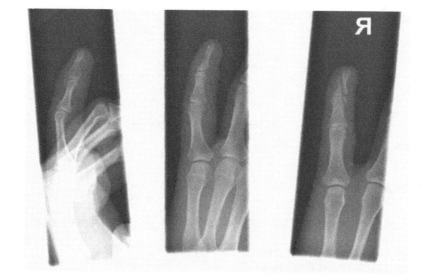

B. Right finger (Figure 1-6): _____

_____

Figure 1-7

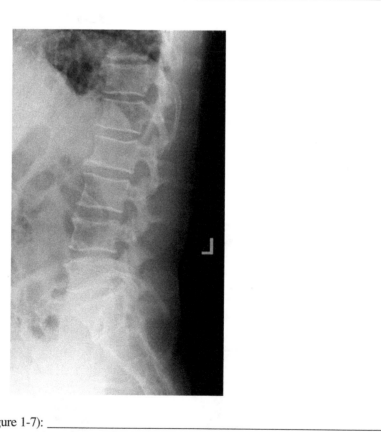

C. Left lateral lumbar vertebrae (Figure 1-7): _____

_____

  Copyright © 2015, 2011, 2006, 1996 by Saunders, an imprint of Elsevier Inc. All rights reserved.

Figure 1-8

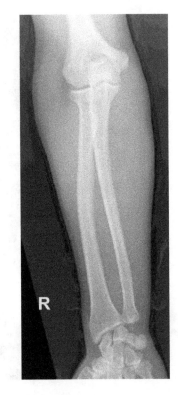

D. AP right forearm (Figure 1-8): _____

_____

Figure 1-9

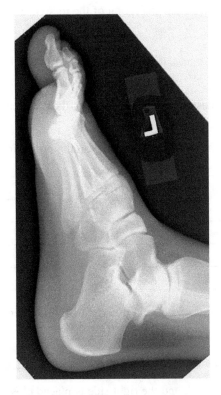

E. Mediolateral left foot (Figure 1-9): _____

_____

Copyright © 2015, 2011, 2006, 1996 by Saunders, an imprint of Elsevier Inc. All rights reserved.   Chapter **1** **Guidelines for Image Analysis**

Figure 1-10

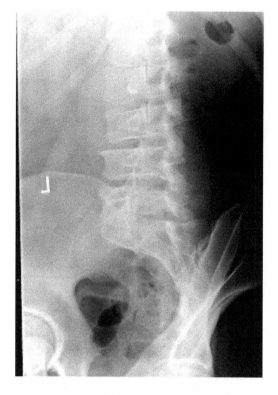

F. AP oblique (LPO) lumbar vertebrae (Figure 1-10): _____

_____

12. When an AP/PA projection or AP/PA oblique projection of the torso is accurately displayed, the patient's right side is on the viewer's _____ side.

13. When using the postprocessing contrast mask feature, only the unexposed areas are masked. _____ (True/False)

14. A projection that has had the contrast mask added and was saved to the PACS can be unmasked. _____ (True/False)

15. List the demographic information that should be displayed on the projection.

    A. _____

    B. _____

    C. _____

    D. _____

    E. _____

    F. _____

16. A. What marker is used for a patient who is placed in a right PA oblique projection (RAO position)?

    _____

    B. Where is the marker placed on the IR in reference to the patient?_____

17. A lateral vertebral projection is requested, and the right side is placed closest to the IR.

    A. What marker is used for a patient in this projection? _____

    B. Where is the marker placed on the IR in reference to the patient?_____

6

Copyright © 2015, 2011, 2006, 1996 by Saunders, an imprint of Elsevier Inc. All rights reserved.

18. Evaluate the following projections for marker placement accuracy.

Figure 1-11

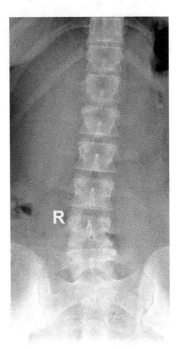

A. AP lumbar vertebrae (Figure 1-11): *Move as far laterally as possible, still collimating correctly*

Figure 1-12

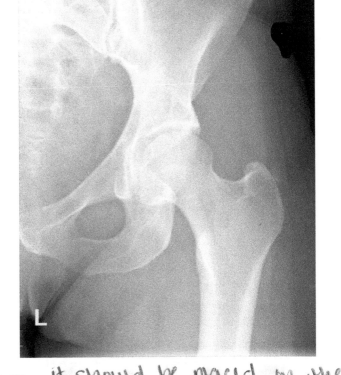

B. AP left hip (Figure 1-12): *It should be placed on the lateral side of the body*

Copyright © 2015, 2011, 2006, 1996 by Saunders, an imprint of Elsevier Inc. All rights reserved.

Chapter **1** **Guidelines for Image Analysis**

Figure 1-13

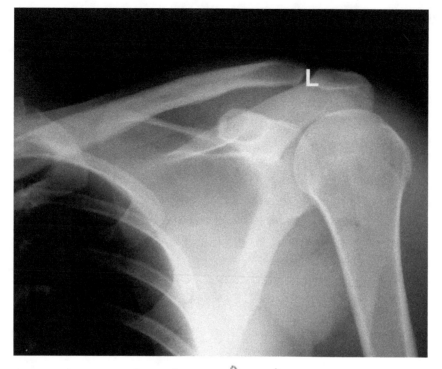

C. AP left shoulder (Figure 1-13): ___move as far laterally as___ ___possible out of the anatomy___

Figure 1-14

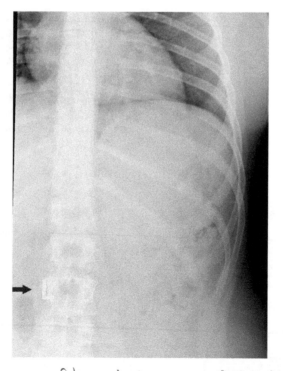

D. AP left lower ribs (Figure 1-14): ___Should be moved to the___ ___top left-lateral side___

  Copyright © 2015, 2011, 2006, 1996 by Saunders, an imprint of Elsevier Inc. All rights reserved.

Figure 1-15

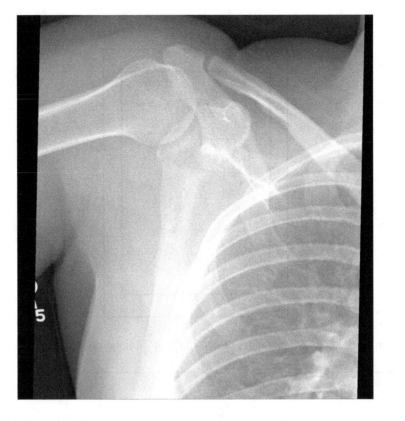

E. AP right scapula (Figure 1-15): _____

_____

19. The markers used in radiography are constructed of (A) ____lead____ and are (B) _radiopaque_ (radiolucent/radiopaque).

20. The marker placed on a lateral projection of the torso or skull represents the side of the patient that is positioned ____Closer to____ (closer to/farther from) the IR.

21. Place an R where the marker should be positioned on the hip diagram in Figure 1-16.

Figure 1-16

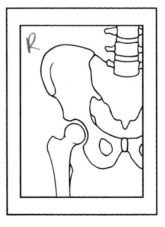

Copyright © 2015, 2011, 2006, 1996 by Saunders, an imprint of Elsevier Inc. All rights reserved.

Chapter **1** **Guidelines for Image Analysis**

22. Place an L where the marker should be positioned on the lateral sacral diagram in Figure 1-17.

Figure 1-17

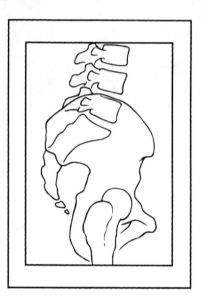

23. How is the projection marked when a patient is placed in an AP oblique projection (LPO or RPO positions)?

_____

_____

24. What procedure is followed when the marker has not been demonstrated within the exposure field but is only faintly seen along its border?

_____

25. The actual area of the IR that is needed to define the VOI is determined by accurate _____

centering and good _____.

26. The smallest possible IR cassette is chosen when using the computer radiography digital system to produce a projection with maximum spatial resolution. _____ *true* _____ (True/False)

27. What is the size of the IR on DR systems?
_____ *14 X 17*

28. Describe why it is necessary to have the IR extend beyond the joint spaces by 1 to 2 inches (2.5 to 5 cm) when imaging long bones, such as the forearm, humerus, lower leg, and femur.
    So the beam doesn't throw the joint off the image receptor

Copyright © 2015, 2011, 2006, 1996 by Saunders, an imprint of Elsevier Inc. All rights reserved.

29. Evaluate the accuracy of the placement of the anatomic structures on the IR in Figure 1-18.

Figure 1-18

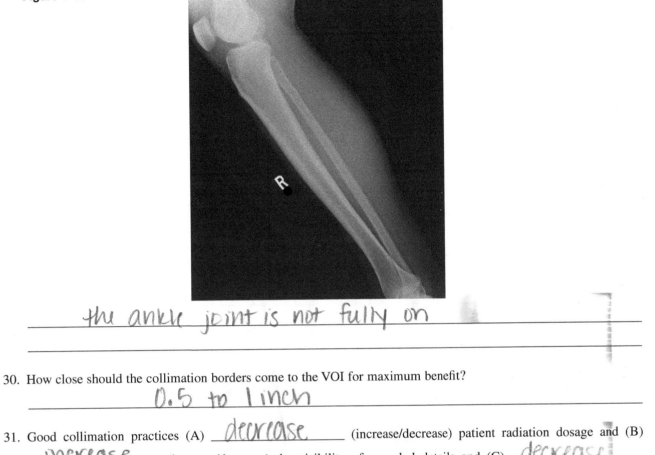

the ankle joint is not fully on

30. How close should the collimation borders come to the VOI for maximum benefit?

0.5 to 1 inch

31. Good collimation practices (A) _decrease_ (increase/decrease) patient radiation dosage and (B) _increase_ (increase/decrease) the visibility of recorded details and (C) _decrease_ (increases/decreases) histogram analysis errors.

32. State where the CR was centered on the projection in Figure 1-19.

Figure 1-19

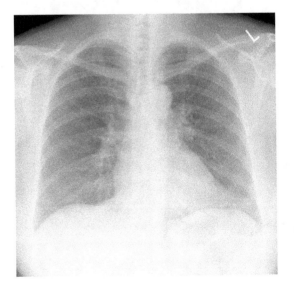

Copyright © 2015, 2011, 2006, 1996 by Saunders, an imprint of Elsevier Inc. All rights reserved.

Chapter **1** **Guidelines for Image Analysis**

33. The collimator's light field that is demonstrated on the patient's abdomen in Figure 1-20 measures 8 × 10 inches (18 × 24 cm). Does this mean that the IR exposure field coverage will be 8 × 10 inches, or should it be larger or smaller?

Figure 1-20

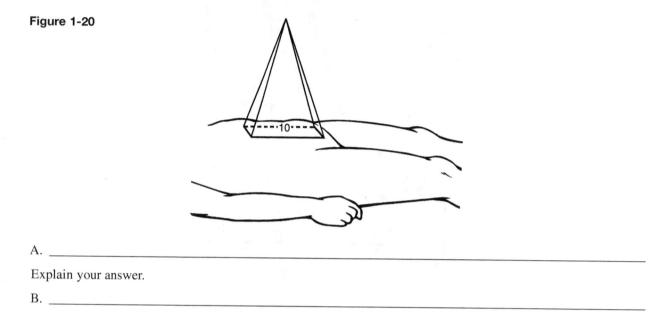

A. _____

Explain your answer.

B. _____

34. Evaluate the following projections for good collimation practices and state how poor CR centering has prevented tighter collimation.

Figure 1-21

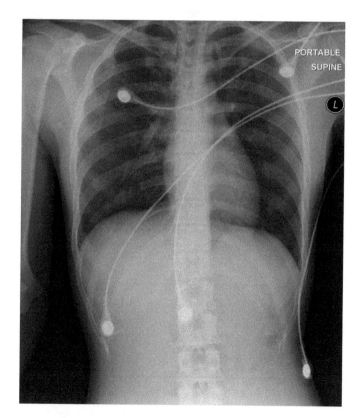

A. Figure 1-21 AP chest _____

Copyright © 2015, 2011, 2006, 1996 by Saunders, an imprint of Elsevier Inc. All rights reserved.

Figure 1-22

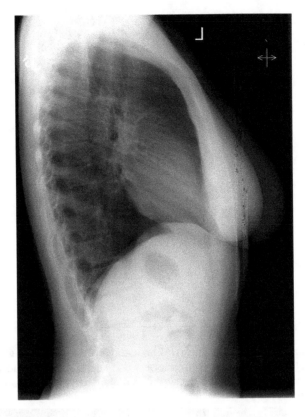

B. Figure 1-22 Lateral chest _____

Figure 1-23

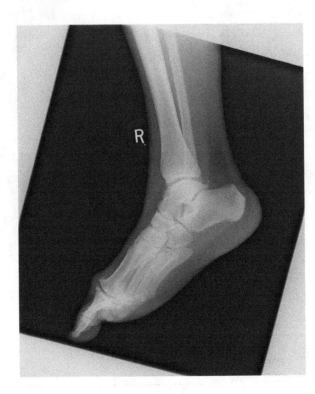

C. Figure 1-23 Lateral foot _____

Copyright © 2015, 2011, 2006, 1996 by Saunders, an imprint of Elsevier Inc. All rights reserved.   Chapter **1   Guidelines for Image Analysis**

Figure 1-24

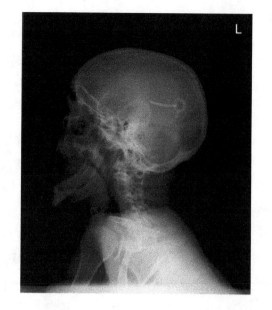

D. Figure 1-24 Lateral skull _____

35. Tighter collimation was obtained on one of the AP clavicular projections in Figure 1-25 with the tube column rotated, and the other was obtained with the collimator head rotated. Indicate below the clavicular projection that was obtained with the tube column rotated and the projection obtained with the collimator head rotated.

Figure 1-25

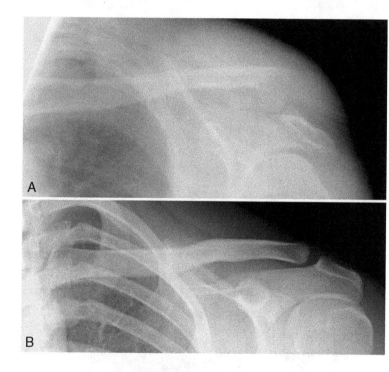

A. Tube column rotation: _____ (A or B)

B. Collimator head rotation: _____ (A or B)

C. Defend your answers to A and B above. _____

_____

Copyright © 2015, 2011, 2006, 1996 by Saunders, an imprint of Elsevier Inc. All rights reserved.

36. Use the lateral knee diagram in Figure 1-26 to answer the following questions.

Figure 1-26

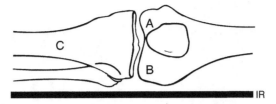

A. If a perpendicular CR was centered to letter A on the knee diagram, where would letter A be positioned in reference to letter B on the resulting radiographic projection?

_____

B. If a perpendicular CR was centered to the letter C on the knee diagram, where would letter A be positioned in reference to letter B on the resulting projection?

(1) _____

Will both letter A and letter B be projected the same distance?

(2) _____ (Yes/No)

Defend your answer.

(3) _____

C. If the CR was angled 15 degrees caudally and centered to letter A on the knee diagram, where would letter A be positioned in reference to letter B on the projection?

(1) _____

How would the projection change if the CR angulation was increased to 45 degrees?

(2) _____

D. If the CR was angled 15 degrees caudally and centered to letter C on the knee diagram, where would letter A be positioned in reference to letter B on the projection?

_____

_____

37. Eight soup cans were arranged on top of a 14 × 17 inch IR as shown in Figures 1-27 and 1-28. A perpendicular CR was centered to the center of the IR. The circles that are demonstrated indicate the bottom of each soup can that is 4 inches (10 cm) tall. Draw a second circle for each of the cans to indicate where the top of the soup can will be located on the resulting projection. You must consider the direction the top of the can will be projected because of diverged beams that will be used to record them and the degree of off-centering from the bottom of the can that will be demonstrated when compared with the other cans.

Figure 1-27   **Figure 1-28**

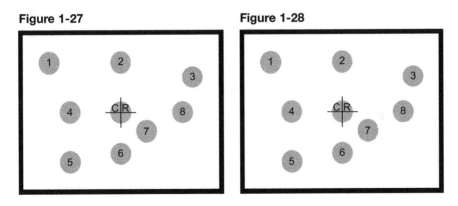

A. On Figure 1-27, draw the circles for an SID of 72 inches (180 cm).
B. On Figure 1-28, draw the circles for an SID of 40 inches (100 cm).

15

Copyright © 2015, 2011, 2006, 1996 by Saunders, an imprint of Elsevier Inc. All rights reserved.

38. The AP chest projection in Figure 1-29 was taken using a 48-inch SID and a perpendicular CR. With this as your reference point, answer the following.

Figure 1-29

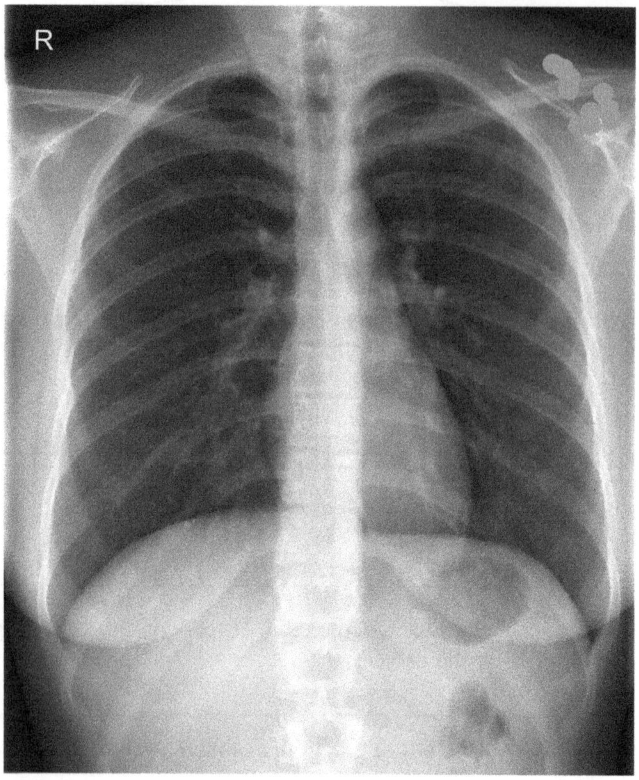

A. If the CR was inadvertently angled 10 degrees toward the right side of the patient, where would the sternoclavicular joints be located in reference to the vertebral column on the resulting AP chest projection?

_____

B. If the CR was angled 10 degrees cephalically, where would the sternoclavicular joints be located in reference to the third thoracic vertebral body?

_____

C. How would your answers to A and B be different if a 72-inch SID were used?

_____

D. How would your answers to A and B be different if the heart shadow were used as your reference point instead of the sternoclavicular joints?

_____

39. To minimize shape distortion on a projection, keep the part positioned (A) _parallel_ (parallel/perpendicular) to the IR and the CR (B) _perp._ (parallel/perpendicular) to both the part and IR.

Copyright © 2015, 2011, 2006, 1996 by Saunders, an imprint of Elsevier Inc. All rights reserved.

40. For the CR, part, and IR setups in the following figures, state the type of shape distortion that will result.

Figure 1-30

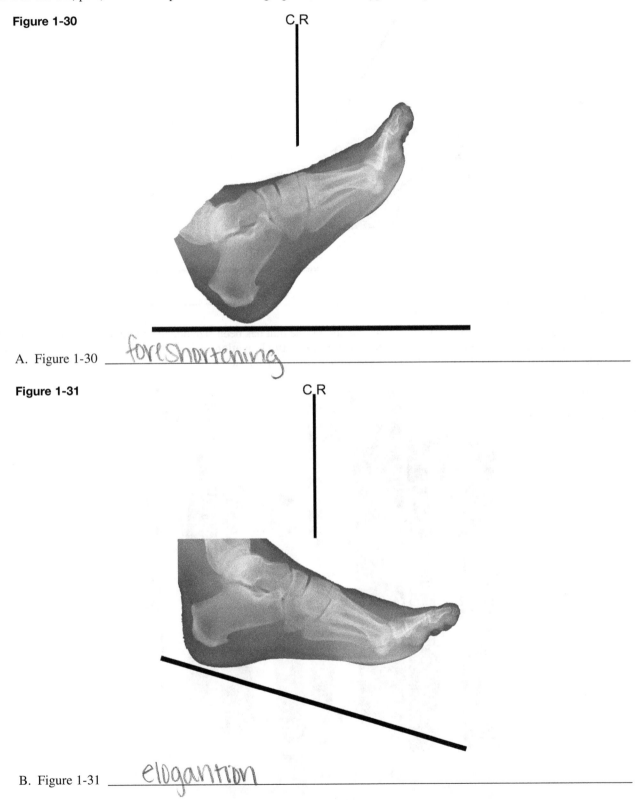

A. Figure 1-30 ___foreshortening___

Figure 1-31

B. Figure 1-31 ___elogantion___

Copyright © 2015, 2011, 2006, 1996 by Saunders, an imprint of Elsevier Inc. All rights reserved.

Chapter **1** **Guidelines for Image Analysis**

Figure 1-32

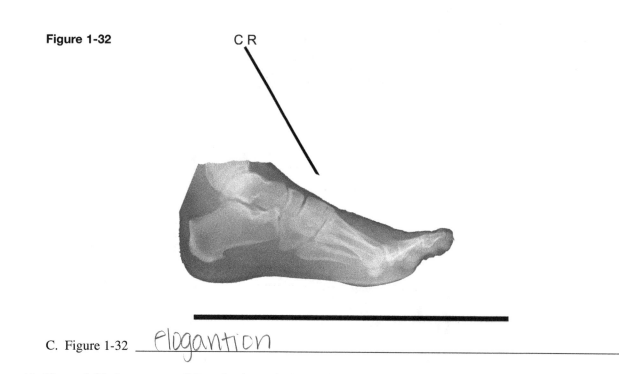

C. Figure 1-32 __elogantion__

41. Figure 1-33 demonstrates AP projections of a humeral bone that has been size and shape distorted. Identify the type of distortion demonstrated on each projection. If you identify elongation or foreshortening, state the aspect of the bone (proximal or distal humerus) that was positioned farther from the IR.

Figure 1-33

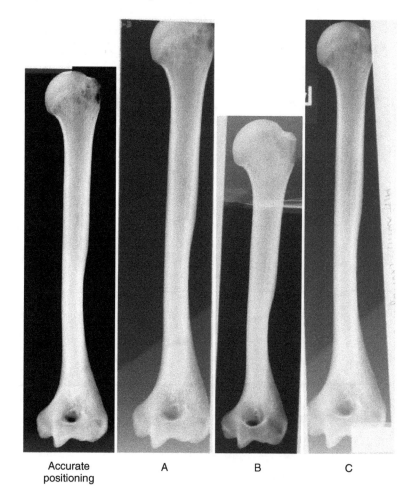

Accurate   A   B   C
positioning

Copyright © 2015, 2011, 2006, 1996 by Saunders, an imprint of Elsevier Inc. All rights reserved.

A. <u>magnification</u>

B. <u>foreshortening - proximal humerus farthest</u>

C. <u>elogation - distal humerus farthest</u>

42. Which of the following images will have the greater part magnification?
    Image 1 was exposed at a 72-inch SID and a 3-inch OID.
    Image 2 was exposed at a 72-inch SID and a 4-inch OID.

43. Which of the following images will have the greater part magnification?
    Image 1 was exposed at a 72-inch SID and a 2-inch OID.
    Image 2 was exposed at a 40-inch SID and a 2-inch OID.

44. List three ways of identifying similarly appearing structures from one another on a projection.

    A. _____

    B. _____

    C. _____

45. If two structures are demonstrated without superimposition on a mispositioned projection and they should be super-imposed on an accurately positioned image of this projection, how does one determine how much to adjust the patient to obtain an optimal projection if both structures move in opposite directions when adjusted?

    A. _____

    If only one structure moved when the patient was adjusted?

    B. _____

46. Estimate the degree of patient obliquity demonstrated in the diagrams in Figure 1-34.

    Figure 1-34

    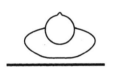   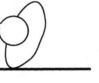   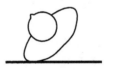

    A. _____ degrees   B. _____ degrees   C. _____ degrees

    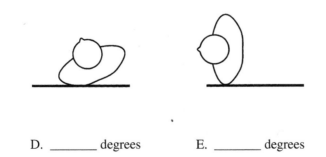

    D. _____ degrees   E. _____ degrees

Copyright © 2015, 2011, 2006, 1996 by Saunders, an imprint of Elsevier Inc. All rights reserved.   Chapter **1**   **Guidelines for Image Analysis**

47. Estimate the degree of flexion demonstrated in the following figures.

Figure 1-35

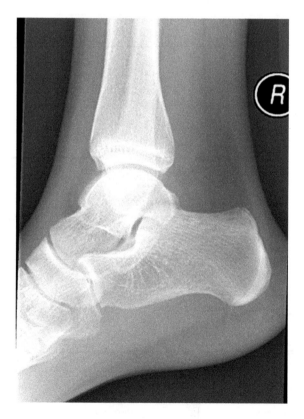

A. _____ degrees (Figure 1-35)

Figure 1-36

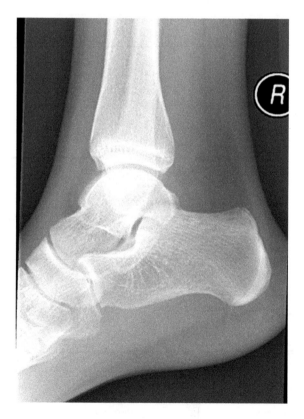

B. _____ degrees (Figure 1-36)

Copyright © 2015, 2011, 2006, 1996 by Saunders, an imprint of Elsevier Inc. All rights reserved.

Figure 1-37

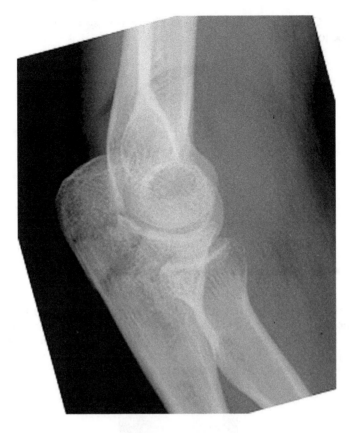

C. _____ degrees (Figure 1-37)

Figure 1-38

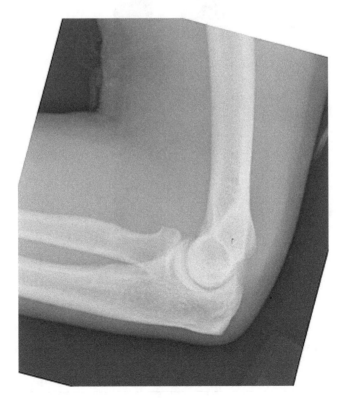

D. _____ degrees (Figure 1-38)

Copyright © 2015, 2011, 2006, 1996 by Saunders, an imprint of Elsevier Inc. All rights reserved.

48. Draw a line to indicate the CR on the AP knee setup in Figure 1-39 so that the resulting AP knee projection will demonstrate an open knee joint space.

Figure 1-39

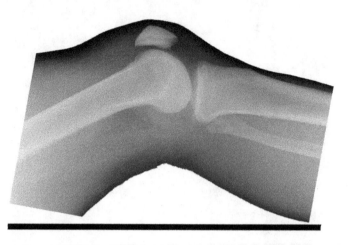

49. Figure 1-40 demonstrates a PA finger projection with closed interphalangeal (IP) joints and foreshortened middle and distal phalanges. The patient was unable to fully extend the finger for the examination. Explain how the central ray and part should be positioned to obtain open IP joints and demonstrate the phalanges without foreshortening.

Figure 1-40

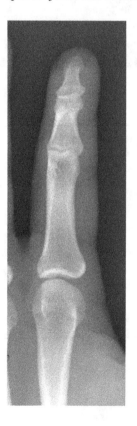

A. _____

Explain how the technologist would have to adjust the CR to obtain open IP joints and nonforeshortened phalanges if the patient was unable to adjust the hand.

B. _____

_____

Copyright © 2015, 2011, 2006, 1996 by Saunders, an imprint of Elsevier Inc. All rights reserved.

50. An angled CR projects the structure situated (A) _____ (closer to/farther from) the IR farther than a structure situated (B) _____ (closer to/farther from) the IR.

51. Figure 1-41 demonstrates an accurately and poorly positioned lateral hand projection. On the poorly positioned projection, the fifth metacarpal (MC) is situated 1 inch (2.5 cm) anterior to the second through fourth MCs. The second through fifth MCs should be superimposed on an optimal lateral hand projection. The physical distance between the second and fifth MCs is 2½ inches (6.25 cm).

Figure 1-41

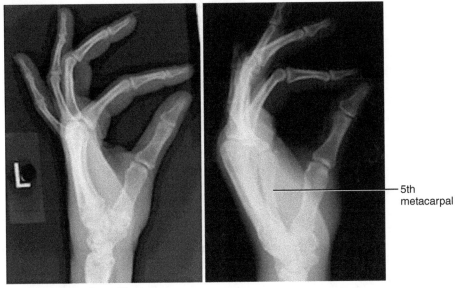

5th metacarpal

Accurate positioning

A. State how and by how much the patient's positioning should be adjusted to obtain an optimal projection. The second and fifth MCs will move in opposite directions from each other when the hand is rotated.

_____

_____

B. State how the CR could be directed toward the hand and the amount of angulation needed to obtain an optimal projection if the patient was unable to adjust positioning.

_____

_____

Copyright © 2015, 2011, 2006, 1996 by Saunders, an imprint of Elsevier Inc. All rights reserved.

52. Figure 1-42 demonstrates an accurately and a poorly positioned lateral knee projection. On the poorly positioned projection, the lateral femoral condyle is situated 2 inches (5 cm) anterior to the medial femoral condyle. The condyles should be superimposed on an optimal lateral knee projection. The physical distance between the femoral condyles is 2½ inches (6.25 cm).

Figure 1-42

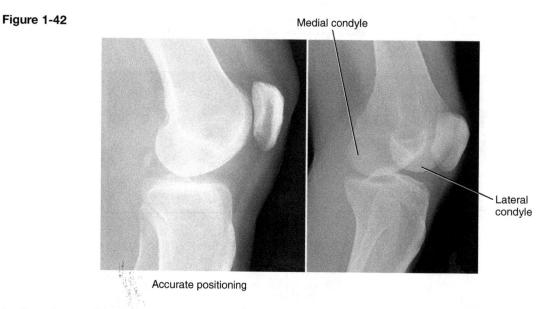

Medial condyle

Lateral condyle

Accurate positioning

A. State how and by how much the patient's positioning could be adjusted to obtain an optimal projection. The lateral and medial condyles will move in opposite directions from each other when the knee is rotated.

_____

B. State how the CR should be directed toward the knee and the amount of angulation needed to obtain an optimal projection if the patient was unable to adjust positioning.

_____

_____

Copyright © 2015, 2011, 2006, 1996 by Saunders, an imprint of Elsevier Inc. All rights reserved.

53. Figure 1-43 demonstrates an accurately and a poorly positioned lateral ankle projection. On the poorly positioned projection, the lateral talar dome is situated ¼ inch (0.6 cm) posterior to the medial dome. The talar domes should be superimposed on an optimal lateral ankle projection. The physical distance between the talar domes is 1 inch (2.5 cm).

Figure 1-43

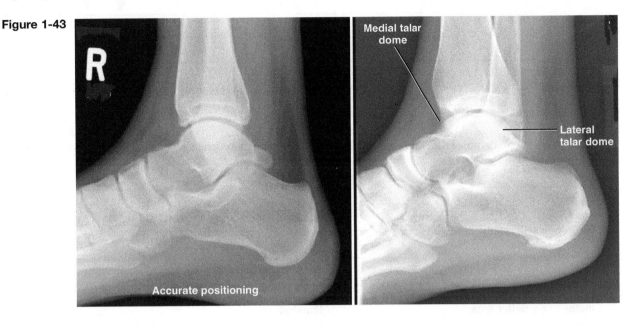

Medial talar dome

Lateral talar dome

Accurate positioning

A. State how and by how much the patient's positioning could be adjusted to obtain an optimal projection. The lateral and medial talar domes will move in opposite directions from each other when the ankle is rotated.

_____

B. State how the CR should be directed toward the ankle and the amount of angulation needed to obtain an optimal projection if the patient was unable to adjust positioning.

_____

54. A (A) ___small___ (large/small) focal spot size is used for fine detail demonstration because a detail that is (B) ___smaller___ (larger/smaller) than the focal spot size used to produce the image will not be demonstrated.

55. A ___longer___ (longer/shorter) SID and a ___shorter___ (longer/shorter) OID will produce the sharpest recorded details on a projection.

56. List four ways that voluntary motion can be controlled.

A. _____

B. _____

C. _____

D. _____

57. How can voluntary and involuntary motion be distinguished from each other on a supine abdominal projection?

_____

_____

_____

Copyright © 2015, 2011, 2006, 1996 by Saunders, an imprint of Elsevier Inc. All rights reserved.

58. State whether the following situations are examples of voluntary or involuntary motions.

    A. The patient was extremely short of breath because of asthma and unable to hold it.

    _____involuntary_____

    B. After being in a car accident, the patient being imaged was unable to stop shaking.

    _____involuntary_____

59. The term _____ is used to describe the spatial resolution of a digital system and refers to the number of details that can be visualized in a set _____.

60. DR system A can demonstrate 5 lp/mm, and DR system B can demonstrate 10 lp/mm. Which system demonstrates the greatest spatial resolution?

    _____

61. An AP pelvis and an AP hip projection were obtained using the same computed radiography system. State which projection will demonstrate the greatest spatial resolution and explain why.

    _____

62. When obtaining a projection using a DR system, greater spatial resolution is obtained when the technologist collimates to a smaller area. _____ (True/False)

63. Gonadal shielding is recommended under which three conditions?

    A. _____

    B. _____

    C. _____

64. What gonadal organs should be shielded on a female patient? _____

65. Draw a shield on the female pelvic diagram in Figure 1-44 to indicate proper shield placement for a female patient.

Figure 1-44

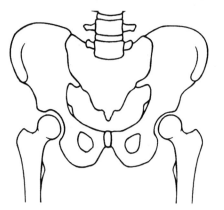

66. Describe how palpable pelvic structures are used to accurately position a flat contact shield on a female patient.

    _____

    _____

Copyright © 2015, 2011, 2006, 1996 by Saunders, an imprint of Elsevier Inc. All rights reserved.

67. Why should the size of the contact shield used for protecting the female patient be seriously considered?

_____

_____

68. What gonadal organs are shielded on a male patient?

A. _____

Where are they located?

B. _____

69. Where is the top of the shield positioned when shielding the male gonadal organs?

_____

70. Draw a shaded shield on the male pelvic diagram in Figure 1-45 to indicate proper shield placement for a male patient.

Figure 1-45

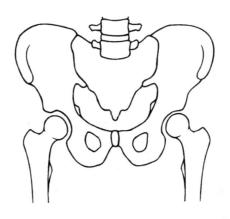

71. Evaluate the female gonadal shielding used on the pelvic projection in Figure 1-46.

Figure 1-46

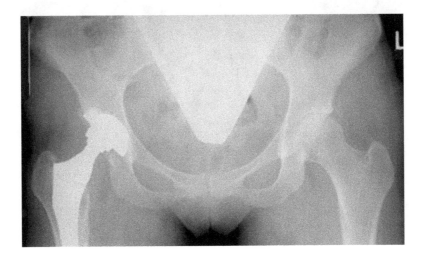

_____

_____

Copyright © 2015, 2011, 2006, 1996 by Saunders, an imprint of Elsevier Inc. All rights reserved.

72. Evaluate the pediatric male gonadal shielding used on the femur projection in Figure 1-47.

Figure 1-47

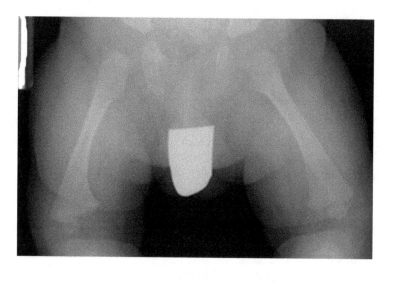

_____

_____

73. Evaluate the pediatric female gonadal shielding used on the pelvic projection in Figure 1-48.

Figure 1-48

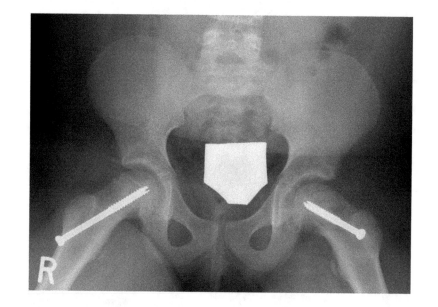

_____

_____

Copyright © 2015, 2011, 2006, 1996 by Saunders, an imprint of Elsevier Inc. All rights reserved.

74. State how to shield a patient who is in a lateral projection.

_____

_____

75. Radiosensitive cells such as the (A) _____, (B) _____, (C) _____, and (D) _____ should be shielded whenever they lie within (E) _____ inches of the primary beam.

76. The projection in Figure 1-49 demonstrates poor radiation protection practices. What type of error is demonstrated?

Figure 1-49

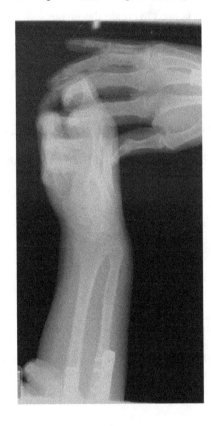

A. _____

How could this examination be taken without this error?

B. _____

77. The technologist sets up for a routine AP abdomen projection on an obese patient using the mobile radiography unit. The resulting SSD is 10 inches (25 cm). Using appropriate radiation protection practices, state how the setup should

be adjusted before exposing the projection. _____

Copyright © 2015, 2011, 2006, 1996 by Saunders, an imprint of Elsevier Inc. All rights reserved.

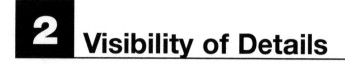

2 Visibility of Details

STUDY QUESTIONS

1. The histogram represents the ___subject contrast___ in the remnant radiation and is determined by the total ___exposure___ that is used to create the image.

2. On a histogram graph, what is identified on the following axes?

   A. x-axis: _____

   B. y-axis: _____

3. The VOI on a histogram graph identifies S1 as the _____ (minimal/maximal) gray shade value.

4. Rank the following in the order each is demonstrated on a histogram, with 1 being farthest to the left on the graph and 5 being farthest to the right.

   __5__ Air/gas

   __2__ Bone

   __1__ Contrast/metal

   __4__ Fat

   __3__ Soft tissue

5. The ___lookup table (LUT)___ represents the ideal histogram for the projection.

6. If the image histogram was positioned farther to the left and was wider than the LUT's histogram, how would the displayed projection differ from that the LUT's histogram represents?

   _____

7. Where is the exposure indicator reading taken from on the histogram after the histogram has been developed?

   _____

8. What are the common causes of poor histogram formation (histogram analysis errors)?

   A. ___wrong body part___

   B. ___CR not to VOI___

   C. ___insufficient collimation___

   D. ___excessive scatter___

   E. ___wrong technical factors___

   F. Computed radiography only: ___more than one image on IR___

   G. Computed radiography only: ___did not cover 30% of IR___

   H. Computed radiography only: ___IP was not erased___

Copyright © 2015, 2011, 2006, 1996 by Saunders, an imprint of Elsevier Inc. All rights reserved.

9. In computed radiography, histogram analysis errors can occur because of the image being improperly centered to the IR or all collimated borders not shown or aligned accurately. Why does this error NOT occur in DR imaging?

_____

10. During the exposure field recognition process in CR imaging, how does the computer identify the VOI?

_____

11. In computed radiography systems, how much of the IP should be covered with anatomy to avoid an EI error?

_____30%_____

Figure 2-1

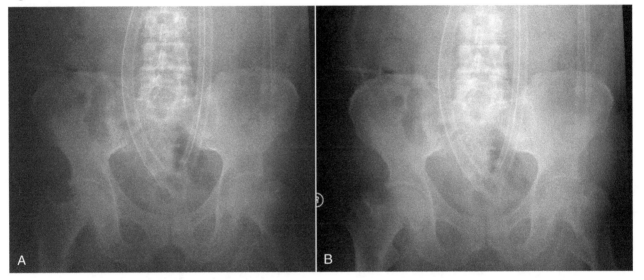

12. Figure 2-1 A and B: Determine which AP abdomen projection was processed under a chest LUT and which was processed under an abdomen LUT.
   (Hint: Look at the contrast of each projection.)

_____

_____

_____

13. List the technical factors that affect the amount of exposure the IR receives.

   A. _____   D. _____

   B. _____   E. _____

   C. _____   F. _____

Copyright © 2015, 2011, 2006, 1996 by Saunders, an imprint of Elsevier Inc. All rights reserved.

14. State how the technologist knows that the technical factors were accurately set after the exposure.

A. _____

_____

B. _____

_____

C. _____

_____

D. _____

_____

15. The IR exposure can be off by a factor of _____ and still create an acceptable image.

16. Quantum noise is demonstrated on a projection by a(n) _grainy_ pattern and indicates _underexposure_.

17. Underexposure to the IR can be identified when:

A. _____

_____

B. _____

_____

C. _____

_____

18. List the steps to follow to determine the technical adjustment to make when an underexposed projection is produced.

A. _____

_____

B. _____

_____

C. _____

_____

19. List the subject contrast differences that cause differential absorption and radiographic contrast.

A. _atomic density_

B. _atomic number_

C. _part thickness_

Copyright © 2015, 2011, 2006, 1996 by Saunders, an imprint of Elsevier Inc. All rights reserved.

20. What is the technical factor that controls subject contrast and contrast resolution? _____

21. Subject contrast can be recovered with digital post-processing techniques. _____ (True/False)

22. Optimal kV has been used for a projection when the cortical outlines of the _____ and _____ bony structures in the VOI are demonstrated.

23. Saturation is demonstrated on a projection when details in the VOI demonstrate a(n) _____ shade and occurs when the IR exposure is _____ times more than the ideal.

24. Overexposure to the IR can be identified when:

    A. _____

    B. _____

    C. _____

25. An AP lumbar vertebrae projection was obtained using the Fuji computed radiography system, 90 kV, and 5 mAs. The resulting projection demonstrated adequate penetration of all structures, quantum noise, and a 600 EI number. How should the technical factors be adjusted before repeating the projection?

    _____

26. An AP shoulder projection was obtained using the Siemens DR system, 80 kV, and 10 mAs. The resulting projection demonstrated adequate penetration of all structures, low contrast, no quantum noise, saturation of the AC joint and lateral clavicle, and a 4000 EI number. What new technical factors should be used for the repeated projection?

    _____

27. An AP pelvis projection was obtained using the Carestream CR system, 70 kV, and 5 mAs. The resulting projection demonstrated a lack of subject contrast at the hip joints, quantum noise, and a 1400 EI number. What new technical factors should be used for the repeated projection?

    _____

28. How can the amount of scatter radiation reaching the IR be controlled?

    A. use a grid

    B. tight collimation

    C. flat contact shield

Copyright © 2015, 2011, 2006, 1996 by Saunders, an imprint of Elsevier Inc. All rights reserved.

Figure 2-2

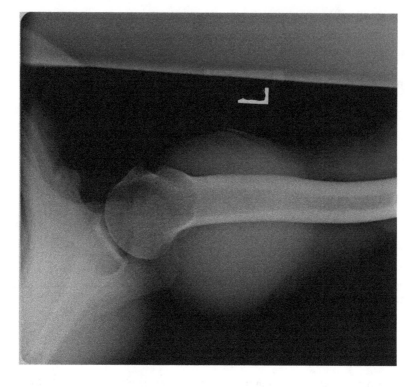

29. Figure 2-2 demonstrates a well-collimated axiolateral (inferosuperior) shoulder projection that demonstrates excessive scatter radiation along the outside of the collimated border. Describe a technique that could be followed to reduce the negative affects of this scatter on the visiblity of the recorded details.

_____

30. Use the original technical factors listed below to determine the new mAs that will be needed to produce an optimal projection if the following changes occurred.
Original Technical Factors: 90 kVp, 80 mAs, 8:1 grid

    A. Nongrid   _____ mAs

    B. 6:1 grid   _____ mAs

    C. 12:1 grid   _____ mAs

    D. 16:1 grid   _____ mAs

31. An optimal AP pelvis projection was obtained in the x-ray department using a 45-inch (113 cm) SID, 80 kVp, and 60 mAs. The next day, the same projection was requested, but because the patient was in traction, the SID needed to be set at 65 inches (163 cm) SID. What should the new mAs be to obtain an optimal projection?

_____

Copyright © 2015, 2011, 2006, 1996 by Saunders, an imprint of Elsevier Inc. All rights reserved.

32. Increasing the OID may result in a significant loss of IR exposure. The amount of loss is dependent on what two factors?

   A. _____

   B. _____

33. When an OID increase causes significant scatter radiation to be diverted from the IR, what technical factor should

    be increased by (A) _____ should be increased by (B) _____ percent for every centimeter of OID increase to compensate for IR exposure loss.

34. State if and by how much the mAs should be adjusted because of increased collimation in the following situations.

   A. A PA chest projection was requested to demonstrate the pulmonary arterial catheter. The technologist used 80 kVp at 3 mAs, and the resulting projection did not visualize the catheter tip in the right atrium. To reduce the effects of scatter radiation and demonstrate the catheter tip, the technologist returns to take a second projection, collimating to the VOI (8 × 10 inches). What technique should be used for the second projection?

      _____

   B. Two PA hand projections were obtained on the same patient's hand. A 10 × 12 inch (25 × 30 cm) IR was needed to include the entire hand on the first projection, and the technique used was 60 kVp at 20 mAs. The second projection was collimated to a 2 × 4 inch (5 × 10 cm) field size to include only the first finger. What technique should be used for the second projection?

      _____

35. Indicate whether the following statements are true (T) or false (F) as they relate to the anode-heel effect by placing a T or F in front of the statement.

   ___F___ A. The anode-heel effect can be used effectively to produce uniform brightness between the toes and foot when obtaining an AP foot projection.

   ___T___ B. To incorporate the anode-heel effect for forearm projections, the wrist is placed at the anode end of the tube.

   ___F___ C. To incorporate the anode-heel effect for lower leg projections, the ankle is placed at the cathode end of the tube.

   ___T___ D. To incorporate the anode-heel effect for an AP thoracic vertebrae, the cephalic end of the patient is placed at the anode end of the tube.

36. What type of patient condition causes the tissues to increase mass density or thickness and become more radi-

    opaque? _____ (additive/destructive)

37. State the technical adjustment needed with the patient condition in the first column and state whether it is an additive or destructive condition, to indicate if the technical adjustment should be increased or decreased by the amount indicated.

	Technical Adjustment	Additive or Destructive
A. Acites	+50% mAs	additive
B. Emphysema	-8% kVp	destructive
C. Pleural effusion	+35% mAs	additive
D. Osteoporosis	-8% kVp	destructive
E. Osteoarthritis	+8% kVp	destructive

Copyright © 2015, 2011, 2006, 1996 by Saunders, an imprint of Elsevier Inc. All rights reserved.

F.	Pneumothorax	-8% kV	destructive
G.	Pneumonia	$+50\%$ mAs	additive
H.	Bowel obstruction	-8% kV	destructive
I.	Osteochondroma	$+8\%$ kV	additive
J.	Rheumatoid arthritis	-8% kV	destructive
K.	Pulmonary edema	$+50\%$ mAs	additive
L.	Cardiomegaly	$+50\%$ mAs	additive

38. Indicate whether the following statements are true (T) or false (F) as they relate to proper AEC usage by placing a T or F in front of the statement.

___T___ A. Set the kV at optimum for the body part being imaged to obtain appropriate part subject contrast.

___F___ B. If the kVp is so low that the part is inadequately penetrated, the exposure (density) control button should be increased to +2.

___T___ C. Exposures taken with an exposure time that is less than the minimum response time will result in an overexposed projection.

___F___ D. The mA station should be increased if the minimum response time halts the exposure before adequate IR exposure is obtained.

___T___ E. The backup time should be set at 150% to 200% of the expected manual exposure time.

___T___ F. If the backup time is set at a time that is too low, the exposure will prematurely stop, resulting in an underexposed projection.

___F___ G. An overexposed projection results when the ionization chamber chosen is located beneath a structure that has a lower atomic number or is thinner or less dense than the VOI.

___T___ H. If the activated ionization chamber is not completely covered by the anatomy, resulting in a portion of the chamber being exposed with a part of the x-ray beam that does not go through the patient, the resulting projection will be underexposed.

___T___ I. Scatter radiation may cause the AEC to terminate prematurely.

___T___ J. The AEC should not be used when the structure above the ionization chamber varies greatly in thickness.

___F___ K. The AEC can be used when radiopaque hardware of prosthetic devices are present as long as the hardware or device is positioned in the center of the chamber.

Copyright © 2015, 2011, 2006, 1996 by Saunders, an imprint of Elsevier Inc. All rights reserved.

39. Evaluate the following projections for proper AEC usage.

Figure 2-3

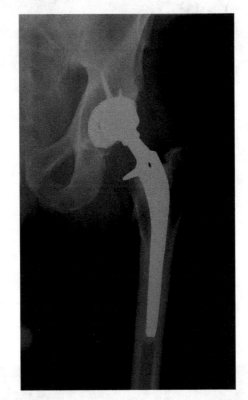

A. AP hip (Figure 2-3) _____

_____

Figure 2-4

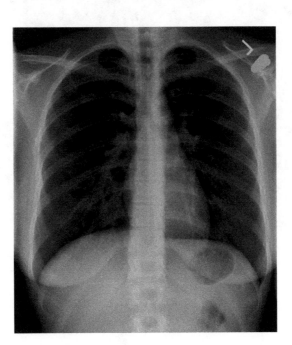

B. PA chest (Figure 2-4) _____

_____

Copyright © 2015, 2011, 2006, 1996 by Saunders, an imprint of Elsevier Inc. All rights reserved.   Chapter **2** **Visibility of Details**

Figure 2-5

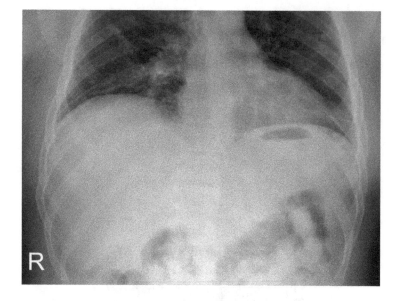

C. AP abdomen, upper projection (Figure 2-5) _____

_____

Figure 2-6

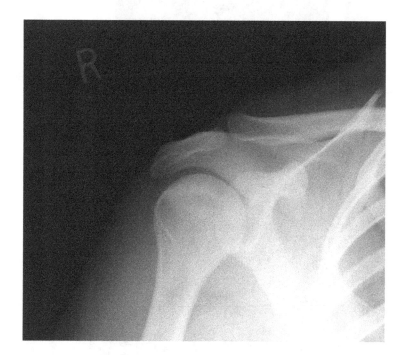

D. AP shoulder (Figure 2-6) _____

_____

Copyright © 2015, 2011, 2006, 1996 by Saunders, an imprint of Elsevier Inc. All rights reserved.

Figure 2-7

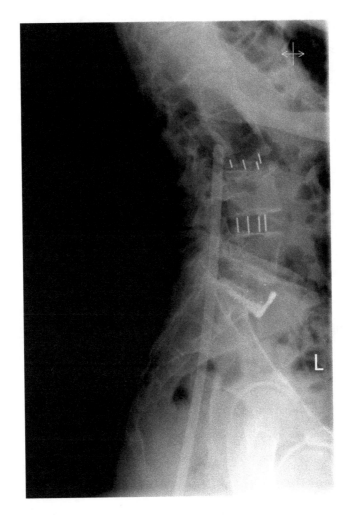

   E. Lateral lumbar vertebrae (Figure 2-7) _____

_____

40. Contrast resolution refers to the degree of difference in _____ levels between adjacent tissues, with _____ (high/low) contrast demonstrating _____ (lesser/greater) difference.

41. Indicate whether projections on patients with the following will display high (H) or low (L) subject contrast.

      _____ A. Strong muscles

      _____ B. Dense bones

      _____ C. Fluid retention caused by disease or injury

      _____ D. Porous bones

      _____ E. High fat

      _____ F. Bones of infants

      _____ G. Obesity

Copyright © 2015, 2011, 2006, 1996 by Saunders, an imprint of Elsevier Inc. All rights reserved.

42. Adjusting the window width changes the (A) _____contrast_____ on the displayed projection, and adjusting the window level changes the (B) _____brightness_____ of the displayed projection.

43. The technologist should window a less than optimal projection and save it to the PACS so the radiologist can display the manipulated projection. _____false_____ (True/False)

44. The contrast mask should be used to improve the appearance of collimation on the projection. _____ (True/False)

45. Describe the following artifact categories.

A. Anatomic artifact: _____

B. Double exposure: _____

C. External artifact: _____

D. Internal artifact: _____

E. Equipment-related artifact: _____

F. Improper film handling and processing artifact: _____

46. State the artifact category for each of the artifacts listed below.

A. A fountain pen is visualized on a PA chest projection. _____

B. A hand is demonstrated on an AP hip projection. _____

C. A prosthesis is demonstrated on an AP shoulder projection. _____

D. Grid cutoff is demonstrated on an axiolateral hip projection. _____

47. Indicate whether the following statements are true (T) or false (F) as they relate to grid cutoff.

A. _____ A projection obtained with a tilted focus grid demonstrates grid cutoff on each side.

B. _____ A projection obtained with the focused grid off centered to the CR demonstrates grid cutoff across the entire projection.

C. _____ A projection obtained with a parallel grid that is inverted demonstrates grid cutoff on each side of the projection.

D. _____ A projection obtained with an off-focused focus grid demonstrates grid cutoff across the entire projection.

48. Grid cutoff resulting from poor grid alignment will be greater on the side the CR is angled (A) _____ (toward/away from), will (B) _____ (increase/decrease) with increased severity of misalignment, and will be more noticeable with (C) _____ (higher/lower) grid ratios.

Copyright © 2015, 2011, 2006, 1996 by Saunders, an imprint of Elsevier Inc. All rights reserved.

Figure 2-8

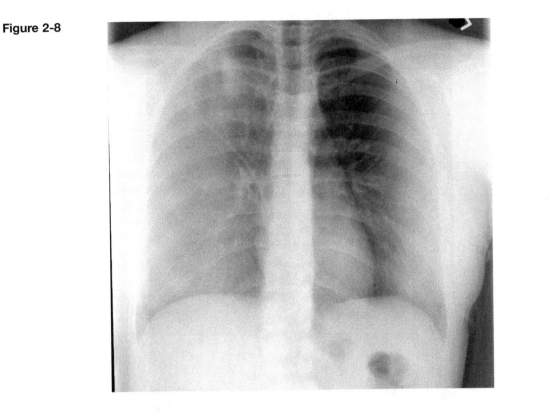

49. State the positioning error that caused the grid alignment arifact that is demonstrated on the PA chest projection in Figure 2-8. _____

50. Evaluate the following projections for phosphor plate handling artifacts. Choose from the options listed.

   1. Dust or dirt   3. Hair

   2. Scratches   4. A solution of some type

Figure 2-9

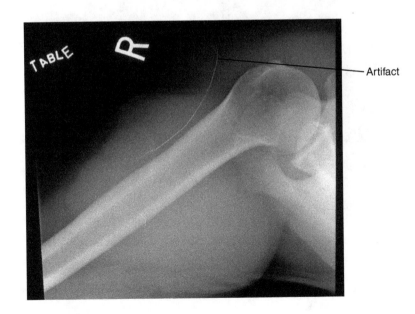

Artifact

   A. _____ Figure 2-9

Copyright © 2015, 2011, 2006, 1996 by Saunders, an imprint of Elsevier Inc. All rights reserved.

Chapter **2** **Visibility of Details**

Figure 2-10

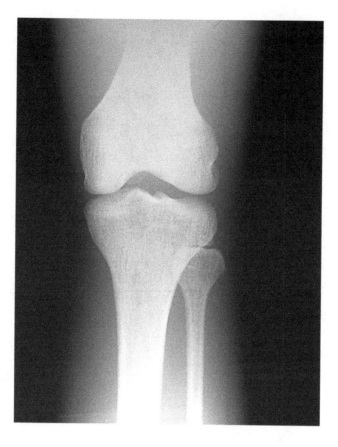

B. _____ Figure 2-10

Figure 2-11

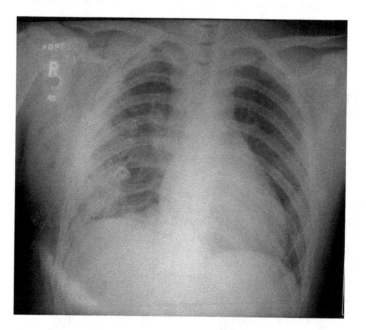

C. _____ Figure 2-11

Copyright © 2015, 2011, 2006, 1996 by Saunders, an imprint of Elsevier Inc. All rights reserved.

67. Complete the statements below referring to adult AP chest projection analysis guidelines.

AP Chest (Supine or Mobile) Projection Analysis Guidelines
▪ (A) _____ thoracic vertebra is at the center of the exposure field.
▪ Distances from vertebral column to (B) _____ are equal, and lengths of the right and left corresponding posterior ribs are equal.
▪ (C) _____ is superimposed by the fourth thoracic vertebra, with 1 inch (2.5 cm) of apical lung field visible above the (D) _____.
▪ Clavicles are positioned on the same (E) _____ plane when possible.
▪ (F) _____ are located outside the lung field, when possible.
▪ (G) _____ posterior ribs are visualized above the diaphragm

68. Why is it important to record the time of day on all mobile chest projections?

_____

69. Why is the degree of patient elevation recorded on all mobile chest projections?

_____

70. Why are air-fluid levels undetectable when the patient is supine?

_____

71. A. Why is it safe to position the computed radiography IR crosswise for almost all mobile AP chest projections on most body types?

_____

   B. Why is it more likely for the lateral edges of the lung field to be clipped if the IR is placed lengthwise for mobile AP chest projections?

_____

72. State how the patient is positioned to prevent rotation on an AP chest projection.

_____

73. How can rotation be identified on an AP chest projection?

_____

74. When the patient's condition allows, the shoulders should be depressed for an AP chest projection. How can this movement be identified on the projection?

_____

75. When an AP chest projection is obtained that demonstrates somewhat vertically appearing clavicles, how can one determine if this appearance is a result of poor CR alignment or poor shoulder positioning?

_____

_____

Copyright © 2015, 2011, 2006, 1996 by Saunders, an imprint of Elsevier Inc. All rights reserved. Chapter **3 Image Analysis of the Chest and Abdomen**

76. When the patient's condition allows, how can the scapulae be drawn from the lung field on an AP supine chest projection?

_____

77. Poor CR alignment on a mobile chest projection will affect the amount of apical lung field demonstrated superior to the clavicles and the contour of the posterior ribs. For each of the following situations, describe the expected change in apical lung visualization and posterior rib contour.

   A. The CR was angled too caudally.

   _____

   B. The CR was angled too cephalically.

   _____

78. How can the CR be adjusted to improve the posterior rib contour and eliminate superimposition of the chin on the apices when imaging a kyphotic patient for an AP chest projection?

_____

79. Why is a 5-degree caudal CR angle used for supine AP chest projections?

_____

80. Why are fewer posterior ribs demonstrated above the diaphragm on a supine AP chest projection than on an upright PA chest projection?

_____

81. How is the patient instructed to breathe to obtain maximum lung aeration?

_____

82. Accurate centering on an AP chest projection is accomplished by centering the CR to the (A) _____

   plane at a level (B) _____ inches inferior to the (C) _____.

83. What anatomic structures are included on an accurately positioned AP chest projection?

_____

For the following descriptions of AP chest projections with poor positioning, state how the patient would have been mispositioned or the CR misaligned for such a projection to result.

84. The left SC joint is visible away from the vertebral column, and the right SC joint is superimposed over the vertebral column (list both the patient and CR mispositioning that could cause this projection).

_____

_____

85. The manubrium is shown superimposed over the fifth thoracic vertebra with more than 1 inch (2.5 cm) of the apical lung field visible above the clavicles and the posterior ribs demonstrate a vertical contour.

_____

_____

 Copyright © 2015, 2011, 2006, 1996 by Saunders, an imprint of Elsevier Inc. All rights reserved.

86. The manubrium is shown superimposed over the third vertebra with less than 1 inch (2.5 cm) of apical lung field visible above the clavicles, and the posterior ribs demonstrate a horizontal contour.

_____

_____

87. A projection of a patient with severe kyphosis demonstrates the chin superimposed over the apical region, and the posterior ribs demonstrate a vertical contour.

_____

_____

For the following AP chest projections with poor positioning, state what anatomic structures are misaligned and how the patient should be repositioned for an optimal projection to be obtained.

Figure 3-28

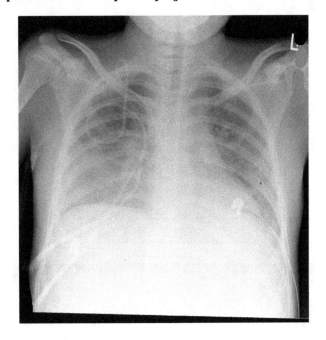

88. (Figure 3-28):

_____

_____

Copyright © 2015, 2011, 2006, 1996 by Saunders, an imprint of Elsevier Inc. All rights reserved.   Chapter **3** **Image Analysis of the Chest and Abdomen**

Figure 3-29

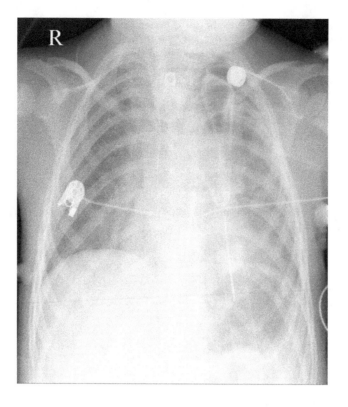

89. (Figure 3-29):

_____

_____

Figure 3-30

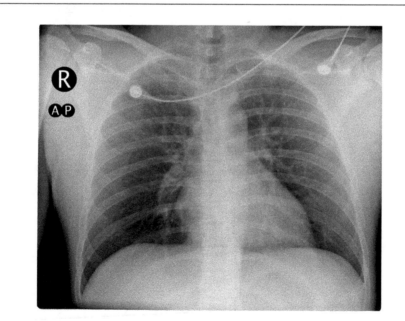

90. (Figure 3-30):

_____

_____

Chapter **3 Image Analysis of the Chest and Abdomen**   Copyright © 2015, 2011, 2006, 1996 by Saunders, an imprint of Elsevier Inc. All rights reserved.

AP or PA Projection (Right or Left Lateral Decubitus Position)

91. Identify the labeled anatomy in Figure 3-31.

Figure 3-31

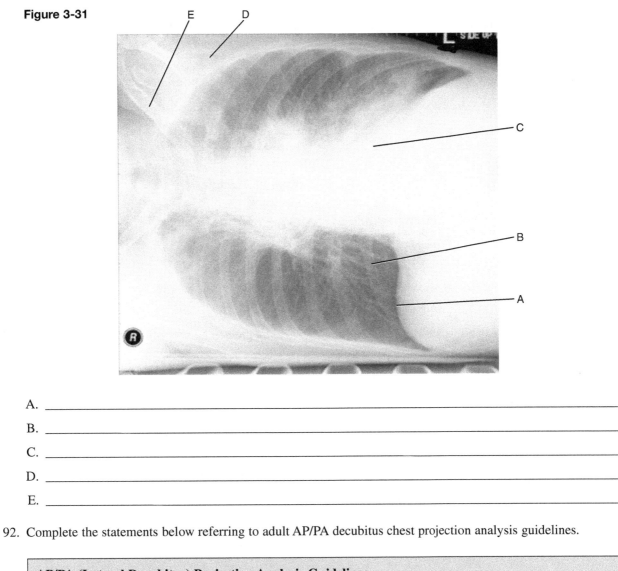

A. _____

B. _____

C. _____

D. _____

E. _____

92. Complete the statements below referring to adult AP/PA decubitus chest projection analysis guidelines.

AP/PA (Lateral Decubitus) Projection Analysis Guidelines

- Arrow or "word" marker identifies the side of the patient positioned (A) _____ from the imaging table or cart.

- (B) _____ thoracic vertebra is at the center of the exposure field.

- Distances from the (C) _____ to the sternal clavicular ends are equal, and lengths of the right and left corresponding posterior ribs are equal.

- The arms, mandible, and lateral borders of the scapulae are situated (D) _____, and lateral aspects of the clavicles are projected upward.

- The manubrium is superimposed by the (E) _____ vertebra, with 1 inch (2.5 cm) of apical lung field visible above the (F) _____.

- At the least nine posterior ribs are visualized above the (G) _____.

Copyright © 2015, 2011, 2006, 1996 by Saunders, an imprint of Elsevier Inc. All rights reserved.   Chapter **3** **Image Analysis of the Chest and Abdomen**

93. The AP/PA (decubitus) projection is primarily performed to confirm the presence of (A) _____ or (B) _____ levels within the pleural cavity.

94. If fluid is present within the pleural cavity on an AP/PA (decubitus) chest projection, where will it be located?

_____

95. For each situation below, state whether a right or left AP/PA decubitus chest projection should be taken.

A. Right pneumothorax: _____

B. Left pleural effusion: _____

96. To avoid rotation on AP/PA (decubitus) chest projections, align the patient's (A) _____, (B) _____, and (C) _____ perpendicular to the cart.

97. Will an AP or PA (decubitus) chest projection demonstrate the sixth and seventh cervical vertebrae without distortion and open intervertebral disk space?

_____

98. The lateral scapular borders are situated outside the lung field when the arms are positioned _____ for an AP/PA (decubitus) chest projection.

99. Chest foreshortening can be avoided on an AP/PA (decubitus) chest projection by positioning the (A) _____ plane (B) _____ (perpendicular/parallel) to the IR.

100. How can the patient be positioned for an AP/PA (decubitus) chest projection to prevent the cart pad from creating an artifact line along the lung field positioned against it?

_____

_____

For the following descriptions of AP/PA (decubitus) chest projections with poor positioning, state how the patient would have been positioned for such a projection to be obtained.

101. Whereas an AP (decubitus) chest projection demonstrates the right SC joint superimposed over the vertebral column, the left SC joint does not demonstrate vertebral superimposition.

_____

102. An AP decubitus chest projection demonstrates the manubrium at the level of the second thoracic vertebra.

_____

Copyright © 2015, 2011, 2006, 1996 by Saunders, an imprint of Elsevier Inc. All rights reserved.

For the following AP/PA (decubitus) chest projections with poor positioning, state what anatomic structures are misaligned and how the patient should be repositioned for an optimal projection to be obtained.

Figure 3-32

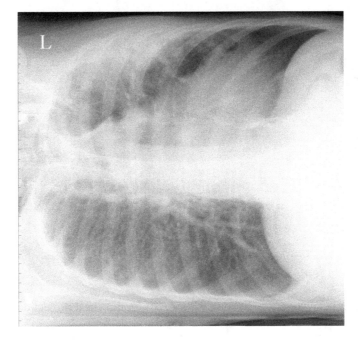

103. (Figure 3-32, AP projection):

_____

_____

Figure 3-33

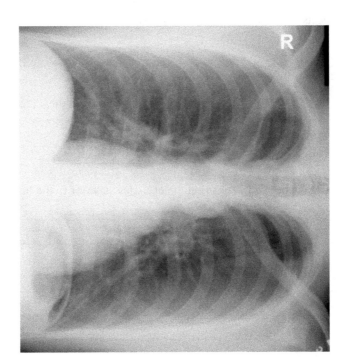

104. (Figure 3-33, AP projection):

_____

_____

Copyright © 2015, 2011, 2006, 1996 by Saunders, an imprint of Elsevier Inc. All rights reserved.   Chapter **3** **Image Analysis of the Chest and Abdomen**

AP Axial Projection (Lordotic Position)

105. Identify the labeled anatomy in Figure 3-34.

Figure 3-34

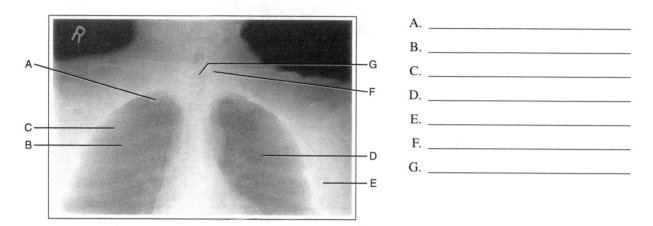

A. _____

B. _____

C. _____

D. _____

E. _____

F. _____

G. _____

106. Complete the statements below referring to adult AP axial (lordotic) chest projection analysis guidelines.

AP Axial (Lordotic) Chest Projection Analysis Guidelines

- (A) _____ lung field is at the center of the exposure field.

- Sternal clavicular ends of clavicles are projected (B) _____ to the lung apices, and posterior and anterior aspects of the first through fourth ribs lie (C) _____ and are nearly superimposed.

- (D) _____ borders of the scapulae are drawn away from the lung field, and the superior angles of scapulae are demonstrated away from lung apices.

- Distances from (E) _____ to the sternal clavicular ends are equal.

---

107. The AP axial chest projection is taken to visualize the _____.

108. Describe three methods that can be used to position the clavicles superior to the lung apices.

A. _____

_____

B. _____

_____

C. _____

_____

Copyright © 2015, 2011, 2006, 1996 by Saunders, an imprint of Elsevier Inc. All rights reserved.

109. An AP axial chest projection with poor positioning demonstrates the clavicles superimposed over the lung apices. What two positional changes can be made to obtain a projection with accurate positioning?

A. _____

B. _____

110. How must the patient be positioned to draw the lateral borders of the scapulae out of the lung field and the superior angles away from the lung apices?

_____

111. How can rotation be identified on an AP axial chest projection?

_____

112. An accurately centered AP axial chest projection is accomplished by centering the CR to the (A) _____

plane halfway between the (B) _____ and (C) _____.

113. What anatomic structures are included on an AP axial chest projection with accurate positioning?

_____

For the following descriptions of AP axial chest projections with poor positioning, state how the patient would have been mispositioned or the CR misaligned for such a projection to be obtained.

114. The clavicles are superimposed over the lung apices, and the anterior ribs appear inferior to their corresponding posterior ribs.

_____

_____

115. The lateral borders of the scapulae are demonstrated within the lung field, and the superior scapular angles are demonstrated within the apical region.

_____

_____

116. The right SC joint superimposes the vertebral column, and the left joint is demonstrated without superimposing the vertebral column.

_____

_____

Copyright © 2015, 2011, 2006, 1996 by Saunders, an imprint of Elsevier Inc. All rights reserved.   Chapter **3** **Image Analysis of the Chest and Abdomen**

For the following lordotic chest projection with poor positioning, state what anatomic structures are misaligned and how the patient should be repositioned for an optimal projection to be obtained.

Figure 3-35

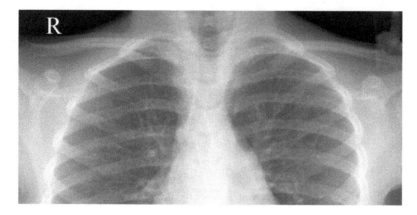

117. (Figure 3-35):

_____

_____

PA Oblique Projection (RAO and LAO Positions)

118. Identify the labeled anatomy in Figure 3-36.

Figure 3-36

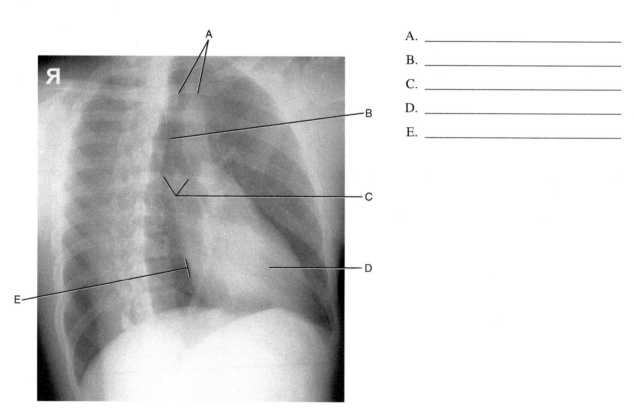

A. _____

B. _____

C. _____

D. _____

E. _____

Copyright © 2015, 2011, 2006, 1996 by Saunders, an imprint of Elsevier Inc. All rights reserved.

119. Complete the statements below referring to adult PA oblique chest projection analysis guidelines.

> **PA Oblique Chest Projection Analysis Guidelines**
>
> - Right and left (A) _____ are at the center of the exposure field.
>
> - (B) _____ are demonstrated without spinal superimposition, with approximately
>   (C) _____ as much lung field demonstrated on one side of the thoracic vertebrae as on the other side.
>
> - (D) _____ is superimposed by the fourth thoracic vertebra, with 1 inch (2.5 cm) of apical lung field visible above the clavicles.
>
> - At least (E) _____ posterior lungs visualized above the diaphragm.

120. What body plane is used to determine if the patient has been adequately rotated for an oblique chest projection?

_____

121. For a left PA oblique (LAO) chest projection, the patient needs to be rotated _____ degrees to demonstrate the heart shadow without vertebral column superimposition.

122. For the AP/PA oblique chest projections indicated below, state which side of the thorax will be best demonstrated.

A. Right AP oblique (RPO): _____

B. Left PA oblique (LAO): _____

123. The right AP oblique chest projection (RPO) corresponds with what PA oblique projection?

_____

124. A PA oblique chest projection with accurate centering is accomplished by centering the CR at a level 7.5 inches (18 cm) inferior to the _____.

125. What anatomic structures are included on a PA oblique chest projection with accurate positioning?

_____

For the following descriptions of PA oblique chest projections with poor positioning, state how the patient would have been mispositioned for such a projection to be obtained.

126. A 45-degree oblique projection demonstrates less than two times the lung field on one side of the thoracic vertebrae than the other side.

_____

127. A 45-degree oblique projection demonstrates more than two times the lung field on one side of the thoracic vertebrae than the other side.

_____

128. A 60-degree LAO projection demonstrates superimposition of the vertebral column and heart shadow.

_____

Copyright © 2015, 2011, 2006, 1996 by Saunders, an imprint of Elsevier Inc. All rights reserved.   Chapter **3 Image Analysis of the Chest and Abdomen**

For the following PA oblique chest projections with poor positioning, state what anatomic structures are misaligned and how the patient should be repositioned for an optimal projection to be obtained.

Figure 3-37

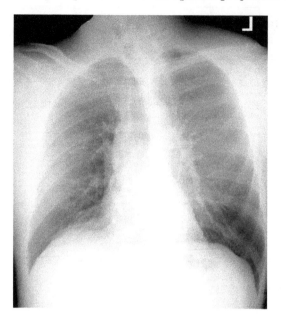

129. (Figure 3-37):

_____

_____

Figure 3-38

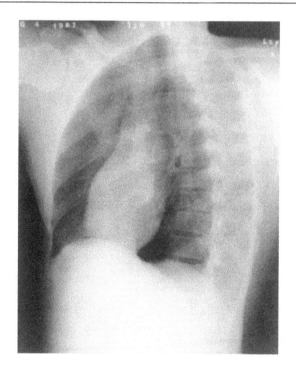

130. (Figure 3-38):

_____

_____

Copyright © 2015, 2011, 2006, 1996 by Saunders, an imprint of Elsevier Inc. All rights reserved.

Pediatric Chest

131. Why do neonatal and infant chest projections demonstrate less projection contrast than adult chest projections?

_____

132. Discuss the importance of the neonate's or infant's face being positioned forward and the cervical vertebrae being in a neutral position when the patient undergoes imaging for endotracheal tube (ET) placement.

_____

Neonate and Infant: AP Projection (Supine or with Mobile X-Ray Unit)

133. Identify the labeled anatomy in Figure 3-39.

Figure 3-39

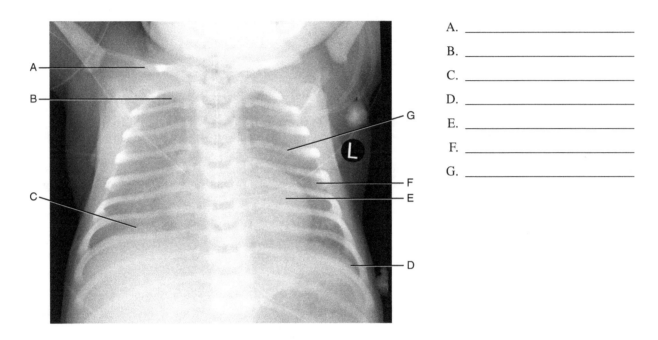

A. _____

B. _____

C. _____

D. _____

E. _____

F. _____

G. _____

134. Complete the statements below referring to neonate and infant AP chest projection analysis guidelines.

Neonate and Infant AP Chest Projection Analysis Guidelines

■ (A) _____ thoracic vertebra is at the center of the exposure field.

■ Distances from the vertebral column to the sternal ends of the clavicles are (B) _____, and the lengths of the right and left corresponding posterior ribs are (C) _____.

■ When a 5-degree caudal CR angle is used, the anterior ribs are projecting (D) _____, and the posterior ribs demonstrate a gentle, (E) _____ bowed contour.

■ Neonate: (F) _____ posterior ribs are demonstrated above the diaphragm, and the lungs demonstrate a fluffy appearance with linear-appearing connecting tissue.

■ Infant: (G) _____ posterior ribs are demonstrated above the diaphragm.

■ (H) _____ does not obscure the airway or apical lung field.

Copyright © 2015, 2011, 2006, 1996 by Saunders, an imprint of Elsevier Inc. All rights reserved.   Chapter **3 Image Analysis of the Chest and Abdomen**

135. Accurate centering is seen on neonatal or infant AP chest projections when a perpendicular CR is centered to the
(A) _____ plane at the level of the (B) _____. The (C) _____
_____ should be included on the projection.

136. What type of distortion is demonstrated when AP neonatal or infant chest projections demonstrate an excessively
lordotic appearance? _____

137. What causes the lungs on a neonatal chest projection to have a fluffy appearance?

_____

138. Explain when the projection should be exposed in the following situations to obtain maximum lung expansion.
   A. Neonate breathing without a ventilator: _____

   _____

   B. Neonate on a high-frequency ventilator: _____

   _____

**For the following descriptions of neonatal or infant AP chest projections with poor positioning, state how the
patient would have been mispositioned or the CR misaligned for such a projection to be obtained.**

139. The right sternal clavicular end is demonstrated farther from the vertebral column than the left sternal clavicular
end, and the right lower posterior ribs are longer than the left. The patient's head is turned toward the right side.

_____

140. The chest demonstrates an excessively lordotic appearance. The anterior ribs are projecting upward, and the posterior ribs are horizontal. The sixth thoracic vertebra is at the center of the projection.

_____

141. Seven posterior ribs are demonstrated above the diaphragm for a neonatal AP chest projection. The patient was on
a conventional ventilator.

_____

142. The patient's chin is superimposed over the airway and apical lung field.

_____

Copyright © 2015, 2011, 2006, 1996 by Saunders, an imprint of Elsevier Inc. All rights reserved.

For the following AP neonatal or infant chest projections with poor positioning, state what anatomic structures are misaligned and how the patient should be repositioned for an optimal projection to be obtained.

Figure 3-40

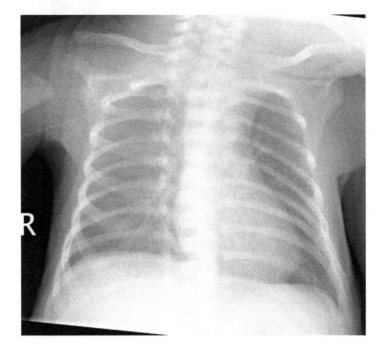

143. (Figure 3-40):

_____

_____

Figure 3-41

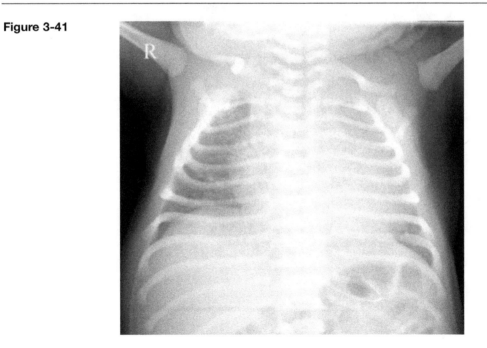

144. (Figure 3-41):

_____

_____

Copyright © 2015, 2011, 2006, 1996 by Saunders, an imprint of Elsevier Inc. All rights reserved.   Chapter **3 Image Analysis of the Chest and Abdomen**

Figure 3-42

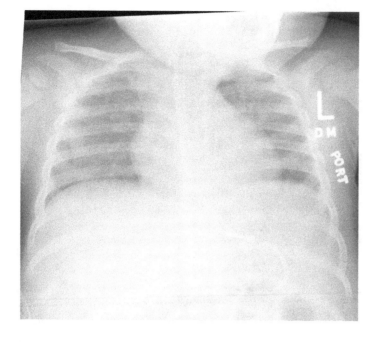

145. (Figure 3-42):

_____

_____

Figure 3-43

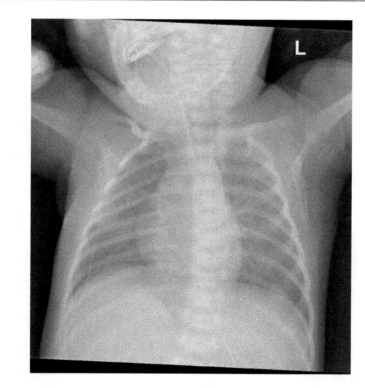

146. (Figure 3-43):

_____

_____

Chapter **3** **Image Analysis of the Chest and Abdomen**   Copyright © 2015, 2011, 2006, 1996 by Saunders, an imprint of Elsevier Inc. All rights reserved.

Child: PA and AP Projections

147. Identify the labeled anatomy in Figure 3-44.

Figure 3-44

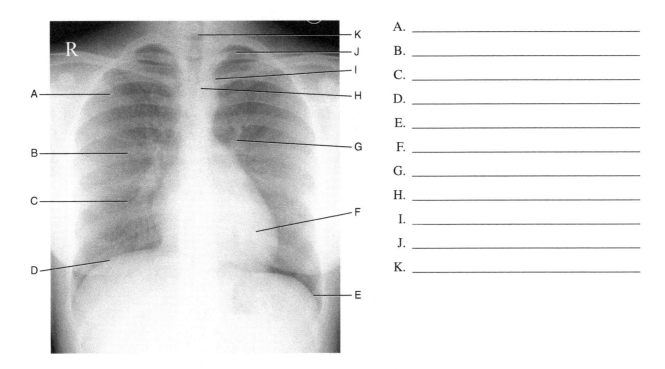

A. _____

B. _____

C. _____

D. _____

E. _____

F. _____

G. _____

H. _____

I. _____

J. _____

K. _____

For the following descriptions of child PA/AP chest projections with poor positioning, state how the patient would have been mispositioned or the central ray misaligned for such a projection to be obtained.

148. Mobile AP projection: The left sternoclavicular end is visualized without vertebral column superimposition, and the vertebral column is superimposed over the right sternal clavicular end.

_____

_____

149. PA projection: Six posterior ribs are demonstrated above the diaphragm.

_____

_____

150. Mobile AP projection: The manubrium is superimposed over the fifth thoracic vertebra, the posterior ribs demonstrate vertical contour, and more than 1 inch (2.5 cm) of apical lung field is visible above the clavicles.

_____

_____

Copyright © 2015, 2011, 2006, 1996 by Saunders, an imprint of Elsevier Inc. All rights reserved.

151. PA projection: The second thoracic vertebra is superimposed over the manubrium.

_____

_____

152. PA projection: The fourth thoracic vertebra is superimposed over the manubrium, and the lateral ends of the clavicles are projecting superiorly.

_____

_____

For the following PA/AP child chest projections with poor positioning, state what anatomic structures are misaligned and how the patient should be repositioned for an optimal projection to be obtained.

Figure 3-45

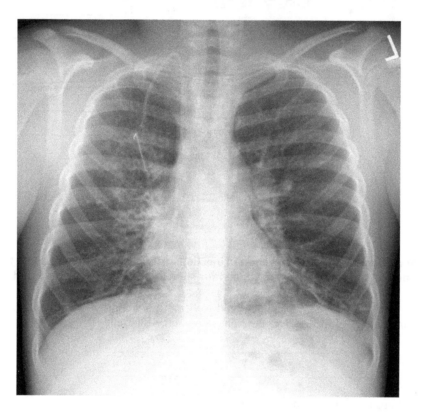

153. (Figure 3-45, PA projection):

_____

_____

Copyright © 2015, 2011, 2006, 1996 by Saunders, an imprint of Elsevier Inc. All rights reserved.

Figure 3-46

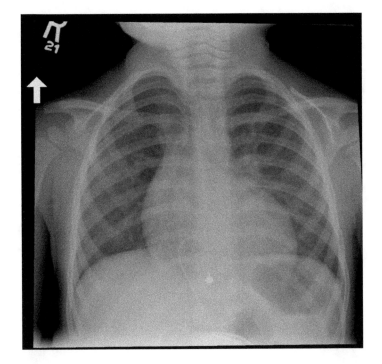

154. (Figure 3-46, PA projection):

_____

_____

Figure 3-47

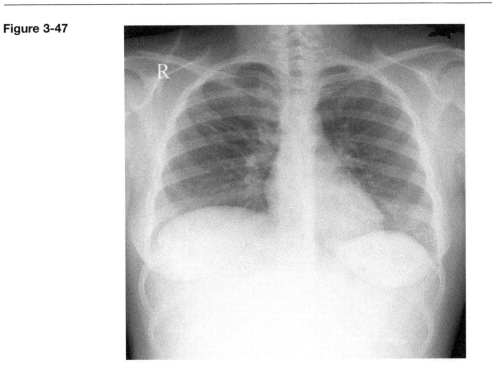

155. (Figure 3-47, PA projection):

_____

_____

Copyright © 2015, 2011, 2006, 1996 by Saunders, an imprint of Elsevier Inc. All rights reserved.

Chapter **3 Image Analysis of the Chest and Abdomen**

Figure 3-48

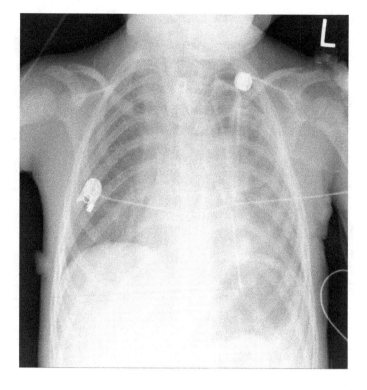

156. (Figure 3-48, AP projection):

_____

_____

Figure 3-49

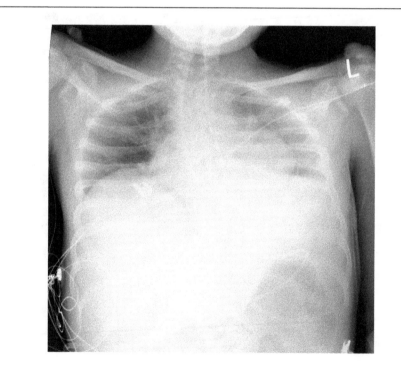

157. (Figure 3-49, AP projection):

_____

_____

     Copyright © 2015, 2011, 2006, 1996 by Saunders, an imprint of Elsevier Inc. All rights reserved.

Neonate and Infant: Cross-Table Lateral Projection (Left Lateral Position)

158. Identify the labeled anatomy in Figure 3-50.

Figure 3-50

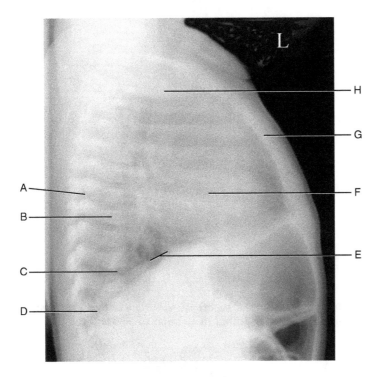

A. _____

B. _____

C. _____

D. _____

E. _____

F. _____

G. _____

H. _____

159. Accurate centering is seen on a neonatal or infant lateral chest projection when the CR is centered to the (A) _____ plane at the level just inferior to the (B) _____. The (C) _____ should be included on the projection.

160. List two reasons why cross-table lateral neonatal chest projections are taken instead of overhead projections.

    A. _____

    B. _____

161. To avoid chest rotation on lateral neonatal and infant chest projections, align an imaginary line connecting the shoulders, the posterior ribs, and the ASISs _____ to the IR.

162. Explain why the 0.5-inch (1.25-cm) posterior rib separation demonstrated on optimally positioned adult lateral chest projections is not demonstrated on neonatal or infant lateral chest projections.

    _____

    _____

Copyright © 2015, 2011, 2006, 1996 by Saunders, an imprint of Elsevier Inc. All rights reserved.

Chapter **3 Image Analysis of the Chest and Abdomen**

For the following descriptions of neonatal or infant lateral chest projections with poor positioning, state how the patient would have been mispositioned or the CR misaligned for such a projection to be obtained.

163. The left posterior ribs are demonstrated posterior to the right posterior ribs.

_____

_____

164. The humeral soft tissue is superimposed over the anterior lung apices.

_____

_____

165. The patient's chin is demonstrated within the collimated field.

_____

_____

166. The hemidiaphragms demonstrate an exaggerated cephalic curvature and are positioned high in the thorax.

_____

_____

For the following neonatal or infant lateral chest projections with poor positioning, state what anatomic structures are misaligned and how the patient should be repositioned for an optimal projection to be obtained.

Figure 3-51

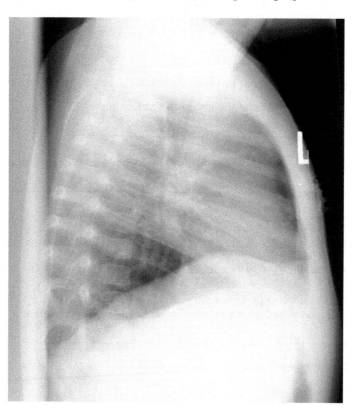

167. (Figure 3-51):

_____

_____

Copyright © 2015, 2011, 2006, 1996 by Saunders, an imprint of Elsevier Inc. All rights reserved.

Figure 3-52

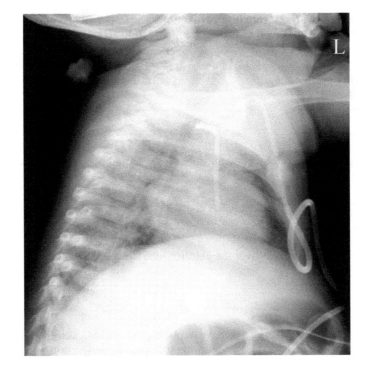

168. (Figure 3-52):

_____

_____

Child: Lateral Projection (Left Lateral Position)

169. Identify the labeled anatomy in Figure 3-53.

Figure 3-53

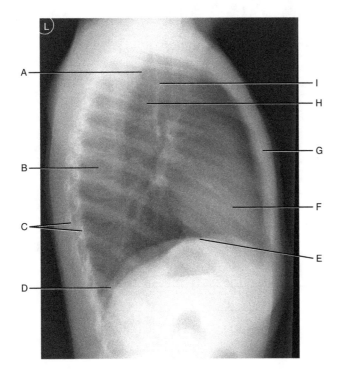

A. _____

B. _____

C. _____

D. _____

E. _____

F. _____

G. _____

H. _____

I. _____

89

Copyright © 2015, 2011, 2006, 1996 by Saunders, an imprint of Elsevier Inc. All rights reserved.

For the following descriptions of child lateral chest projections with poor positioning, state how the patient would have been mispositioned or the CR misaligned for such a projection to be obtained.

170. More than 0.5 inch (1.25 cm) of separation is demonstrated between the posterior ribs. The gastric air bubble is adjacent to the posteriorly located lung.

    _____

    _____

171. The hemidiaphragms demonstrate an exaggerated cephalic curve, and they do not cover the entire eleventh thoracic vertebra.

    _____

    _____

172. The humeral soft tissue is superimposed over the anterior lung apices.

    _____

    _____

For the following lateral child chest projections with poor positioning, state what anatomic structures are misaligned and how the patient should be repositioned for an optimal projection to be obtained.

Figure 3-54

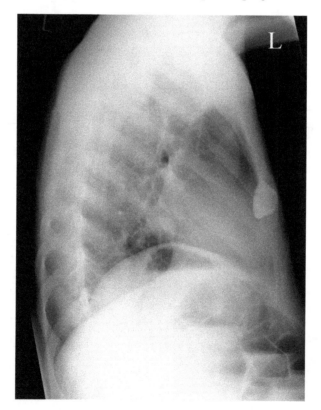

173. (Figure 3-54):

    _____

    _____

Copyright © 2015, 2011, 2006, 1996 by Saunders, an imprint of Elsevier Inc. All rights reserved.

Figure 3-55

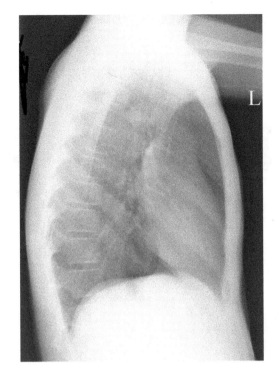

174. (Figure 3-55):

_____

_____

Figure 3-56

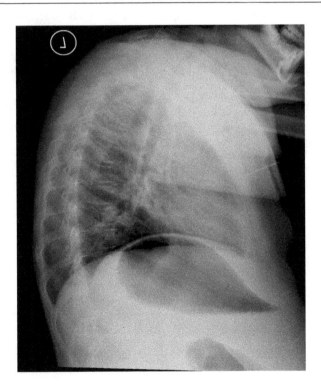

175. (Figure 3-56):

_____

_____

Copyright © 2015, 2011, 2006, 1996 by Saunders, an imprint of Elsevier Inc. All rights reserved.   Chapter **3 Image Analysis of the Chest and Abdomen**

Neonate and Infant: AP Projection (Right or Left Lateral Decubitus Projection)

176. Identify the labeled anatomy in Figure 3-57.

Figure 3-57

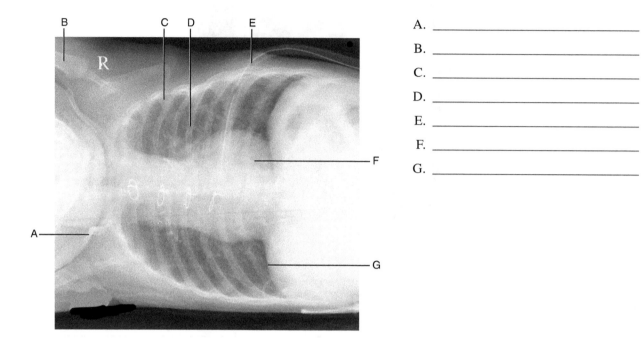

A. _____

B. _____

C. _____

D. _____

E. _____

F. _____

G. _____

177. Complete the statements below referring to neonate and infant AP (decubitus) chest projection analysis guidelines.

Neonate and Infant AP (Decubitus) Chest Projection Analysis Guidelines

- (A) _____ vertebra is at the center of the exposure field.

- Distances from the (B) _____ to the sternal ends of the clavicles are equal, and the lengths of the right and left corresponding posterior ribs are equal.

- The chin and arms are situated outside the lung field, and the lateral aspects of the (C)

  _____ are projected upward.

- With the posterior surface resting against IR, each upper anterior rib is demonstrated (D)

  _____ to its corresponding posterior rib.

- (E) _____ posterior ribs are demonstrated above the diaphragm, and the lungs demonstrate a fluffy appearance with linear-appearing connecting tissue.

- Lung field positioned against the bed or cart is demonstrated without superimposition of the bed or cart pad.

- (F) _____ plane is seen without lateral tilting.

Copyright © 2015, 2011, 2006, 1996 by Saunders, an imprint of Elsevier Inc. All rights reserved.

AP Projection (Left Lateral Decubitus Position)

226. Identify the labeled anatomy in Figure 3-79.

Figure 3-79

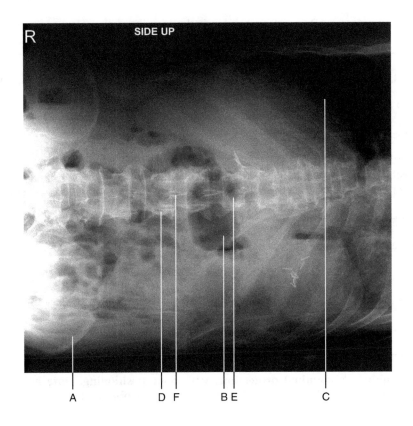

A. _____

B. _____

C. _____

D. _____

E. _____

F. _____

227. Complete the statements below referring to adult AP (decubitus) abdomen projection analysis guidelines.

AP (Decubitus) Abdomen Projection Analysis Guidelines

■ Spinous processes are aligned with the midline of the (A) _____, and the distance from the pedicles to the (B) _____ is the same on both sides. The sacrum is centered within the inlet of pelvis and is aligned with the symphysis pubis.

■ Diaphragm domes are located superior to the (C) _____ posterior ribs.

■ (D) _____ lumbar vertebra is at the center of the exposure field.

---

228. A patient's requisition requests that an AP (decubitus) abdominal projection be taken to rule out ascites. Describe how to determine the technique factors to use for this patient.

_____

_____

Copyright © 2015, 2011, 2006, 1996 by Saunders, an imprint of Elsevier Inc. All rights reserved.

229. For an AP (decubitus) abdominal projection, the (A) _____ side of the patient is positioned against the imaging table or cart. Why is this side chosen? (B) _____

_____

230. Placing a pillow between the patient's knees for an AP (decubitus) abdominal projection will prevent

_____.

231. To obtain optimal intraperitoneal air demonstration, the patient should remain in the decubitus position for (A) _____ minutes before the AP (decubitus) projection is taken. Why is this time delay necessary?

(B) _____

232. Intraperitoneal air is most often found beneath the (A) _____ on an AP (decubitus) abdominal projection with proper positioning. Describe the shape of a patient's body that will result in the intraperitoneal air being demonstrated over the right iliac wing on a properly positioned AP (decubitus) abdominal

projection. (B) _____

233. What respiration is used for an AP (decubitus) abdominal projection?

_____

234. What anatomic structures are included on an AP (decubitus) abdominal projection with accurate positioning?

_____

_____

For the following descriptions of AP (decubitus) abdominal projections with poor positioning, state how the patient would have been mispositioned or the CR misaligned for such a projection to be obtained.

235. The projection demonstrates a greater distance from the left lumbar vertebral pedicles to the spinous processes than the right pedicles to the spinous processes.

_____

236. The projection demonstrates the upper abdominal region with equal distances from the vertebral pedicles to the spinous processes on each side, and the lower abdominal region demonstrates the sacrum and symphysis pubis without alignment. The sacrum is rotated toward the left pelvic inlet.

_____

_____

237. The projection demonstrates a clipped right diaphragmatic dome.

_____

  Copyright © 2015, 2011, 2006, 1996 by Saunders, an imprint of Elsevier Inc. All rights reserved.

For the following AP (decubitus) abdominal projection with poor positioning (Figure 3-80), state what anatomic structures are misaligned and how the patient should be repositioned for an optimal projection to be obtained.

Figure 3-80

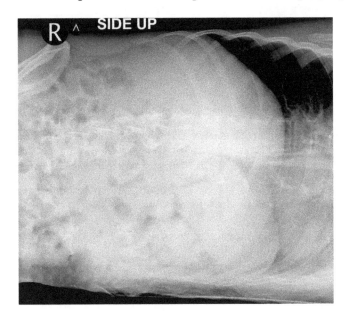

238. (Figure 3-80):

_____

_____

Neonate and Infant: AP Projection

239. Identify the labeled anatomy in Figure 3-81.

Figure 3-81

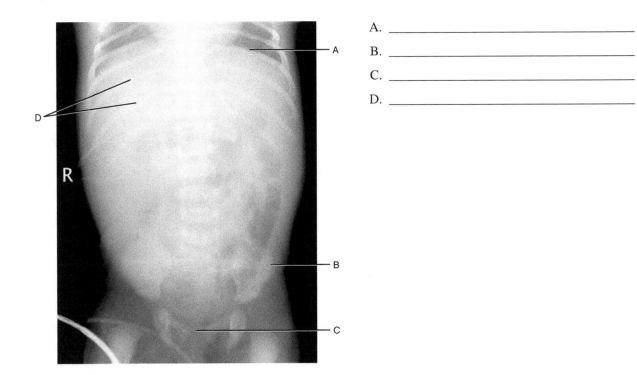

A. _____

B. _____

C. _____

D. _____

Copyright © 2015, 2011, 2006, 1996 by Saunders, an imprint of Elsevier Inc. All rights reserved.

240. Complete the statements below referring to neonate and infant AP abdomen projection analysis guidelines.

AP Abdomen Projection Analysis Guidelines
■ Diaphragm domes are superior to the (A) _____ posterior rib.
■ (B) _____ vertebra is at the center of the exposure field.

241. To accurately center a neonatal and infant AP abdominal projection, the CR is centered to the (A) _____

plane at a level (B) _____ inches (C) _____ to the (D) _____.

For the following descriptions of neonatal or infant AP abdominal projections with poor positioning, state how the patient would have been mispositioned or the CR misaligned for such a projection to be obtained.

242. The diaphragm is not included on the projection.

_____

243. The patient's upper vertebral column is tilted toward the left side.

_____

244. The left inferior posterior ribs are longer than the posterior ribs on the right side.

_____

245. The right iliac wing is wider than the left wing.

_____

246. The diaphragm is at the level of the ninth posterior rib.

_____

Copyright © 2015, 2011, 2006, 1996 by Saunders, an imprint of Elsevier Inc. All rights reserved.

For the following AP neonatal or infant abdominal projections with poor positioning, state what anatomic structures are misaligned and how the patient should be repositioned for an optimal projection to be obtained.

Figure 3-82

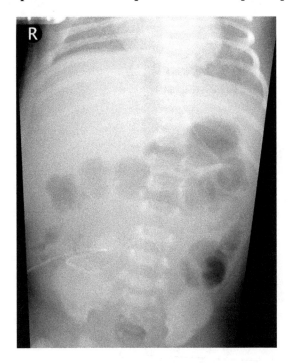

247. (Figure 3-82):

_____

_____

Figure 3-83

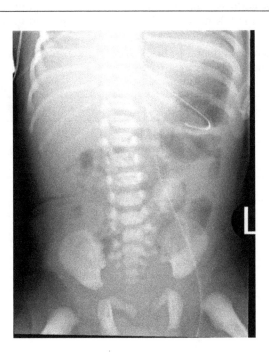

248. (Figure 3-83):

_____

_____

Copyright © 2015, 2011, 2006, 1996 by Saunders, an imprint of Elsevier Inc. All rights reserved. Chapter **3 Image Analysis of the Chest and Abdomen**

Child: AP Projection

249. Identify the labeled anatomy in Figure 3-84.

Figure 3-84

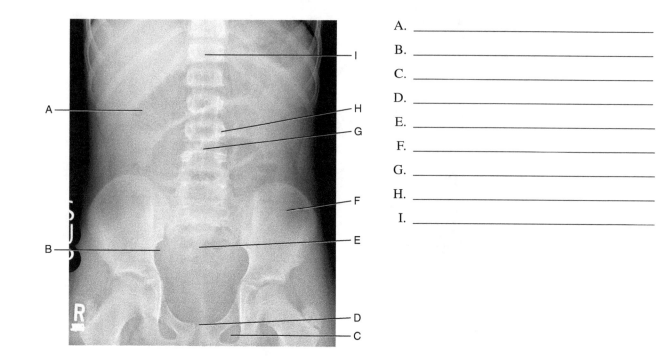

A. _____

B. _____

C. _____

D. _____

E. _____

F. _____

G. _____

H. _____

I. _____

For the following descriptions of child AP abdominal projections with poor positioning, state how the patient would have been mispositioned or the CR misaligned for such a projection to be obtained.

250. The distance from the right lumbar vertebral pedicles to the spinous processes is greater than the distance from the left pedicles to the spinous processes.

_____

_____

251. The left inferior posterior ribs are longer than the right, and the left iliac wing is wider than the right.

_____

_____

Copyright © 2015, 2011, 2006, 1996 by Saunders, an imprint of Elsevier Inc. All rights reserved.

For the following AP child abdominal projections with poor positioning, state what anatomic structures are misaligned and how the patient should be repositioned for an optimal projection to be obtained.

Figure 3-85

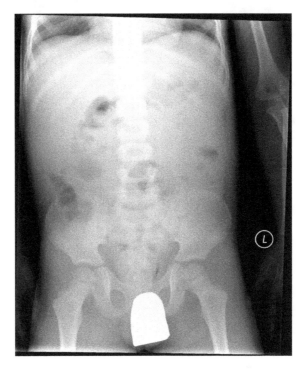

252. (Figure 3-85, supine abdomen):

_____

_____

Figure 3-86

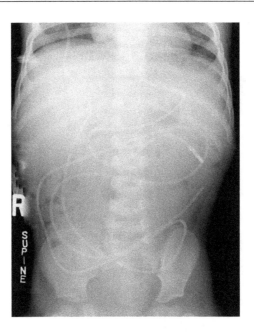

253. (Figure 3-86, supine abdomen):

_____

_____

Copyright © 2015, 2011, 2006, 1996 by Saunders, an imprint of Elsevier Inc. All rights reserved. Chapter **3** **Image Analysis of the Chest and Abdomen**

Figure 3-87

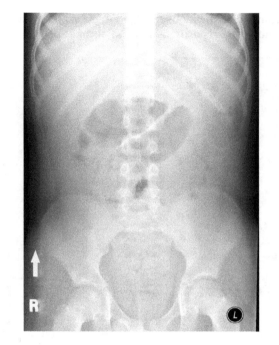

254. (Figure 3-87, upright abdomen):

_____

_____

Neonate and Infant: AP Projection (Left Lateral Decubitus Position)

255. Identify the labeled anatomy in Figure 3-88.

Figure 3-88

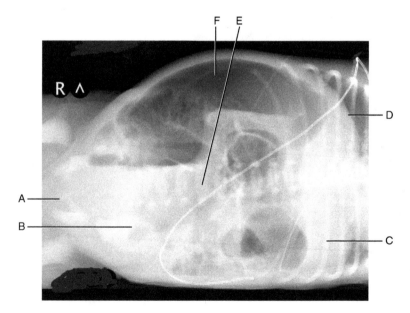
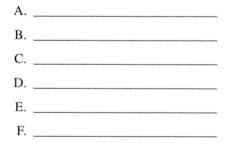

A. _____

B. _____

C. _____

D. _____

E. _____

F. _____

Chapter **3 Image Analysis of the Chest and Abdomen**   Copyright © 2015, 2011, 2006, 1996 by Saunders, an imprint of Elsevier Inc. All rights reserved.

256. Explain why the left side of the patient is placed adjacent to the bed or cart when the patient is positioned for neonatal or infant AP (decubitus) abdomen projections.

_____

_____

257. For a neonatal and infant AP (decubitus) abdominal projection, a horizontal CR is centered to the (A) _____ plane at a level (B) _____ inches (C) _____ to the (D) _____.

For the following descriptions of neonatal or infant left AP (decubitus) abdominal projections with poor positioning, state how the patient would have been mispositioned or the CR misaligned for such a projection to be obtained.

258. The left iliac wing is narrower than the right iliac wing.

_____

_____

259. The diaphragm is not included on the projection.

_____

_____

260. The right posterior ribs are longer than the posterior ribs on the left side.

_____

_____

For the following neonatal or infant left AP (decubitus) abdominal projections with poor positioning, state what anatomic structures are misaligned and how the patient should be repositioned for an optimal projection to be obtained.

Figure 3-89

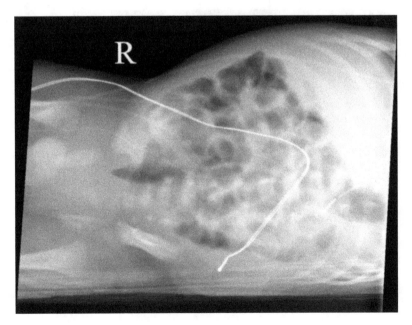

261. (Figure 3-89):

_____

_____

Copyright © 2015, 2011, 2006, 1996 by Saunders, an imprint of Elsevier Inc. All rights reserved.   Chapter **3 Image Analysis of the Chest and Abdomen**

Figure 3-90

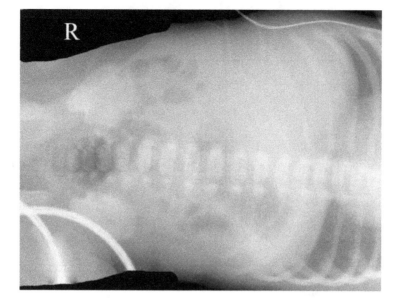

262. (Figure 3-90):

_____

_____

Child: AP Projection (Left Lateral Decubitus Position)

263. Identify the labeled anatomy in Figure 3-91.

Figure 3-91

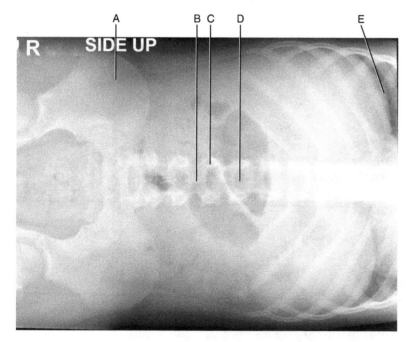

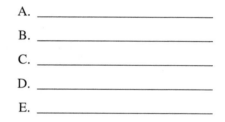

A. _____

B. _____

C. _____

D. _____

E. _____

    Copyright © 2015, 2011, 2006, 1996 by Saunders, an imprint of Elsevier Inc. All rights reserved.

Figure 3-92

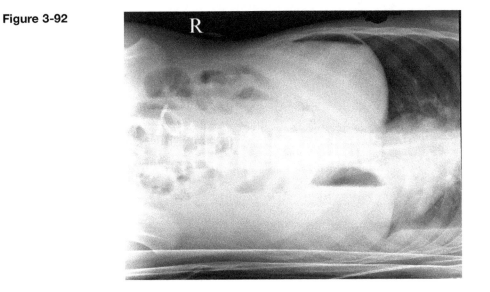

264. Identify the patient condition demonstrated on the projection in Figure 3-92.

_____

For the following descriptions of child AP (decubitus) abdominal projections with poor positioning, state how the patient would have been mispositioned or the CR misaligned for such a projection to be obtained.

265. The distance from the left lumbar vertebral pedicles to the spinous processes is greater than that from the right pedicles to the spinous processes.

_____

_____

For the following child AP (decubitus) projections with poor positioning, state what anatomic structures are misaligned and how the patient should be repositioned for an optimal projection to be obtained.

Figure 3-93

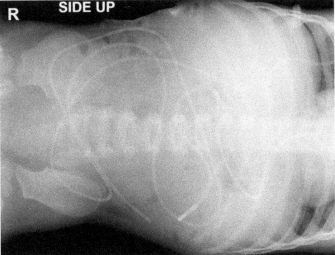

266. (Figure 3-93):

_____

_____

119

Copyright © 2015, 2011, 2006, 1996 by Saunders, an imprint of Elsevier Inc. All rights reserved.

4 Image Analysis of the Upper Extremity

STUDY QUESTIONS

1. Complete Figure 4-1

   Figure 4-1

Upper Extremity Technical Data				
Projection	kV	Grid	mAs	**SID**
Finger				
Thumb				
Hand				
Wrist				
Forearm				
Elbow				
Humerus				
Pediatric				

 Copyright © 2015, 2011, 2006, 1996 by Saunders, an imprint of Elsevier Inc. All rights reserved.

Finger: PA Projection

2. Identify the labeled anatomy in Figure 4-2.

Figure 4-2

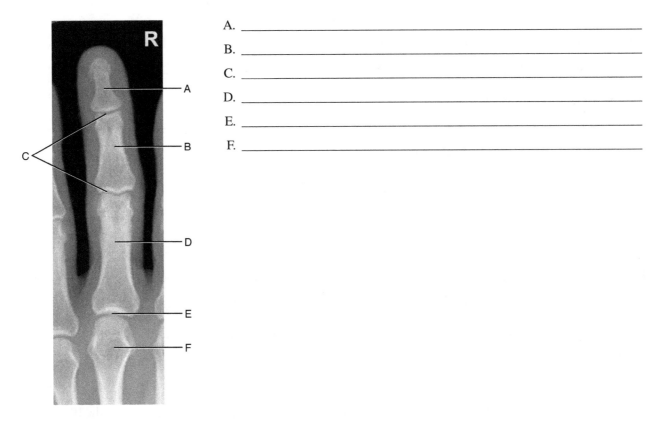

A. _____

B. _____

C. _____

D. _____

E. _____

F. _____

3. Complete the statements below referring to PA finger projection analysis guidelines.

PA Finger Projection Analysis Guidelines
■ Soft tissue width and the midshaft concavity are (A) _equal_ on both sides of phalanges.
■ IP and (B) _MCP_ joints are demonstrated as open spaces, and the phalanges are seen without foreshortening.
■ The (C) _PIP_ joint is at the center of the exposure field.
■ The entire digit and half of the (D) _metacarpal_ are included within the collimated field.

4. A finger projection has been requested for a patient with severe rheumatoid arthritis. The patient has a ring on the affected finger that cannot be removed. What procedure should be followed?

_____

_____

5. To prevent finger rotation on a PA finger projection, the hand should be positioned _flat_ against the IR.

Copyright © 2015, 2011, 2006, 1996 by Saunders, an imprint of Elsevier Inc. All rights reserved.

6. In which direction is the finger most frequently rotated when rotation occurs on a PA finger projection?

A. _____

Why?

B. _____

7. On a rotated PA projection, the side of the finger that is rolled (A) _farther_ (farther from/closer to) the IR will demonstrate the greatest phalangeal midshaft concavity and the (B) _greatest_ soft tissue thickness.

8. Which of the finger MCs is the longest?

_____

9. Which of the finger MCs is the shortest?

_____

10. How is the patient positioned for a PA finger projection to prevent soft tissue overlap of adjacent fingers onto the affected finger?

Spreading the fingers apart

11. To accomplish open joint spaces on a PA finger projection, the CR must be aligned (A) _perp._ (perpendicular/parallel) to the joint space, and the IR must be aligned (B) _parallel_ to the joint space.

12. If the finger is flexed for the PA projection, the joint spaces will be (A) _____, and the phalanges will be (B) _____.

13. On a patient whose finger is flexed, open IP joint spaces can be obtained by (A) _____ the hand and elevating the proximal MCs until the joint of interest is aligned (B) _____ to the IR.

14. Accurate CR centering is seen on a PA finger projection by centering a (A) _____ CR to the (B) _____ joint.

15. Included within the exposure field on a PA finger projection with accurate positioning are the (A) _____ and half of the (B) _____.

16. Accurate transverse collimation has been obtained when the collimated borders are _____.

For the following descriptions of PA finger projections with poor positioning, state how the patient would have been mispositioned for such a projection to be obtained.

17. The projection demonstrates unequal soft tissue width and midshaft concavity on each side of the phalanges. The side of the phalanges with the least amount of concavity is facing the longest finger MC.

_____

Copyright © 2015, 2011, 2006, 1996 by Saunders, an imprint of Elsevier Inc. All rights reserved.

18. The projection demonstrates closed IP and MCP joints, and the distal and middle phalanges are foreshortened.

For the following PA finger projections with poor positioning, state what anatomic structures are misaligned and how the patient should be repositioned for an optimal projection to be obtained.

Figure 4-3

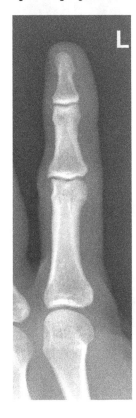

19. (Figure 4-3): _The finger is slightly obliqued causing more concavity & tissue on one side. Fix by: slightly rotating finger back, so its flat on the IR._

Copyright © 2015, 2011, 2006, 1996 by Saunders, an imprint of Elsevier Inc. All rights reserved.

Figure 4-4

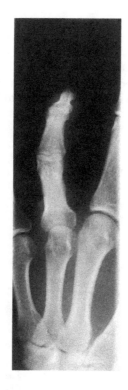

20. (Figure 4-4): _____

_____

_____

_____

Finger: PA Oblique Projection

21. Identify the labeled anatomy in Figure 4-5.

Figure 4-5

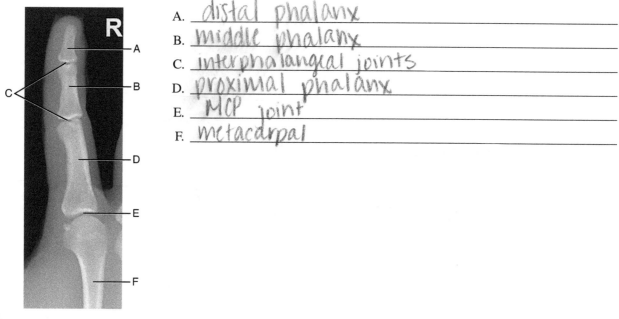

A. _distal phalanx_

B. _middle phalanx_

C. _interphalangeal joints_

D. _proximal phalanx_

E. _MCP joint_

F. _metacarpal_

124

Copyright © 2015, 2011, 2006, 1996 by Saunders, an imprint of Elsevier Inc. All rights reserved.

22. Complete the statements below referring to PA oblique finger projection analysis guidelines.

> **PA Oblique Finger Projection Analysis Guidelines**
> - (A) _Twice_ as much soft tissue width is demonstrated on one side of the digit as on the other side, and more (B) _concavity_ is seen on one aspect of the phalangeal midshafts than the others.
> - IP and MCP joints are demonstrated as (C) _open spaces_, and the phalanges are not foreshortened.
> - The (D) _PIP_ joint is at the center of the exposure field.

23. The affected finger is rotated _____degrees from the PA projection for a PA oblique finger projection.

24. In which direction are the hand and finger rotated for a PA oblique projection when imaging the third through fifth fingers?

    A. _____

    For the second finger?

    B. _____

    Why is the second finger rotated differently?

    C. _____

25. To obtain open IP and MCP joint spaces, the finger needs to be fully (A) _extended_ and positioned (B) _parallel_ to the IR.

26. When imaging the third and fourth fingers, why is it often necessary to position a sponge beneath the distal phalanx?
    to prevent finger from tilting towards the IR

27. Accurate CR centering on a PA oblique finger projection is accomplished by centering a (A) _____ CR to the (B) _____ joint.

28. What anatomic structures are included on a PA oblique finger projection with accurate positioning?
    entire digit and half of the metacarpal

For the following descriptions of PA oblique finger projections with poor positioning, state how the patient would have been mispositioned for such a projection to be obtained.

29. The soft tissue width and midshaft concavity are nearly equal on each side of the digit.

    _____

30. More than twice as much soft tissue width is present on one side of the phalanges as on the other. One aspect of the midshafts of the phalanges is concave, and the other aspect is slightly convex.
    the finger was obliqued too much

31. The projection demonstrates closed IP joint spaces, and the distal and middle phalanges are foreshortened.
    the finger was bent towards the IR

Copyright © 2015, 2011, 2006, 1996 by Saunders, an imprint of Elsevier Inc. All rights reserved. Chapter **4** **Image Analysis of the Upper Extremity**

For the following PA oblique finger projections with poor positioning, state what anatomic structures are misaligned and how the patient should be repositioned for an optimal projection to be obtained.

Figure 4-6

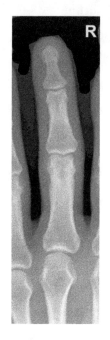

32. (Figure 4-6, third digit): _____

_____

_____

Figure 4-7

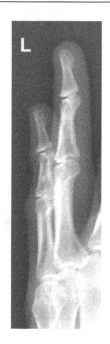

33. (Figure 4-7, fourth digit): _____

_____

_____

Copyright © 2015, 2011, 2006, 1996 by Saunders, an imprint of Elsevier Inc. All rights reserved.

Figure 4-8

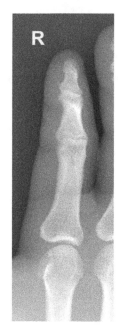

34. (Figure 4-8, second digit): _____

_____

_____

Finger: Lateral Projection

35. Identify the labeled anatomy in Figure 4-9.

Figure 4-9

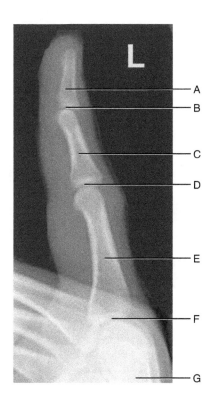

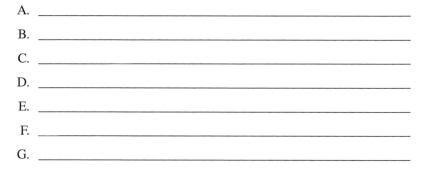

A. _____

B. _____

C. _____

D. _____

E. _____

F. _____

G. _____

Copyright © 2015, 2011, 2006, 1996 by Saunders, an imprint of Elsevier Inc. All rights reserved.

36. Complete the statements below referring to lateral finger projection analysis guidelines.

Lateral Finger Projection Analysis Guidelines
■ (A) _anterior_ surface of the middle and proximal phalanges demonstrate midshaft concavity, and the (B) _posterior_ surfaces show slight convexity.
■ (C) _IP joints_ are demonstrated as open spaces, and the phalanges are not foreshortened.
■ (D) _PIP joints_ is at the center of the exposure field.

37. How many degrees from the PA projection should the finger be rotated for a lateral finger projection with accurate positioning? _____

38 For each of the following fingers, state how the hand is rotated (internally/externally) from the PA projection to place the finger in a lateral projection.

   A. Second finger: _____

   B. Third finger:_____

   C. Fourth finger: _____

   D. Fifth finger: _____

39. What determines how the hand is rotated for the previous question?

   _____

40 How is the hand positioned for a lateral finger projection to prevent soft tissue overlap of the adjacent fingers onto the affected finger and to best demonstrate the affected finger's proximal phalanx?

   _____

41. What anatomic structures are included on a lateral finger projection with accurate positioning?

   _____

Chapter **4** **Image Analysis of the Upper Extremity**   Copyright © 2015, 2011, 2006, 1996 by Saunders, an imprint of Elsevier Inc. All rights reserved.

42. Describe the positioning error that is demonstrated on the projection in Figure 4-10.

Figure 4-10

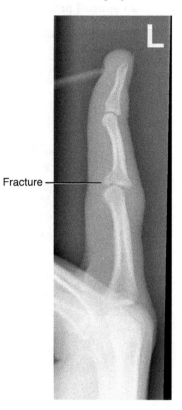

Fracture

_____

_____

For the following descriptions of lateral finger projections with poor positioning, state how the patient would have been mispositioned for such a projection to be obtained.

43. The proximal phalanges of the unaffected fingers overlap the proximal phalanx of the affected finger.

_____

44. Concavity is demonstrated on both sides of the middle and proximal phalangeal midshafts.

_____

45. The IP joint spaces are closed, and the phalanges are foreshortened.

_____

Copyright © 2015, 2011, 2006, 1996 by Saunders, an imprint of Elsevier Inc. All rights reserved.   Chapter **4**   **Image Analysis of the Upper Extremity**

For the following lateral finger projections with poor positioning, state what anatomic structures are misaligned and how the patient should be repositioned for an optimal projection to be obtained.

Figure 4-11

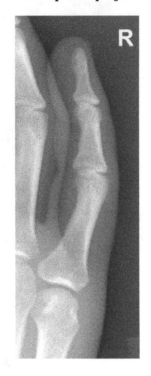

46. (Figure 4-11): _____

_____

_____

Figure 4-12

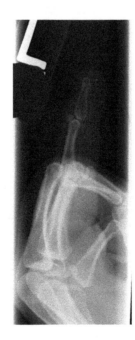

47. (Figure 4-12): _____

_____

_____

 Copyright © 2015, 2011, 2006, 1996 by Saunders, an imprint of Elsevier Inc. All rights reserved.

Thumb: AP Projection

48. Identify the labeled anatomy in Figure 4-13.

Figure 4-13

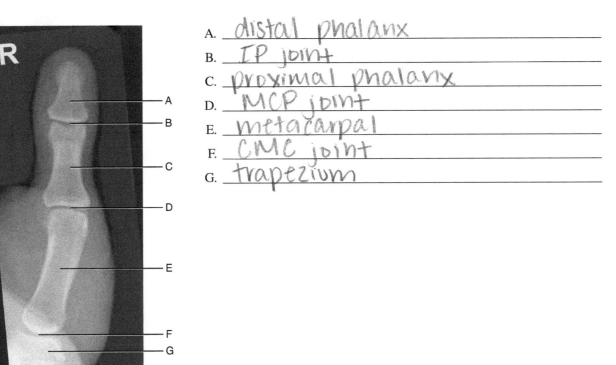

A. _distal phalanx_
B. _IP joint_
C. _proximal phalanx_
D. _MCP joint_
E. _metacarpal_
F. _CMC joint_
G. _trapezium_

49. Complete the statements below referring to AP thumb projection analysis guidelines.

AP Thumb Projection Analysis Guidelines

- (A) _concavity_ on both sides of phalanges and MC midshafts is equal. Equal (B) _soft tissue_ width on each side of phalanges.

- IP, MCP, and CM joints are demonstrated as (D) _open spaces_, and the phalanges are not foreshortened.

- Superimposition of the (E) _medial palm_ soft tissue over the proximal first MC and the CM joint is minimal.

- (F) _MCP joint_ is at the center of the exposure field.

---

50. For the thumb to be positioned in an AP projection, the hand is (A) _____ (internally/externally) rotated, and the thumbnail is positioned (B) _____ against the IR.

51. When the thumb is rotated away from an AP projection, the amount of phalangeal midshaft concavity increases on the side positioned _____ (farther/closer) from/to the IR.

52. To obtain open joint spaces on an AP thumb projection, the thumb is fully _____ and the CR is accurately aligned and centered to the thumb.

Copyright © 2015, 2011, 2006, 1996 by Saunders, an imprint of Elsevier Inc. All rights reserved.

Chapter **4**   **Image Analysis of the Upper Extremity**

53. How is the hand positioned to prevent the medial palm soft tissue and possibly the fourth and fifth MCs from being superimposed over the proximal MC?

_____

54. Accurate CR centering on an AP thumb projection is accomplished by centering a (B) _____ CR to the

(C) _____ joint.

55. List the anatomic structures that are included within the collimated field on an AP thumb projection with accurate positioning.

_____whole digit, MC joint, 3 CM joint_____

For the following descriptions of AP thumb projections with poor positioning, state how the patient would have been mispositioned for such a projection to be obtained.

56. The soft tissue width and the concavity of the phalangeal and MC midshafts on each side are not equal. The side demonstrating the more concavity is facing toward the second through fifth digits, and the thumbnail is facing away from the second through fifth digits.

_____

57. The projection demonstrates a foreshortened distal phalanx and a closed DIP joint space.

_____

58. The fifth MC and the medial palm soft tissue are superimposed over the proximal first MC and CM joints.

_____

For the following AP thumb projections with poor positioning, state what anatomic structures are misaligned and how the patient should be repositioned for an optimal projection to be obtained.

Figure 4-14

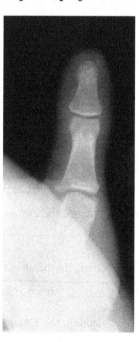

59. (Figure 4-14): _____
_____The palm is superimposing the MC 3 CM joints._____
_____Pull back whole hand w/ other hand to prevent._____

Chapter **4** **Image Analysis of the Upper Extremity**   Copyright © 2015, 2011, 2006, 1996 by Saunders, an imprint of Elsevier Inc. All rights reserved.

Figure 4-15

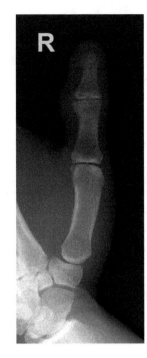

60. (Figure 4-15): _____

_____

_____

Thumb: Lateral Projections

61. Identify the labeled anatomy in Figure 4-16.

Figure 4-16

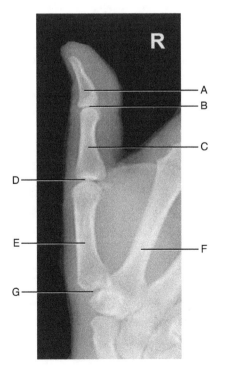

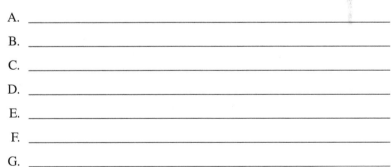

A. _____

B. _____

C. _____

D. _____

E. _____

F. _____

G. _____

Copyright © 2015, 2011, 2006, 1996 by Saunders, an imprint of Elsevier Inc. All rights reserved.   Chapter **4**   **Image Analysis of the Upper Extremity**

62. Complete the statements below referring to lateral thumb projection analysis guidelines.

Lateral Thumb Projection Analysis Guidelines

- (A) _anterior_ aspect of the proximal phalanx and MC demonstrates midshaft concavity, and the (B) _posterior_ aspect of the proximal phalanx and MC demonstrates slight convexity.
- The IP, MCP, and CM joints are demonstrated as (C) _open spaces_ and the phalanges are not foreshortened.
- The proximal first MC is only slightly superimposed by the proximal (D) _2nd_ MC.
- (E) _MCP joint_ is at the center of the exposure field.

63. To obtain a lateral projection of the thumb, rest the hand flat against the IR and then _____ it until the thumb rolls into a lateral projection.

64. Abducting the thumb will decrease the amount of _____ superimposition of the CM joint.

65. Accurate CR centering on a lateral thumb projection is accomplished by centering a (A) _____ CR to the

(B) _____ joint.

66. List the anatomic structures that are included within the collimated field on a lateral thumb projection with accurate positioning.

_____

For the following descriptions of lateral thumb projections with poor positioning, state how the patient would have been mispositioned for such a projection to be obtained.

67. The projection does not demonstrate a lateral projection. The second and third proximal MCs are superimposed over the first proximal MC.

_____

68. The projection does not demonstrate a lateral position. The anterior and posterior aspects of the proximal phalanx and MC midshafts demonstrate concavity. The first proximal MC is demonstrated without superimposition of the second and third proximal MCs.

_____

Copyright © 2015, 2011, 2006, 1996 by Saunders, an imprint of Elsevier Inc. All rights reserved.

For the following lateral thumb projections with poor positioning, state what anatomic structures are misaligned and how the patient should be repositioned for an optimal projection to be obtained.

Figure 4-17

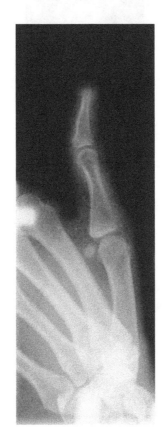

69. (Figure 4-17): _____

_____

_____

Copyright © 2015, 2011, 2006, 1996 by Saunders, an imprint of Elsevier Inc. All rights reserved.   Chapter **4** **Image Analysis of the Upper Extremity**

Figure 4-18

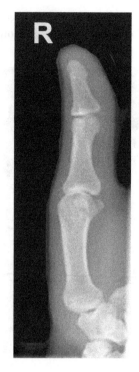

70. (Figure 4-18): _____

_____

_____

Thumb: PA Oblique Projection

71. Identify the labeled anatomy in Figure 4-19.

Figure 4-19

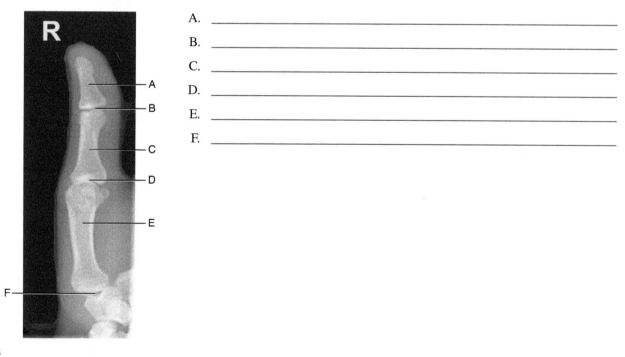

A. _____

B. _____

C. _____

D. _____

E. _____

F. _____

Copyright © 2015, 2011, 2006, 1996 by Saunders, an imprint of Elsevier Inc. All rights reserved.

72. Complete the statements below referring to PA oblique thumb projection analysis guidelines.

PA Oblique Thumb Projection Analysis Guidelines
■ (A) _twice_ as much soft tissue, and more phalangeal and MC midshaft concavity are present on the side of the thumb next to the fingers than on the other side.
■ The IP, MCP, and CM joints are demonstrated as open spaces, and the (B) _phalanges_ are not foreshortened.
■ (C) _MCP joint_ is at the center of the exposure field.

73. The affected thumb is rotated _____ degrees for accurate positioning for a PA oblique thumb projection.

74. The thumb is placed in a PA oblique projection when the hand is (A) _____, and the palm surface is placed

    (B) _____ against the IR.

75. What anatomic structures are included on a PA oblique thumb projection with accurate positioning?

    _____

For the following description of a PA oblique thumb projection with poor positioning, state how the patient would have been mispositioned for such a projection to be obtained.

76. The midshafts of the proximal phalanx and MC demonstrate slight convexity on the posterior surfaces and concavity on the anterior surfaces.

    _____

Copyright © 2015, 2011, 2006, 1996 by Saunders, an imprint of Elsevier Inc. All rights reserved.   Chapter **4**   **Image Analysis of the Upper Extremity**

For the following PA oblique thumb projections with poor positioning, state what anatomic structures are misaligned and how the patient should be repositioned for an optimal projection to be obtained.

Figure 4-20

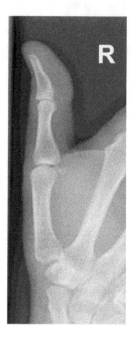

77. (Figure 4-20): _____

_____

_____

Figure 4-21

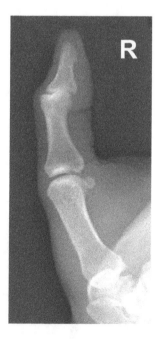

78. (Figure 4-21): _____

_____

_____

Chapter **4**   **Image Analysis of the Upper Extremity**   Copyright © 2015, 2011, 2006, 1996 by Saunders, an imprint of Elsevier Inc. All rights reserved.

Hand: PA Projection

79. Identify the labeled anatomy in Figure 4-22.

Figure 4-22

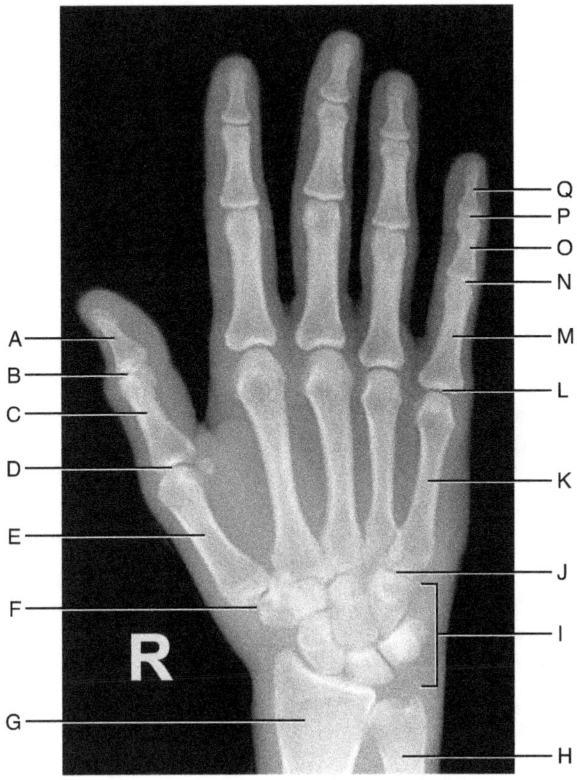

A. _____

B. _____

C. _____

D. _____

E. _____

F. _____

G. _____

H. _____

I. _____

J. _____

K. _____

L. _____

M. _____

N. _____

O. _____

P. _____

Q. _____

80. Complete the statements below referring to PA hand projection analysis guidelines.

PA Hand Projection Analysis Guidelines

- Soft tissue outlines of the second through fifth phalanges are uniform, the distance between the (A) __MC heads__ is equal, and the same midshaft concavity is seen on both sides of the (B) __phalanges__ and MCs of the second through fifth digits.
- (C) __IP__, __MCP__, and __CM__ joints are demonstrated as open spaces, and the phalanges are not foreshortened. The thumb demonstrates a 45-degree oblique projection.
- (D) __3rd   MCP__ is at the center of the exposure field.

81. To obtain a PA hand projection, (A) _____ the hand and place it (B) _____ against the IR.

82. What changes in the joint spaces, phalanges, and MCs would be expected on a PA hand projection if the hand is in a flexed position when it is taken?

_____

Copyright © 2015, 2011, 2006, 1996 by Saunders, an imprint of Elsevier Inc. All rights reserved.

83. How will the position of the first digit change if the hand is flexed for a PA hand projection?

_____

84. What anatomic structures are included on an accurately collimated PA hand projection?

_____

For the following descriptions of PA hand projections with poor positioning, state how the patient would have been mispositioned for such a projection to be obtained.

85. The projection demonstrates superimposed third through fifth MC heads and unequal midshaft concavity of the phalanges and MCs.

_____

For the following PA hand projections with poor positioning, state what anatomic structures are misaligned and how the patient should be repositioned for an optimal projection to be obtained.

Figure 4-23

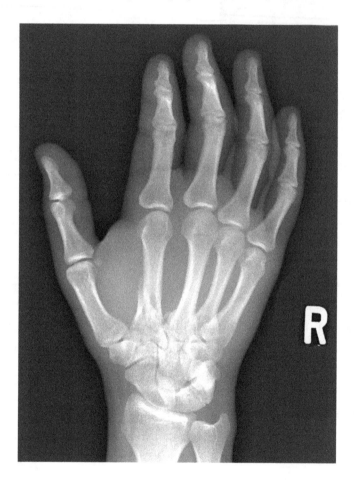

86. (Figure 4-23): _____

_____

_____

    Copyright © 2015, 2011, 2006, 1996 by Saunders, an imprint of Elsevier Inc. All rights reserved.

Figure 4-24

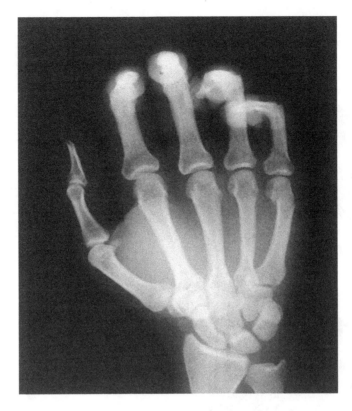

87. (Figure 4-24): _____

_____

_____

88. The PA hand projection in Figure 4-23 demonstrates a proximal second MC fracture. If the patient could not move the hand from this position, how should the CR and IR be adjusted to obtain an optimal PA projection of this fractured MC?

_____

_____

Copyright © 2015, 2011, 2006, 1996 by Saunders, an imprint of Elsevier Inc. All rights reserved.

Hand: PA Oblique Projection

89. Identify the labeled anatomy in Figure 4-25.

Figure 4-25

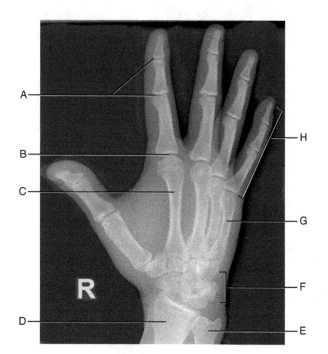

A. _____

B. _____

C. _____

D. _____

E. _____

F. _____

G. _____

H. _____

90. Complete the statements below referring to PA oblique hand projection analysis guidelines.

<table>
<tr><td>PA Oblique Hand Projection Analysis Guidelines</td></tr>
</table>

- Each of the second through fifth MC midshafts demonstrate more concavity on one side than on the other and have varying amounts of space between them. The (A) _____1st & 2nd_____ MC heads are not superimposed, and the (B) _____3rd-5th._____ MC heads are slightly superimposed, and a slight space is present between the (C) _____4th & 5th_____ MC midshafts.
- (D) _____3rd MCP_____ is at the center of the exposure field.

91. The hand is rotated (A) _____ degrees (B) _____ (internally/externally) from the PA projection for a PA oblique hand projection.

92. Why is it important to view the hand and not the wrist when determining the degree of hand obliquity to use for a PA oblique hand projection?

_____

93. How must the fingers be positioned to demonstrate open IP and MCP joints on a PA oblique hand projection?

_____

94. What anatomic structures are included on an accurately collimated PA oblique hand projection?

_____

142

Copyright © 2015, 2011, 2006, 1996 by Saunders, an imprint of Elsevier Inc. All rights reserved.

For the following descriptions of PA oblique hand projections with poor positioning, state how the patient would have been mispositioned for such a projection to be obtained.

95. The MC heads are demonstrated without superimposition, and the spaces between the MC midshafts are nearly equal.

_____

96. The third through fifth MC midshafts are superimposed.

_____

For the following PA oblique hand projections with poor positioning, state what anatomic structures are misaligned and how the patient should be repositioned for an optimal projection to be obtained.

Figure 4-26

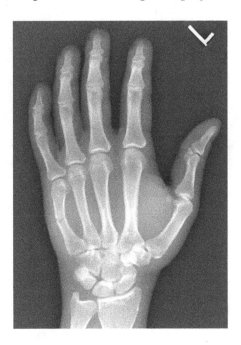

97. (Figure 4-26): _____

_____

_____

Copyright © 2015, 2011, 2006, 1996 by Saunders, an imprint of Elsevier Inc. All rights reserved.

Figure 4-27

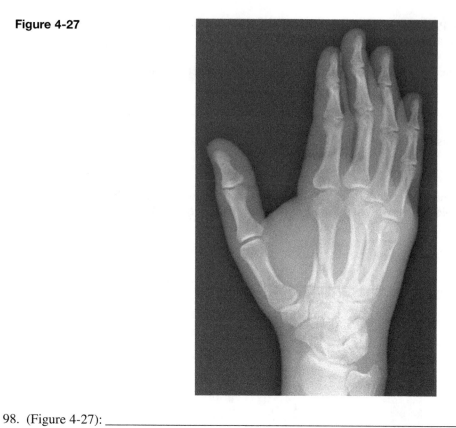

98. (Figure 4-27): _____

_____

_____

99. The PA oblique hand projection in Figure 4-26 demonstrates a midshaft fifth MC fracture. If the patient could not move the hand to adequately position it in a PA oblique projection, how should the CR and IR be adjusted for an optimal PA oblique projection to be obtained?

_____

_____

_____

100. The PA oblique hand projection in Figure 4-27 demonstrates a proximal second MC fracture. If the patient could not move the hand to adequately position it in a PA oblique projection, how should the CR and IR be adjusted for an optimal PA oblique projection to be obtained?

_____

_____

_____

  Copyright © 2015, 2011, 2006, 1996 by Saunders, an imprint of Elsevier Inc. All rights reserved.

Hand: Lateral "Fan" Projection (Lateromedial)

101. Identify the labeled anatomy in Figure 4-28.

Figure 4-28

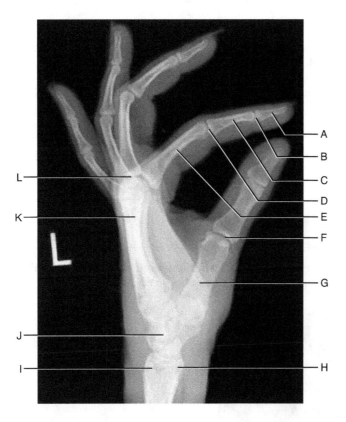

A. _____

B. _____

C. _____

D. _____

E. _____

F. _____

G. _____

H. _____

I. _____

J. _____

K. _____

L. _____

102. Complete the statements below referring to lateral hand projection analysis guidelines.

Lateral Hand Projection Analysis Guidelines
■ The second through (A) _____5th_____ digits are separated, demonstrating little superimposition of the proximal bony or soft tissue structures.
■ The second through (B) _____5th_____ MCs are superimposed.
■ (C) ___MCP joints___ are at the center of the exposure field.

103. Why is it difficult to demonstrate the phalanges and MCs simultaneously on a fan lateral hand projection?

_____

104. For a fan lateral hand projection, the digits are most effectively fanned by drawing the second and third fingers

(A) _____ (anteriorly/posteriorly) and the fourth and fifth fingers (B) _____ (anteriorly/
posteriorly).

105. In what projection or position will the first digit be placed for accurate positioning for a lateral hand projection?

_____

Copyright © 2015, 2011, 2006, 1996 by Saunders, an imprint of Elsevier Inc. All rights reserved.   Chapter **4**   **Image Analysis of the Upper Extremity**

106. How should the thumb be positioned to obtain open joint spaces and demonstrate the phalanges without foreshortening on a lateral hand projection?

depress thumb so it's parallel w/ the IR

107. What anatomic structures are included on an accurately collimated lateral hand projection?

whole hand, carpals, & 1 inch. of forearm

For the following descriptions of lateral hand projections with poor positioning, state how the patient would have been mispositioned for such a projection to be obtained.

108. The second through fifth MC midshafts are demonstrated without superimposition. The shortest MC is demonstrated anterior to the other MCs.

_____

109. The second through fifth MC midshafts are demonstrated without superimposition. The longest MC is demonstrated anterior to the other MCs.

_____

110. The projection demonstrates superimposed MCs and superimposed digits.

_____

For the following lateral hand projections with poor positioning, state what anatomic structures are misaligned and how the patient should be repositioned for an optimal projection to be obtained.

Figure 4-29

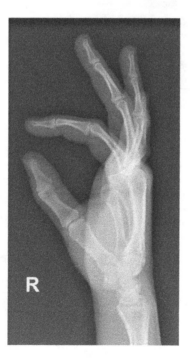

111. (Figure 4-29): _____

_____

_____

Chapter **4** **Image Analysis of the Upper Extremity**   Copyright © 2015, 2011, 2006, 1996 by Saunders, an imprint of Elsevier Inc. All rights reserved.

Figure 4-30

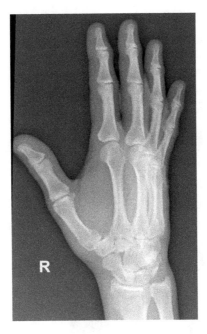

112. (Figure 4-30): _____

_____

_____

Figure 4-31

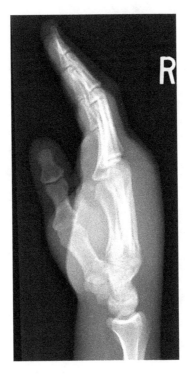

113. (Figure 4-31): _____

_____

_____

Copyright © 2015, 2011, 2006, 1996 by Saunders, an imprint of Elsevier Inc. All rights reserved.

Chapter **4   Image Analysis of the Upper Extremity**

Wrist: PA Projection

114. Identify the labeled anatomy in Figure 4-32.

Figure 4-32

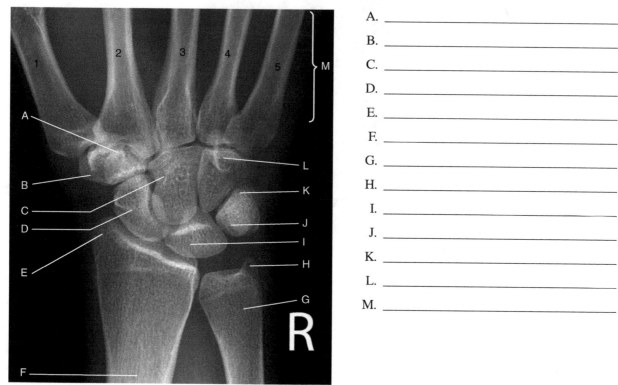

A. _____

B. _____

C. _____

D. _____

E. _____

F. _____

G. _____

H. _____

I. _____

J. _____

K. _____

L. _____

M. _____

115. Complete the statements below referring to PA wrist projection analysis guidelines.

PA Wrist Projection Analysis Guidelines
■ (A) _Scaphoid_ fat stripe is demonstrated.
■ Radial and ulnar styloids are at the extreme lateral and medial edges, respectively, of each bone. (B) _radioulnar_ articulation is open, and superimposition of the MC bases is limited.
■ Anterior and posterior margins of the distal radius are within (C) _.25_ inch of each other.
■ (D) _2nd–5th_ CM joint spaces are open. Scaphoid is only slightly foreshortened, and the lunate is trapezoidal.
■ Long axes of the third MC and the (E) _midforearm_ are aligned with the long axis of the collimated field.
■ (F) _carpal bones_ are at the center of the exposure field.

116. Describe the shape and location of the scaphoid fat stripe. _____

_____

117. Why is the visualization of the scaphoid fat stripe important on a PA wrist projection?

_____

Chapter **4** **Image Analysis of the Upper Extremity**   Copyright © 2015, 2011, 2006, 1996 by Saunders, an imprint of Elsevier Inc. All rights reserved.

118. To demonstrate the ulnar styloid in profile, the elbow is placed in a/an (A) _____ projection, and the humerus is positioned (B) _____ with the IR.

119. The (A) _____ (anterior/posterior) margin of the distal radius is demonstrated distal to the (B) _____ (anterior/posterior) margin on a PA wrist projection with accurate positioning.

120. How is the forearm positioned for a PA wrist projection to obtain open radioscaphoid and radiolunate joint spaces?

_____

121. How is a patient with large muscular or thick proximal forearms positioned for a PA wrist projection to prevent demonstrating an excessive amount of the radial articular surface? _____

122. How is the patient positioned for a PA wrist projection to obtain open second through fifth CM joint spaces?

_____

123. When the hand is placed on a flat surface, the wrist will be (A) _____ (flexed/extended), causing the distal scaphoid to shift (B) _____ (anteriorly/posteriorly).

124. When the fifth MC and ulna are aligned with the long axis of the collimation field for a PA wrist projection, the distal scaphoid shifts (A) _____ (anteriorly/posteriorly) and is (B) _____ (foreshortened/ elongated), and the lunate moves (C) _____ (medially/laterally).

125. The distal scaphoid shifts _____ (anteriorly/posteriorly) when the wrist is ulnar-deviated.

126. Accurate CR centering on a PA wrist projection is accomplished by centering a _____ CR to the wrist.

127. What anatomic structures are included on an accurately collimated PA wrist projection?

_____

128. How should one center the CR and collimate differently when a PA wrist projection is ordered with the request that more than one fourth of the distal forearm be included?

_____

For the following descriptions of PA wrist projections with poor positioning, state how the patient would have been mispositioned for such a projection to be obtained.

129. The ulnar styloid is not demonstrated in profile.

_____

130. The laterally located carpal and MC joints are demonstrated as open spaces, and the medially located carpals and MCs are superimposed, closing the medially located carpal joints. The radioulnar joint is closed, and the radial styloid is not in profile.

_____

131. The laterally located carpals and MCs are superimposed, the pisiform and hamate hook are well demonstrated, and the radioulnar joint is closed.

_____

Copyright © 2015, 2011, 2006, 1996 by Saunders, an imprint of Elsevier Inc. All rights reserved.   Chapter **4**   **Image Analysis of the Upper Extremity**

132. The posterior margin of the distal radius has been projected too far distal to the anterior margin.

133. The scaphoid is foreshortened and demonstrates a signet ring configuration, the CM joints are obscured, and the lunate is triangular and properly positioned distal to the radius.

134. The scaphoid is elongated, the second through fourth MCs are superimposed over the CM joints, and the lunate is triangular and properly positioned distal to the radius.

    The hand was overflexed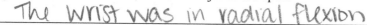

135. The scaphoid is foreshortened, the lunate is positioned mostly distal to the ulna, the third MC is not aligned with the long axis of the midforearm, and the CM joints are open.

    The wrist was in radial flexion

136. The scaphoid is elongated, the lunate is entirely positioned distal to the radius, and the third MC is not aligned with the long axis of the midforearm.

For the following PA wrist projections with poor positioning, state what anatomic structures are misaligned and how the patient should be repositioned for an optimal projection to be obtained.

Figure 4-33

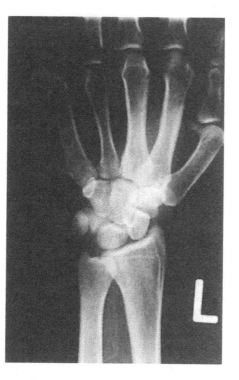

137. (Figure 4-33): *lateral carpals are superimposed and radioulnar articulation closed. Fix by externally rotating hand and wrist.*

Chapter **4** **Image Analysis of the Upper Extremity**   Copyright © 2015, 2011, 2006, 1996 by Saunders, an imprint of Elsevier Inc. All rights reserved.

Figure 4-34

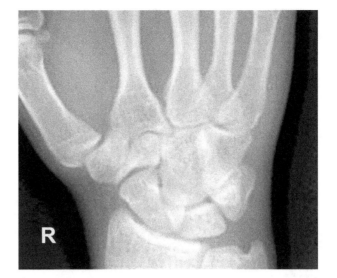

138. (Figure 4-34): <u>medial carpals superimposed and radioulnar</u> <u>articulation closed. Fix by: internally rotating</u> <u>hand and wrist.</u>

Figure 4-35

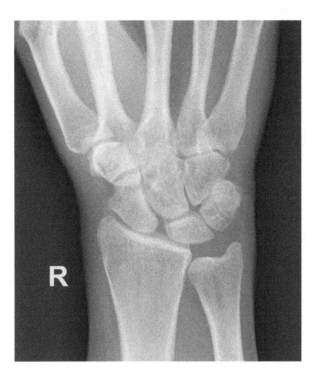

139. (Figure 4-35): _____

_____

_____

Copyright © 2015, 2011, 2006, 1996 by Saunders, an imprint of Elsevier Inc. All rights reserved.

Chapter **4** **Image Analysis of the Upper Extremity**

Figure 4-36

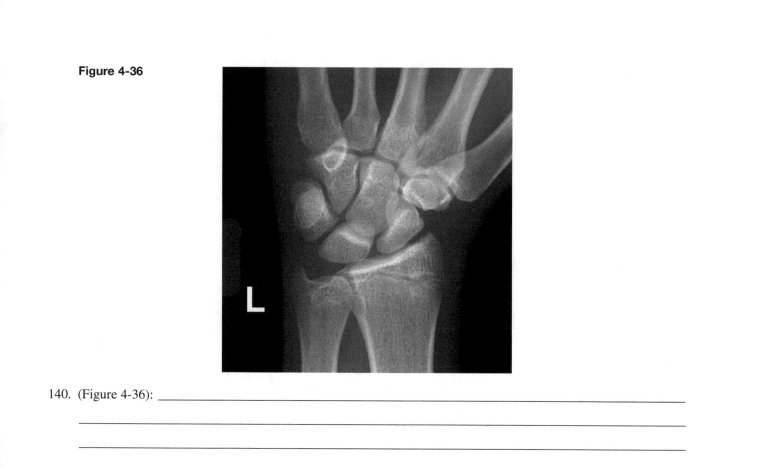

140. (Figure 4-36): _____

_____

_____

     Copyright © 2015, 2011, 2006, 1996 by Saunders, an imprint of Elsevier Inc. All rights reserved.

Wrist: PA Oblique Projection

141. Identify the labeled anatomy in Figure 4-37.

Figure 4-37

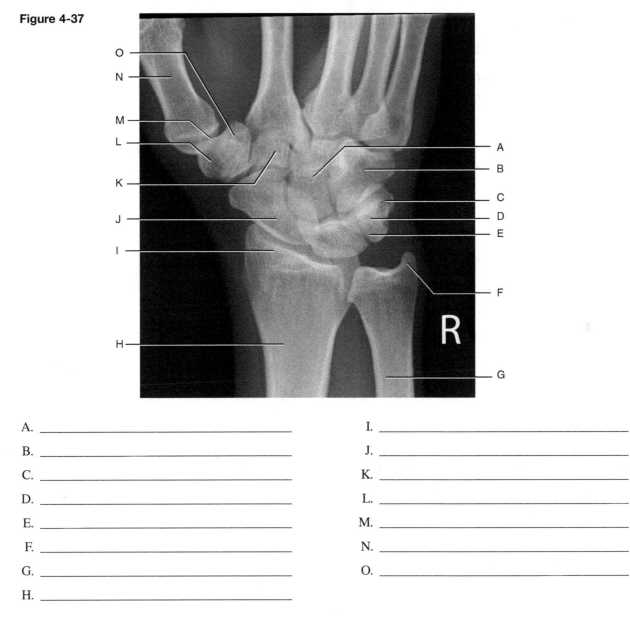

A. _____

B. _____

C. _____

D. _____

E. _____

F. _____

G. _____

H. _____

I. _____

J. _____

K. _____

L. _____

M. _____

N. _____

O. _____

142. Complete the statements below referring to PA oblique wrist projection analysis guidelines.

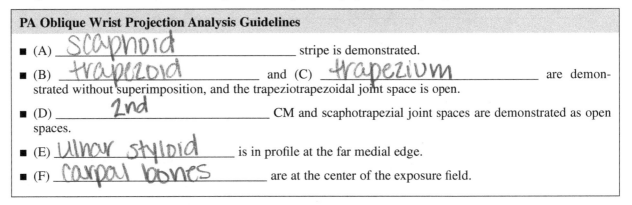

PA Oblique Wrist Projection Analysis Guidelines

- (A) _Scaphoid_ stripe is demonstrated.
- (B) _trapezoid_ and (C) _trapezium_ are demonstrated without superimposition, and the trapeziotrapezoidal joint space is open.
- (D) _2nd_ CM and scaphotrapezial joint spaces are demonstrated as open spaces.
- (E) _ulnar styloid_ is in profile at the far medial edge.
- (F) _carpal bones_ are at the center of the exposure field.

153

Copyright © 2015, 2011, 2006, 1996 by Saunders, an imprint of Elsevier Inc. All rights reserved.

143. What routine degree of patient wrist rotation is required for a PA oblique wrist projection?

A. _____

As a routine, should the wrist be internally or externally rotated from a PA projection?

B. _____

144. For a PA projection of the wrist, the trapezoid and trapezium are superimposed. Which of these carpal bones is located anteriorly?

_____

145. The long axes of which two anatomic structures should be aligned when positioning the patient for a PA oblique wrist projection to ensure that no radial or ulnar deviation will result?

A. _____

B. _____

146. If the forearm is positioned parallel with the IR for a PA oblique wrist projection, how is the distal radius demonstrated on the resulting projection?

_____

147. On a PA oblique wrist projection with accurate positioning, the radioulnar joint space is closed. Which surface of the radius is superimposed over the ulna? _____ (anterior/posterior)

148. Accurate CR centering on a PA oblique wrist projection is accomplished by centering a _____ CR to the wrist.

149. What anatomic structures are included on an accurately collimated PA oblique wrist projection?

_____

For the following descriptions of PA oblique wrist projections with poor positioning, state how the patient would have been mispositioned for such a projection to be obtained.

150. The trapezoid and trapezium demonstrate slight superimposition, obscuring the trapeziotrapezoidal joint space, and trapezoid-capitate superimposition is minimal.

_____

151. The scaphoid is foreshortened, and the scaphoid is situated next to the radius.

_____

152. The posterior margin of the distal radius is more than 1⁄4 inch (0.6 cm) proximal to the anterior margin.

_____

 Copyright © 2015, 2011, 2006, 1996 by Saunders, an imprint of Elsevier Inc. All rights reserved.

For the following PA oblique wrist projections with poor positioning, state what anatomic structures are mis-aligned and how the patient should be repositioned for an optimal projection to be obtained.

Figure 4-38

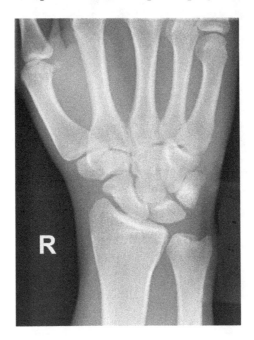

153. (Figure 4-38):_____

_____

_____

Figure 4-39

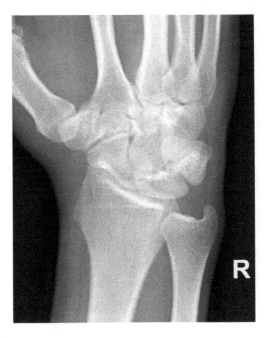

154. (Figure 4-39): _____

_____

_____

Copyright © 2015, 2011, 2006, 1996 by Saunders, an imprint of Elsevier Inc. All rights reserved. Chapter **4** **Image Analysis of the Upper Extremity**

Figure 4-40

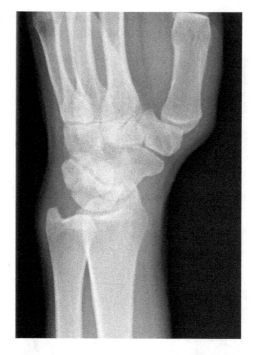

155. (Figure 4-40):_____
_____
_____

Figure 4-41

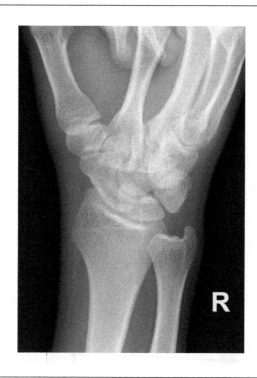

156. (Figure 4-41):_____
_____
_____

     Copyright © 2015, 2011, 2006, 1996 by Saunders, an imprint of Elsevier Inc. All rights reserved.

Wrist: Lateral Projection (Lateromedial)

157. Identify the labeled anatomy in Figure 4-42.

Figure 4-42

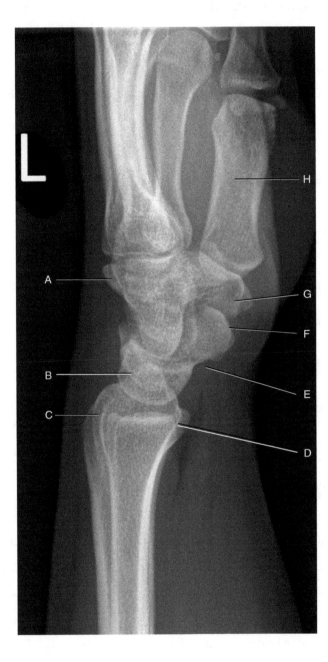

A. _____

B. _____

C. _____

D. _____

E. _____

F. _____

G. _____

H. _____

Copyright © 2015, 2011, 2006, 1996 by Saunders, an imprint of Elsevier Inc. All rights reserved.

Chapter **4**   **Image Analysis of the Upper Extremity**

158. Complete the statements below referring to lateral wrist projection analysis guidelines.

Lateral Wrist Projection Analysis Guidelines
■ (A) _pronator_ fat stripe is demonstrated.
■ (B) _anterior_ aspects of the distal scaphoid and pisiform are aligned, and the distal radius and ulna are superimposed.
■ (C) _distal_ aspect of the distal scaphoid and pisiform are aligned.
■ The second through fifth MCs are placed at a (D) _10-15_ -degree angle with the anterior plane of the wrist.
■ The thumb is parallel with the (E) _forearm_ .
■ Ulnar styloid is demonstrated in profile (F) _posteriorly_ .
■ (G) _trapezium_ is demonstrated without superimposition of the first MC.

159. Describe the shape and location of the pronator fat stripe that is demonstrated on a lateral wrist projection with accurate positioning.

_____

_____

160. Why is the visualization of the pronator fat stripe on a lateral wrist projection of importance?

_____

161. Which side of the wrist is placed against the IR for a routine lateral wrist projection?

A. _ulnar_ _____ (radial/ulnar)

What projection is this?

B. _lateromedial_ _____

In this projection, is the pisiform or distal scaphoid positioned closer to the IR?

C. _pisiform_ _____

162. How are the hand and forearm aligned to prevent radial or ulnar deviation of the wrist for a lateral wrist projection?

third MC & forearm parallel to IR
and in same plane

163. Ulnar deviation of the wrist causes the distal scaphoid to be demonstrated (A) _____ (proximal/distal) to the

pisiform, and radial deviation causes the distal scaphoid to be demonstrated (B) _____ (proximal/distal) to the pisiform on a lateral wrist projection.

164. If a patient with large muscular or thick proximal forearms is positioned without hanging the proximal forearm off

the IR or imaging table, what type of wrist deviation will result? _____

165. For a lateral wrist projection, how is the patient positioned so that the wrist is in a neutral position without extension or flexion?

_____

Copyright © 2015, 2011, 2006, 1996 by Saunders, an imprint of Elsevier Inc. All rights reserved.

166. For a lateral wrist projection, how are the humerus and elbow positioned to demonstrate the ulnar styloid in profile?

_____

167. For a lateral wrist projection, how are the humerus and elbow positioned to demonstrate the ulnar styloid projecting distal to the midline of the ulnar head?

_____

168. Which of the elbow and humeral positions described in the previous two questions demonstrates the ulna closer to the lunate on the resulting lateral wrist projection? _____

169. How is the patient positioned to prevent the first MC from being superimposed over the trapezium? _____

_____

170. Accurate CR centering on a lateral wrist projection is accomplished by centering a(n) _____ CR to the wrist.

171. What anatomic structures are included on an accurately collimated lateral wrist projection?_____

_____

172. State whether the elbow was positioned in an AP or lateral projection for the wrist projections in figure 4-43.

Figure 4-43

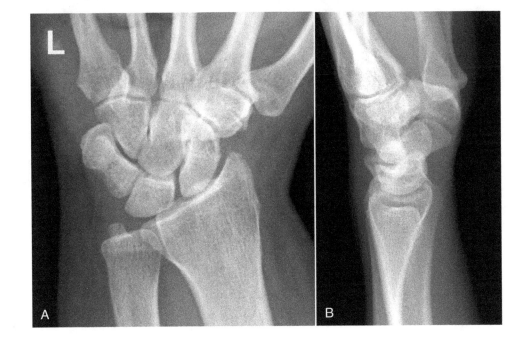

A. _____

B. _____

For the following descriptions of lateral wrist projections with poor positioning, state how the patient would have been mispositioned for such a projection to be obtained.

173. The pisiform is demonstrated anterior to the scaphoid, and the ulna is demonstrated anterior to the radius.

_____

Copyright © 2015, 2011, 2006, 1996 by Saunders, an imprint of Elsevier Inc. All rights reserved.   Chapter **4**   **Image Analysis of the Upper Extremity**

174. The distal scaphoid is demonstrated distal to the pisiform.

_____

175. The ulnar styloid is projecting distal to the midline of the ulnar head. (In some facilities, this may not be considered poor positioning.)

_____

176. The first proximal MC is superimposed over the trapezium.

_____

For the following lateral wrist projections with poor positioning, identify the anatomic structures that are misaligned, state how the patient should be repositioned for an optimal projection to be obtained, and describe the position of the ulnar styloid.

Figure 4-44

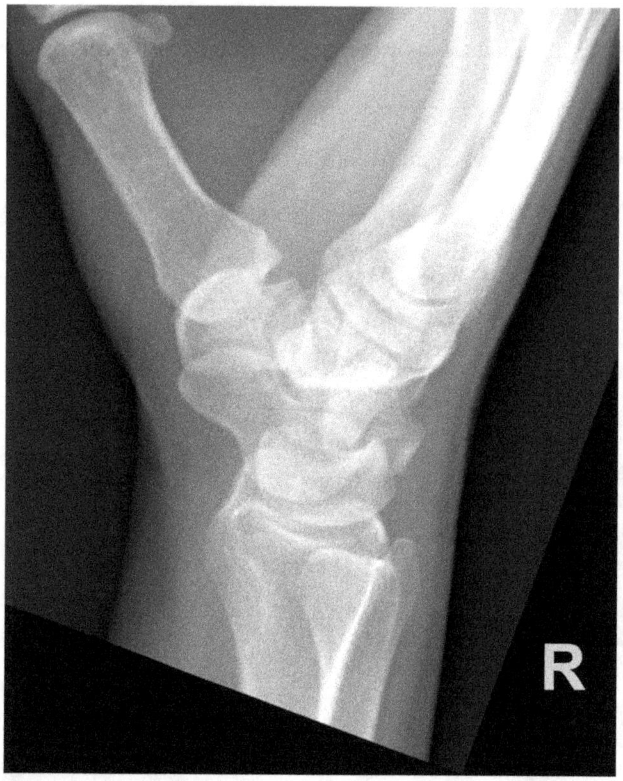

177. (Figure 4-44): _hand is under rotated, fix by: externally rotating hand._

Ulnar styloid: _in profile_ _____ (Profile/midline of ulnar head)

Copyright © 2015, 2011, 2006, 1996 by Saunders, an imprint of Elsevier Inc. All rights reserved.

Figure 4-45

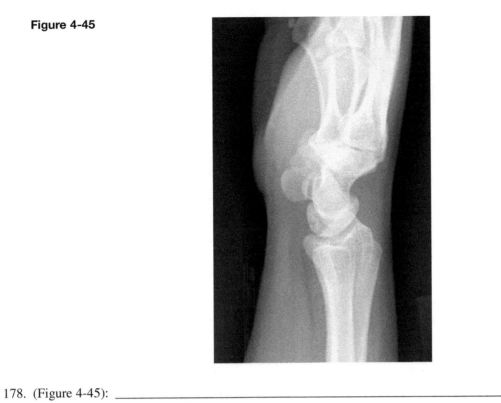

178. (Figure 4-45): _____

_____

Ulnar styloid: _____ (Profile/midline of ulnar head)

Figure 4-46

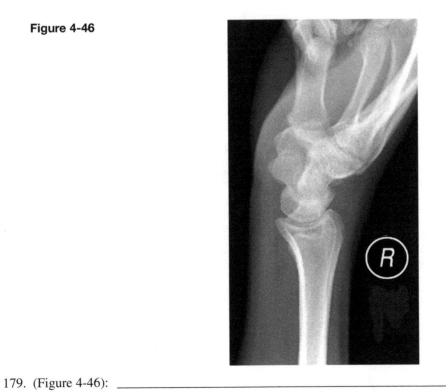

179. (Figure 4-46): _____

_____

Ulnar styloid: _____ (Profile/midline of ulnar head)

161

Copyright © 2015, 2011, 2006, 1996 by Saunders, an imprint of Elsevier Inc. All rights reserved.

Figure 4-47

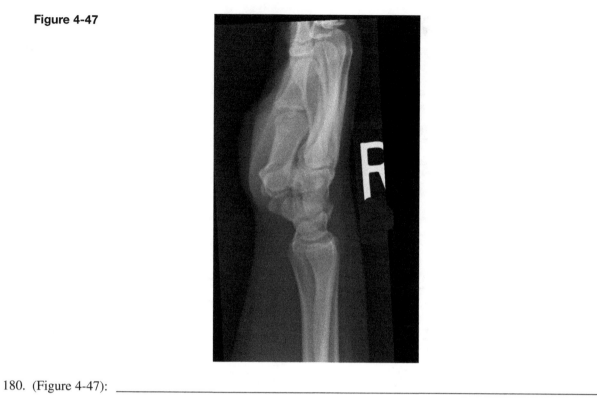

180. (Figure 4-47): _____

_____

Ulnar styloid: _____ (Profile/midline of ulnar head)

Figure 4-48

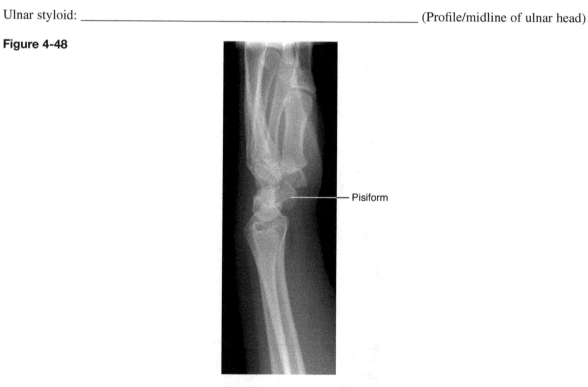

— Pisiform

181. (Figure 4-48): _____

_____

Ulnar styloid: _____ (Profile/midline of ulnar head)

Copyright © 2015, 2011, 2006, 1996 by Saunders, an imprint of Elsevier Inc. All rights reserved.

182. (Figure 4-49) Because of the distal forearm fracture, the patient was unable to externally rotate the arm enough to obtain an accurately position the wrist in a lateral projection. How should the CR have been adjusted from perpendicular to obtain accurate positioning?

Figure 4-49

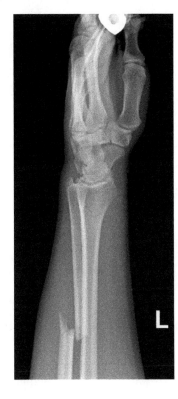

Wrist: Ulnar-Deviation, PA Axial Projection (Scaphoid)

183. Identify the labeled anatomy in Figure 4-50.

Figure 4-50

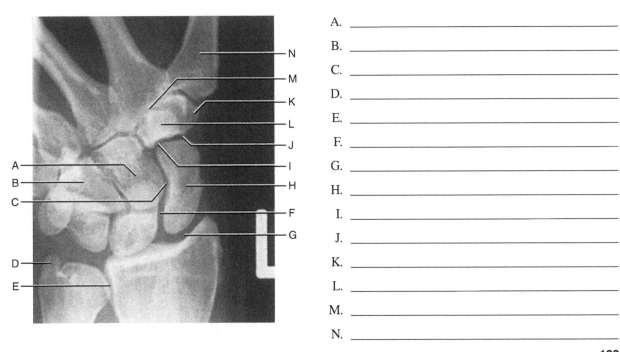

A. _____

B. _____

C. _____

D. _____

E. _____

F. _____

G. _____

H. _____

I. _____

J. _____

K. _____

L. _____

M. _____

N. _____

Copyright © 2015, 2011, 2006, 1996 by Saunders, an imprint of Elsevier Inc. All rights reserved. Chapter **4** **Image Analysis of the Upper Extremity**

184. Complete the statements below referring to PA axial (scaphoid) wrist projection analysis guidelines.

> **PA Axial (Scaphoid) Wrist Projection Analysis Guidelines**
>
> - (A) __Scaphoid__ fat stripe is demonstrated.
> - (B) _____ and scaphotrapezoidal joint spaces are open.
> - Long axis of the (C) _____ and the radius are aligned.
> - Radioscaphoid, (D) _____, and scapholunate joints are open.
> - Ulnar styloid is in profile (E) _____.
> - (F) _____ is at the center of the exposure field.

185. Sufficient ulnar deviation of the wrist has been accomplished in the PA axial projection when the long axis of the (A) __first MC__ and (B) __the radius__ are aligned and the lunate is positioned distal to the (C) __radius__.

186. Why does ulnar deviation of the wrist increase the demonstration of the scaphoid?

_____

187. For a PA axial projection, how is the patient positioned to obtain open scaphocapitate and scapholunate joint spaces?

_____

188. If the wrist is adequately ulnar-deviated for the PA axial projection, how much and in what direction is the CR angled if a fracture of the scaphoid waist is suspected? _____

_____

189. What CR angulation is used if the patient is unable to adequately ulnar-deviate for a PA axial wrist projection?

A. _____

Why is this adjustment needed?

B. _____

190. Where do most fractures occur on the scaphoid? _____

191. How is the CR angle adjusted for a PA axial wrist projection if a fracture of the distal scaphoid is suspected?

A. _____

If a proximal scaphoid fracture is suspected?

B. _____

192. If the CR is not aligned parallel with the fracture site for a PA axial wrist projection, will the fracture line be visible?

_____ (Yes/No)

193. How is the patient positioned for a PA axial wrist projection to obtain an open radioscaphoid joint space?

_____

Copyright © 2015, 2011, 2006, 1996 by Saunders, an imprint of Elsevier Inc. All rights reserved.

For the following descriptions of lateral forearm projections with poor positioning, state how the patient would have been mispositioned for such a projection to be obtained.

241. The pisiform is demonstrated anterior to the distal scaphoid, and the ulna is anterior to the radius. The proximal forearm demonstrates accurate positioning.

_____

242. The pisiform is visible posterior to the distal scaphoid, and the distal surface of the capitulum is demonstrated proximal to the distal surfaces of the medial trochlea.

_____

_____

243. The ulnar styloid is projecting distal to the midline of the ulnar head.

_____

244. The projection demonstrates the radial tuberosity in profile anteriorly.

_____

245. The radial head is demonstrated too far posterior on the coronoid process. The distal forearm demonstrates accurate positioning.

_____

For the following lateral forearm projection with poor positioning, state what anatomic structures are misaligned and how the patient should be repositioned for an optimal projection to be obtained.

Figure 4-66

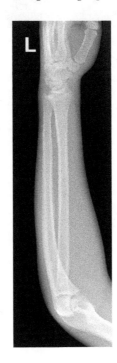

246. (Figure 4-66): _____

_____

_____

_____

Copyright © 2015, 2011, 2006, 1996 by Saunders, an imprint of Elsevier Inc. All rights reserved.   Chapter **4** **Image Analysis of the Upper Extremity**

247. The lateral forearm projection in Figure 4-67 demonstrates a distal radial fracture. The patient's arm was externally rotated as far as possible. How should the CR and IR be adjusted for an optimal lateral forearm projection to be obtained?

Figure 4-67

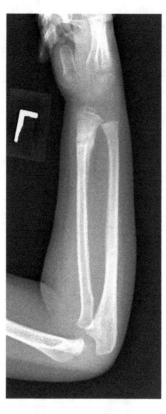

_____

_____

_____

_____

Copyright © 2015, 2011, 2006, 1996 by Saunders, an imprint of Elsevier Inc. All rights reserved.

Elbow: AP Projection

248. Identify the labeled anatomy in Figure 4-68.

Figure 4-68

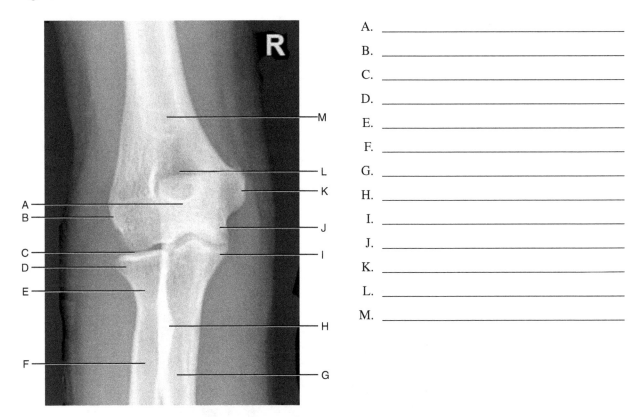

A. _____

B. _____

C. _____

D. _____

E. _____

F. _____

G. _____

H. _____

I. _____

J. _____

K. _____

L. _____

M. _____

249. Complete the statements below referring to AP elbow projection analysis guidelines.

AP Elbow Projection Analysis Guidelines

- Medial and lateral humeral epicondyles are demonstrated in (A) _profile_ .
- One-eighth of the (B) _radial head_ superimposes the proximal ulna.
- Radial tuberosity is in profile (C) _medially_ , and the radius and ulna are parallel.
- The elbow joint is (D) _open_ .
- (E) _elbow joint_ is at the center of the exposure field.

250. If the humeral epicondyles are accurately positioned for an AP elbow projection, what other structure can be manipulated to change the degree of radial tuberosity visualization?

_____

251. What two aspects of the positioning procedure need to be accurately set up to demonstrate the elbow joint space as an open space on an AP elbow projection?

A. _____

B. _____

Copyright © 2015, 2011, 2006, 1996 by Saunders, an imprint of Elsevier Inc. All rights reserved.

Chapter **4** **Image Analysis of the Upper Extremity**

252. A poorly positioned AP elbow projection demonstrates a closed elbow joint space. How can one determine if this closure was a result of poor CR placement or elbow flexion? _____

_____

_____

253. How is the patient positioned for an AP elbow projection if the elbow is unable to extend at least 30 degrees?

_____

254. Accurate CR centering on an AP elbow projection is accomplished by centering a (A) _____ CR

(B) _____ (C) _____ to the medial epicondyle

255. What anatomic structures are included on an accurately collimated AP elbow projection?

_____

256. What patient condition is demonstrated on the projection in Figure 4-69?

Figure 4-69

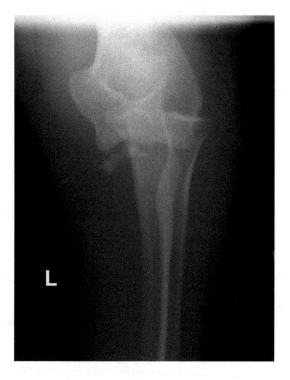

_____

_____

_____

Copyright © 2015, 2011, 2006, 1996 by Saunders, an imprint of Elsevier Inc. All rights reserved.

For the following descriptions of AP elbow projections with poor positioning, state how the patient would have been mispositioned for such a projection to be obtained.

257. The radial head superimposes approximately half of the ulna.

_____

258. The projection demonstrates the radius crossing over the ulna, and the radial tuberosity is not shown in profile.

_____

259. The projection demonstrates a foreshortened proximal forearm and a closed capitulum–radial joint space.

_____

For the following AP elbow projections with poor positioning, state what anatomic structures are misaligned and how the patient should be repositioned for an optimal projection to be obtained.

Figure 4-70

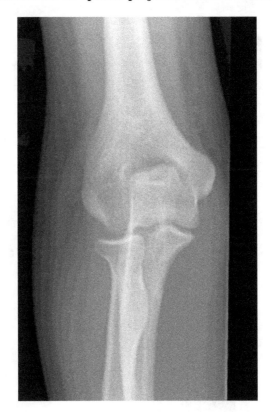

260. (Figure 4-70): _____

_____

_____

_____

Copyright © 2015, 2011, 2006, 1996 by Saunders, an imprint of Elsevier Inc. All rights reserved.

Figure 4-71

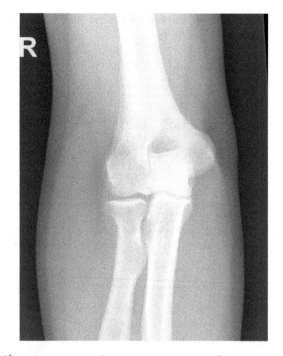

261. (Figure 4-71): <u>The elbow is too much externally rotated, showing the separation of the radioulnar articulation. Fix by slightly internally rotating whole arm.</u>

Figure 4-72

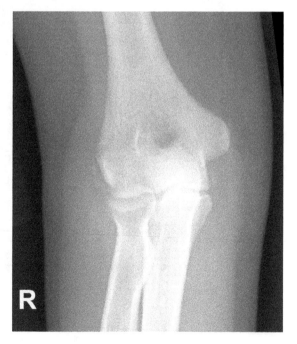

262. (Figure 4-72): _____

_____

_____

_____

 Copyright © 2015, 2011, 2006, 1996 by Saunders, an imprint of Elsevier Inc. All rights reserved.

263. The AP projection in Figure 4-73 demonstrates a proximal radial fracture. If the patient could not move the arm to adequately position it for an AP projection, how should the CR and IR be adjusted for an optimal AP elbow projection to be obtained?

Figure 4-73

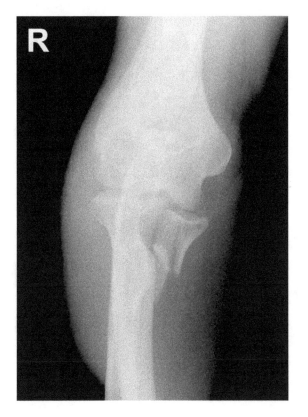

_____

_____

_____

Copyright © 2015, 2011, 2006, 1996 by Saunders, an imprint of Elsevier Inc. All rights reserved.   Chapter **4** **Image Analysis of the Upper Extremity**

264. The AP projection in Figure 4-74 demonstrates a distal forearm fracture that prevented the patient from internally rotating the arm the needed amount to obtain an accurate AP elbow projection. How should the CR and IR be adjusted to obtain an optimal projection?

Figure 4-74

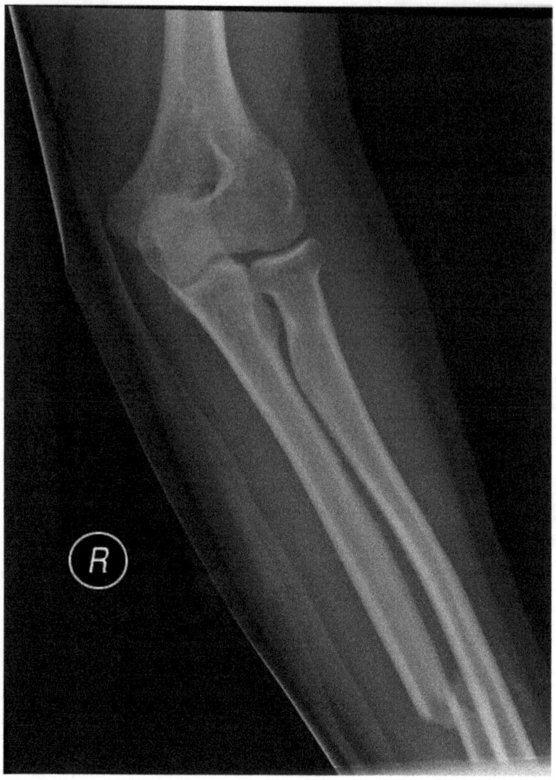

_____

_____

_____

Chapter **4** **Image Analysis of the Upper Extremity**   Copyright © 2015, 2011, 2006, 1996 by Saunders, an imprint of Elsevier Inc. All rights reserved.

Elbow: AP Oblique Projections (Internal and External Rotation)

265. Identify the labeled anatomy in Figure 4-75.

Figure 4-75

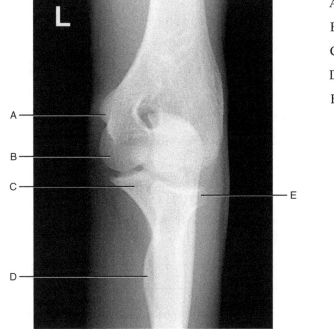

A. _____

B. _____

C. _____

D. _____

E. _____

266. Identify the labeled anatomy in Figure 4-76

Figure 4-76

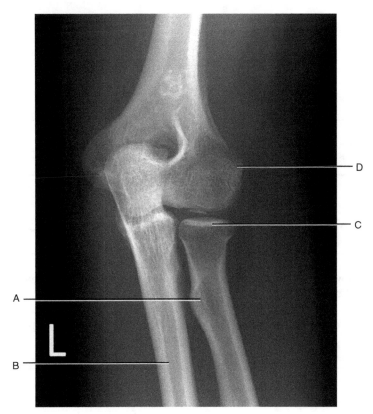

A. _____

B. _____

C. _____

D. _____

Copyright © 2015, 2011, 2006, 1996 by Saunders, an imprint of Elsevier Inc. All rights reserved.

267. Complete the statements below referring to AP oblique elbow projection analysis guidelines.

AP Oblique Elbow Projection Analysis Guidelines
Medial oblique:
■ The coronoid process, trochlear notch, and (A) *trochlea* are in profile.
■ (B) _____ is open.
■ Three-quarters of the (C) *radial head* superimposes the ulna.
Lateral oblique:
■ The radial head and (D) *capitulum* are in profile.
■ (E) *ulna* is demonstrated without radial head, neck, and tuberosity superimposition.
■ (F) *elbow joint* is at the center of the exposure field.

268. An AP oblique elbow projection with poor positioning demonstrates a closed capitulum–radial joint space. List two possible positioning problems that might have resulted in this projection.

A. _____

B. _____

269. State whether the forearm or humerus should be placed parallel with the IR to best demonstrate the anatomy listed below in a patient whose arm will not fully extend.

A. Coronoid: _____

B. Radial head: _____

C. Medial trochlea: _____

D. Capitulum: _____

E. Capitulum-radial joint: _____

270. What is the degree of elbow rotation used for AP oblique projections?

_____

271. Accurate CR centering on an AP oblique elbow projection is accomplished by centering a (A) _____ CR to the elbow joint located at a level (B) _____ distal to the (C) _____ _____.

272. What anatomic structures are included on an AP oblique elbow projection with accurate positioning?_____

_____

For the following descriptions of AP oblique elbow projections with poor positioning, state how the patient would have been mispositioned for such a projection to be obtained.

273. The externally rotated AP (lateral) oblique projection demonstrates a closed capitulum–radial joint space. The olecranon is positioned outside the olecranon fossa, and the radial articulating surface is demonstrated.

_____

Copyright © 2015, 2011, 2006, 1996 by Saunders, an imprint of Elsevier Inc. All rights reserved.

274. On the internally rotated AP (medial) oblique projection, the radial head is demonstrated lateral to the coronoid process, without complete superimposition of the ulna, and the proximal aspect of the olecranon is not demonstrated in profile.

_____

275. On the internally rotated AP (medial) oblique projection, a portion of the radial head is demonstrated anterior to the coronoid process without complete superimposition of the ulna.

_____

276. On the externally rotated AP (lateral) oblique projection, a portion of the radial head and tuberosity is superimposed over the ulna.

_____

277. On the externally rotated AP (lateral) oblique projection, the coronoid is superimposed over a portion of the radial neck, and the radial head and tuberosity are free of superimposition. The radial tuberosity is not demonstrated in profile.

_____

For the following AP oblique elbow projections with poor positioning, state what anatomic structures are misaligned and how the patient should be repositioned for an optimal projection to be obtained.

Figure 4-77

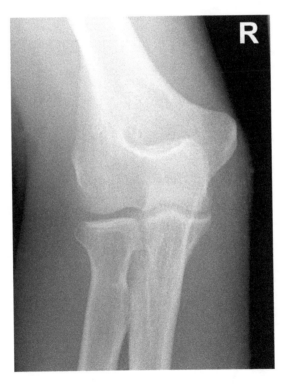

278. (Figure 4-77, Lateral oblique): _____

_____

_____

_____

Copyright © 2015, 2011, 2006, 1996 by Saunders, an imprint of Elsevier Inc. All rights reserved.

Figure 4-78

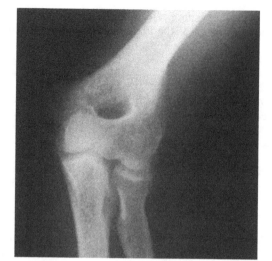

279. (Figure 4-78, Lateral oblique): _____

_____

_____

_____

Figure 4-79

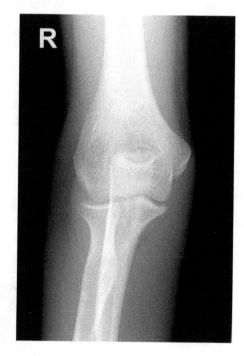

280. (Figure 4-79, Medial oblique): _____

_____

_____

_____

Copyright © 2015, 2011, 2006, 1996 by Saunders, an imprint of Elsevier Inc. All rights reserved.

Figure 4-80

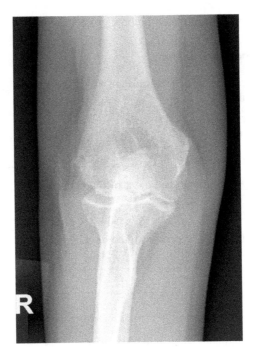

281. (Figure 4-80, Medial oblique): _____

_____

_____

_____

Elbow: Lateral Projection (Lateromedial)

282. Identify the labeled anatomy in Figure 4-81.

Figure 4-81

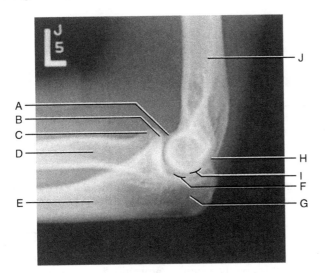

A. _____

B. _____

C. _____

D. _____

E. _____

F. _____

G. _____

H. _____

I. _____

J. _____

Copyright © 2015, 2011, 2006, 1996 by Saunders, an imprint of Elsevier Inc. All rights reserved.

283. Complete the statements below referring to lateral elbow projection analysis guidelines.

> **Lateral Elbow Projection Analysis Guidelines**
>
> - The distal humerus demonstrates three concentric arcs, which are formed by the (A) _trochlear sulcus_ capitulum, and medial trochlea.
> - The elbow joint is open, and the distal and (B) _anterior_ surfaces of the radial head and the coronoid process are aligned.
> - The radial tuberosity is not demonstrated in (C) _profile_.
> - (D) _elbow joint_ is at the center of the exposure field.

284. List the three soft tissue fat pads that may be demonstrated on a lateral elbow projection and describe their locations.

A. _____

B. _____

C. _____

Displacement of these pads may indicate what to the reviewer?

D. _____

285. Why is it important to flex the elbow 90 degrees for a lateral elbow projection? _____
_____posterior fat pad shown & olecranon out of its fossa_____

286. What three anatomic structures form the three concentric arcs on a lateral elbow projection with accurate positioning?

A. _____

B. _____

C. _____

Which of these arcs is the smallest?

D. _____

Which is the largest?

E. _____

How will improper alignment of these arcs affect the elbow joint space?

F. _____

287. A lateral elbow projection with poor positioning demonstrates the radial head positioned posterior on the coronoid process. How would the capitulum and medial trochlea be misaligned on this projection?

_____
_____

288. The distal forearm was positioned too low for a lateral elbow projection. What will be the relationship between the radial head and coronoid and the capitulum and medial trochlea on the resulting projection?

_____
_____

Copyright © 2015, 2011, 2006, 1996 by Saunders, an imprint of Elsevier Inc. All rights reserved.

289. A lateral elbow projection with poor positioning demonstrates the capitulum too far posterior to the medial trochlea. How will the radial head and coronoid be aligned on this projection?

_____

290. The proximal humerus was positioned lower than the distal humerus on a lateral elbow projection. What will be the relationship between the radial head and coronoid and the capitulum and medial trochlea on the resulting projection?

_____

291. The position of the radial tuberosity on a lateral elbow projection is determined by the position of the hand and wrist. For the following positions, describe the location of the radial tuberosity.

   A. Lateral hand and wrist: _____

   B. Supinated hand and wrist: _____

   C. Pronated hand and wrist: _____

   Which of the radial tuberosity positions above is the desired position for an accurate lateral elbow projection?

   D. _____

292. Accurate CR centering on a lateral elbow projection is accomplished by centering a (A) _____ CR to the elbow joint located (B) _____ inch (C) _____ to the lateral humeral epicondyle.

293. What anatomic structures are included on a lateral elbow projection with accurate positioning?_____

_____

For the following descriptions of lateral elbow projections with poor positioning, state how the patient would have been mispositioned for such a projection to be obtained.

294. The olecranon is positioned within the olecranon fossa, and the posterior fat pad is demonstrated proximal to the olecranon process.

_____

295. The radial tuberosity is positioned in profile anteriorly.

_____

296. The radial head is positioned posterior on the coronoid process, and the distal surface of the capitulum is demonstrated distal to the distal surface of the medial trochlea.

_____

297. The radial head is positioned anterior on the coronoid process, and the distal surface of the capitulum is proximal to the distal surface of the medial trochlea.

_____

298. The radial head is distal to the coronoid process, and the capitulum appears anterior to the medial trochlea.

_____

299. The radial head is proximal to the coronoid process, and the capitulum appears posterior to the medial trochlea.

_____

Copyright © 2015, 2011, 2006, 1996 by Saunders, an imprint of Elsevier Inc. All rights reserved.   Chapter **4**   **Image Analysis of the Upper Extremity**

For the following lateral elbow projections with poor positioning, state what anatomic structures are misaligned and how the patient should be repositioned for an optimal projection to be obtained.

Figure 4-82

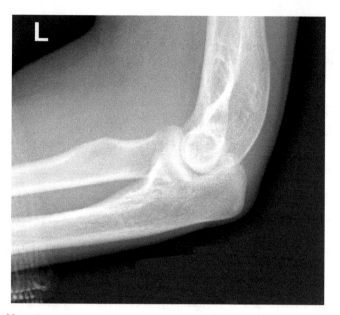

300. (Figure 4-82): _Capitulum is posterior to the trochlea. Depress distal forearm until the epicondyles are perp. to the IR and put lower arm in a true lateral position._

Figure 4-83

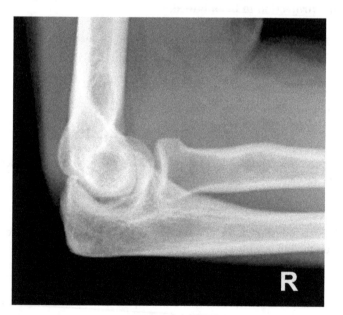

301. (Figure 4-83): _____

_____

_____

_____

Copyright © 2015, 2011, 2006, 1996 by Saunders, an imprint of Elsevier Inc. All rights reserved.

Figure 4-84

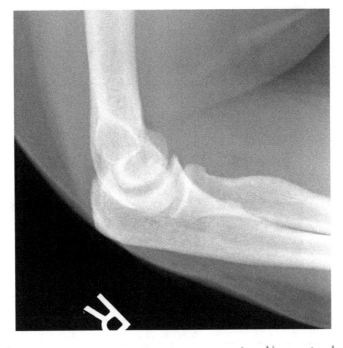

302. (Figure 4-84): <u>Capitulum is anterior and distal to the</u> <u>trochlea. Arm is not fully 90°.</u> <u>Fix by: elevate distal forearm, place epicondyles</u> <u>perp to IR, & flex elbow to 90°.</u>

Figure 4-85

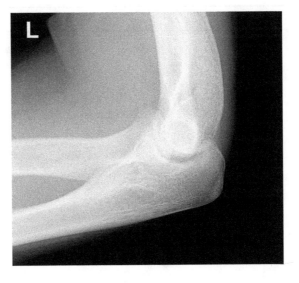

303. (Figure 4-85): _____

_____

_____

_____

Copyright © 2015, 2011, 2006, 1996 by Saunders, an imprint of Elsevier Inc. All rights reserved. Chapter **4   Image Analysis of the Upper Extremity**

Figure 4-86

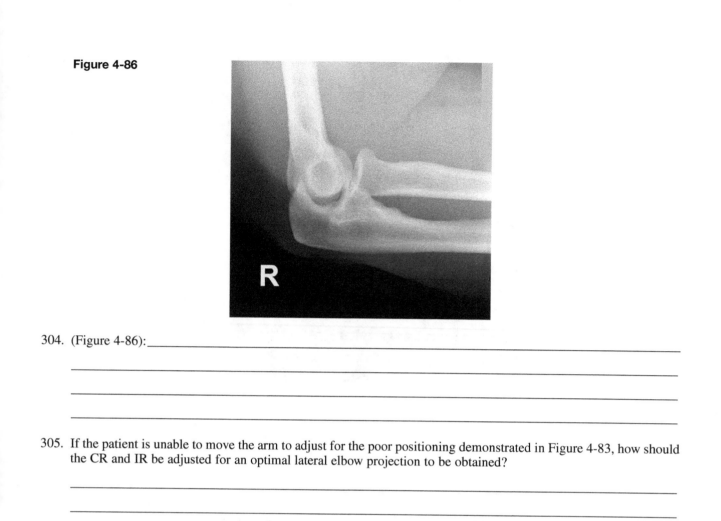

R

304. (Figure 4-86): _____

_____

_____

_____

305. If the patient is unable to move the arm to adjust for the poor positioning demonstrated in Figure 4-83, how should the CR and IR be adjusted for an optimal lateral elbow projection to be obtained?

_____

_____

_____

  Copyright © 2015, 2011, 2006, 1996 by Saunders, an imprint of Elsevier Inc. All rights reserved.

306. (Figure 4-87) The patient is unable to adjust positioning. How should the CR and IR be adjusted for an optimal lateral elbow projection to be obtained?

Figure 4-87

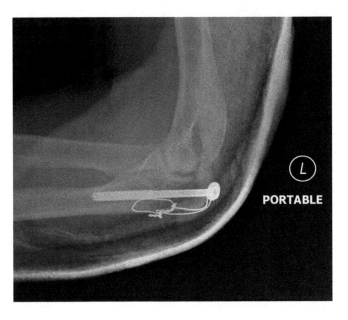

_____

_____

_____

Elbow: Axiolateral Projection (Coyle Method)

307. Identify the labeled anatomy in Figure 4-88.

Figure 4-88

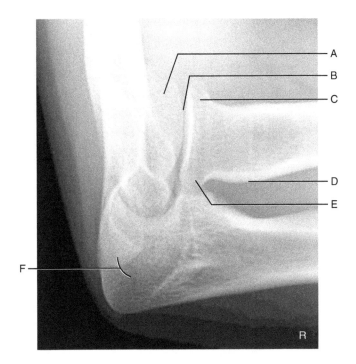

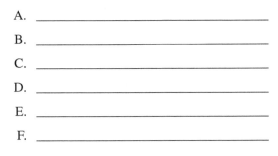

A. _____

B. _____

C. _____

D. _____

E. _____

F. _____

195

Copyright © 2015, 2011, 2006, 1996 by Saunders, an imprint of Elsevier Inc. All rights reserved.

308. Complete the statements below referring to axiolateral elbow projection analysis guidelines.

Axiolateral Elbow Projection Analysis Guidelines
■ The capitulum is (A) _____ to the medial trochlea.
■ The radial head superimposes only the tip of the (B)_____.
■ (C) _____ surfaces of the capitulum and medial trochlea are nearly aligned.
■ (D) _____ surfaces of the radial head and coronoid process are aligned.
■ (E) _____ is at the center of the exposure field.

309. In what position is the elbow placed to obtain the axiolateral projection of the elbow?

_____

310. The position of the distal forearm for an axiolateral projection affects the relationship of what anatomic elbow structures?

_____

_____

311. How can one determine from the projection if the forearm was elevated too high for the axiolateral elbow projection?

_____

_____

312. An axiolateral elbow projection with poor positioning demonstrates the radial head distal to the coronoid process. What is the relationship of the capitulum and medial trochlea on such a projection?

_____

313. To accurately separate the arcs of the distal humerus, an imaginary line connecting the humeral epicondyles is

positioned (A) _____ to the IR, and a(n) (B)_____-degree CR angulation is directed (C) _____. Will this

angle cause the radial head or coronoid to project farther proximally? (D) _____ Will this angle cause

the medial trochlea or capitulum to project farther proximally? (E) _____

314. What anatomic structure can be used to determine the portion of the radial head that is positioned in profile on an axiolateral elbow projection?

_____

315. For each of the following wrist projections, list the location of the radial tuberosity and the aspect of the radial head surface that are demonstrated in profile.

A. PA wrist:_____

B. Lateral wrist: _____

Copyright © 2015, 2011, 2006, 1996 by Saunders, an imprint of Elsevier Inc. All rights reserved.

316. State which aspects of the radial head surface is demonstrated in profile on the projection in Figure 4-89.

A. Anterior _____

B. Posterior _____

Figure 4-89

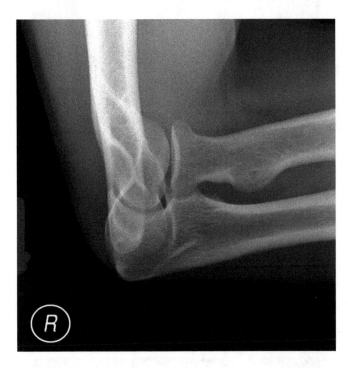

317. Accurate CR centering on an axiolateral elbow projection is accomplished by centering the CR to the

_____.

318. What anatomic structures are included on an axiolateral elbow projection with accurate positioning?

_____

For the following descriptions of axiolateral elbow projections with poor positioning, state how the patient would have been mispositioned for such a projection to be obtained.

319. The capitulum–radial joint space is closed, the radial head is demonstrated proximal to the coronoid process, and the capitulum is demonstrated too far posterior to the medial trochlea.

_____

Copyright © 2015, 2011, 2006, 1996 by Saunders, an imprint of Elsevier Inc. All rights reserved. Chapter **4** **Image Analysis of the Upper Extremity**

For the following axiolateral elbow projections with poor positioning, state what anatomic structures are misaligned and how the patient should be repositioned for an optimal projection to be obtained.

Figure 4-90

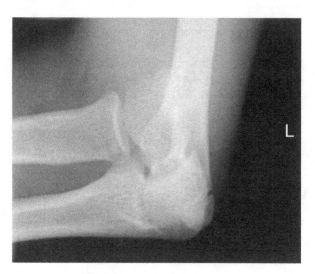

320. (Figure 4-90): _____

_____

_____

_____

Figure 4-91

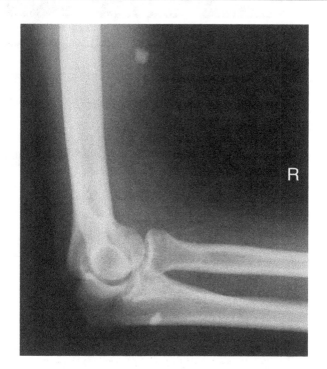

321. (Figure 4-91):_____

_____

_____

_____

Copyright © 2015, 2011, 2006, 1996 by Saunders, an imprint of Elsevier Inc. All rights reserved.

322. The axiolateral elbow projection in Figure 4-92 demonstrates a radial head fracture. Even though the projection was obtained with a 45-degree CR angle the radial head is not anterior enough to the coronoid, nor is the capitulum proximal enough to the medial trochlea, indicating poor patient positioning. If the patient could not move the arm from this position, how should the CR be adjusted to obtain an optimal capitulum–radial head projection?

Figure 4-92

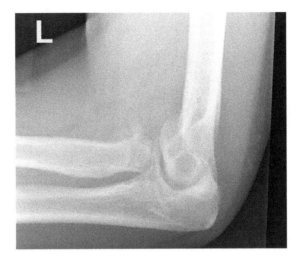

323. The patient was accurately positioned for the axiolateral elbow projection in Figure 4-93, but the CR was poorly aligned with the elbow, causing less than optimal anatomic relationships. Describe how the CR was aligned with the elbow to cause these results.

Figure 4-93

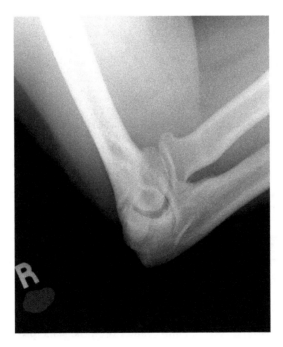

Copyright © 2015, 2011, 2006, 1996 by Saunders, an imprint of Elsevier Inc. All rights reserved.

Humerus: AP Projection

324. Identify the labeled anatomy in Figure 4-94.

Figure 4-94

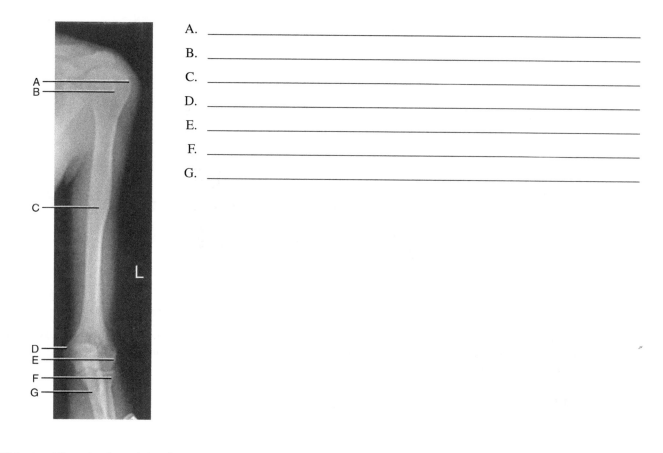

A. _____

B. _____

C. _____

D. _____

E. _____

F. _____

G. _____

325. An AP projection of the distal humerus has been obtained when _____ of the radial head superimposes the ulna.

326. On an AP proximal humeral projection with accurate positioning, the (A) _____ tubercle is demonstrated laterally in profile, the (B) _____ is demonstrated medially in profile, and the (C) _____ is visible approximately halfway between the greater tubercle and the humeral head.

327. If an AP humeral projection is ordered for a patient with a suspected proximal humeral fracture, why is it important not to externally rotate the arm?

A. _____

How can the ordered procedure still be performed without adjusting the arm position?

B. _____

328. An AP humeral projection is ordered for a patient with a humerus that is longer than 17 inches (43 cm). How should the arm be aligned with the IR to include the entire humerus on the same projection?

_____

Copyright © 2015, 2011, 2006, 1996 by Saunders, an imprint of Elsevier Inc. All rights reserved.

329. Why is it necessary to have the IR and collimator light field extend beyond the shoulder and elbow joints when imaging the humerus in the AP projection?

_____

330. Describe how the shoulder and elbow joints can be located to ensure that the IR extends beyond each for an AP humeral projection.

A. Shoulder: _____

B. Elbow: _____

331. On an AP humeral projection with accurate positioning, the _____ is centered within the collimated field.

332. What anatomic structures are included on an AP humeral projection with accurate positioning?

_____

For the following descriptions of AP humeral projections with poor positioning, state how the patient would have been mispositioned for such a projection to be obtained.

333. The projection demonstrates the ulna without radial head and tuberosity superimposition.

_____

For the following AP humeral projections with poor positioning, state what anatomic structures are misaligned and how the patient should be repositioned for an optimal projection to be obtained.

Figure 4-95

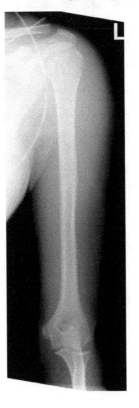

334. (Figure 4-95): _____

_____

_____

_____

Copyright © 2015, 2011, 2006, 1996 by Saunders, an imprint of Elsevier Inc. All rights reserved.   Chapter **4   Image Analysis of the Upper Extremity**

Figure 4-96

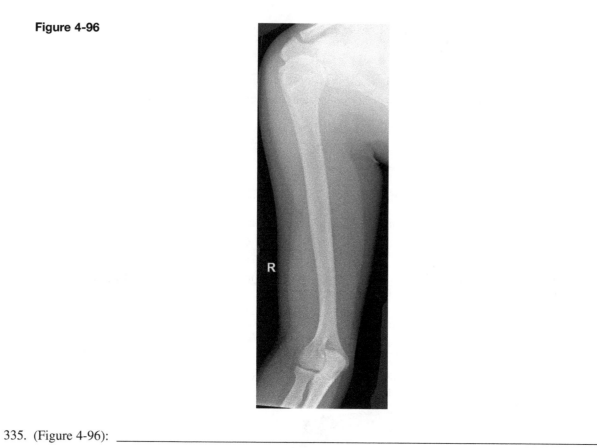

335. (Figure 4-96): _____

_____

_____

_____

 Copyright © 2015, 2011, 2006, 1996 by Saunders, an imprint of Elsevier Inc. All rights reserved.

Humerus: Lateral Projection

336. Is the projection demonstrated in Figure 4-97 a mediolateral or lateromedial projection?

_____

Figure 4-97

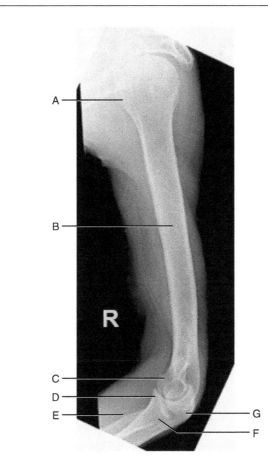

337. Identify the labeled anatomy in Figure 4-97.

A. _____

B. _____

C. _____

D. _____

E. _____

F. _____

G. _____

Copyright © 2015, 2011, 2006, 1996 by Saunders, an imprint of Elsevier Inc. All rights reserved.

Figure 4-98

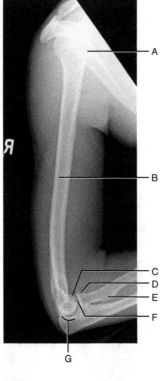

338. Identify the labeled anatomy in Figure 4-98.

A. _____

B. _____

C. _____

D. _____

E. _____

F. _____

G. _____

339. A lateral humeral projection with accurate positioning demonstrates the (A) _____ tubercle in profile (B) _____ (medially/laterally).

340. When positioning the patient for a lateral humeral projection, the (A) _____ should be internally rotated until an imaginary line connecting the (B) _____ is positioned perpendicular to the IR.

341. List two alternative projections that can be used to position the humerus in the lateral projection in a patient with a suspected fractured proximal humerus.

A. _____

B. _____

342. On a lateral humeral projection with accurate positioning, the _____ is centered within the collimated field.

343. What anatomic structures are included on a lateral humeral projection with accurate positioning?

both joints, the humerus, 3 lateral soft tissue

          Copyright © 2015, 2011, 2006, 1996 by Saunders, an imprint of Elsevier Inc. All rights reserved.

For the following lateral humeral projections with poor positioning, state what anatomic structures are misaligned and how the patient should be repositioned for an optimal projection to be obtained.

Figure 4-99

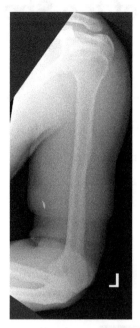

344. (Figure 4-99): Greater tubercle in profile & epicondyles not superimposed. Fix by: internally rotate arm until epicondyles are perp. to IR.

Figure 4-100

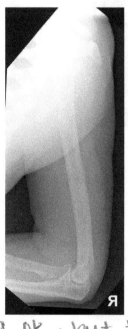

345. (Figure 4-100): Positioning ok, but torso obstructing proximal forearm. Fix by: rotating torso into a PA projection

205

Copyright © 2015, 2011, 2006, 1996 by Saunders, an imprint of Elsevier Inc. All rights reserved.

5 Image Analysis of the Shoulder

STUDY QUESTIONS

1. Routine shoulder projections are obtained using (A)_____ kV and (B)_____ SID.

2. When should a grid be used for the inferosuperior axial projection?

_____

Shoulder: AP Projection
3. Identify the labeled anatomy on Figure 5-1.

Figure 5-1

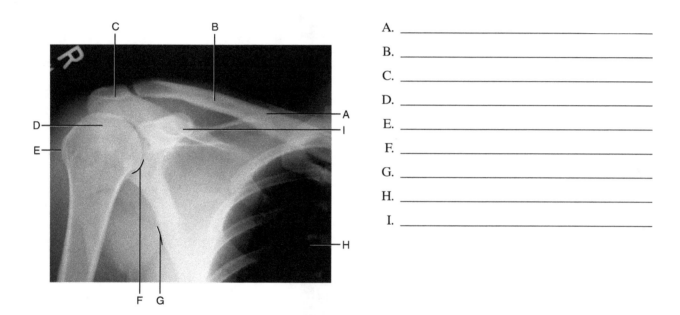

A. _____

B. _____

C. _____

D. _____

E. _____

F. _____

G. _____

H. _____

I. _____

4. Complete the statements below referring to AP shoulder projection analysis guidelines.

AP Shoulder Projection Analysis Guidelines
■ The scapular body demonstrates minimal transverse foreshortening, and (A) __1/2__ of the scapular body is visualized without thorax superimposition.
■ The clavicle is demonstrated with minimal longitudinal foreshortening, with the medial clavicular end positioned adjacent to the (B) _Vertebral column_
■ The superior scapular angle is superimposed by the (C) _____.

Copyright © 2015, 2011, 2006, 1996 by Saunders, an imprint of Elsevier Inc. All rights reserved.

- Neutral humerus: (D) _____ tubercle partially seen in profile laterally and the humeral head is partially seen in profile (E) _____.

- Externally rotated humerus: greater tubercle in profile (F) _____ and humeral head in profile (G) _____.

- Internally rotated humerus: (H) _____ tubercle in profile medially and humeral head superimposed by the greater tubercle.

5. How is the patient positioned to prevent rotation on an AP shoulder projection?

_____

6. What is the degree of scapular body obliquity on an AP shoulder projection?

A. _____

What portion of the scapula is situated anteriorly?

B. _____

7 A nondislocated shoulder demonstrates slight superimposition of the humeral head and glenoid cavity

8. Which shoulder dislocation is the most common? _____ (anterior/posterior)

9. How is the patient positioned to demonstrate the scapular body without longitudinal foreshortening on an AP shoulder projection?

_____

10. If the scapula is longitudinally foreshortened, the superior scapular angle is projected inferiorly or superiorly to the

_____.

11. How can longitudinal scapular foreshortening be reduced when obtaining an AP shoulder projection on a patient with kyphosis?

_____

12. The lateral humeral epicondyle is aligned with the (A) _____ tubercle, and the medial epicondyle

is aligned with the (B) _____ of the proximal humerus.

13. State how the humeral epicondyles are positioned in reference to the IR to place the anatomic structures as described on the following AP shoulder projections.

A. Greater tubercle is partially in profile laterally: ___45°_____

B. Lesser tubercle is in profile medially: ___perpendicular_____

C. Greater tubercle is in profile laterally: ___parallel_____

D. Humeral head is in profile medially: ___parallel_____

14. How is the patient's arm positioned for an AP shoulder projection if a shoulder dislocation or humeral fracture is suspected?

_____

Copyright © 2015, 2011, 2006, 1996 by Saunders, an imprint of Elsevier Inc. All rights reserved.

15. Accurate CR centering on an AP shoulder projection is accomplished by centering a(n) (A)_____

    CR 1 inch (2.5 cm) (B) _____ to the coracoid process.

16. What anatomic structures are demonstrated within the exposure field on an AP shoulder projection with accurate collimation?

    _____

For the following descriptions of AP shoulder projections with poor positioning, state how the patient would have been mispositioned for such a projection to be obtained.

17. The glenoid cavity is nearly in profile with only a small amount of the articulating surface demonstrated, the superolateral border of the scapula is superimposed by the thorax, and the medial clavicular end has been rolled away from the vertebral column.

    _____

    _____

18. The scapular body is drawn from beneath the thorax and is transversely foreshortened, the glenoid cavity is demonstrated on end, and the medial clavicular end is superimposed over the vertebral column.

    _____

    _____

19. The superior scapular angle is demonstrated superior to the clavicle, and the acromion process and humeral head demonstrate no superimposition.

    _____

    _____

20. A neutral shoulder projection demonstrates the greater tubercle in profile laterally and the humeral head in profile medially.

    _____

    _____

21. A neutral shoulder projection demonstrates the lesser tubercle in profile medially.

    _____

    _____

Copyright © 2015, 2011, 2006, 1996 by Saunders, an imprint of Elsevier Inc. All rights reserved.

For the following AP shoulder projections with poor positioning, state what anatomic structures are misaligned and how the patient should be repositioned for an optimal projection to be obtained.

Figure 5-2

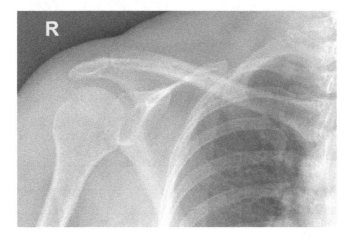

22. (Figure 5-2): _____

_____

_____

Figure 5-3

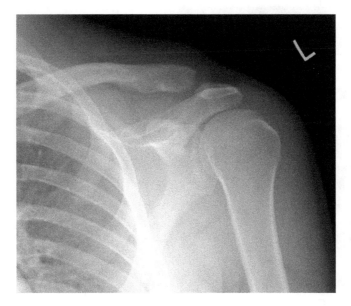

23. (Figure 5-3): _____

_____

_____

Copyright © 2015, 2011, 2006, 1996 by Saunders, an imprint of Elsevier Inc. All rights reserved.   Chapter **5** **Image Analysis of the Shoulder**

Figure 5-4

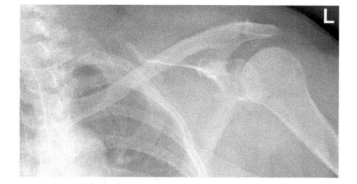

24. (Figure 5-4): _____

_____

_____

Shoulder: Inferosuperior Axial Projection

25. Identify the labeled anatomy in Figure 5-5.

Figure 5-5

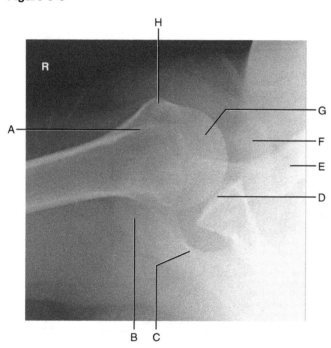

A. _____

B. _____

C. _____

D. _____

E. _____

F. _____

G. _____

H. _____

Copyright © 2015, 2011, 2006, 1996 by Saunders, an imprint of Elsevier Inc. All rights reserved.

26. Complete the statements below referring to inferosuperior axial shoulder projection analysis guidelines.

> **Inferosuperior Axial Shoulder Projection Analysis Guidelines**
>
> ■ The inferior and superior margins of the (A) _____ are nearly superimposed, demonstrating an open glenohumeral joint space.
>
> ■ The lateral edge of the coracoid process base is aligned with the (B) _____ glenoid cavity margin.
>
> ■ The epicondyles are parallel with floor: (C) _____ in profile anteriorly.
>
> ■ The epicondyles at a 45-degree angle with floor: (D) _____ in partial profile anteriorly and the posterolateral aspect of the humeral head in profile (E) _____. The (F) _____ is at the center of the exposure field.

27. Humeral abduction of the arm is obtained by combined movements of the (A) _____ and (B) _____.

28. On a patient who has no trouble abducting the humerus to a 90-degree angle with the body, the glenoid cavity is placed at a _____ angle with the lateral body surface.

29. How should the angle between the lateral body surface and the CR be adjusted if the patient can abduct the humerus to only a 45-degree angle with the body?

    A. _____

    Why is this change required?

    B. _____

    _____

30. How is the IR positioned for an inferosuperior axial shoulder projection?

    _____

    _____

31. Describe the anatomic structures of the proximal humerus that are demonstrated anteriorly and posteriorly in profile on an inferosuperior axial shoulder projection when the humerus is positioned as stated below.

    A. Arm externally rotated until the humeral epicondyles are at a 45-degree angle with the floor:

    _____

    _____

    B. Arm externally rotated until the humeral epicondyles are perpendicular to the floor:

    _____

    _____

    C. Arm externally rotated until the humeral epicondyles are parallel with the floor:

    _____

32. Accurate CR centering on an inferiorsuperior axial shoulder projection is accomplished by centering a (A) __horizontal__ CR to the midaxillary region at the same transverse level as the (B) __coracoid process__.

Copyright © 2015, 2011, 2006, 1996 by Saunders, an imprint of Elsevier Inc. All rights reserved.

33. What anatomic structures are included on an inferosuperior axial shoulder projection with accurate positioning?

glenoid cavity, coracoid process, scapular spine, acromion,
3 1/3 of proximal humerus

34. For an inferosuperior axial shoulder, elevation of the shoulder on a sponge or washcloth prevents clipping of the

_____ aspect of the humerus and shoulder.

35. Lateral neck flexion and turning the face away from the affected shoulder prevents clipping of the _____.

36. How were the humeral epicondyles positioned for the following inferosuperior axial shoulder projections?

Figure 5-6

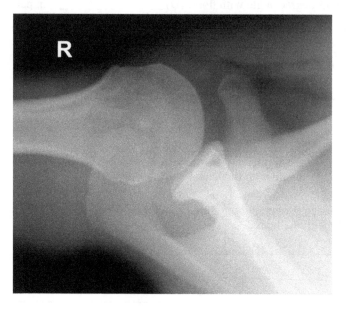

A. (Figure 5-6): _____

Figure 5-7

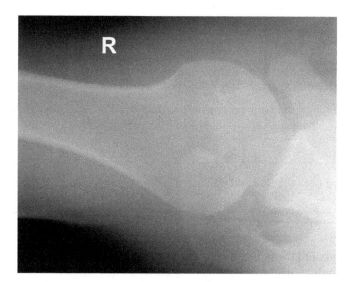

B. (Figure 5-7): _____

Chapter **5** **Image Analysis of the Shoulder**   Copyright © 2015, 2011, 2006, 1996 by Saunders, an imprint of Elsevier Inc. All rights reserved.

For the following descriptions of inferosuperior axial shoulder projections with poor positioning, state how the patient would have been mispositioned or the CR aligned for such a projection to be obtained.

37. The glenohumeral joint space is obscured, and the inferior glenoid cavity is demonstrated lateral to the coracoid process base.

_____

38. The glenohumeral joint space is obscured, and the inferior glenoid cavity is demonstrated medial to the lateral edge of the coracoid process base.

_____

39. The greater tubercle is demonstrated in profile posteriorly.

_____

40. The acromion process, scapular spine, and posterior aspect of the proximal humerus were not included on the projection.

_____

For the following inferosuperior axial shoulder projections with poor positioning, state what anatomic structures are misaligned and how the patient should be repositioned for an optimal projection to be obtained.

Figure 5-8

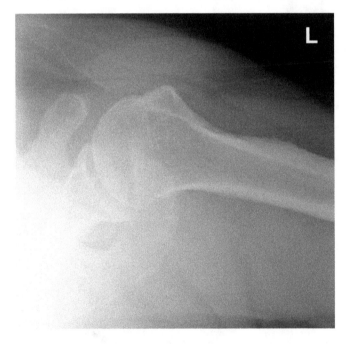

41. (Figure 5-8): _____

_____

_____

Copyright © 2015, 2011, 2006, 1996 by Saunders, an imprint of Elsevier Inc. All rights reserved.

Figure 5-9

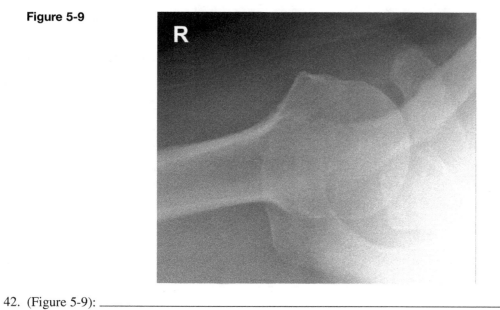

42. (Figure 5-9): _____

_____

_____

Figure 5-10

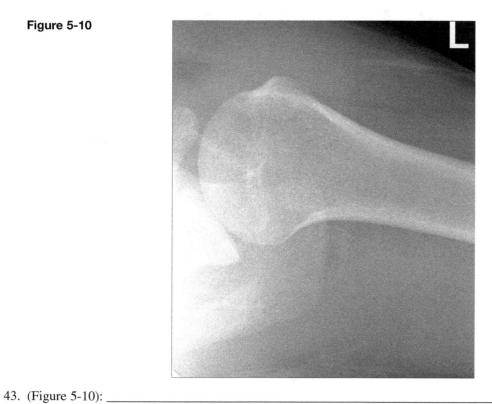

43. (Figure 5-10): _____

_____

_____

Copyright © 2015, 2011, 2006, 1996 by Saunders, an imprint of Elsevier Inc. All rights reserved.

Shoulder: AP Oblique Projection (Grashey Method)

44. Identify the labeled anatomy in Figure 5-11.

Figure 5-11

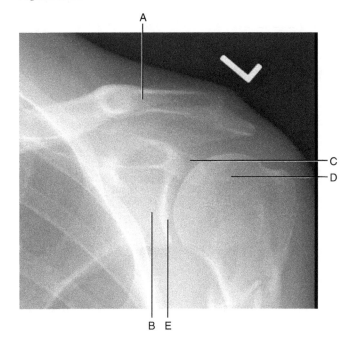

A. _____

B. _____

C. _____

D. _____

E. _____

45. Complete the statements below referring to AP oblique shoulder projection analysis guidelines.

AP Oblique (Grashey Method) Projection Analysis Guidelines
■ The glenoid cavity is demonstrated (A) _____, and the glenohumeral joint space is (B) _____.
■ The lateral coracoid process superimposing humeral head by about (C) _____.
■ The superior margin of the (D) _____ is aligned with the superior margin of the (E) _____.
■ The (F) _____ is at the center of the exposure field.

Copyright © 2015, 2011, 2006, 1996 by Saunders, an imprint of Elsevier Inc. All rights reserved.

46. The (A)_____and (B) _____ joints function coopera-
tively to allow the shoulder to be protracted.

47. The scapular body is positioned parallel with the IR for the AP oblique shoulder projection by aligning an imaginary

line connecting the (A) _____ and (B) _____ perpendicular to the IR.

48. A 45-degree oblique is routinely used for the AP oblique shoulder projection. List three situations in which the patient
requires more than 45 degrees of obliquity to obtain an AP oblique shoulder projection with accurate positioning.

   A. _____

   B. _____

   C. _____

49. How is the clavicle positioned on an AP oblique shoulder projection with accurate rotation that was exposed with
the patient recumbent?

   _____

50. Accurate CR centering on an AP oblique shoulder projection is accomplished by centering a (A)_____

   CR to the (B) _____.

51. What anatomic structures are demonstrated within the collimated field on an AP oblique shoulder projection with
accurate positioning?

   _____

**For the following descriptions of AP oblique shoulder projections with poor positioning, state how the patient
would have been mispositioned for such a projection to be obtained.**

52. The glenohumeral joint space is closed, approximately ½ inch (1.25 cm) of the coracoid process is superimposed
over the humeral head, and the clavicle demonstrates excessive transverse foreshortening.

   _____

53. The glenohumeral joint space is closed, the lateral tip of the coracoid process is not superimposed over the humeral
head, and the clavicle demonstrates little foreshortening.

   _____

54. Recumbent patient: the glenohumeral joint is closed, and the clavicle is superimposed over the scapular neck.

   _____

55. The superior margin of the coracoid process is demonstrated superior to the superior margin of the glenoid cavity.

   _____

 Copyright © 2015, 2011, 2006, 1996 by Saunders, an imprint of Elsevier Inc. All rights reserved.

For the following AP oblique shoulder projections with poor positioning, state what anatomic structures are misaligned and how the patient should be repositioned for an optimal projection to be obtained.

Figure 5-12

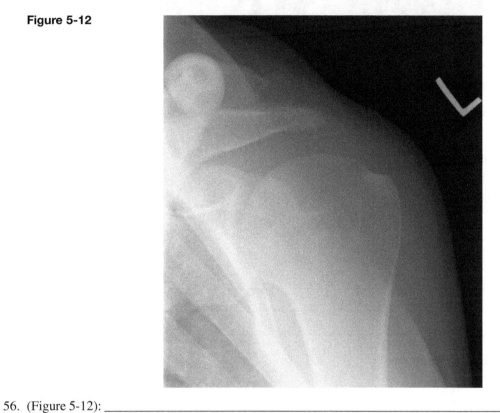

56. (Figure 5-12): _____

_____

_____

Copyright © 2015, 2011, 2006, 1996 by Saunders, an imprint of Elsevier Inc. All rights reserved.

Figure 5-13

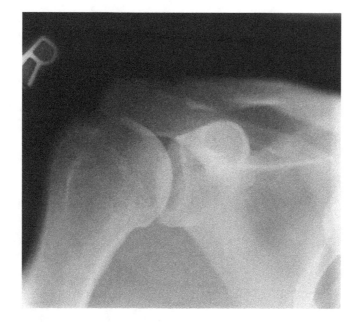

57. (Figure 5-13): _____

_____

_____

Shoulder: PA Oblique Projection (Scapular Y)

58. Identify the labeled anatomy in Figure 5-14.

Figure 5-14

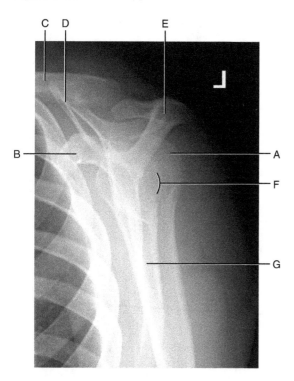

A. _____

B. _____

C. _____

D. _____

E. _____

F. _____

G. _____

Copyright © 2015, 2011, 2006, 1996 by Saunders, an imprint of Elsevier Inc. All rights reserved.

59. Complete the statements below referring to PA oblique (scapular Y) shoulder projection analysis guidelines.

PA Oblique (Scapular Y) Shoulder Projection Analysis Guidelines
■ The lateral and vertebral scapular borders are (A) _____.
■ The scapular body and the (B) _____ and (C) _____ form a Y.
■ The clavicle and (D) _____ are visualized at the same transverse level.
■ The (E) _____ is at the center of the exposure field.

60. The scapular body is placed in a lateral position for the PA oblique shoulder projection by rotating the patient until an imaginary line drawn between the (A) _____ and (B) _____ is aligned parallel with the IR.

61. List two indications for ordering the PA oblique (scapular Y) projection:

   A. _____

   B. _____

62. For a PA oblique shoulder projection, the patient is rotated toward the (A) _____ (affected/unaffected) shoulder. For an AP oblique shoulder projection, the patient is rotated toward the (B) _____ (affected/unaffected) shoulder.

63. How can one distinguish the medial and lateral scapular borders from each other on a PA oblique shoulder projection with poor positioning?

   _____

64. Where are the humeral head and shaft positioned in respect to the scapula on a nondislocated PA oblique shoulder projection?

   _____

65. If the patient's shoulder is dislocated, should the Y formation desired on the PA oblique shoulder projection be visualized? _____ (Yes/No)

66. Where is the humeral head positioned on the AP oblique shoulder projection if the shoulder is dislocated anteriorly?

   A. _____

   _____

   If the shoulder is dislocated posteriorly?

   B. _____

   _____

67. How can the patient be positioned to prevent longitudinal foreshortening of the scapula on a PA oblique shoulder projection?

   _____

   _____

Copyright © 2015, 2011, 2006, 1996 by Saunders, an imprint of Elsevier Inc. All rights reserved.

68. What spinal condition results in longitudinal scapular foreshortening on a PA oblique shoulder projection?

A. _____

How can the CR be adjusted to offset this foreshortening when obtaining a PA oblique projection?

B. _____

69. Accurate CR centering on a PA oblique shoulder projection is accomplished by centering a(n) (A) _____ CR to the (B) _____ border of the scapula halfway between the (C) _____ and (D) _____.

70. What anatomic structures are demonstrated on a PA oblique shoulder projection with accurate positioning?

_____

_____

For the following descriptions of PA oblique shoulder projections with poor positioning, state how the patient would have been mispositioned for such a projection to be obtained.

71. The vertebral and lateral borders of the scapular body are demonstrated without superimposition, the lateral scapular border is demonstrated next to the ribs, and the medial border appears laterally.

_____

_____

72. The lateral and medial borders of the scapula are demonstrated without superimposition, the thicker scapular border is demonstrated laterally, and the thinner scapular border is demonstrated next to the ribs.

_____

_____

73. The scapular body, acromion process, and coracoid process demonstrate a Y formation, but the superior scapular angle is demonstrated superior to the clavicle.

_____

_____

Copyright © 2015, 2011, 2006, 1996 by Saunders, an imprint of Elsevier Inc. All rights reserved.

For the following AP oblique shoulder projections with poor positioning, state what anatomic structures are misaligned and how the patient should be repositioned for an optimal projection to be obtained.

Figure 5-15

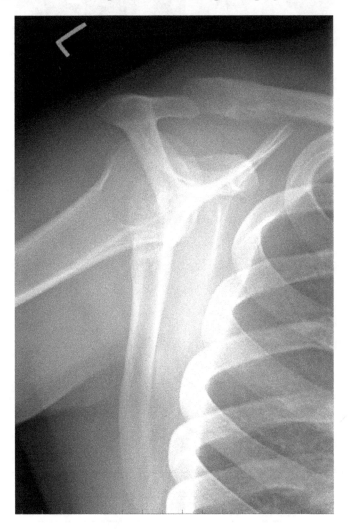

74. (Figure 5-15): _____

_____

_____

Copyright © 2015, 2011, 2006, 1996 by Saunders, an imprint of Elsevier Inc. All rights reserved.

Figure 5-16

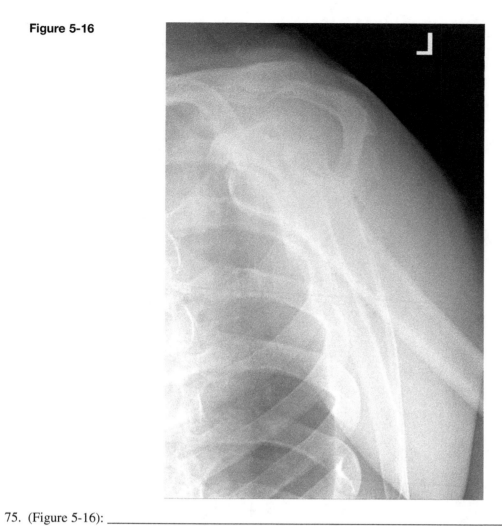

75. (Figure 5-16): _____

_____

_____

Copyright © 2015, 2011, 2006, 1996 by Saunders, an imprint of Elsevier Inc. All rights reserved.

Figure 5-17

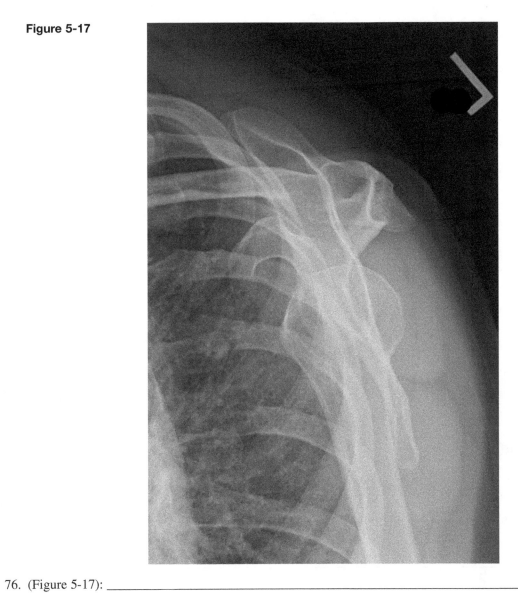

76. (Figure 5-17): _____

_____

_____

Copyright © 2015, 2011, 2006, 1996 by Saunders, an imprint of Elsevier Inc. All rights reserved.

Figure 5-18

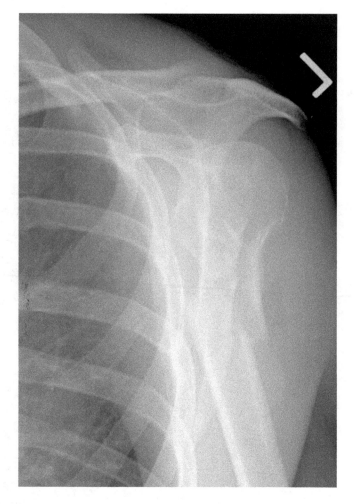

77. (Figure 5-18, trauma): _____

_____

_____

     Copyright © 2015, 2011, 2006, 1996 by Saunders, an imprint of Elsevier Inc. All rights reserved.

Proximal Humerus: AP Axial Projection (Stryker "Notch" Method)

78. Identify the labeled anatomy in Figure 5-19.

   Figure 5-19

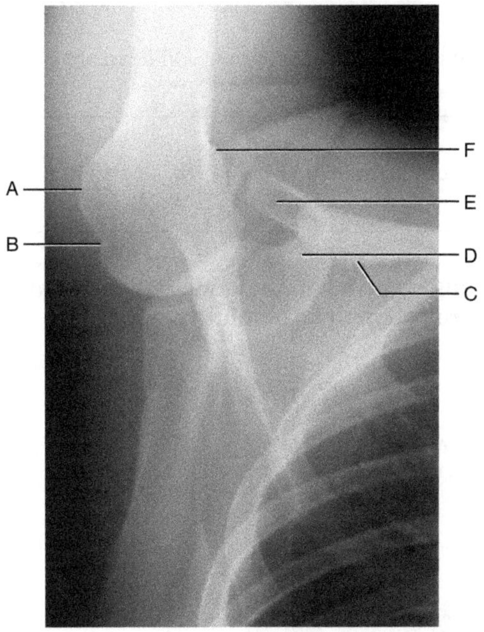

   A. _____

   B. _____

   C. _____

   D. _____

   E. _____

   F. _____

79. Complete the statements below referring to AP axial (Stryker notch) shoulder projection analysis guidelines.

AP Axial (Stryker "Notch" Method) Shoulder Projection Analysis Guidelines
■ The coracoid process is situated directly lateral to the (A) _____ of the clavicle.
■ The (B) _____ aspect of the humeral head is in profile laterally, and the greater and lesser tubercles are seen in partial profile.
■ The (C) _____ is superimposed over the lateral clavicle.
■ The (D) _____ is at the center of the exposure field.

80. The AP axial shoulder projection is performed to diagnose the presence of the (A) _____ defect of the shoulder. When present, the defect is demonstrated on the (B) _____ aspect of the humeral head.

81. For the AP axial shoulder projection, the affected arm is abducted until the humerus is (A) _____, and then the elbow is flexed and the palm of the hand is placed (B) _____.

82. Accurate CR centering on an AP axial projection is accomplished when the CR is centered to the

   _____.

83. What anatomic structures are demonstrated on an AP axial projection with accurate positioning?

   _____

Copyright © 2015, 2011, 2006, 1996 by Saunders, an imprint of Elsevier Inc. All rights reserved. Chapter **5 Image Analysis of the Shoulder**

For the following descriptions of AP axial shoulder projections with poor positioning, state how the patient would have been mispositioned for such a projection to be obtained.

84. The coracoid process is seen inferior to the clavicle, and the humeral shaft demonstrates increased foreshortening.

_____

85. The lesser tubercle is seen in profile medially, but the greater tubercle and posterolateral humeral head are obscured.

_____

86. The posterolateral humeral head is obscured, and the humeral shaft demonstrates increased foreshortening.

_____

For the following AP axial shoulder projections with poor positioning, state what anatomic structures are misaligned and how the patient should be repositioned for an optimal projection to be obtained.

Figure 5-20

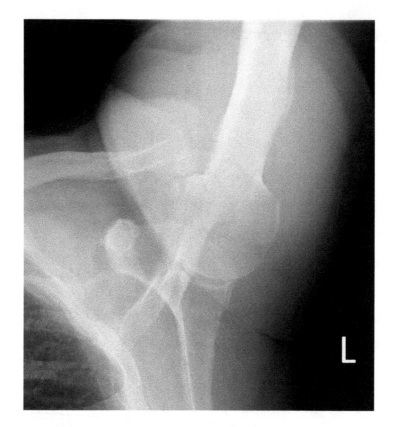

87. (Figure 5-20): _____

_____

_____

Copyright © 2015, 2011, 2006, 1996 by Saunders, an imprint of Elsevier Inc. All rights reserved.

Figure 5-21

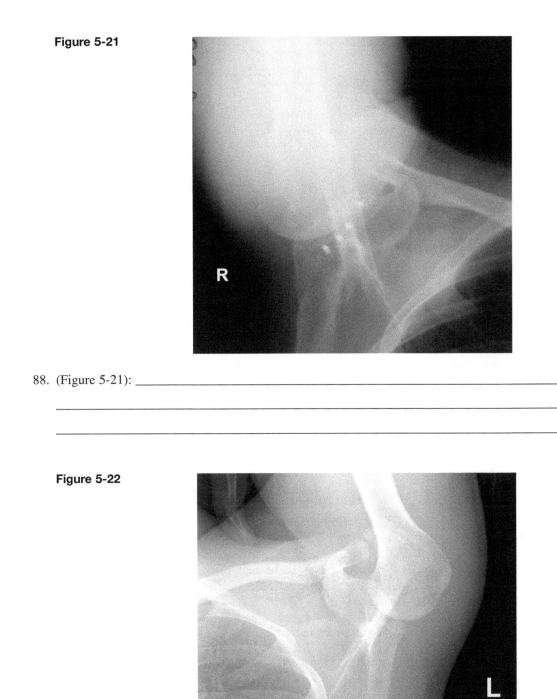

88. (Figure 5-21): _____

_____

_____

Figure 5-22

89. (Figure 5-22): _____

_____

_____

Copyright © 2015, 2011, 2006, 1996 by Saunders, an imprint of Elsevier Inc. All rights reserved.

Supraspinatus "Outlet": Tangential Projection (Neer Method)

90. Identify the labeled anatomy in Figure 5-23.

Figure 5-23

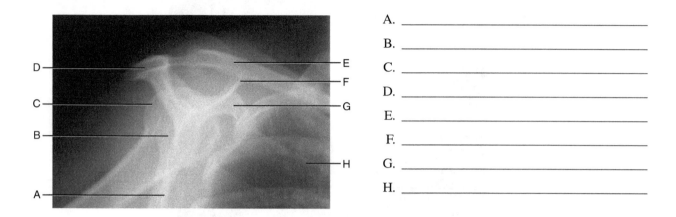

A. _____

B. _____

C. _____

D. _____

E. _____

F. _____

G. _____

H. _____

91. Complete the statements below referring to tangential supraspinatus outlet projection analysis guidelines.

> **Tangential "Outlet" Projection Analysis Guidelines**
>
> - The lateral and vertebral scapular borders are (A) _____.
>
> - The (B) _____, (C) _____, and (D) _____
>   form a Y, with the glenoid cavity demonstrated on end.
>
> - The lateral clavicle and acromion process form a smooth continuous arch, the superior scapular angle is at the
>   level of the (E) _____ and is positioned about ½ inch (1.25 cm) inferior to the
>   (F) _____.
>
> - The (G) _____ is at the center of the exposure field.

92. Should the tangential outlet projection be obtained with the patient placed in an AP or PA oblique projection to demonstrate the least scapular magnification and the greatest scapular detail?

_____

93. Allowing the arm to dangle freely instead of abducted and flexed for the tangential outlet projection requires

_____ (less/more) patient obliquity to obtain accurate positioning.

94. The tangential outlet projection is taken to identify spurs and osteophyte formation on the _____ surfaces of the lateral clavicle and acromion angle.

95. Accurate CR placement on a tangential outlet shoulder projection is accomplished when the CR is angled

(A) _____ and centered to the (B) _____.

96. What anatomic structures should be included within the collimated field?

_____

Copyright © 2015, 2011, 2006, 1996 by Saunders, an imprint of Elsevier Inc. All rights reserved.

For the following descriptions of tangential outlet shoulder projections with poor positioning, state how the patient would have been mispositioned for such a projection to be obtained.

97. The vertebral and lateral borders of the scapular body are demonstrated without superimposition, the lateral scapular border is demonstrated next to the ribs, and the medial border appears laterally.

_____

98. The lateral clavicle and acromion process are demonstrated less than ½ inch (1.25 cm) superior to the humeral head and supraspinous fossa, and the superior scapular spine appears superior to the clavicle.

_____

For the following tangential outlet shoulder projections with poor positioning, state what anatomic structures are misaligned and how the patient should be repositioned for an optimal projection to be obtained.

Figure 5-24

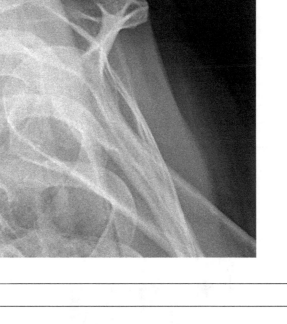

99. (Figure 5-24): _____

_____

_____

_____

Copyright © 2015, 2011, 2006, 1996 by Saunders, an imprint of Elsevier Inc. All rights reserved.

Figure 5-25

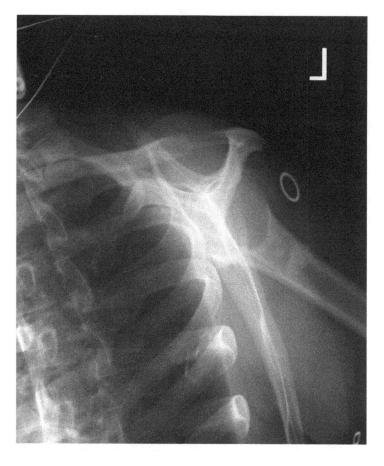

100. (Figure 5-25): _____

_____

_____

Clavicle: AP Projection

101. Identify the labeled anatomy in Figure 5-26.

Figure 5-26

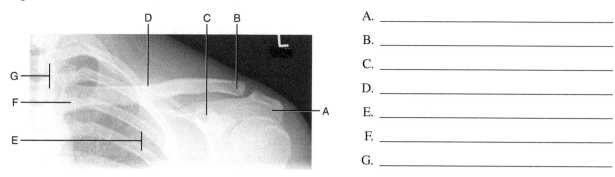

A. _____

B. _____

C. _____

D. _____

E. _____

F. _____

G. _____

Copyright © 2015, 2011, 2006, 1996 by Saunders, an imprint of Elsevier Inc. All rights reserved.

102 Complete the statements below referring to AP clavicle projection analysis guidelines.

> **AP Clavicle Projection Analysis Guidelines**
>
> ■ The medial clavicular end lies next to the (A) _____ of the vertebral column.
>
> ■ The clavicle and (B) _____ are visualized at the same
>
>   (C) _____ level.
>
> ■ The (D) _____ is at the center of the exposure field.

103. How can the technologist position the patient to prevent rotation on an AP clavicular projection?

_____

104. Accurate CR centering on an AP clavicular is accomplished by centering a(n) (A) _____ CR to the

(B) _____.

105. What anatomic structures are demonstrated on an AP clavicular projection with accurate positioning?

_____

For the following descriptions of AP clavicular projections with poor positioning, state how the patient would have been mispositioned for such a projection to be obtained.

106. The medial clavicular end is superimposed over the vertebral column, and the vertebral border of the scapula is positioned away from the thoracic cavity.

_____

107. The medial clavicular end is placed 1 inch (2.5 cm) away from the vertebral column, and the lateral border of the scapula is mostly superimposed by the thoracic cavity.

_____

108. The lateral clavicular end is superimposed over the scapular spine, and the superior scapular angle is projected above the midclavicle.

_____

Copyright © 2015, 2011, 2006, 1996 by Saunders, an imprint of Elsevier Inc. All rights reserved.

For the following AP clavicular projections with poor positioning, state what anatomic structures are misaligned and how the patient should be repositioned for an optimal projection to be obtained.

Figure 5-27

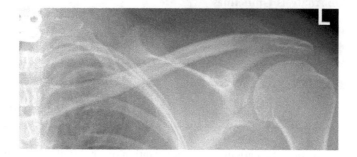

109. (Figure 5-27): _____

_____

_____

Figure 5-28

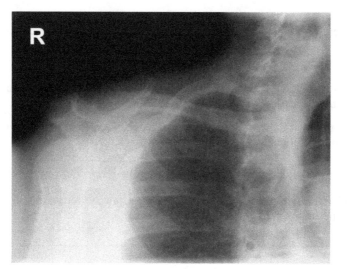

110. (Figure 5-28): _____

_____

_____

Copyright © 2015, 2011, 2006, 1996 by Saunders, an imprint of Elsevier Inc. All rights reserved.

Clavicle: AP Axial Projection (Lordotic Position)

111. Identify the labeled anatomy in Figure 5-29.

Figure 5-29

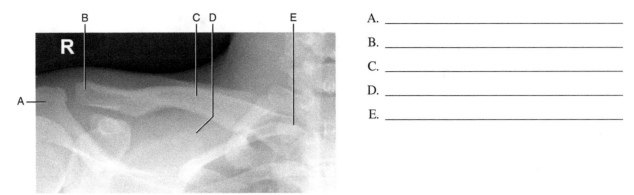

A. _____

B. _____

C. _____

D. _____

E. _____

112. Complete the statements below referring to AP axial clavicle projection analysis guidelines.

<table>
<tr><td>AP Axial Clavicle Projection Analysis Guidelines</td></tr>
</table>

- The medial (A) _____ end lies next to the lateral edge of the vertebral column.

- The superior scapular angle is visualized 0.5 inch (B) _____ to the clavicle.

- The medial end of clavicle is superimposed over the (C) _____ rib.

- The middle and lateral thirds of clavicle are seen superior to the (D) _____ and the clavicle bows upwardly.

- The (E) _____ is at the center of the exposure field.

113. What are the degree and direction of CR angulation used for the AP axial clavicular projection?

_____

114. Where do most fractures of the clavicle occur?

_____

115. What anatomic structures are demonstrated on an AP axial clavicular projection with accurate positioning?

_____

For the following descriptions of AP axial clavicular projections with poor positioning, state how the patient would have been mispositioned or the central ray aligned for such a projection to be obtained.

116. The medial clavicular end is drawn away from the vertebral column, the vertebral and lateral borders of the scapula are superimposed by the thoracic cavity, and the clavicle is longitudinally foreshortened.

_____

117. The lateral and middle thirds of the clavicle are superimposed over the scapula.

_____

233

Copyright © 2015, 2011, 2006, 1996 by Saunders, an imprint of Elsevier Inc. All rights reserved.

For the following AP axial clavicular projection with poor positioning, state what anatomic structures are misaligned and how the patient should be repositioned for an optimal projection to be obtained.

Figure 5-30

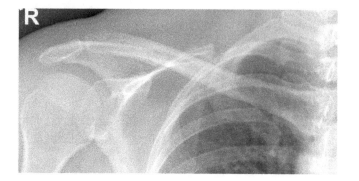

118. (Figure 5-30): _____

_____

_____

AC Joint: AP Projection

119. Identify the labeled anatomy in Figure 5-31.

Figure 5-31

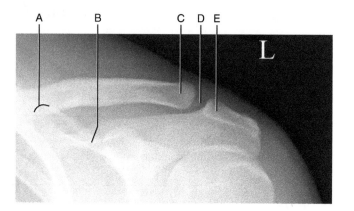

A. _____

B. _____

C. _____

D. _____

E. _____

120. Complete the statements below referring to AP acromioclavicular joint projection analysis guidelines.

> **AP Acromioclavicular Joint Projection Analysis Guidelines**
>
> ■ Weight-bearing projection displays a (A) _____ marker to indicate that the projection
> was taken (B) _____. The lateral clavicle is (C) _____, and about 1/8 inch (0.3 cm) of space is present between the lateral clavicle and acromial apex.
>
> ■ The lateral clavicle demonstrates minimal (D) _____ superimposition.
>
> ■ The (E)_____ is at the center of the exposure field.

Copyright © 2015, 2011, 2006, 1996 by Saunders, an imprint of Elsevier Inc. All rights reserved.

121. Why are weight- and non–weight-bearing AP AC joint projections often requested?

_____

_____

122. How is an AC ligament injury identified on an AP AC joint projection?

_____

_____

123. How much weight does the patient hold in each arm for the weight-bearing AC joint projection?

_____

124. What anatomic structures are demonstrated on an AP AC joint projection with accurate positioning?

_____

125. Why is it necessary to place the CR at the same location when weight- and non–weight-bearing projections are requested?

_____

For the following description of an AP AC joint projection with poor positioning, state how the patient would have been mispositioned for such a projection to be obtained.

126. The left AC joint is closed, and the scapular body demonstrates an increased amount of thoracic superimposition.

_____

For the following AC joint projection with poor positioning, state what anatomic structures are misaligned and how the patient should be repositioned for an optimal projection to be obtained.

Figure 5-32

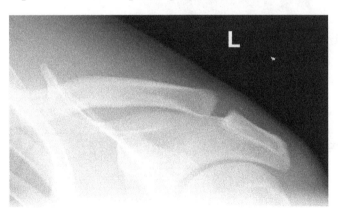

127. (Figure 5-32):  _____

_____

_____

Copyright © 2015, 2011, 2006, 1996 by Saunders, an imprint of Elsevier Inc. All rights reserved.

Scapula: AP Projection

128. Identify the labeled anatomy in Figure 5-33.

Figure 5-33

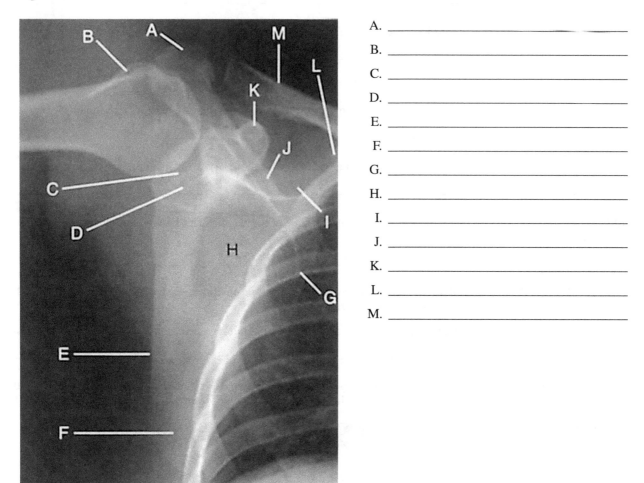

A. _____

B. _____

C. _____

D. _____

E. _____

F. _____

G. _____

H. _____

I. _____

J. _____

K. _____

L. _____

M. _____

129. Complete the statements below referring to AP Scapula projection analysis guidelines.

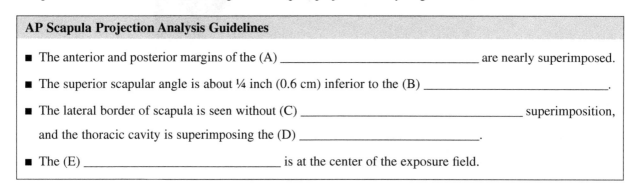

AP Scapula Projection Analysis Guidelines

- The anterior and posterior margins of the (A) _____ are nearly superimposed.

- The superior scapular angle is about ¼ inch (0.6 cm) inferior to the (B) _____.

- The lateral border of scapula is seen without (C) _____ superimposition, and the thoracic cavity is superimposing the (D) _____.

- The (E) _____ is at the center of the exposure field.

130. Even though the AP thickness is approximately the same across the scapula, why is the brightness level not uniform across the scapula?

_____

_____

 Copyright © 2015, 2011, 2006, 1996 by Saunders, an imprint of Elsevier Inc. All rights reserved.

131. If a breathing technique cannot be used for the AP scapular projection, what respiration should be used?

_____

132. What degree of scapular rotation is demonstrated when the patient is positioned in an AP projection with the humerus resting against the side?

A. _____

Which scapular dimension is foreshortened in this position?

B. _____

133. How is the patient's arm positioned for an AP projection of the scapula?

A. _____

What effect does this positioning have on the shoulder when the projection is obtained with the patient in a supine position?

B. _____

What effect does the positioning have on the visualization of the glenoid cavity on an AP scapular projection?

C. _____

134. What scapular dimension is foreshortened when the patient's midcoronal plane is poorly positioned? _____

_____

135. Accurately CR centering on an AP scapular projection is accomplished by centering a (A) _____

CR (B) _____ inches (C) _____ to the palpable coracoid process.

136. What anatomic structures are included on an AP scapular projection with accurate positioning?

_____

For the following descriptions of AP scapular projections with poor positioning, state how the patient would have been mispositioned for such a projection to be obtained.

137. The glenoid cavity is not in profile, and approximately 0.5 inch (1 cm) of it is demonstrated. _____

_____

138. A projection of a patient who was very mobile demonstrates the inferior scapular angle and inferolateral scapular border with thoracic cavity superimposition.

_____

Copyright © 2015, 2011, 2006, 1996 by Saunders, an imprint of Elsevier Inc. All rights reserved.

For the following AP scapular projections with poor positioning, state what anatomic structures are misaligned and how the patient should be repositioned for an optimal projection to be obtained.

Figure 5-34

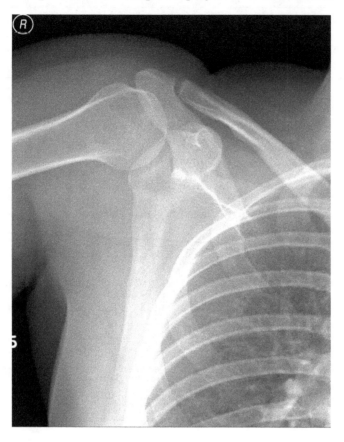

139. (Figure 5-34): _____

_____

_____

Copyright © 2015, 2011, 2006, 1996 by Saunders, an imprint of Elsevier Inc. All rights reserved.

Figure 5-35

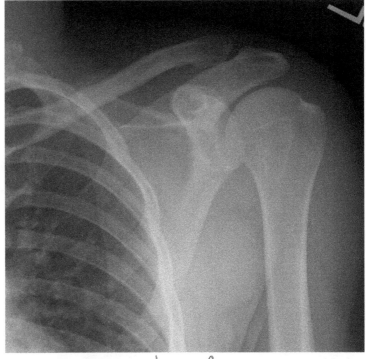

140. (Figure 5-35): Inferolateral border of scapula superimposed, β superior angle superimposed by clavicle. Fix by: abduct humerus 90° from body

Scapula: Lateral Projection (Lateromedial or Mediolateral)

141. Identify the labeled anatomy in Figure 5-36.

Figure 5-36

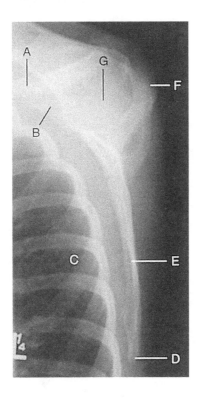

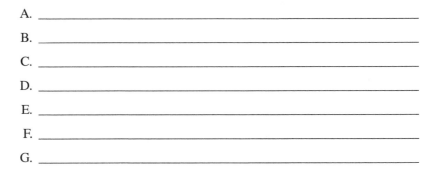

A. _____

B. _____

C. _____

D. _____

E. _____

F. _____

G. _____

239

Copyright © 2015, 2011, 2006, 1996 by Saunders, an imprint of Elsevier Inc. All rights reserved.

142. Complete the statements below referring to lateral scapula projection analysis guidelines.

Lateral Scapula Projection Analysis Guidelines
■ The superior scapular angle and (A) _____ arc on the same transverse plane.
■ The lateral and vertebral scapular borders are (B) _____.
■ The (C) _____ is at the center of the exposure field.

143. The lateral scapula is positioned with the patient placed in an AP or PA oblique projection. For the AP oblique projection, the patient is rotated (A) _____ (toward/away from) the affected scapula and for the PA oblique projection, the patient is rotated (B) _____ the affected scapula.

144. What patient positioning procedure determines the degree of obliquity needed to place the scapula in a lateral position?

_____

145. How is rotation identified on a lateral scapular projection with poor positioning?

_____

146. Most scapular fractures occur at the (A) _____ and (B) _____ of the scapula.

147. What humeral position with respect to the body places the long axis of the scapula parallel with the IR for a lateral scapular projection?

_____

_____

148. What humeral position with respect to the body places the lateral border of the scapula parallel with the IR for a lateral scapular projection?

_____

_____

149. The higher the humerus is elevated for a lateral scapular projection, the (A)_____ (more/less) the patient needs to be rotated to obtain accurate positioning. Why? (B) _____

150. What anatomic structures are included on a lateral scapular projection with accurate positioning?

_____

_____

Copyright © 2015, 2011, 2006, 1996 by Saunders, an imprint of Elsevier Inc. All rights reserved.

For the following descriptions of lateral scapular projections with poor positioning, state how the patient would have been mispositioned for such a projection to be obtained.

151. The lateral and vertebral borders of the scapula are demonstrated without superimposition, the thick border is next to the ribs, and the thin border is demonstrated laterally.

_____

152. The lateral and vertebral borders of the scapula are demonstrated without superimposition, the lateral border is demonstrated laterally, and the vertebral border appears next to the ribs.

_____

_____

For the following lateral scapular projections with poor positioning, state what anatomic structures are misaligned and how the patient should be repositioned for an optimal projection to be obtained.

Figure 5-37

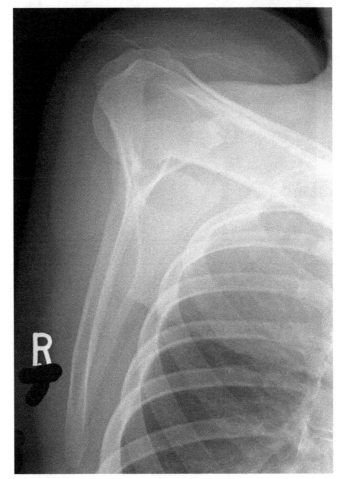

153. (Figure 5-37): lateral and vertebral borders are not superimposed. Fix by increase pt rotation to make more lateral.

Copyright © 2015, 2011, 2006, 1996 by Saunders, an imprint of Elsevier Inc. All rights reserved.

Chapter **5 Image Analysis of the Shoulder**

Figure 5-38

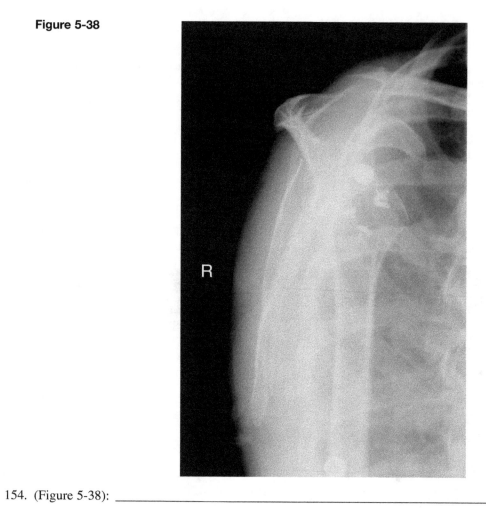

R

154. (Figure 5-38): _____

_____

_____

Copyright © 2015, 2011, 2006, 1996 by Saunders, an imprint of Elsevier Inc. All rights reserved.

6 | Image Analysis of the Lower Extremity

STUDY QUESTIONS

1. State the kV range for the following projections.

   A. Lateral ankle: _____

   B. Grid, AP Knee: _____

   C. AP femur: _____

2. Match the term with its definition.

   _____ A. Abductor tubercle   1. Partial dislocation

   _____ B. Dorsiflex   2. Sole of foot

   _____ C. Intermalleolar line   3. Located posteriorly on medial femoral condyle

   _____ D. Lateral mortise   4. Act of moving toes and forefoot downward

   _____ E. Plantar   5. Lateral side of knee joint is narrower

   _____ F. Plantarflexion   6. Opening between the calcaneus and talus

   _____ G. Subluxation   7. Line connecting medial and lateral malleoli

   _____ H. Tarsi sinus   8. Medial side of knee joint narrower

   _____ I. Valgus deformity   9. Act of moving toes and forefoot upward

   _____ J. Varus deformity   10. Tibiofibular joint

Copyright © 2015, 2011, 2006, 1996 by Saunders, an imprint of Elsevier Inc. All rights reserved.

Toe: AP Axial Projection

3. Identify the labeled anatomy in Figure 6-1.

Figure 6-1

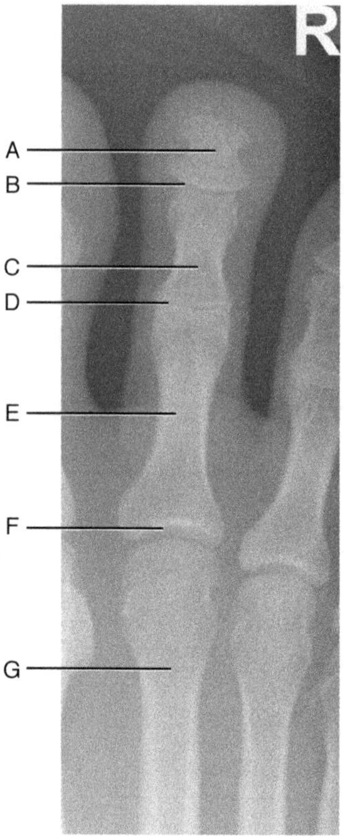

A. _____

B. _____

C. _____

D. _____

E. _____

F. _____

G. _____

4. Complete the statements below referring to AP axial toe projection analysis guidelines.

AP Axial Toe(s) Projection Analysis Guidelines
■ The (A) _soft tissue_ width and midshaft (B) _concavity_ are equal on both sides of phalanges.
■ The (C) _IP_ and (D) _MTP_ joints are open, and the phalanges are seen without fore-shortening.
■ The (E) _MTP_ joint is at the center of the exposure field for a toe projection and (F)_3rd_ MTP joint is at the center when all toes are imaged.

5. If the toe is medially rotated for a right AP axial toe projection, the (A) _lateral_ (medial/lateral) side of the toe demonstrates the greatest soft tissue width, and the (B) _lateral_ side demonstrates the greatest phalangeal midshaft concavity.

6. To obtain open joint spaces on an AP axial toe projection, align the CR (A) _____ to the joint space and align the joint space (B) _____ to the IR.

7. What anatomic structures are included on an AP axial toe projection with accurate positioning?

_____

 Copyright © 2015, 2011, 2006, 1996 by Saunders, an imprint of Elsevier Inc. All rights reserved.

For the following descriptions of AP axial toe projections with poor positioning, state how the patient would have been mispositioned for such a projection to be obtained.

8. The phalanges demonstrate more soft tissue width on the medial toe surface than the lateral surface.

   _____

9. The IP and MTP joint spaces are closed, and the phalanges are foreshortened.

   _____

For the following AP axial toe projections with poor positioning, state what anatomic structures are misaligned and how the patient should be repositioned for an optimal projection to be obtained.

Figure 6-2

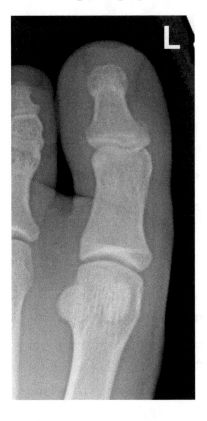

10. (Figure 6-2): _____

    _____

    _____

    _____

Copyright © 2015, 2011, 2006, 1996 by Saunders, an imprint of Elsevier Inc. All rights reserved. Chapter **6** **Image Analysis of the Lower Extremity**

Toe: AP Oblique Projection

11. Identify the labeled anatomy in Figure 6-3.

Figure 6-3

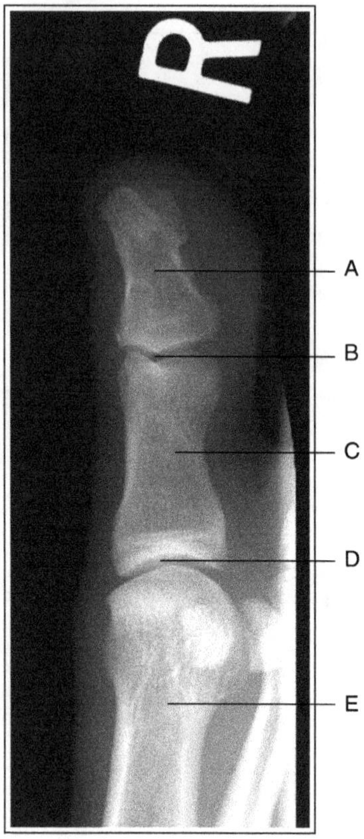

A. _____

B. _____

C. _____

D. _____

E. _____

12. Complete the statements below referring to AP oblique toe projection analysis guidelines.

AP Oblique Toe(s) Projection Analysis Guidelines
■ (A) _Twice_ as much soft tissue width and more phalangeal and metatarsal concavity are present on the side of the digit rotated (B) _away_ the IR.
■ The (C) _IP_ and (D) _MTP_ joint(s) are open, and the phalanges are demonstrated without foreshortening.
■ (E) _MTP_ joint is at the center of the exposure field for a toe projection and third MTP joint is at the center when all toes are imaged.

13. What degree of patient toe obliquity is used for an AP oblique toe projection?

A. _____

How is the accuracy of the degree of toe obliquity identified on an AP oblique toe projection?

B. _____

 Copyright © 2015, 2011, 2006, 1996 by Saunders, an imprint of Elsevier Inc. All rights reserved.

14. In what direction are the foot and toe rotated for a first through third AP oblique toe projection?

    A. _____

    For a fourth through fifth AP oblique toe projection?

    B. _____

    Why are the patient's foot and toe rotated differently for these examinations?

    C. _____

15. The patient was unable to fully extend the toe for an AP oblique toe projection. What will the resulting projection demonstrate if a perpendicular CR was used for this patient?

    _____

16. What anatomic structures are included on an AP oblique toe projection with accurate positioning?

    _____

17. To ensure that half of the affected toe's metatarsal is included on an AP oblique toe projection, the longitudinally collimated field should extend 2 inches (5 cm) proximal to the _____.

For the following descriptions of AP oblique toe projections with poor positioning, state how the patient would have been mispositioned for such a projection to be obtained.

18. The soft tissue width demonstrated on each side of the phalanges is nearly equal.

    _____

19. The proximal phalanx demonstrates more concavity on the posterior aspect than on the anterior aspect.

    _____

20. The IP and MTP joint spaces are obscured and the phalanges foreshortened.

    _____

Copyright © 2015, 2011, 2006, 1996 by Saunders, an imprint of Elsevier Inc. All rights reserved.

For the following AP oblique toe projections with poor positioning, state what anatomic structures are misaligned and how the patient should be repositioned for such a projection to be obtained.

Figure 6-4

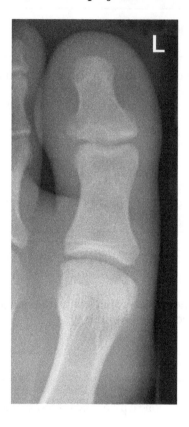

21. (Figure 6-4): _____

_____

_____

_____

   Copyright © 2015, 2011, 2006, 1996 by Saunders, an imprint of Elsevier Inc. All rights reserved.

Figure 6-5

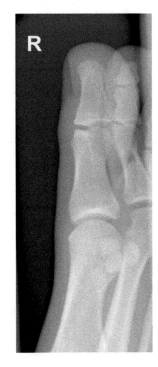

22. (Figure 6-5): _____

_____

_____

_____

Figure 6-6

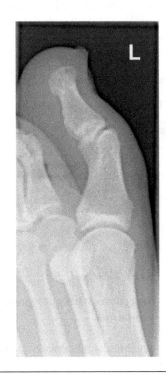

23. (Figure 6-6): _____

_____

_____

_____

Copyright © 2015, 2011, 2006, 1996 by Saunders, an imprint of Elsevier Inc. All rights reserved.   Chapter **6**   **Image Analysis of the Lower Extremity**

Toe: Lateral Projection

24. Identify the labeled anatomy in Figure 6-7.

Figure 6-7

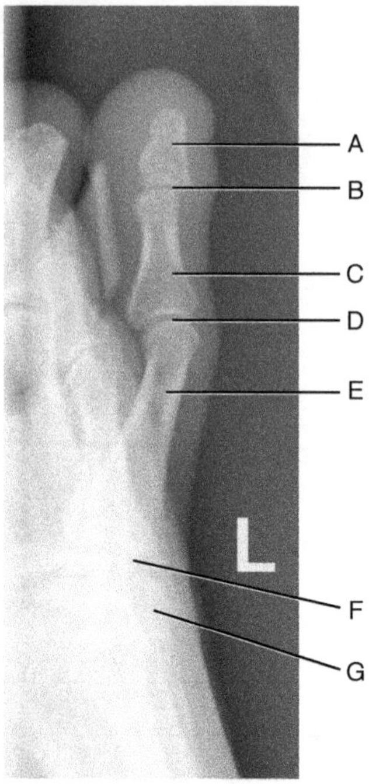

A. _____

B. _____

C. _____

D. _____

E. _____

F. _____

G. _____

25. Complete the statements below referring to lateral toe projection analysis guidelines.

Lateral Toe Projection Analysis Guidelines
■ (A) ___posterior___ surface of the proximal phalanx demonstrates more concavity than the (B) ___anterior___ surface, and the condyles of the proximal phalanx are superimposed.
■ The (C) ___PIP___ joint is at the center of the exposure field.

26. To position the toe in a lateral projection, the foot is rotated (A) _____ (medially/laterally) when the first, second, and third toes are imaged and (B) _____ (medially/laterally) when the fourth and fifth toes are imaged.

27. What anatomic structures are included on a lateral toe projection with accurate positioning?

_____

For the following descriptions of lateral toe projections with poor positioning, state how the patient would have been mispositioned for such a projection to be obtained.

28. The proximal phalanx demonstrates nearly equal midshaft concavity, the condyles of the proximal phalanx and the MT heads are demonstrated without superimposition.

_____

 Copyright © 2015, 2011, 2006, 1996 by Saunders, an imprint of Elsevier Inc. All rights reserved.

29. The proximal phalanx demonstrates nearly equal midshaft concavity, the condyles of the proximal phalanx are shown without superimposition, and the MT heads are superimposed.

30. Soft tissue and bony overlap of unaffected digits onto the affected digit is present.

unaffected digits were not pulled away

For the following lateral toe projections with poor positioning, state what anatomic structures are misaligned and how the patient should be repositioned for an optimal projection to be obtained.

Figure 6-8

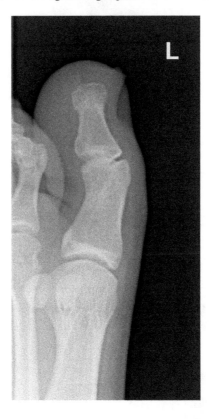

31. (Figure 6-8): _____

_____

_____

_____

Copyright © 2015, 2011, 2006, 1996 by Saunders, an imprint of Elsevier Inc. All rights reserved.

Figure 6-9

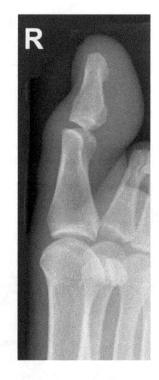

32. (Figure 6-9): _____

_____

_____

_____

Foot: AP Axial Projection (Dorsoplantar Projection)

33. Identify the labeled anatomy in Figure 6-10.

Figure 6-10

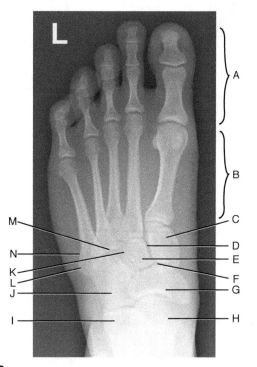

A. _____

B. _____

C. _____

D. _____

E. _____

F. _____

G. _____

H. _____

I. _____

J. _____

K. _____

L. _____

M. _____

N. _____

Copyright © 2015, 2011, 2006, 1996 by Saunders, an imprint of Elsevier Inc. All rights reserved.

34. Complete the statements below referring to AP axial foot projection analysis guidelines.

AP Axial Foot Projection Analysis Guidelines
■ Joint space between the (A) __1st__ and (B) __2nd__ cuneiforms is open, and about (C) __1/3__ of the talus is superimposing the calcaneus.
■ (D) __TMT__ and navicular–cuneiform joint spaces are open.
■ (E) __base of 3rd__ metatarsal base is at the center of the exposure field.

35. For an AP axial foot projection, equal pressure is placed on the (A) _____ foot surface and the (B) _____, (C) _____, and (D) _____ should remain aligned.

36. Will medial or lateral foot rotation result in the talus moving away from the calcaneus?

_____

37. Will medial or lateral foot rotation result in increased superimposition of the MT bases?

_____

38. A (A) _____ degree proximal CR angulation is required for an AP axial foot projection to demonstrate open TMT joint spaces. Is a higher degree of CR angulation needed in a patient with a low medial longitudinal arch or a high medial longitudinal arch? (B) _____

39. What anatomic structures are included on an AP axial foot projection with accurate positioning?

_____

For the following descriptions of AP axial foot projections with poor positioning, state how the patient or CR would have been mispositioned for such a projection to be obtained.

40. The joint space between the medial and intermediate cuneiforms is closed, the navicular is demonstrated in profile, and more than one-third of the talus superimposes the calcaneus.

_____

41. The joint space between the medial and intermediate cuneiforms is closed, the calcaneus is demonstrated without talar superimposition, and the MT bases demonstrate decreased superimposition.

_____

42. The TMT and navicular–cuneiform joint spaces are obscured.

_____

Copyright © 2015, 2011, 2006, 1996 by Saunders, an imprint of Elsevier Inc. All rights reserved.

For the following AP axial foot projections with poor positioning, state what anatomic structures are misaligned and how the patient should be repositioned for an optimal projection to be obtained.

Figure 6-11

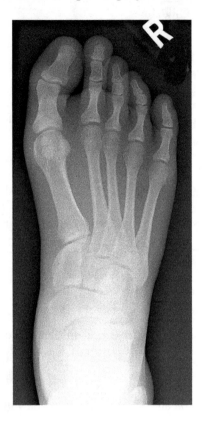

43. (Figure 6-11): _____

_____

_____

_____

 Copyright © 2015, 2011, 2006, 1996 by Saunders, an imprint of Elsevier Inc. All rights reserved.

Figure 6-12

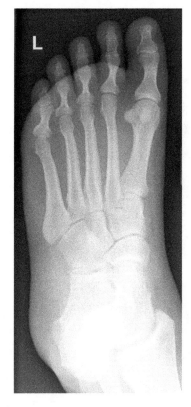

44. (Figure 6-12): _foot is obliqued, joint spaces closed between cuniforms, & calcaneus not superimposed by 1/3 of talus. Fix rotate foot laterally & place flat on IR._

Copyright © 2015, 2011, 2006, 1996 by Saunders, an imprint of Elsevier Inc. All rights reserved.

Chapter **6** **Image Analysis of the Lower Extremity**

Foot: AP Oblique Projection (Medial Rotation)

45. Identify the labeled anatomy in Figure 6-13.

Figure 6-13

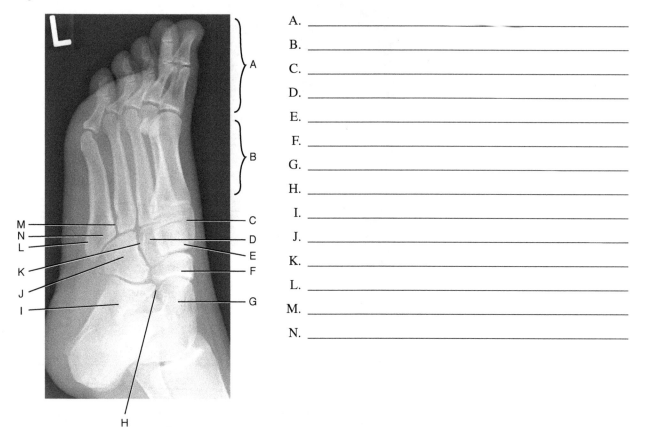

A. _____

B. _____

C. _____

D. _____

E. _____

F. _____

G. _____

H. _____

I. _____

J. _____

K. _____

L. _____

M. _____

N. _____

46. Complete the statements below referring to AP oblique foot projection analysis guidelines.

AP Oblique Foot Projection Analysis Guidelines
■ The (A) _cuboid-cuneiform_ and the (B) _2-5_ intermetatarsal joints spaces are open.
■ Tarsi sinus and (C) _5th_ metatarsal tuberosity are visualized.
■ (D) _3rd_ base is at the center of the exposure field.

47. An AP oblique foot projection is obtained by rotating the patient 30 to 60 degrees _____ (medially/laterally).

48. The degree of foot obliquity needed for an AP oblique foot projection varies according to the height of the medial longitudinal arch. What degree of obliquity is used in a patient with a high medial longitudinal arch?

A. _____

In a patient with a low medial longitudinal arch?

B. _____

On a patient with an average medial longitudinal arch?

C. _____

 Copyright © 2015, 2011, 2006, 1996 by Saunders, an imprint of Elsevier Inc. All rights reserved.

49. View the AP oblique foot projection in Figure 6-13. State whether the patient has a high or low medial longitudinal arch.

A. _____

How did you determine this?

B. _____

50. View the lateral foot projections in Figures 6-15 and 6-17. State which projection was obtained from the patient with the higher medial longitudinal arch.

A. _____

How did you determine this difference?

B. _____

51. As a foot is rotated medially from an AP projection, the first MT base rotates (A) _____ (over/beneath) the (B) _____ MT base and the second through third MT heads move (C) _____ (closer to/farther away from) one another.

52. Is the fourth MT tubercle or the fifth MT located more posteriorly when the foot is overrotated for an AP oblique foot projection?

A. _____

When the foot is medially rotated more than needed for an AP oblique foot projection with accurate positioning, will the fourth MT tubercle be superimposed over the fifth MT or will the fifth MT be superimposed over the fourth MT?

B. _____

_____

53. What anatomic structures are demonstrated within the collimated field on an AP oblique foot projection with accurate positioning?

_____

For the following descriptions of AP oblique foot projections with poor positioning, state how the patient would have been mispositioned for such a projection to be obtained.

54. The lateral cuneiform–cuboid, navicular–cuboid, and third through fifth intermetatarsal spaces are closed, and the fourth MT tubercle is demonstrated without fifth MT superimposition.

_____

55. The lateral cuneiform–cuboid, navicular–cuboid, and intermetatarsal joint spaces are closed, and the fifth MT is superimposed over the fourth MT tubercle.

_____

Copyright © 2015, 2011, 2006, 1996 by Saunders, an imprint of Elsevier Inc. All rights reserved.

For the following AP oblique foot projection with poor positioning, state what anatomic structures are misaligned and how the patient should be repositioned for an optimal projection to be obtained.

Figure 6-14

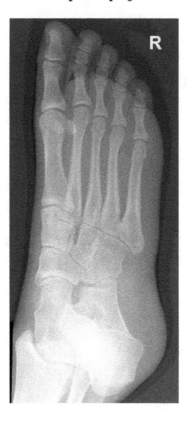

56. (Figure 6-14): _____

_____

_____

_____

Foot: Lateral Projection (Mediolateral and Lateromedial)

57. Identify the labeled anatomy in Figure 6-15.

Figure 6-15

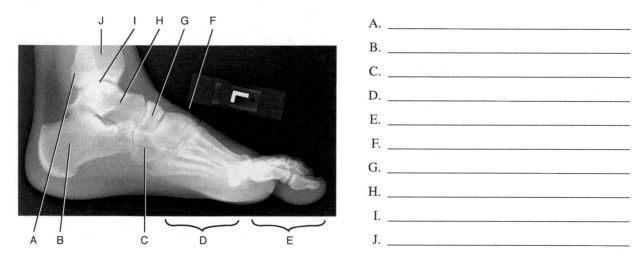

A. _____

B. _____

C. _____

D. _____

E. _____

F. _____

G. _____

H. _____

I. _____

J. _____

Copyright © 2015, 2011, 2006, 1996 by Saunders, an imprint of Elsevier Inc. All rights reserved.

58. Complete the statements below referring to lateral foot projection analysis guidelines.

> **Lateral Foot Projection Analysis Guidelines**
>
> - Contrast and density are adequate to demonstrate the (A) _____anterior_____ and (B) _____posterior_____ fat pads.
> - Talar domes are superimposed, the (C) _____tibiotalar_____ joint is open, and the distal fibula is superimposed by the posterior half of the distal tibia.
> - The long axis of the foot is positioned at a (D) _____90°_____ angle with the lower leg.
> - (E)_____distal tarsals_____ are at the center of the exposure field.

59. Which surface of the foot is positioned against the IR for a mediolateral projection of the foot? _____lateral_____

60. List the two soft tissue fat pads that should be demonstrated on a lateral foot projection, and describe their locations.

    A. _____

    B. _____

61. How is the lower leg placed to obtain a lateral foot projection with accurate positioning?

    _____

62. How is the foot positioned with the lower leg and IR to obtain a lateral foot projection with accurate positioning?

    A. Lower leg: _____

    B. IR: _____

63. A lateral foot projection was requested for a patient with a large upper thigh that prevented the lower leg from aligning parallel with the imaging table when the patient was positioned. If the projection was obtained with the patient positioned in this manner, how would this poor positioning be identified on the resulting projection?

    A. _____

    How is the positioning setup adjusted in this situation before the projection is obtained?

    B. _____

64. The height of the medial longitudinal arch can be determined on a lateral foot projection with accurate positioning by measuring the amount of cuboid that appears (A) _____ to the (B) _____.

65. The average foot projection demonstrates approximately _____ inch of the cuboid posterior to the navicular.

66. In a patient with a low medial foot arch, (A) _____ (more/less) of the cuboid will be demonstrated posterior to the navicular, and in a patient with a high medial foot arch, (B) _____ (more/less) will be demonstrated.

67. The actual height of the medial foot arch on a lateral foot projection is accurate only when the _____ are superimposed.

68. Misalignment of the talar domes can be caused by poor (A) _____ or (B) _____ positioning.

Copyright © 2015, 2011, 2006, 1996 by Saunders, an imprint of Elsevier Inc. All rights reserved.

69. If the distal tibia is positioned farther from the imaging table than the proximal tibia for a lateral foot projection, the

   (A) _____ (lateral/medial) dome is demonstrated (B) _____ to the (C) _____ (lateral/medial) talar dome and the medial foot arch appears (D) _____ (higher/lower) on the resulting projection.

70. If the proximal tibia is positioned farther from the imaging table than the distal tibia for a lateral foot projection, the

   (A) _lateral_ dome is demonstrated (B) _superior_ to the (C) _medial_ talar dome, and the medial foot arch appears (D) _lower_ (higher/lower) on the resulting projection.

71. If a lateral foot projection with poor positioning demonstrates an obscured tibiotalar joint space, one talar dome proximal to the other, and the navicular superimposed over most of the cuboid, which dome is proximal? _lateral_

72. If the calcaneus is positioned too close to the IR and the forefoot is raised off the IR for a lateral foot projection, the

   (A) _____ talar dome is demonstrated (B) _____ to the (C) _____ talar dome, and the fibula is demonstrated too far (D) _____ on the tibia.

73. If the forefoot is positioned too close to the IR and the calcaneus is elevated off the IR for a lateral foot projection,

   the (A) _medial_ talar dome is demonstrated (B) _anterior_ to the (C) _lateral_ talar dome, and the fibula is demonstrated too far (D) _posterior_ on the tibia.

74. Why is it important to dorsiflex the foot to a 90-degree angle with the lower leg?

   A. _____

   B. _____

   C. _____

75. Against what aspect of the foot is the IR placed for a standing lateromedial projection of the foot?

   A. _____

   What surface (medial/lateral) of the foot is aligned parallel with the IR for a lateromedial projection of the foot with accurate positioning?

   B. _____

76. If a standing lateromedial projection of the foot with poor positioning demonstrates one talar dome posterior to the other talar dome and the fibula is situated too far posterior on the tibia, how should the patient's position be adjusted for an optimal projection to be obtained?

   _____

77. Accurate CR centering on a lateral foot projection is accomplished by centering a (A) _____ CR to the foot midline at the level of the (B) _____.

78. What anatomic structures are included on a lateral foot projection with accurate positioning?

   _____

Copyright © 2015, 2011, 2006, 1996 by Saunders, an imprint of Elsevier Inc. All rights reserved.

For the following descriptions of mediolateral foot projections with poor positioning, state how the patient would have been mispositioned for such a projection to be obtained.

79. The tibiotalar joint space is obscured, one talar dome is demonstrated proximal to the other dome, and the navicular is superimposed over most of the cuboid.

_____

80. The tibiotalar joint space is obscured, one talar dome is demonstrated proximal to the other dome, and more than ½ inch (1.25 cm) of the cuboid appears posterior to the navicular.

_____

81. The tibiotalar joint is obscured, one talar dome is demonstrated anterior to the other dome, and the fibula is demonstrated too posterior on the tibia.

_____

82. The tibiotalar joint is obscured, one talar dome is demonstrated anterior to the other dome, and the fibula is demonstrated too anterior on the tibia.

_____

For the following lateral foot projections with poor positioning, state what anatomic structures are misaligned and how the patient should be repositioned for an optimal projection to be obtained.

Figure 6-16

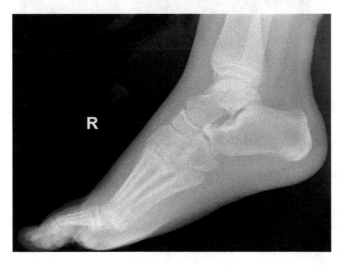

83. (Figure 6-16): _____

_____

_____

_____

Copyright © 2015, 2011, 2006, 1996 by Saunders, an imprint of Elsevier Inc. All rights reserved.   Chapter **6** **Image Analysis of the Lower Extremity**

Figure 6-17

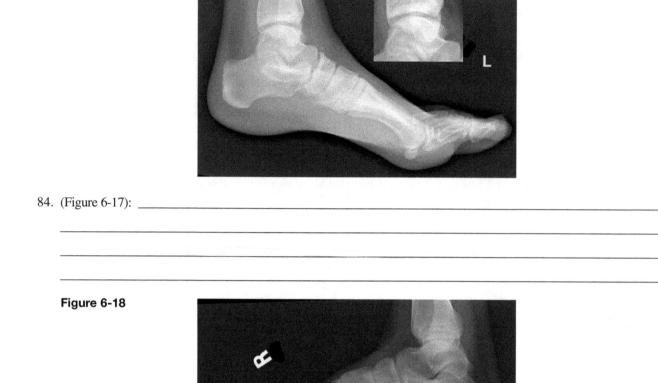

84. (Figure 6-17): _____

_____

_____

_____

Figure 6-18

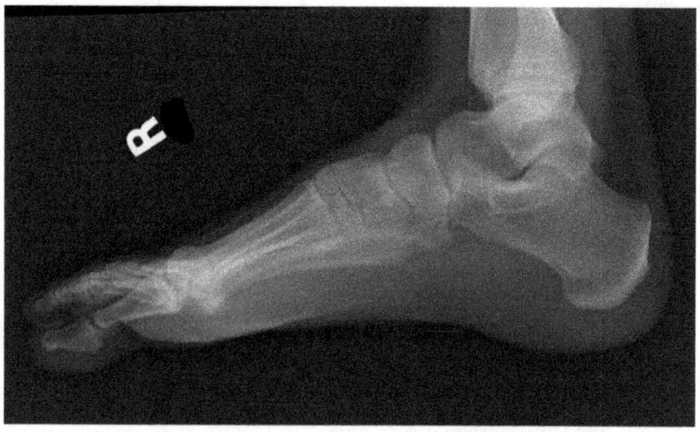

85. (Figure 6-18, lateromedial projection, average medial arch):

_____

_____

_____

Copyright © 2015, 2011, 2006, 1996 by Saunders, an imprint of Elsevier Inc. All rights reserved.

Figure 6-19

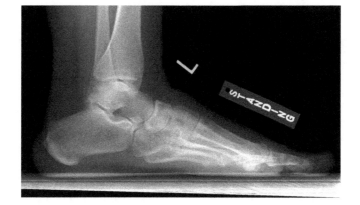

86. (Figure 6-19, lateromedial projection)

   <u>fib. too posterior ß medial dome anterior to</u>
   <u>lateral dome. Fix: internally rotate leg</u>

Calcaneus: Axial Projection (Plantodorsal)

87. Identify the labeled anatomy in Figure 6-20.

Figure 6-20

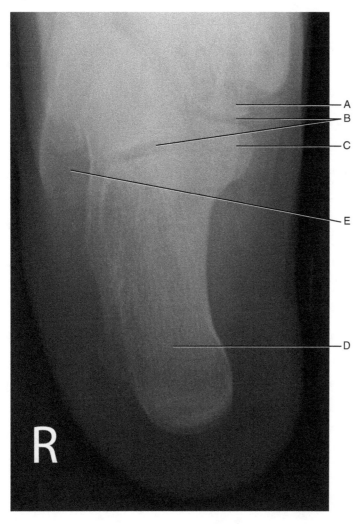

A. talus
B. talocal caneal joint
C. Sustentaculum tali
D. tuberosity
E. base of 5th MT

Copyright © 2015, 2011, 2006, 1996 by Saunders, an imprint of Elsevier Inc. All rights reserved.   Chapter **6**   **Image Analysis of the Lower Extremity**

88. Complete the statements below referring to axial calcaneus projection analysis guidelines.

Axial Calcaneus Projection Analysis Guidelines
■ The (A) _____ joint is open, and the calcaneal tuberosity is demonstrated without distortion.
■ The second through fourth distal MTs are not demonstrated on the (B) _____ or (C) _____ aspects of the foot, respectively.
■ The (D) _____ is at the center of the exposure field.

89. To obtain an axial calcaneal projection with accurate positioning, position the foot (A) _____ and direct a

(B) _____-degree proximal CR angulation toward the (C) _____ foot surface.

90. When the CR and foot are accurately aligned, the CR is aligned (A) _____ to the talocalcaneal joint

space and (B) _____ to the calcaneal tuberosity.

91. If an axial calcaneal projection is requested for a patient who is unable to dorsiflex the foot to a vertical position, how is the positioning setup adjusted before the projection is obtained?

A. _____

How is the setup changed if the patient dorsiflexed the foot beyond the vertical position?

B. _____

92. What anatomic structures can be used to estimate the CR angulation needed when the patient is unable to dorsiflex the foot into a vertical position?

_____

93. How is the patient positioned to prevent calcaneal tilting?

A. _____

How is calcaneal tilting identified on an axial calcaneal projection with poor positioning?

B. _____

94. Accurate CR centering on an axial calcaneal projection is accomplished by centering the CR to the midline of the

foot at the level of the _____.

95. What anatomic structures are included on an axial calcaneal projection with accurate positioning?

_____

For the following descriptions of axial calcaneal projections with poor positioning, state how the patient would have been mispositioned for such a projection to be obtained.

96. The talocalcaneal joint space is obscured, and the calcaneal tuberosity is foreshortened. The standard 40-degree angulation was used.

___foot not dorsiflexed_____

Copyright © 2015, 2011, 2006, 1996 by Saunders, an imprint of Elsevier Inc. All rights reserved.

97. The first MT is demonstrated medially.

_____

98. The fourth and fifth MTs are demonstrated laterally.

_____

For the following axial calcaneal projection with poor positioning, state what anatomic structures are misaligned and how the patient should be repositioned for an optimal projection to be obtained.

Figure 6-21

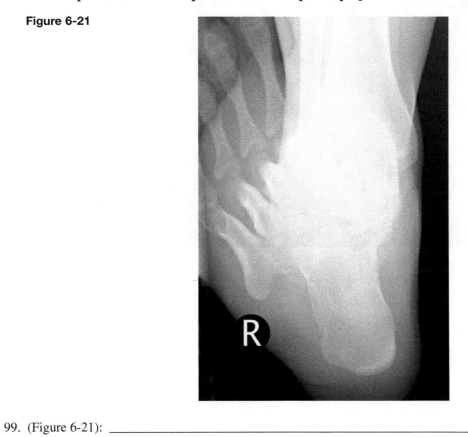

99. (Figure 6-21): _____

_____

_____

_____

Copyright © 2015, 2011, 2006, 1996 by Saunders, an imprint of Elsevier Inc. All rights reserved.   Chapter **6**   **Image Analysis of the Lower Extremity**

Figure 6-22

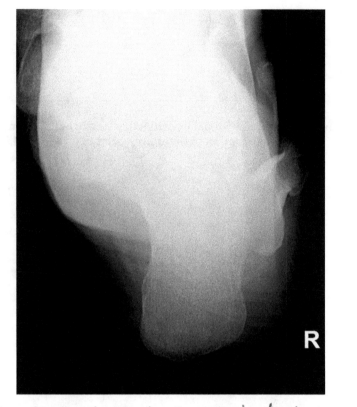

100. (Figure 6-22): _talocalcanial joint obscured $\bar{c}$ tuberosity foreshortened. Fix: dorsiflex foot or increase CR angle._

   Copyright © 2015, 2011, 2006, 1996 by Saunders, an imprint of Elsevier Inc. All rights reserved.

Figure 6-23

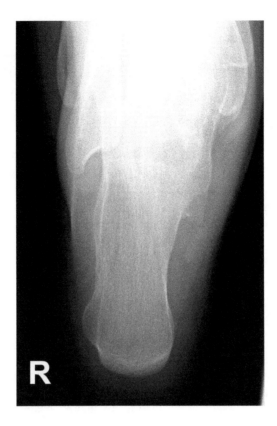

101. (Figure 6-23): _____

_____

_____

_____

Calcaneus: Lateral Projection (Mediolateral)

102. Identify the labeled anatomy in Figure 6-24.

Figure 6-24

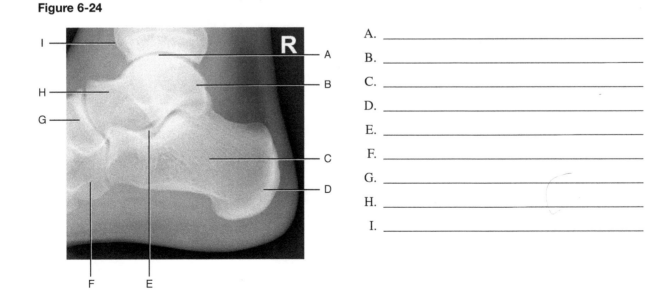

A. _____

B. _____

C. _____

D. _____

E. _____

F. _____

G. _____

H. _____

I. _____

Copyright © 2015, 2011, 2006, 1996 by Saunders, an imprint of Elsevier Inc. All rights reserved.

103. Complete the statements below referring to lateral calcaneus projection analysis guidelines.

Lateral Calcaneus Projection Analysis Guidelines

- The talar domes are superimposed, the tibiotalar joint space is open, and the distal fibula is superimposed by the (A) _____ half of the distal tibia.

- The long axis of the foot is positioned at a 90-degree angle with the (B) _____.

- The (C) _____ is at the center of the exposure field.

---

104. How is the lower leg positioned to obtain a lateral calcaneal projection with accurate positioning?

_____

105. How is the foot positioned with the lower leg and IR to obtain a lateral calcaneal projection with accurate positioning?

A. Lower leg: _____

B. IR: _____

106. A calcaneal foot projection was requested for a patient with a large upper thigh that prevented the lower leg from aligning parallel with the imaging table when the patient was positioned. If the projection was obtained with the patient positioned in this manner, how would this poor positioning be identified on the resulting projection?

_____

107. The height of the medial longitudinal arch is determined on a lateral calcaneal projection with accurate positioning by measuring the amount of cuboid that appears (A) _____ to the (B) _____.

108. The average calcaneal projection demonstrates approximately _____ inch of the cuboid posterior to the navicular.

109. If the distal tibia is positioned farther from the imaging table than the proximal tibia for a lateral calcaneal projection, the (A) _____ dome is demonstrated (B) _____ to the (C) _____ talar dome, and the medial longitudinal foot arch appears (D) _____ (higher/lower) on the resulting projection.

110. If the calcaneus is positioned too close to the IR and the forefoot is raised off the IR for a lateral calcaneal projection, the (A) _____ talar dome is demonstrated (B) _____ to the (C) _____ talar dome, and the fibula is demonstrated too far (D) _____ on the tibia.

111. Accurate CR centering on a lateral calcaneal projection is accomplished by centering a (A) _____ CR 1 inch (2.5 cm) (B) _____ to the (C) _____.

112. What anatomic structures are included on a lateral calcaneal projection with accurate positioning?

_____

Copyright © 2015, 2011, 2006, 1996 by Saunders, an imprint of Elsevier Inc. All rights reserved.

For the following descriptions of lateral calcaneal projections with poor positioning, state how the patient would have been mispositioned for such a projection to be obtained.

113. The tibiotalar joint space is obscured, one talar dome is demonstrated proximal to the other, and the navicular bone is superimposed over most of the cuboid.

_____

114. The tibiotalar joint is obscured, one talar dome is demonstrated anterior to the other dome, and the fibula is demonstrated too posterior on the tibia.

_____

For the following axial calcaneal projections with poor positioning, state what anatomic structures are misaligned and how the patient should be repositioned for an optimal projection to be obtained.

Figure 6-25

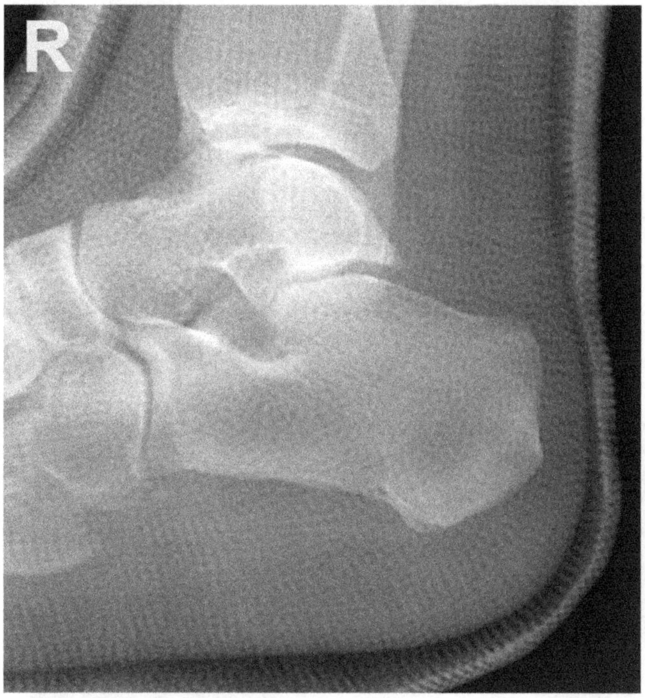

115. (Figure 6-25): _____

_____

_____

_____

Copyright © 2015, 2011, 2006, 1996 by Saunders, an imprint of Elsevier Inc. All rights reserved.

Figure 6-26

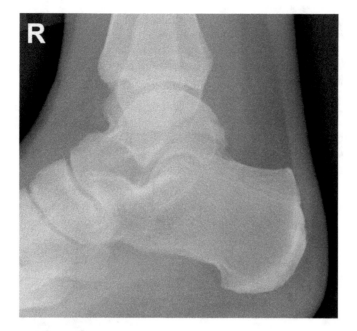

116. (Figure 6-26): _____

_____

_____

_____

Figure 6-27

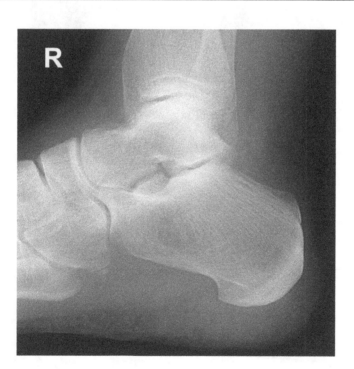

117. (Figure 6-27): _____

_____

_____

_____

Chapter **6** **Image Analysis of the Lower Extremity**   Copyright © 2015, 2011, 2006, 1996 by Saunders, an imprint of Elsevier Inc. All rights reserved.

Ankle: AP Projection

118. Identify the labeled anatomy in Figure 6-28.

Figure 6-28

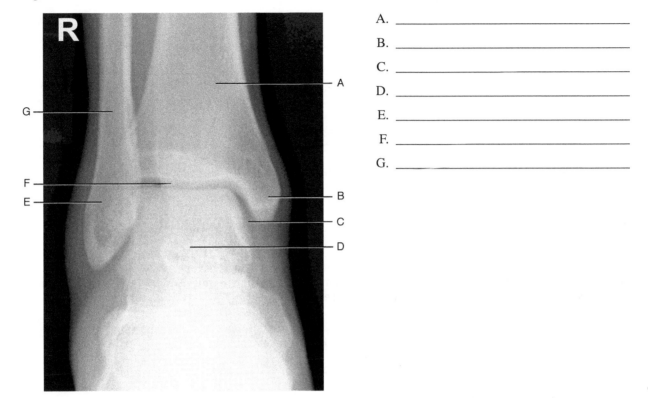

A. _____

B. _____

C. _____

D. _____

E. _____

F. _____

G. _____

119. Complete the statements below referring to AP ankle projection analysis guidelines.

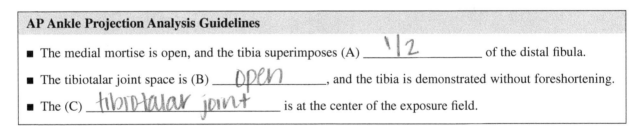

AP Ankle Projection Analysis Guidelines

- The medial mortise is open, and the tibia superimposes (A) _____1/2_____ of the distal fibula.
- The tibiotalar joint space is (B) ____open____, and the tibia is demonstrated without foreshortening.
- The (C) ____tibiotalar joint____ is at the center of the exposure field.

120. The ankle joint is located at the same level as what palpable anatomic structure?

_____

121. Is the distal fibula superimposed by the tibia or is the tibia superimposed by the distal fibula on an AP ankle projection?

_____

122. The intermalleolar line is at what angle with the IR when the patient is accurately positioned for an AP ankle projection?

_____15° – 20°_____

Copyright © 2015, 2011, 2006, 1996 by Saunders, an imprint of Elsevier Inc. All rights reserved.

Chapter **6**   **Image Analysis of the Lower Extremity**

123. The patient's leg was laterally rotated for an AP ankle projection. How can this mispositioning be identified on an AP ankle projection?

_____

_____

124. How is the patient positioned for an AP ankle projection to obtain an open ankle joint space?

_____

125. The CR was centered proximal to the ankle joint space for an AP ankle projection. How is this mispositioning identified on an AP ankle projection?

_____

126. Accurate CR centering on an AP ankle projection is accomplished by centering a(n) (A) _____ CR to

the ankle midline at the level of the (B) _____.

127. What anatomic structures are included on an AP ankle projection with accurate positioning?

_____

For the following descriptions of AP ankle projections with poor positioning, state how the patient would have been mispositioned for such a projection to be obtained.

128. The medial mortise is obscured, the tibia and talus demonstrate increased superimposition of the fibula, and the posterior aspect of the medial malleolus is situated medial to the anterior aspect.

_____

129. The tibiotalar joint is closed, and the anterior tibial margin has been projected into the joint space.

_____

 Copyright © 2015, 2011, 2006, 1996 by Saunders, an imprint of Elsevier Inc. All rights reserved.

For the following AP ankle projection with poor positioning, state what anatomic structures are misaligned and how the patient should be repositioned for an optimal projection to be obtained.

Figure 6-29

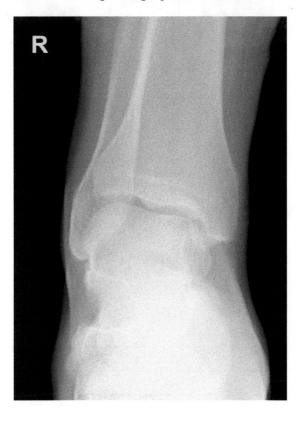

130. (Figure 6-29): _____

_____

_____

_____

Copyright © 2015, 2011, 2006, 1996 by Saunders, an imprint of Elsevier Inc. All rights reserved.

Figure 6-30

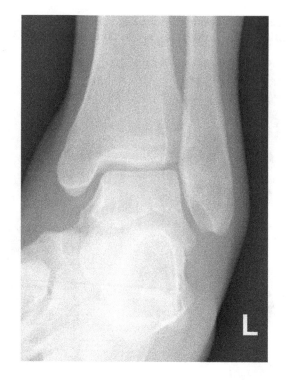

131. (Figure 6-30): _____

_____

_____

_____

Ankle: AP Oblique Projection (Medial Rotation)

132. Identify the labeled anatomy in Figure 6-31.

Figure 6-31

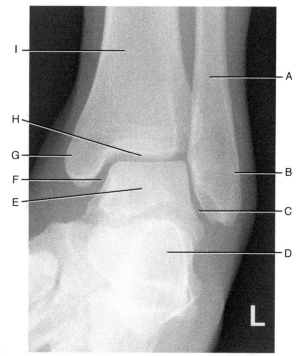

A. fibula

B. lateral malleolus

C. lateral mortise

D. calcaneus

E. talus

F. medial mortise

G. medial malleolus

H. tibiotalar joint

I. tibia

274

Copyright © 2015, 2011, 2006, 1996 by Saunders, an imprint of Elsevier Inc. All rights reserved.

133. Complete the statements below referring to AP oblique ankle projection analysis guidelines.

> **AP Oblique Ankle Projection Analysis Guidelines**
>
> - Mortise (15–20 degree) oblique: Distal fibula is demonstrated without (A) __talar__ superimposition, demonstrating an open (B) __lateral__ mortise, and the lateral and medial malleoli are in profile. The tibia superimposes one-fourth of the (C) __distal fibula__.
> - 45-degree oblique: The fibula is seen without (D) __tibial__ superimposition, and the tarsi sinus is demonstrated.
> - The calcaneus is visualized (E) __distal__ to the lateral mortise and fibula.
> - The (F) __tibiotalar joint__ is at the center of the exposure field.

134. Approximately how much ankle obliquity is needed for a mortise AP oblique ankle projection with accurate positioning?

A. __15-20°__

In which direction is the patient's leg rotated?

B. __medially__

135. How is the patient positioned to obtain an open tibiotalar joint space on an AP oblique ankle projection with accurate positioning?

__leg parallel to IR__

136. How is the patient positioned to demonstrate the calcaneus distal to the lateral mortise and fibula on an AP oblique ankle projection?

_____

137. Accurate CR centering on an AP oblique ankle projection is accomplished by centering a (A) _____ CR to the ankle midline at the level of the (B) _____.

138. What anatomic structures are included on an AP ankle projection with accurate positioning?

_____

For the following descriptions of AP oblique ankle projections with poor positioning, state how the patient would have been mispositioned for such a projection to be obtained.

139. Mortise oblique: The lateral and medial mortises are closed, and the tarsal sinus is demonstrated.

_____

140. 45-degree oblique: The lateral and medial mortises are closed, the fibula is demonstrated without tibial superimposition, and the tarsal sinus is demonstrated.

_____

141. Mortise oblique: The tibiotalar joint space is expanded, the anterior tibial margin is projected superior to the posterior margin, and the tibial articulating surface is demonstrated.

_____

142. 45-degree oblique: The calcaneus is obscuring the distal aspect of the lateral mortise and the distal fibula.

_____

Copyright © 2015, 2011, 2006, 1996 by Saunders, an imprint of Elsevier Inc. All rights reserved.

For the following AP oblique ankle projections with poor positioning, state what anatomic structures are misaligned and how the patient should be repositioned for an optimal projection to be obtained.

Figure 6-32

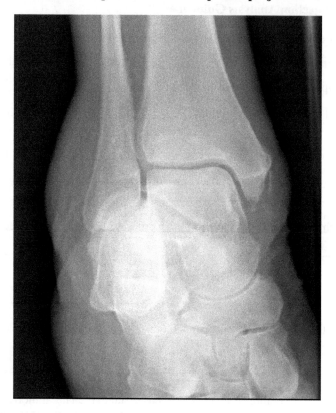

143. (Figure 6-32, mortise oblique): _____

_____

_____

_____

   Copyright © 2015, 2011, 2006, 1996 by Saunders, an imprint of Elsevier Inc. All rights reserved.

Figure 6-33

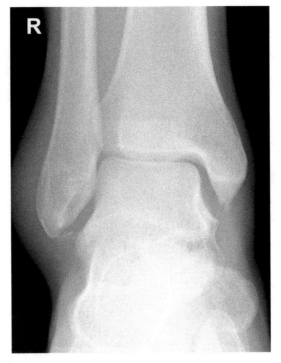

144. (Figure 6-33, mortise oblique): _____

_____

_____

_____

Figure 6-34

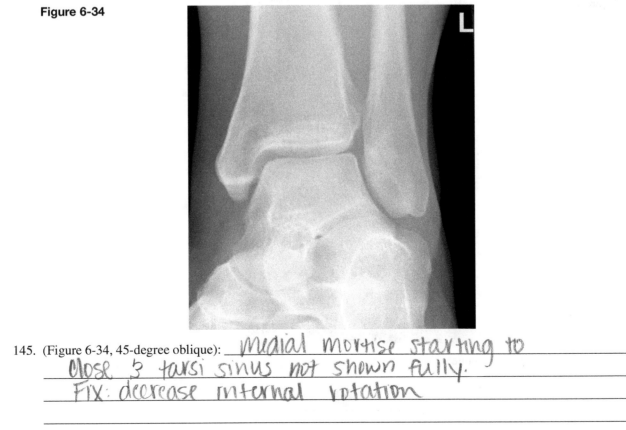

145. (Figure 6-34, 45-degree oblique): _Medial mortise starting to_
close 3 tarsi sinus not shown fully.
Fix: decrease internal rotation

_____

277

Copyright © 2015, 2011, 2006, 1996 by Saunders, an imprint of Elsevier Inc. All rights reserved.

Figure 6-35

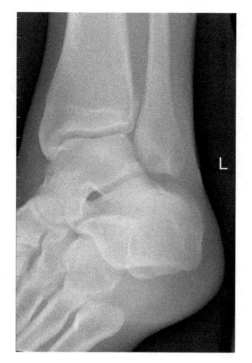

146. (Figure 6-35, 45-degree oblique): _____

_____

_____

_____

Figure 6-36

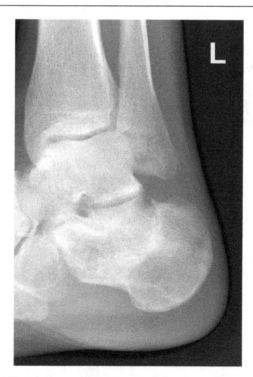

147. (Figure 6-36, 45-degree oblique): _____

_____

_____

_____

  Copyright © 2015, 2011, 2006, 1996 by Saunders, an imprint of Elsevier Inc. All rights reserved.

Figure 6-37

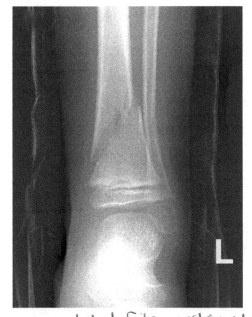

148. (Figure 6-37, trauma, 45-degree oblique): ___tib/fib articulation not___ ___open, can't seen tarsal sinus, & calcaneus___ ___not distal to lateral mortise. Fix. angle___ ___CR medially.___

Ankle: Lateral Projection (Mediolateral)

149. Identify the labeled anatomy in Figure 6-38.

Figure 6-38

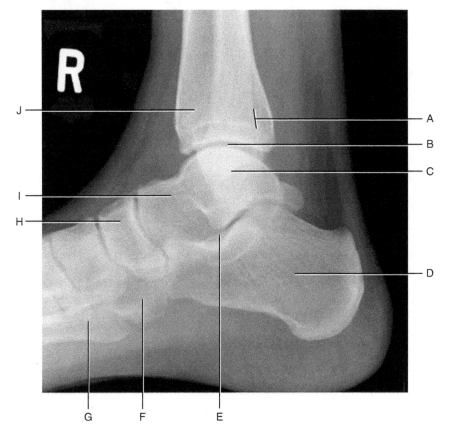

A. _____

B. _____

C. _____

D. _____

E. _____

F. _____

G. _____

H. _____

I. _____

J. _____

Copyright © 2015, 2011, 2006, 1996 by Saunders, an imprint of Elsevier Inc. All rights reserved.

150. Complete the statements below referring to lateral ankle projection analysis guidelines.

> **Lateral Ankle Projection Analysis Guidelines**
>
> - The talar domes are superimposed, the tibiotalar joint is (A) _open_, and the distal fibula is superimposed by the posterior half of the (B) _tibia_.
> - The long axis of the foot is positioned at a 90-degree angle with the (C) _lower leg_.
> - The (D) _tibiotalar joint_ is at the center of the exposure field.

151. To obtain a lateral ankle projection with accurate positioning, the patient's leg is extended, the lower leg is positioned (A) _____ to the imaging table, and the foot is dorsiflexed with its (B) _____ surface aligned parallel to the IR.

152. Accurate lower leg positioning for a lateral ankle projection ensures accurate _____ alignment of the talar domes.

153. If the proximal lower leg is positioned farther from the imaging table than the distal tibia for a lateral ankle projection, the (A) _____ dome is demonstrated (B) _____ to the (C) _____ talar dome, and the longitudinal foot arch appears (D) _____ on the resulting projection.

154. Accurate lateral foot surface positioning for a lateral ankle projection ensures proper (A) _____ and (B) _____ alignment of the talar domes.

155. If the forefoot is positioned too close to the IR and the calcaneus is raised off the IR for a lateral ankle projection, the (A) _____ talar domes are demonstrated (B) _____ to the (C) _____ talar dome, and the fibula is demonstrated too far (D) _____ on the tibia.

156. Accurate CR centering on a lateral ankle projection is accomplished by centering a(n) (A) _____ CR to the (B) _____.

157. What anatomic structures are included on a lateral ankle projection with accurate positioning?

_____

158. What is a Jones fracture?

_____

159. Why should the transversely collimated field remain open to include 1 inch (2.5 cm) of the fifth MT base?

_____

For the following descriptions of lateral ankle projections with poor positioning, state how the patient would have been mispositioned for such a projection to be obtained.

160. Average longitudinal arch: The tibiotalar joint space is obscured, one talar dome is demonstrated proximal to the other dome, and more than ½ inch (1.25 cm) of the cuboid appears posterior to the navicular.

distal lower leg was elevated

161. The tibiotalar joint is obscured, one talar dome is demonstrated anterior to the other dome, and the fibula is demonstrated too anterior on the tibia.

_____

Copyright © 2015, 2011, 2006, 1996 by Saunders, an imprint of Elsevier Inc. All rights reserved.

For the following lateral ankle projections with poor positioning, state what anatomic structures are misaligned and how the patient should be repositioned for an optimal projection to be obtained.

Figure 6-39

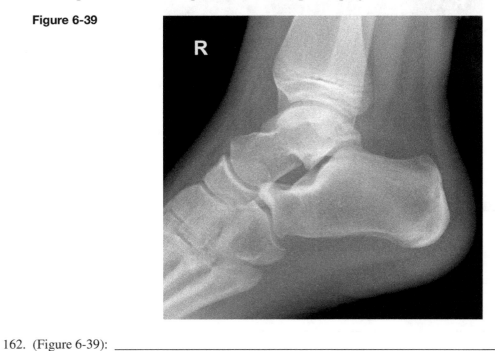

162. (Figure 6-39): _____

_____

_____

_____

Figure 6-40

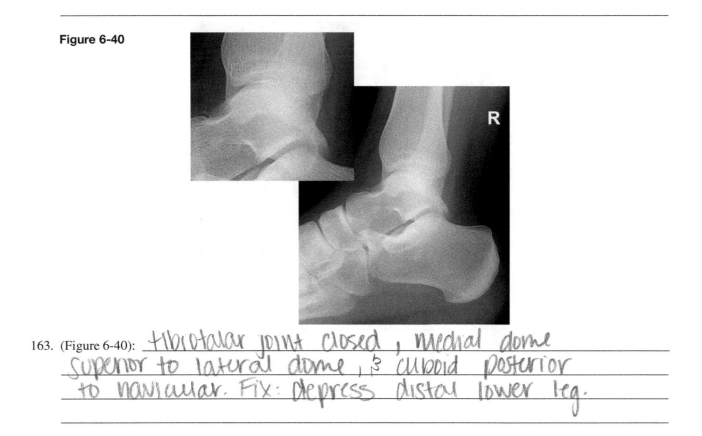

163. (Figure 6-40): tibiotalar joint closed, medial dome superior to lateral dome, & cuboid posterior to navicular. Fix: depress distal lower leg.

281

Copyright © 2015, 2011, 2006, 1996 by Saunders, an imprint of Elsevier Inc. All rights reserved.

Figure 6-41

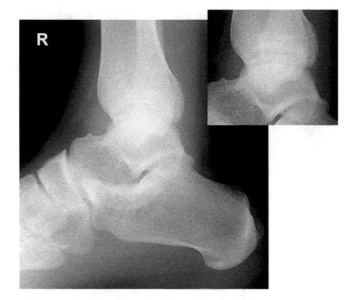

164. (Figure 6-41): _____

_____

_____

_____

Figure 6-42

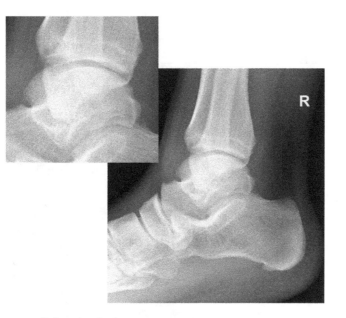

165. (Figure 6-42, trauma, lateromedial projection): _____

_____

_____

_____

    Copyright © 2015, 2011, 2006, 1996 by Saunders, an imprint of Elsevier Inc. All rights reserved.

Figure 6-43

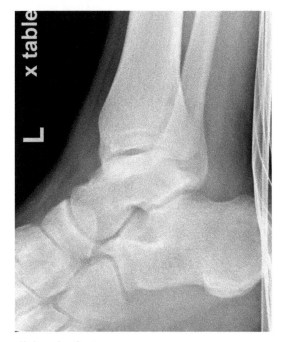

166. (Figure 6-43, trauma, lateromedial projection): _____

_____

_____

_____

Figure 6-44

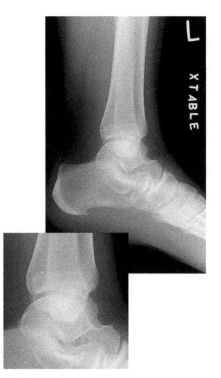

167. (Figure 6-44, trauma, lateromedial projection): _____

_____

_____

_____

Copyright © 2015, 2011, 2006, 1996 by Saunders, an imprint of Elsevier Inc. All rights reserved.   Chapter **6**   **Image Analysis of the Lower Extremity**

Figure 6-45

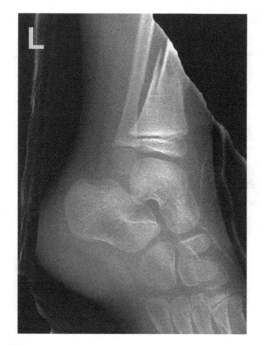

168. (Figure 6-45, trauma, lateromedial projection): _____

_____

_____

_____

Lower Leg: AP Projection

169. Identify the labeled anatomy in Figure 6-46.

Figure 6-46

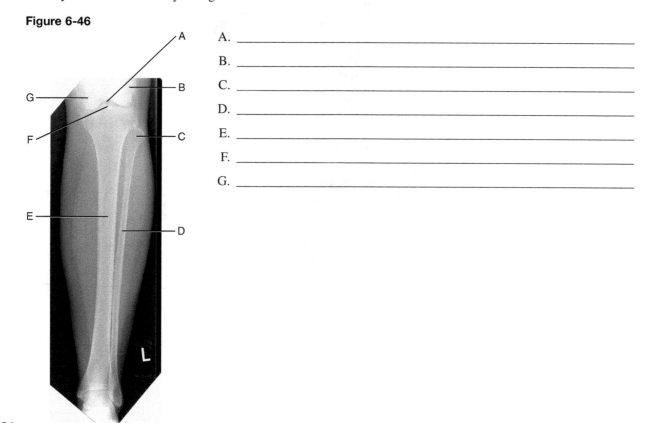

A. _____

B. _____

C. _____

D. _____

E. _____

F. _____

G. _____

   Copyright © 2015, 2011, 2006, 1996 by Saunders, an imprint of Elsevier Inc. All rights reserved.

170. Complete the statements below referring to AP lower leg projection analysis guidelines.

AP Lower Leg Projection Analysis Guidelines
▪ The tibia superimposes (A) _____1/4_____ of the fibular head and (B) _____1/2_____ of the distal tibia.
▪ The fibular midshaft is (C) _____free_____ of tibial superimposition.
▪ The knee and tibiotalar joint spaces are (D) _____Closed_____.
▪ The (E) _____tibial midshaft_____ is at the center of the exposure field.

171. How should the lower leg be positioned with respect to the x-ray tube to take advantage of the anode-heel effect?

_____

172. Describe how the tibia and fibula on an AP lower leg projection are misaligned at the knee and ankle if the leg is internally rotated.

A. Knee: _____

B. Ankle: _____

173. A patient from the emergency department is unable to position the ankle and knee in an AP projection simultaneously for an AP lower leg projection. If the area of interest is closer to the knee joint, how should the leg be positioned for the projection?

_____

174. Are the femorotibial and tibiotalar joint spaces closed on an AP lower leg projection with accurate positioning?

A. _____ (Yes/No)

B. Explain how the divergence of the x-ray beam used to record these two joints affects their openness.

175. Why is it necessary for the IR to extend at least 1 inch (2.5 cm) beyond the ankle and knee joints when the lower leg is positioned in an AP projection?

_____

176. The ankle joint is located at the level of the (A) _____, and the knee joint is located 1 inch (2.5 cm)

(B) _____ to the (C) _____.

177. The _____ is centered to the collimated field on an AP lower leg projection with accurate positioning.

178. What anatomic structures are included on an AP lower leg projection with accurate positioning?

_____

For the following descriptions of AP lower leg projections with poor positioning, state how the patient would have been mispositioned for such a projection to be obtained.

179. The medial mortise is closed, and the tibia and talus demonstrate excessive fibular superimposition.

_____

180. The distal fibula is free of talar superimposition, and the proximal fibula is free of tibial superimposition.

_____

Copyright © 2015, 2011, 2006, 1996 by Saunders, an imprint of Elsevier Inc. All rights reserved.

For the following AP lower leg projection with poor positioning, state what anatomic structures are misaligned and how the patient should be repositioned for an optimal projection to be obtained.

Figure 6-47

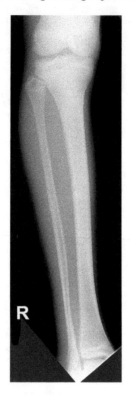

181. (Figure 6-47): _____

_____

_____

_____

Chapter **6** **Image Analysis of the Lower Extremity**   Copyright © 2015, 2011, 2006, 1996 by Saunders, an imprint of Elsevier Inc. All rights reserved.

Lower Leg: Lateral Projection (Mediolateral)

182. Identify the labeled anatomy in Figure 6-48.

Figure 6-48

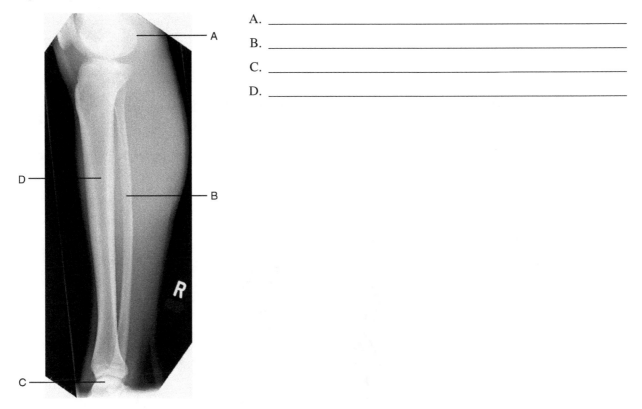

A. _____

B. _____

C. _____

D. _____

183. Complete the statements below referring to lateral lower leg projection analysis guidelines.

Lateral Lower Leg Projection Analysis Guidelines
■ The tibia superimposes (A) _____1∕2_____ of the fibular head, and the (B) _posterior_ aspects of the distal tibia and fibula are aligned.
■ The fibular (C) _midshaft_ is free of tibial superimposition.
■ The (D) _tibial midshaft_ is at the center of the exposure field.

184. Describe the anatomic relationship of the tibia and fibula at the knee, midshaft, and ankle on a lateral lower leg projection with accurate positioning.

A. Knee: _____

B. Midshaft: _____

C. Ankle: _____

185. How does the relationship between the tibia and fibula at the knee and ankle described in the previous question change if the patient's medial femoral epicondyle is rotated anterior to the lateral epicondyle for the projection?

A. Knee: _____

B. Ankle: _____

Copyright © 2015, 2011, 2006, 1996 by Saunders, an imprint of Elsevier Inc. All rights reserved.

Chapter **6** **Image Analysis of the Lower Extremity**

186. To ensure that the ankle and knee joints are included on a lateral lower leg projection, how far should the IR and longitudinally collimated field extend beyond the them?

_____

187. The _____ is centered to the collimated field on a lateral lower leg projection with accurate positioning.

188. What anatomic structures are included on a lateral lower leg projection with accurate positioning?

_____

For the following descriptions of lateral lower leg projections with poor positioning, state how the patient would have been mispositioned for such a projection to be obtained.

189. The distal fibula is situated too far anterior on the tibia, the medial talar dome is posterior to the lateral dome, and the fibular head and midshaft are superimposed by the tibia.

_____

For the following lateral lower leg projections with poor positioning, state what anatomic structures are misaligned and how the patient should be repositioned for an optimal projection to be obtained.

Figure 6-49

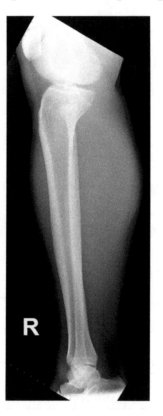

190. (Figure 6-49): _____

_____

_____

_____

     Copyright © 2015, 2011, 2006, 1996 by Saunders, an imprint of Elsevier Inc. All rights reserved.

Figure 6-50

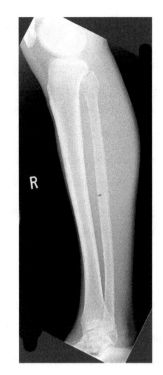

191. (Figure 6-50): _____

_____

_____

_____

Knee: AP Projection

192. Identify the labeled anatomy in Figure 6-51.

Figure 6-51

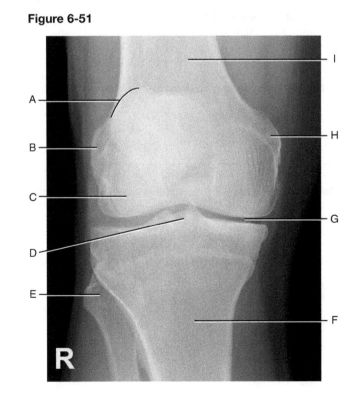

A. _____

B. _____

C. _____

D. _____

E. _____

F. _____

G. _____

H. _____

I. _____

289

Copyright © 2015, 2011, 2006, 1996 by Saunders, an imprint of Elsevier Inc. All rights reserved.

193. Complete the statements below referring to AP knee projection analysis guidelines.

AP Knee Projection Analysis Guidelines

- The medial and lateral femoral epicondyles are in (A) ___profile___, the femoral condyles are symmetrical, the intercondylar eminence is centered within the intercondylar fossa, and the tibia is superimposed over (B) ___1/2___ of the fibular head.

- The knee joint space is open, the anterior and posterior distal tibial margins are aligned, and the fibular head is demonstrated approximately ½ inch (1.25 cm) distal to the (C) ___tibial plateau___.

- The patella lies just (D) ___proximal___ to the patellar surface of the femur and is situated slightly (E) ___lateral___ to the knee midline.

- The (F) ___knee joint___ is at the center of the exposure field.

---

194. A grid is used for a knee projection if the patient's knee measures more than _____ cm.

195. An AP knee projection is obtained by placing the patient supine with the knee (A) _____ and leg (B) _____ rotated until the femoral epicondyles are placed at (C) _____ from the IR.

196. Is the proximal tibia superimposed over the proximal fibula or is the proximal fibula superimposed over the proximal tibia when the knee is in an AP projection?

_____

197. If the knee is rotated from an AP projection, will the femoral condyle positioned closer to or farther away from the IR appear larger on the resulting projection?

198. If the patient's leg is not internally rotated to accurately position the femoral epicondyles, how will the appearances of the femoral condyles and the alignment of the tibia and fibula change?

_____

199. How is the CR aligned with the femorotibial joint space and tibial plateau to demonstrate them as open spaces on an AP knee projection?

200. Describe the slope of the tibial plateau.

_____

201. Why is it necessary to vary the degree of CR angulation for AP knee projections in patients with different upper thigh and buttock thicknesses?

_____

202. Should the patient's abdominal thickness be included in the anterior superior iliac spine (ASIS)-to-imaging table measurement obtained for a patient undergoing AP knee imaging? _____ (Yes/No)

Copyright © 2015, 2011, 2006, 1996 by Saunders, an imprint of Elsevier Inc. All rights reserved.

203. What CR angulation is used when obtaining an AP knee projection in a patient with a large (24 cm) ASIS-to-imaging table measurement?

A. _____

When imaging a patient with a small (18 cm) ASIS-to-imaging table measurement?

B. _____

204. If the wrong CR angle is used for an AP knee projection, the shape of the fibular head and its proximity to the tibial plateau change from that demonstrated on an AP knee projection in which an accurate CR angle was used. For each situation that follows, state the change that occurs.

A. CR angled too cephalically: _____

B. CR angled too caudally: _____

205. Which knee compartment on an AP knee projection is the narrower when a valgus deformity is present?

A. _____

When a varus deformity is present?

B. _____

206. What deformity is demonstrated in Figure 6-52?

Figure 6-52

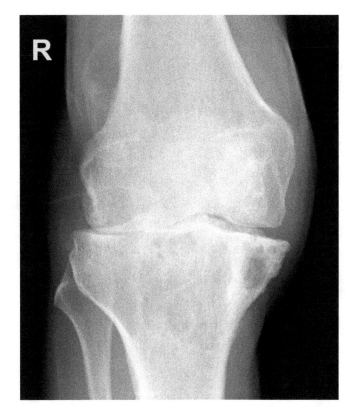

Copyright © 2015, 2011, 2006, 1996 by Saunders, an imprint of Elsevier Inc. All rights reserved.

Chapter **6** **Image Analysis of the Lower Extremity**

207. An AP knee projection is requested for a patient who is unable to fully extend the knee. The technologist angled the CR until it was perpendicular to the anterior surface of the lower leg and obtained a 10-degree cephalic angle. How is this angle adjusted to align the CR parallel with the tibial plateau and obtain an open femorotibial joint?

_____

208. When the knee is flexed, the patella shifts (A) _____ (proximally/distally) and (B) _____

(medially/laterally) onto the patellar surface of the femur and then (C) _____ (medially/laterally) onto the intercondylar fossa.

209. Match the following degrees of knee flexion with the patella location.

A. 10 degrees: 1. Between the patellar surface and intercondylar fossa

B. 20 degrees: 2. Superior to the patella surface

C. 60 degrees: 3. On the patellar surface

210. Accurate CR centering on an AP knee projection is accomplished by centering the CR (A) _____ inch

(B) _____ to the palpable (C) _____.

211. What anatomic structures are included on an AP knee projection with accurate positioning?

_____

For the following descriptions of AP knee projections with poor positioning, state how the patient or CR would have been mispositioned for such a projection to be obtained.

212. The medial femoral condyle appears larger than the lateral condyle, and the head, neck, and shaft of the fibula are almost entirely superimposed by the tibia.

_____

213. The lateral femoral condyle appears larger than the medial condyle, and the tibia demonstrates very little superimposition of the fibular head.

_____

214. The femorotibial joint space is obscured, the tibial plateau is demonstrated, and the fibular head is foreshortened and demonstrated more than ½ inch (1.25 cm) distal to the tibial plateau.

_____

215. The medial femorotibial joint space is closed, and the fibular head is elongated and demonstrated less than ½ inch (1.25 cm) distal to the tibial plateau.

_____

Copyright © 2015, 2011, 2006, 1996 by Saunders, an imprint of Elsevier Inc. All rights reserved.

For the following AP knee projections with poor positioning, state what anatomic structures are misaligned and how the patient should be repositioned for an optimal projection to be obtained.

Figure 6-53

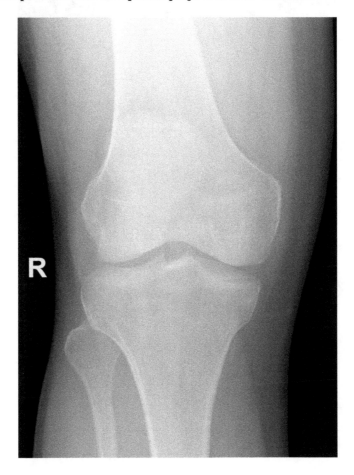

216. (Figure 6-53): _____

_____

_____

_____

Copyright © 2015, 2011, 2006, 1996 by Saunders, an imprint of Elsevier Inc. All rights reserved.   Chapter **6**   **Image Analysis of the Lower Extremity**

Figure 6-54

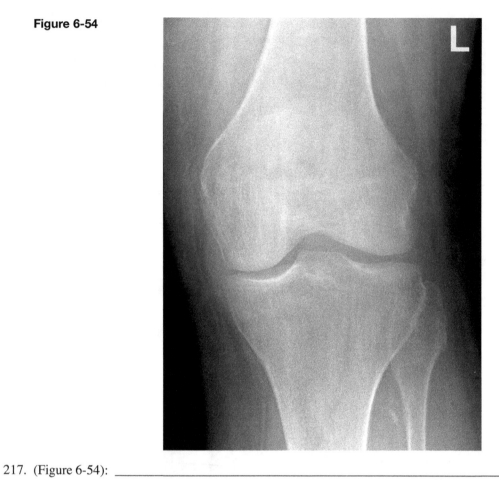

217. (Figure 6-54): _____

_____

_____

_____

   Copyright © 2015, 2011, 2006, 1996 by Saunders, an imprint of Elsevier Inc. All rights reserved.

Figure 6-55

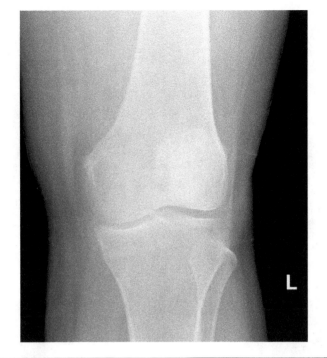

218. (Figure 6-55): _____
_____
_____
_____

Figure 6-56

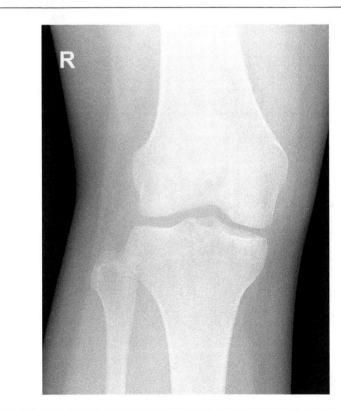

219. (Figure 6-56):_____
_____
_____
_____

Copyright © 2015, 2011, 2006, 1996 by Saunders, an imprint of Elsevier Inc. All rights reserved. Chapter **6** **Image Analysis of the Lower Extremity**

Figure 6-57

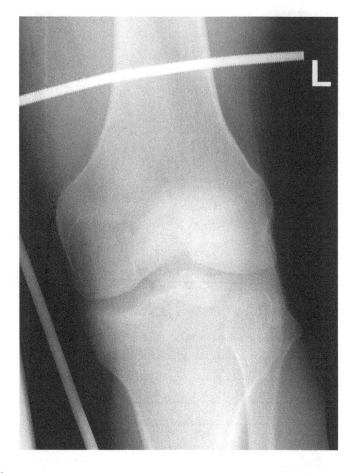

220. (Figure 6-57, trauma): _____

_____

_____

_____

Copyright © 2015, 2011, 2006, 1996 by Saunders, an imprint of Elsevier Inc. All rights reserved.

Figure 6-58

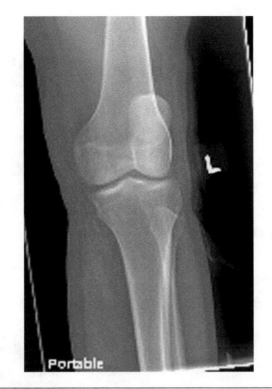

221. (Figure 6-58, trauma): _____
_____
_____
_____

Copyright © 2015, 2011, 2006, 1996 by Saunders, an imprint of Elsevier Inc. All rights reserved.

Figure 6-59

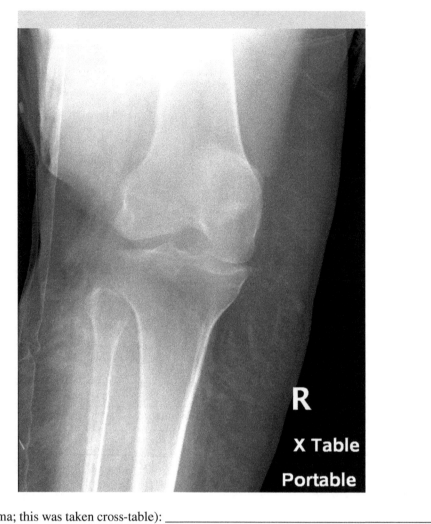

222. (Figure 6-59, trauma; this was taken cross-table): _____

_____

_____

_____

 Copyright © 2015, 2011, 2006, 1996 by Saunders, an imprint of Elsevier Inc. All rights reserved.

Knee: AP Oblique Projection (Medial and Lateral Rotation)

223. Identify the labeled anatomy in Figure 6-60.

Figure 6-60

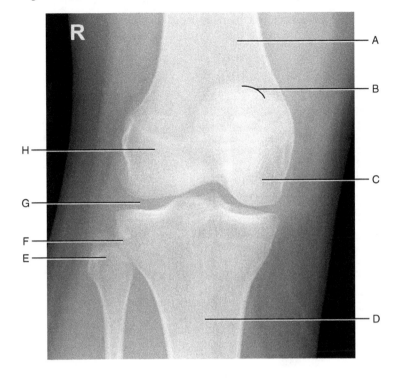

A. _____
B. _____
C. _____
D. _____
E. _____
F. _____
G. _____
H. _____

224. Identify the labeled anatomy in Figure 6-61.

Figure 6-61

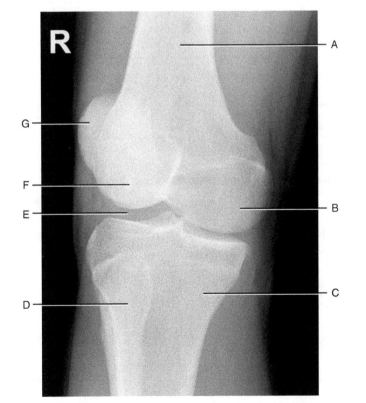

A. _____
B. _____
C. _____
D. _____
E. _____
F. _____
G. _____

Copyright © 2015, 2011, 2006, 1996 by Saunders, an imprint of Elsevier Inc. All rights reserved.

225. Complete the statements below referring to AP oblique knee projection analysis guidelines.

AP Oblique Knee Projection Analysis Guidelines

- The knee joint space is open, the anterior and posterior condylar margins of the tibia are superimposed, and the fibular head is approximately ½ inch (1.25 cm) (A) _____ to the (B) _____ .

- Medial oblique: The fibular head is seen free of (C) _____ superimposition, and the lateral femoral condyle is in profile without superimposing the medial condyle.

- Lateral oblique: The fibular head is aligned with the (D) _____ edge of the tibia, and the medial femoral condyle is in profile without superimposing the lateral condyle.

- The (E) _____ is at the center of the exposure field.

---

226. For AP oblique knee projections, an imaginary line drawn between the femoral epicondyles should form a(n) _____-degree angle with the IR.

227. How can one determine from an internally rotated AP oblique knee projection that the knee was overrotated?

_____

228. How can one determine if an externally rotated AP oblique knee projection was overrotated?

_____

229. What degree of CR angulation is used for a laterally rotated AP oblique knee projection on a patient whose ASIS-to-imaging table measurement is 12 cm?

    A. _____

Why is it common to need a cephalic angle for the medially (internally) AP oblique knee projection?

    B. _____

Why is it common to need a caudal angle for the lateral (externally) AP oblique knee projection?

    C. _____

230. The CR is centered to the (A) _____ at the level of the (B) _____ for AP oblique knee projections.

231. What anatomic structures are included on an oblique knee projection with accurate positioning?

_____

For the following descriptions of AP oblique knee projections with poor positioning, state how the patient or CR would have been mispositioned for such a projection to be obtained.

232. On an internally rotated knee projection, the tibia is partially superimposed over the fibular head.

_____

233. On an externally rotated knee projection, the lateral femoral condyle is superimposed over the medial condyle, and the fibula is located in the center of the tibia.

_____

300

Copyright © 2015, 2011, 2006, 1996 by Saunders, an imprint of Elsevier Inc. All rights reserved.

234. On an externally rotated knee projection, the fibula is not entirely superimposed by the tibia.

_____

235. On an internally rotated knee projection, the femorotibial joint space is obscured, and the fibular head is foreshortened and demonstrated more than ½ inch (1.25 cm) distal to the tibial plateau.

_____

For the following AP oblique knee projections with poor positioning, state what anatomic structures are misaligned and how the patient should be repositioned for an optimal projection to be obtained.

Figure 6-62

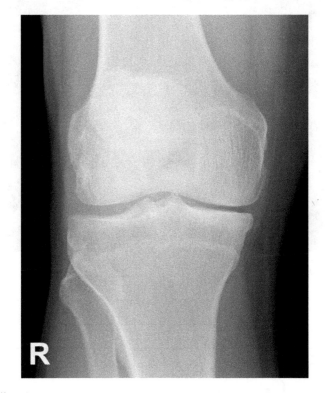

236. (Figure 6-62 medial oblique): _____

_____

_____

_____

Copyright © 2015, 2011, 2006, 1996 by Saunders, an imprint of Elsevier Inc. All rights reserved.

Figure 6-63

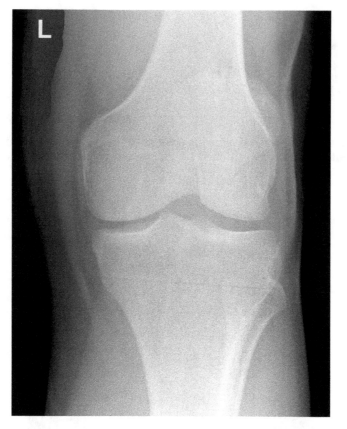

237. (Figure 6-63, lateral oblique): _____

_____

_____

_____

 Copyright © 2015, 2011, 2006, 1996 by Saunders, an imprint of Elsevier Inc. All rights reserved.

Figure 6-64

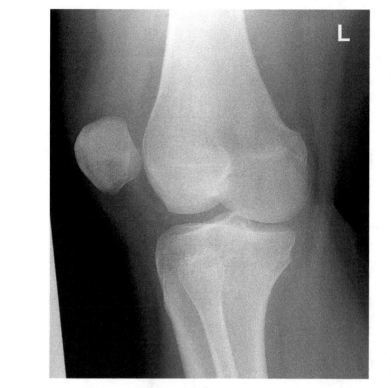

238. (Figure 6-64, lateral oblique): _____

_____

_____

_____

Copyright © 2015, 2011, 2006, 1996 by Saunders, an imprint of Elsevier Inc. All rights reserved.

Knee: Lateral Projection (Mediolateral)

239. Identify the labeled anatomy in Figure 6-65.

Figure 6-65

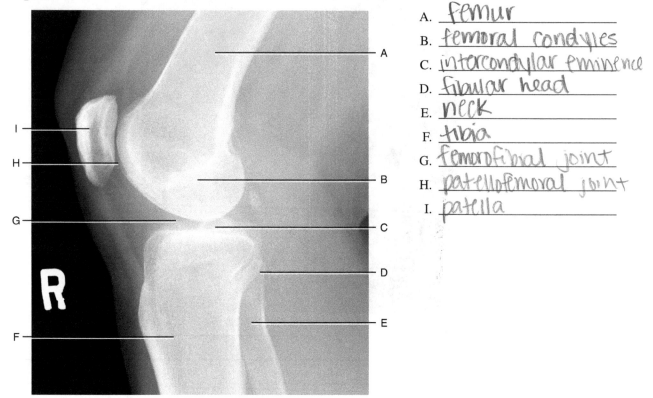

A. femur

B. femoral condyles

C. intercondylar eminence

D. fibular head

E. neck

F. tibia

G. femorofibial joint

H. patellofemoral joint

I. patella

240. Complete the statements below referring to lateral knee projection analysis guidelines.

Lateral Knee Projection Analysis Guidelines
■ Contrast and density are adequate to demonstrate the (A) suprapatellar fat pad.
■ The patella is situated (B) proximal to the patellar surface of the femur and the patellofemoral joint is open.
■ The distal articulating surfaces of the medial and lateral (C) femoral condyles are aligned, and the knee joint space is open.
■ The anterior and posterior surfaces of the medial and lateral femoral condyles are aligned, and the tibia is superimposes one-half of the (D) fibular head.
■ The (E) knee joint is at the center of the exposure field.

241. Why can a joint effusion diagnosis be made when evaluating a lateral knee projection if the knee is flexed less than 20 degrees but become difficult to make when the knee is flexed more than 20 degrees?

Because it forces the patella in coming in contact w/ the patellar surface

Chapter **6** **Image Analysis of the Lower Extremity**   Copyright © 2015, 2011, 2006, 1996 by Saunders, an imprint of Elsevier Inc. All rights reserved.

242. When a patient is erect, the distal femoral condylar surfaces are aligned (A) _____ to the floor, and the femoral shaft inclines (B) _____ approximately (C) _____ degrees. A patient who demonstrates the greatest femoral inclination will have a (D) _____ (wide/narrow) pelvis and (E) _____ (long/short) femoral shaft length.

243. When the average patient is placed in a recumbent lateral position for a lateral knee projection, the femoral shaft inclination displayed in the erect position is reduced, causing the (A) _____ condyle to be projected (B) _____ to the (C) _____ condyle.

244. To obtain superimposed distal femoral condylar surfaces when imaging the average patient for a lateral knee projection, a(n) (A) _____-degree cephalic CR angulation is used to shift the (B) _____ condyle anteriorly and proximally. The CR angulation is (C) _____ (increased/reduced) when imaging a patient with a narrow pelvis and long femora.

245. State two methods of distinguishing the medial femoral condyle from the lateral femoral condyle on a lateral knee projection with poor positioning.

    A. _____

    B. _____

246. When is it necessary to use a cephalic CR angulation for a cross-table lateral knee projection in a patient in a supine position?

    _____

    _____

247. What is the relationship between the tibia and the fibular head on a lateral knee projection with accurate positioning if superimposed condyles were obtained by aligning the femoral epicondyles perpendicular to the IR and directing the CR across the femur to project the medial condyle anteriorly and proximally?

    A. _____

    How will this relationship change if superimposed condyles are obtained by rolling the patient's patella approximately ¼ inch (0.6 cm) closer to the IR and directing the CR toward the femur so it only moves the medial condyle proximally?

    B. _____

248. Why is the medial condyle shifted more than the lateral condyle when the degree of CR angulation is adjusted?

    _____

249. If the medial condyle is demonstrated anterior to the lateral condyle on a lateral knee projection with poor positioning, what will the tibia and fibular relationship be?

    _____ not Superimposed _____

250. If the lateral condyle is demonstrated anterior to the medial condyle on a lateral knee projection with poor positioning, what will the tibia and fibular relationship be?

    _____

251. Accurate CR centering on a lateral knee projection is accomplished by centering the CR to the midline of the knee at a level (A) _____ inch (B) _____ to the palpable (C) _____ .

Copyright © 2015, 2011, 2006, 1996 by Saunders, an imprint of Elsevier Inc. All rights reserved.

252. What anatomic structures are included on a lateral knee projection with accurate positioning?

¼ distal femur & prox. tib/fib

For the following descriptions of lateral knee projections with poor positioning, state how the patient or CR would have been mispositioned for such a projection to be obtained.

253. The patient's patella is in contact with the patellar surface of the femur, and the suprapatellar fat pads are obscured.

_____

254. The distal articulating surfaces of the femoral condyles are demonstrated without superimposition. The condyle that has the adductor tubercle attached to it is demonstrated approximately ¼ inch (0.6 cm) distal to the other condyle.

_____

255. The distal articulating surfaces of the femoral condyles are demonstrated without superimposition. The condyle that has the flattest distal surface is demonstrated approximately ½ inch (1.25 cm) distal to the other condyle.

_____

256. The anterior and posterior aspects of the femoral condyles are demonstrated without superimposition. The medial condyle is demonstrated posteriorly.

_____

257. The anterior and posterior aspects of the femoral condyles are demonstrated without superimposition. The medial condyle is demonstrated anteriorly.

_____

Copyright © 2015, 2011, 2006, 1996 by Saunders, an imprint of Elsevier Inc. All rights reserved.

For the following lateral knee projections with poor positioning, state what anatomic structures are misaligned and how the patient should be repositioned for an optimal projection to be obtained.

Figure 6-66

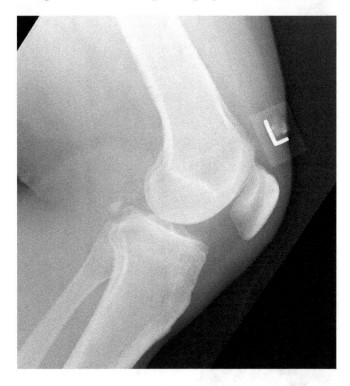

258. (Figure 6-66): _____

_____

_____

_____

Copyright © 2015, 2011, 2006, 1996 by Saunders, an imprint of Elsevier Inc. All rights reserved.

Chapter **6** **Image Analysis of the Lower Extremity**

Figure 6-67

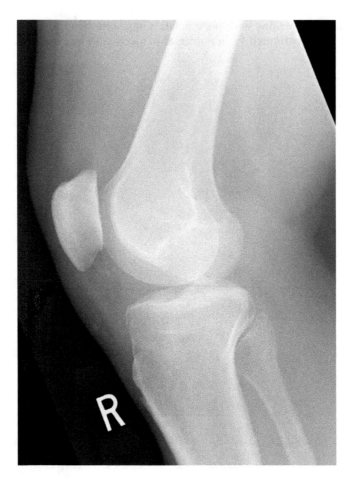

259. (Figure 6-67): _____
_____
_____
_____

      Copyright © 2015, 2011, 2006, 1996 by Saunders, an imprint of Elsevier Inc. All rights reserved.

Figure 6-68

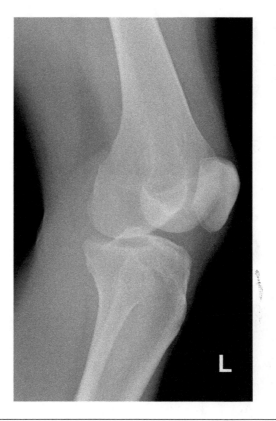

260. (Figure 6-68): _____

_____

_____

_____

Copyright © 2015, 2011, 2006, 1996 by Saunders, an imprint of Elsevier Inc. All rights reserved.   Chapter **6** **Image Analysis of the Lower Extremity**

Figure 6-69

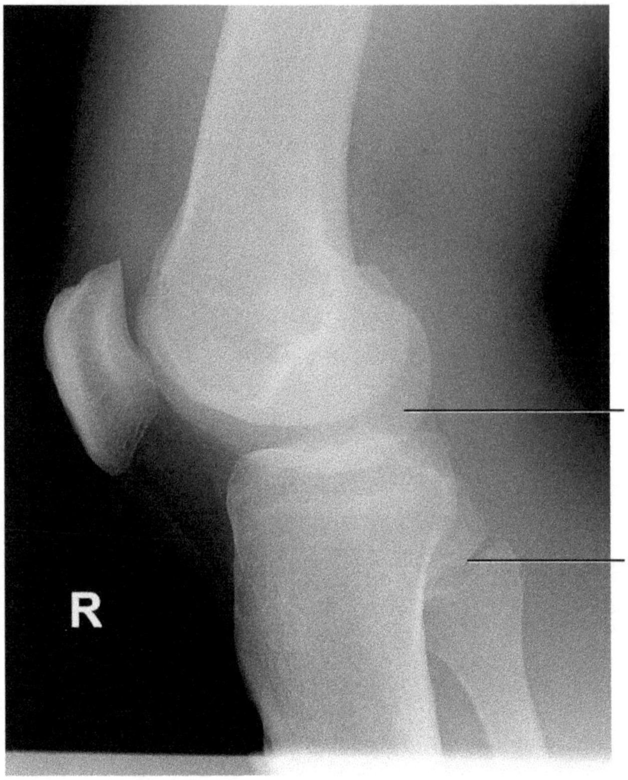

Lateral condyle

Tibiofibular joint

R

261. (Figure 6-69): _____

_____

_____

_____

  Copyright © 2015, 2011, 2006, 1996 by Saunders, an imprint of Elsevier Inc. All rights reserved.

Figure 6-70

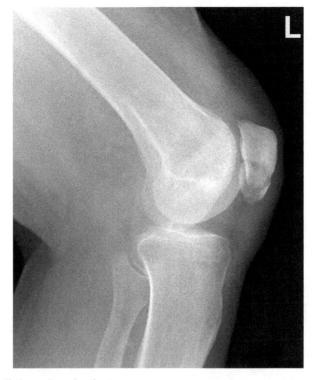

262. (Figure 6-70, trauma, mediolateral projection): _____

_____

_____

_____

Figure 6-71

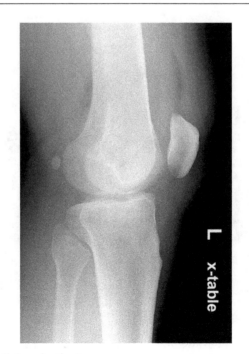

263. (Figure 6-71, trauma, lateromedial projection): _____

_____

_____

_____

Copyright © 2015, 2011, 2006, 1996 by Saunders, an imprint of Elsevier Inc. All rights reserved.

Figure 6-72

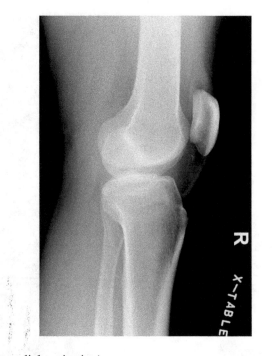

264. (Figure 6-72, trauma, lateromedial projection): _____

_____

_____

_____

Figure 6-73

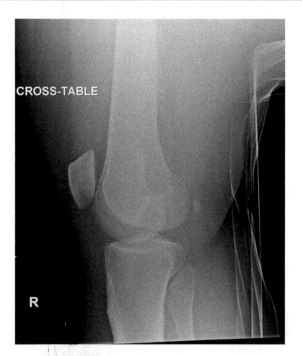

265. (Figure 6-73, trauma, lateromedial projection): _____

_____

_____

_____

Copyright © 2015, 2011, 2006, 1996 by Saunders, an imprint of Elsevier Inc. All rights reserved.

Intercondylar Fossa: PA Axial Projection (Holmblad Method)

266. Identify the labeled anatomy in Figure 6-74.

Figure 6-74

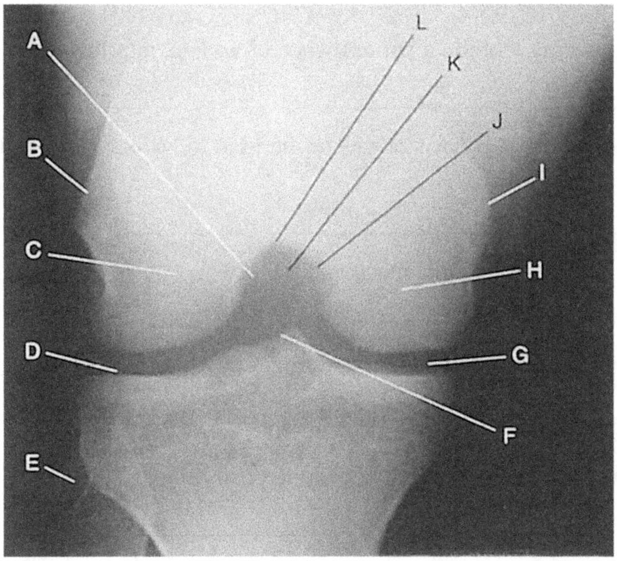

A. _____

B. _____

C. _____

D. _____

E. _____

F. _____

G. _____

H. _____

I. _____

J. _____

K. _____

L. _____

267. Complete the statements below referring to PA axial (Holmblad method) knee projection analysis guidelines.

PA Axial (Holmblad Method) Knee Projection Analysis Guidelines
■ The medial and lateral surfaces of the intercondylar fossa and the femoral epicondyles are in profile, and the (A) _____1/2_____ of the fibular head superimposes the proximal tibia.
■ The proximal surface of the intercondylar fossa is in (B) _____profile_____, and the patellar apex is demonstrated (C) _____proximal_____ to the intercondylar fossa.
■ The knee joint space is (D) _____open_____, and the tibial plateau and intercondylar eminence and the tubercles are in profile. The fibular head is demonstrated approximately ½ inch (1.25 cm) (E) _____distal_____ to the tibial plateau.
■ The (F) _____ICF_____ is at the center of the exposure field.

268. How are the femur and foot positioned to demonstrate superimposed medial and lateral intercondylar fossa surfaces on a PA axial knee projection?

A. Femur: _incline medially 10-15°_

B. Foot: _perp. to table_

269. Which direction does the patella move when the patient is positioned for a PA axial knee projection and the heel is rotated as indicated below?

A. Internally: _laterally_

B. Externally: _medially_

270. To superimpose the proximal surfaces of the intercondylar fossa in the PA axial knee position, position the patient's femur at (A) _____ degrees from vertical or (B) _____ degrees from the imaging table.

Copyright © 2015, 2011, 2006, 1996 by Saunders, an imprint of Elsevier Inc. All rights reserved.

271. If the knee is flexed more than needed to superimpose the proximal surfaces of the intercondylar fossa, is the patella demonstrated proximally or distally to where it is demonstrated on an AP axial knee projection with accurate positioning?

_____

272. What is the relationship of the tibial plateau to the imaging table in a patient whose foot is plantarflexed?

A. _____

How is the patient positioned for the anterior and posterior condylar margins of the tibia to be superimposed on a PA axial knee projection?

B. _____

This positioning also demonstrates an open (C) _____ joint space and the (D) _____ and (E) _____ without foreshortening.

273. Accurate CR centering on a PA axial knee projection is accomplished by centering a (A) _____ CR

to the midline of the knee at a level (B) _____ inch distal to the palpable (C) _____.

274. What anatomic structures are included on a PA axial knee projection with accurate positioning?

_____

For the following descriptions of PA axial (Holmblad method) knee projections with poor positioning, state how the patient would have been mispositioned for such a projection to be obtained.

275. The medial and lateral aspects of the intercondylar fossa are demonstrated without superimposition, and the patella is situated laterally.

_____

276. The medial and lateral aspects of the intercondylar fossa are demonstrated without superimposition, the patella is situated medially, and the tibia is demonstrated without fibular head superimposition.

_____

277. The proximal surfaces of the intercondylar fossa are demonstrated without superimposition, and the patella is positioned within the intercondylar fossa.

_____

278. The proximal surfaces of the intercondylar fossa are demonstrated without superimposition, and the patella is positioned too far proximal to the intercondylar fossa.

_____

279. The femorotibial joint is obscured, and the tibial plateau is demonstrated.

_____

Copyright © 2015, 2011, 2006, 1996 by Saunders, an imprint of Elsevier Inc. All rights reserved.

For the following PA axial (Holmblad method) knee projections with poor positioning, state what anatomic structures are misaligned and how the patient should be repositioned for an optimal projection to be obtained.

Figure 6-75

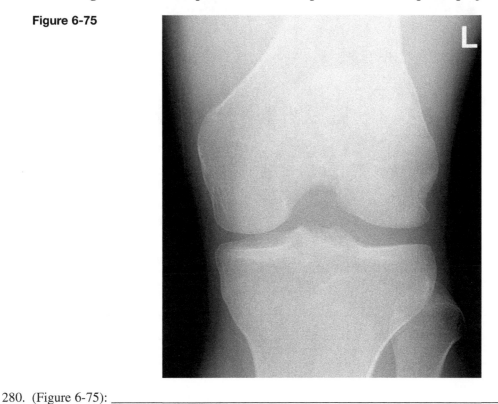

280. (Figure 6-75): _____

_____

_____

_____

Copyright © 2015, 2011, 2006, 1996 by Saunders, an imprint of Elsevier Inc. All rights reserved.   Chapter **6   Image Analysis of the Lower Extremity**

Figure 6-76

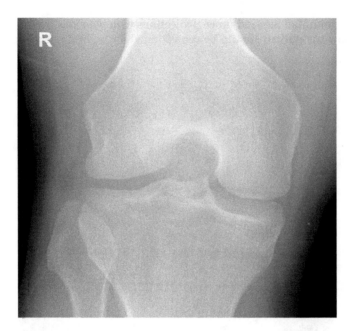

281. (Figure 6-76): _____

_____

_____

_____

Figure 6-77

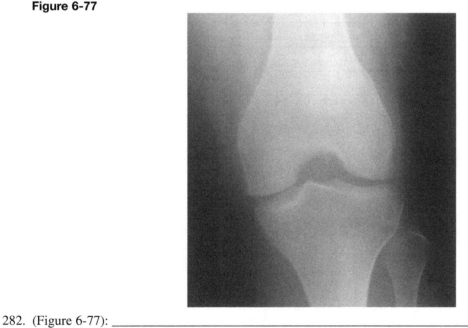

282. (Figure 6-77): _____

_____

_____

_____

Copyright © 2015, 2011, 2006, 1996 by Saunders, an imprint of Elsevier Inc. All rights reserved.

Intercondylar Fossa: AP Axial Projection (Béclere Method)

283. Identify the labeled anatomy in Figure 6-78.

Figure 6-78

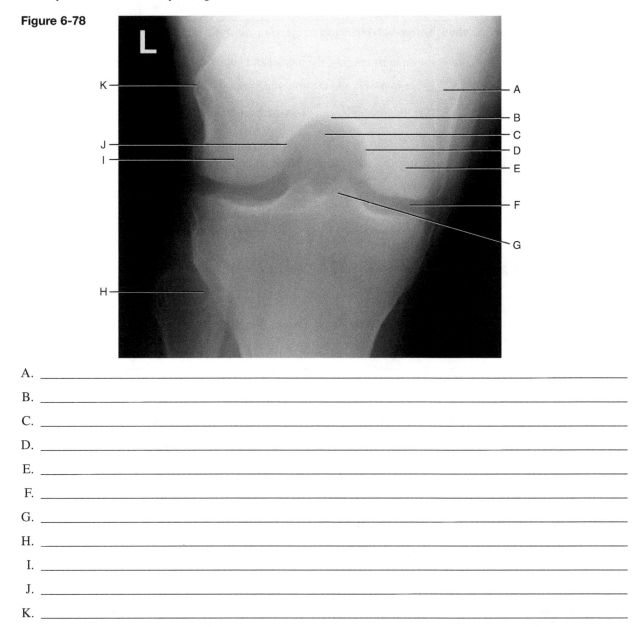

A. _____

B. _____

C. _____

D. _____

E. _____

F. _____

G. _____

H. _____

I. _____

J. _____

K. _____

Copyright © 2015, 2011, 2006, 1996 by Saunders, an imprint of Elsevier Inc. All rights reserved.

Chapter **6** **Image Analysis of the Lower Extremity**

284. Complete the statements below referring to AP axial (Béclere method) intercondylar fossa projection analysis guidelines.

AP Axial (Béclere Method) Intercondylar Fossa Projection Analysis Guidelines

- The intercondylar fossa is shown in its entirety, the medial and lateral surfaces of the intercondylar fossa, and the (A) _femoral epicondyles_ are in profile and the tibia superimposes half of the (B) _fib. head_.
- The proximal surface of the intercondylar fossa is in profile, and the patellar apex is demonstrated (C) _proximal_ to the fossa.
- The knee joint space is open, the intercondylar eminence and tubercles are in profile, and the fibular head is demonstrated approximately (D) _1/2_ inch distal to the tibial plateau.
- The (E) _ICF_ is at the center of the exposure field.

285. How is the knee positioned to superimpose the medial and lateral surfaces on the PA axial projection?

_____

286. How are the CR and the patient positioned to obtain a projection that demonstrates the proximal surfaces of the intercondylar fossa in profile?

A. CR: _____

B. Patient: _____

287. For an open knee joint space and demonstration of the intercondylar eminence and tubercles in profile, the (A) _____ and (B) _____ must be aligned parallel with each other.

288. Accurate CR centering on an AP axial projection is accomplished by first positioning the CR (A) _____ with the anterior lower leg surface; then (B) _____ the obtained angulation by 5 degrees and centering the CR 1 inch (2.5 cm) distal to the (C) _____.

289. What anatomic structures are included on an AP axial knee projection with accurate positioning?

_____

For the following descriptions of AP axial (Béclere method) knee projections with poor positioning, state how the patient would have been mispositioned for such a projection to be obtained.

290. The medial and lateral aspects of the intercondylar fossa are not superimposed, the lateral femoral condyle is wider than the lateral condyle, and the fibular head demonstrates decreased tibial superimposition.

_____

291. The medial and lateral aspects of the intercondylar fossa are not superimposed, the medial femoral condyle is wider than the medial condyle, and the fibular head demonstrates increased tibial superimposition.

_____

292. The proximal surfaces of the intercondylar fossa are not superimposed, and the patellar apex is demonstrated within the intercondylar fossa.

_____

Copyright © 2015, 2011, 2006, 1996 by Saunders, an imprint of Elsevier Inc. All rights reserved.

293. The proximal surfaces of the intercondylar fossa are not superimposed, and the patellar apex is demonstrated proximal to the intercondylar fossa.

_____

294. The knee joint space is closed, and the fibular head is shown less than ½ inch (1.25 cm) distal to the tibial plateau.

_____

295. The knee joint space is closed, and the fibular head is shown more than ½ inch (1.25 cm) distal to the tibial plateau.

_____

For the following AP axial (Béclere method) knee projections with poor positioning, state what anatomic structures are misaligned and how the patient should be repositioned for an optimal projection to be obtained.

Figure 6-79

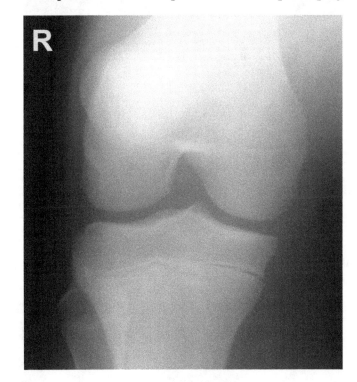

296. (Figure 6-79): _____

_____

_____

_____

Copyright © 2015, 2011, 2006, 1996 by Saunders, an imprint of Elsevier Inc. All rights reserved.

Chapter **6**   **Image Analysis of the Lower Extremity**

Figure 6-80

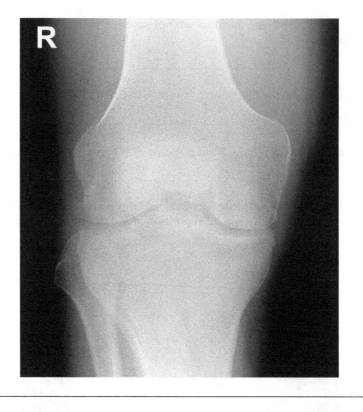

297. (Figure 6-80): _____

_____

_____

_____

Patella and Patellofemoral Joint: Tangential Projection (Merchant Method)

298. Identify the labeled anatomy in Figure 6-81.

Figure 6-81

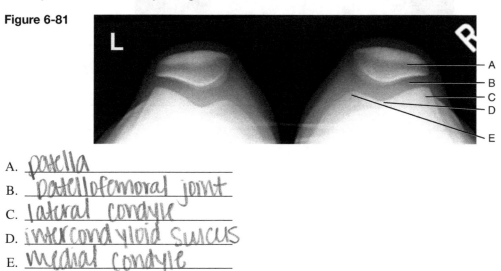

A. <u>patella</u>

B. <u>patellofemoral joint</u>

C. <u>lateral condyle</u>

D. <u>intercondyloid sulcus</u>

E. <u>medial condyle</u>

Copyright © 2015, 2011, 2006, 1996 by Saunders, an imprint of Elsevier Inc. All rights reserved.

299. Complete the statements below referring to tangential (Merchant method) patella projection analysis guidelines.

Tangential (Merchant Method) Patella and Patellofemoral Joint Projection Analysis Guidelines
■ The patellae, anterior femoral condyles, and intercondylar sulci are seen superiorly, and the (A) __lateral__ femoral condyle demonstrates slightly more height than the (B) __medial__ condyle.
■ The patellofemoral joint spaces are (C) __open__ with no superimposition of the upper anterior thigh soft tissue, patellae, or tibial tuberosities.
■ A point midway between the (D) __patellofemoral joints__ is at the center of the exposure field.

300. Why is a grid not required for a tangential projection knee projection?

_____

301. How are the legs positioned to prevent rotation on a tangential knee projection?

_____

302. How do the positions of the patellae and femoral condyles change when the knees are in external rotation for a tangential knee projection?

A. Patellae: _____

B. Femoral condyles: _____

303. The tangential knee projection is most often obtained to demonstrate what patient condition?

A. _____

How is this condition demonstrated on a tangential knee projection with accurate positioning?

B. _____

How can one distinguish this condition from rotation on a tangential knee projection?

C. _____

304. Why is it important for the patient to relax the quadriceps femoris muscles for the tangential knee projection?

_____

305. How are the femurs positioned to obtain a tangential knee projection with accurate positioning?

_____

306. Where are the posterior knee curves positioned with respect to the axial viewer for a tangential knee projection with accurate positioning?

_____

307. How is the positioning setup for a tangential knee projection adjusted when imaging a patient with large posterior calves?

A. _____

If this positioning setup is not changed, what anatomic misalignment appears on the resulting projection?

B. _____

Copyright © 2015, 2011, 2006, 1996 by Saunders, an imprint of Elsevier Inc. All rights reserved.

308. What are the standard direction and degree of CR angulation used for the tangential knee projection?

_____

309. What is the sum of the CR angle and the angle of the axial viewer for all tangential knee projections?

_____

310. Why is a 72-inch (183 cm) SID used for the tangential projection?

_____

311. What anatomic structures are included on a tangential knee projection with accurate positioning?

_____

For the following descriptions of tangential knee projections with poor positioning, state how the patient would have been mispositioned for such a projection to be obtained.

312. The patellae are demonstrated directly above the intercondylar sulci and rotated laterally. The medial femoral condyles demonstrate more height than the lateral condyles.

_____

313. Soft tissue from the patient's anterior thighs has been projected onto the patellae and patellofemoral joint spaces.

_____

314. The patellae are resting against the intercondylar sulci, obscuring the patellofemoral joint spaces.

_____

315. The tibial tuberosities are demonstrated within the patellofemoral joint spaces. The patient's calves were not large.

_____

For the following tangential (axial) knee projections with poor positioning, state what anatomic structures are misaligned and how the patient should be repositioned for an optimal projection to be obtained.

Figure 6-82

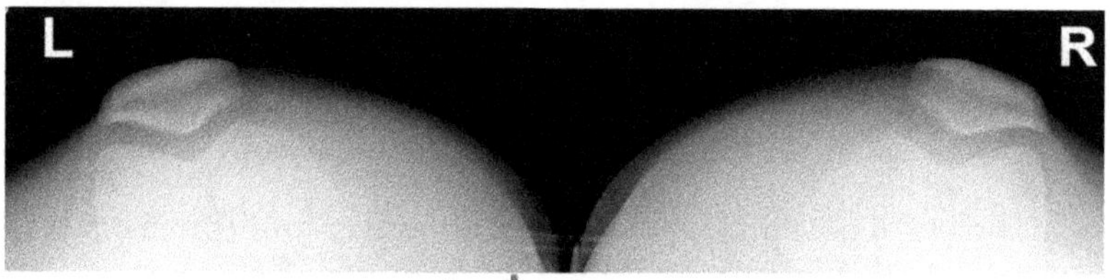

316. (Figure 6-82): _legs are rotated laterally_
fix: internally rotate legs

_____

_____

Copyright © 2015, 2011, 2006, 1996 by Saunders, an imprint of Elsevier Inc. All rights reserved.

Figure 6-83

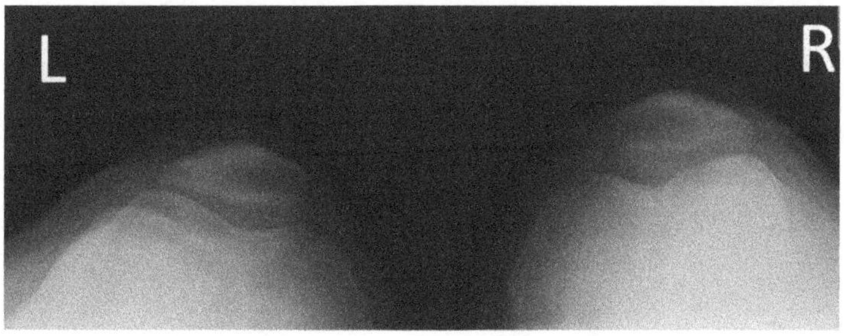

317. (Figure 6-83): _____
_____
_____
_____

Figure 6-84

318. (Figure 6-84): _____
_____
_____
_____

Figure 6-85

319. (Figure 6-85): _____
_____
_____
_____

Copyright © 2015, 2011, 2006, 1996 by Saunders, an imprint of Elsevier Inc. All rights reserved.

Femur: AP Projection

320. Identify the labeled anatomy in Figure 6-86.

Figure 6-86

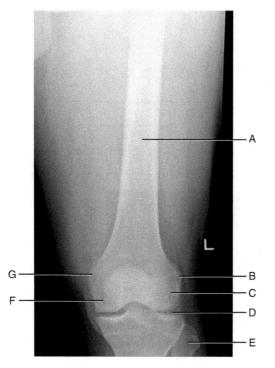

A. _____

B. _____

C. _____

D. _____

E. _____

F. _____

G. _____

321. Identify the labeled anatomy in Figure 6-87.

Figure 6-87

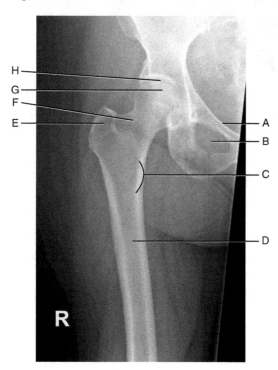

A. _____

B. _____

C. _____

D. _____

E. _____

F. _____

G. _____

H. _____

Copyright © 2015, 2011, 2006, 1996 by Saunders, an imprint of Elsevier Inc. All rights reserved.

322. Complete the statements below referring to AP distal femur projection analysis guidelines.

AP Distal Femur Projection Analysis Guidelines

■ The medial and lateral epicondyles are in (A) __profile__, the femoral condyles are symmetrical in shape, and the tibia is superimposes one-half of the (B) __fib. head__.

■ The (C) __femoral shaft__ is at the center of the exposure field.

---

323. Complete the statements below referring to AP proximal femur projection analysis guidelines.

AP Proximal Femur Projection Analysis Guidelines

■ The ischial spine is aligned with the (A) __pelvic brim__, and the obturator foramen is open.

■ The femoral neck is demonstrated without foreshortening, the (B) __greater__ trochanter is in profile laterally, and the (C) __lesser__ trochanter is completely superimposed by the proximal femur.

■ The (D) __femoral shaft__ is at the center of the exposure field.

---

324. How is the femur positioned with respect to the x-ray tube for an AP femoral projection to take advantage of the anode-heel effect?

_____

325. Why is it necessary to include all the femoral soft tissue when imaging the femur?

_____

326. An AP distal femur is obtained by placing the patient in a (A) _____ position with the knee (B) _____ and leg (C) _____ rotated until the femoral epicondyles are at equal distances from the IR.

327. Should the technologist rotate a patient with a suspected fractured femur in an attempt to position the leg in an AP projection?

A. _____ (Yes/No)

Justify your answer.

B. _____

328. Accurate CR centering on a distal femoral projection is accomplished by positioning the lower IR edge approximately (A) _____ inches below the (B) _____ joint.

329. What anatomic structures are included on an AP distal femur projection with accurate positioning?

_____

Copyright © 2015, 2011, 2006, 1996 by Saunders, an imprint of Elsevier Inc. All rights reserved.

330. How can the patient be positioned to prevent pelvic rotation on an AP proximal femur projection?

_____

331. How are the femoral epicondyles positioned for an AP proximal femur projection?

A. _____

How will this positioning demonstrate the femoral neck and greater trochanter on the resulting projection?

B. _____

332. On an AP proximal femur projection with accurate positioning, the (A) _____ is centered within the exposure field. This is accomplished by placing the upper IR edge at the level of the (B) _____.

333. What anatomic structures are included on an AP proximal femur projection with accurate positioning?

_____

For the following descriptions of AP femoral projections with poor positioning, state how the patient would have been mispositioned for such a projection to be obtained.

334. Distal femur: The medial femoral condyle appears larger than the lateral condyle, and the intercondylar eminence is not centered within the intercondylar fossa.

_____

335. Proximal femur: The affected side's obturator foramen is narrowed, and the iliac spine is demonstrated without pelvic brim superimposition.

_____

336. Proximal femur: The affected side's obturator foramen is open, and the ischial spine is not aligned with the pelvic brim but is demonstrated closer to the acetabulum.

_____

337. Proximal femur: The femoral neck is partially foreshortened, and the lesser trochanter is demonstrated in profile.

_____

Copyright © 2015, 2011, 2006, 1996 by Saunders, an imprint of Elsevier Inc. All rights reserved.

For the following AP femoral projections with poor positioning, state what anatomic structures are misaligned and how the patient should be repositioned for an optimal projection to be obtained.

Figure 6-88

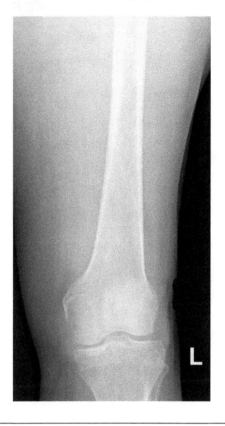

338. (Figure 6-88, distal femur): _____

_____

_____

_____

Copyright © 2015, 2011, 2006, 1996 by Saunders, an imprint of Elsevier Inc. All rights reserved.

Figure 6-89

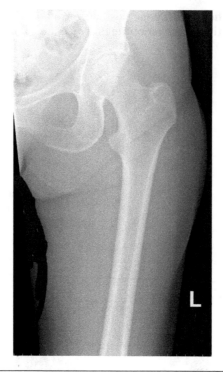

339. (Figure 6-89, proximal femur): _____

_____

_____

_____

Femur: Lateral Projection (Mediolateral)

340. Identify the labeled anatomy in Figure 6-90.

Figure 6-90

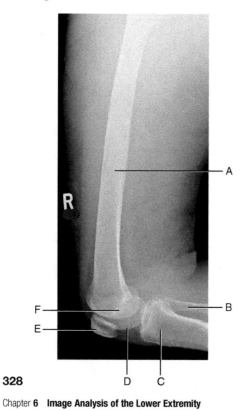

A. _____

B. _____

C. _____

D. _____

E. _____

F. _____

Copyright © 2015, 2011, 2006, 1996 by Saunders, an imprint of Elsevier Inc. All rights reserved.

341. Identify the labeled anatomy in Figure 6-91.

Figure 6-91

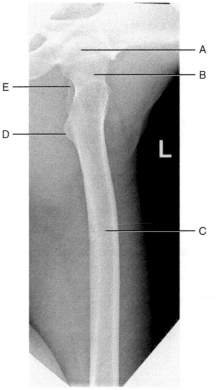

A. _____

B. _____

C. _____

D. _____

E. _____

342. Identify the labeled anatomy in Figure 6-92.

Figure 6-92

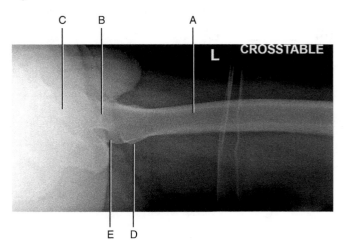

A. _____

B. _____

C. _____

D. _____

E. _____

Copyright © 2015, 2011, 2006, 1996 by Saunders, an imprint of Elsevier Inc. All rights reserved.

343. Complete the statements below referring to lateral distal femur projection analysis guidelines.

> **Lateral Proximal Distal Femur Projection Analysis Guidelines**
>
> ■ Anterior and posterior margins of the (A) _____medial_____, and (B) _lateral_ con-dyles are aligned.
> ■ The (C) __femoral shaft__ is at the center of the exposure field.

344. Complete the statements below referring to lateral proximal femur projection analysis guidelines.

> **Lateral Proximal Femur Projection Analysis Guidelines**
>
> ■ The lesser trochanter is in profile (A) __medially__, and the femoral neck and head are superimposed over the (B) _greater trochanter_.
> ■ The femoral shaft is seen without foreshortening, the femoral neck is demonstrated on end, and the (C) __greater__ trochanter is demonstrated at the same transverse level as the femoral head.
> ■ The (D) __femoral shaft__ is at the center of the exposure field.

345. A lateral distal femur projection is obtained by rotating the patient onto the (A) _____ (medial/lateral) aspect of the affected femur until an imaginary line connecting the femoral epicondyles is aligned (B) _____ to the IR.

346. How is a lateral distal femur projection obtained in a patient with a known or suspected femur fracture?

_____

347. Accurate CR centering on a lateral distal femur projection is accomplished by placing the lower IR edge approximately (A) _____ inches below the (B) _____.

348. What anatomic structures are included on a lateral distal femur projection with accurate positioning?

_____

349. How is the patient positioned to place the lesser trochanter in profile and the greater trochanter beneath the femoral neck on a lateral proximal femur projection?

_____

350. How is the patient positioned for a lateral proximal femur projection to demonstrate the femoral shaft without foreshortening and the femoral neck on end?

_____

351. What position is performed to demonstrate a lateral proximal femur when a fracture is suspected or known to be present?

_____

352. On a lateral proximal femoral projection with accurate positioning, the (A) _____ is centered within the collimated field. This is accomplished by positioning the upper IR edge at the level of the (B) _____.

330

    Copyright © 2015, 2011, 2006, 1996 by Saunders, an imprint of Elsevier Inc. All rights reserved.

353. What anatomic structures are included on a lateral proximal femoral projection with accurate positioning?

_____

For the following descriptions of lateral femoral projections with poor positioning, state how the patient would have been mispositioned for such a projection to be obtained.

354. Distal femur: The anterior and posterior surfaces of the medial and lateral femoral condyles are demonstrated without alignment. The medial condyle is posterior to the lateral condyle.

_____

355. Proximal femur: The greater trochanter is demonstrated medially (next to the ischial tuberosity), and the lesser trochanter is obscured.

_____

356. Proximal femur: The greater trochanter is demonstrated laterally, and the lesser trochanter is obscured.

_pelvis under-rotated & condyles not perp._____

For the following lateral femoral projections with poor positioning, state what anatomic structures are misaligned and how the patient should be repositioned for an optimal projection to be obtained.

Figure 6-93

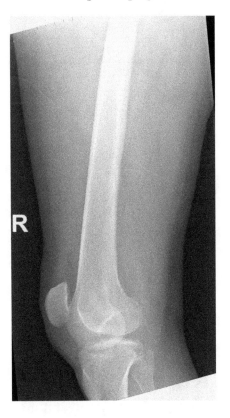

357. (Figure 6-93, distal femur): _____

_____

_____

_____

Copyright © 2015, 2011, 2006, 1996 by Saunders, an imprint of Elsevier Inc. All rights reserved.   Chapter **6** **Image Analysis of the Lower Extremity**

Figure 6-94

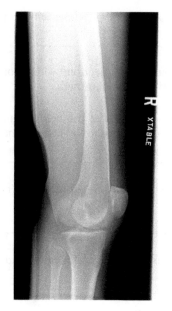

358. (Figure 6-94, trauma lateromedial distal femur): _____

_____

_____

_____

Figure 6-95

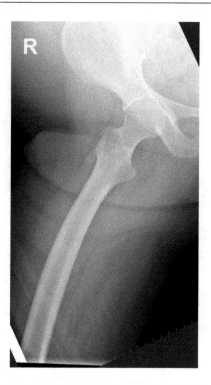

359. (Figure 6-95, proximal femur): _____

_____

_____

_____

  Copyright © 2015, 2011, 2006, 1996 by Saunders, an imprint of Elsevier Inc. All rights reserved.

Figure 6-96

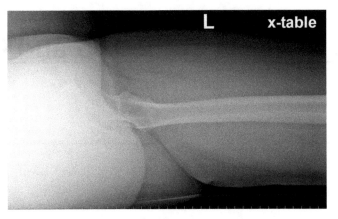

360. (Figure 6-96, proximal femur): _____

_____

_____

_____

Figure 6-97

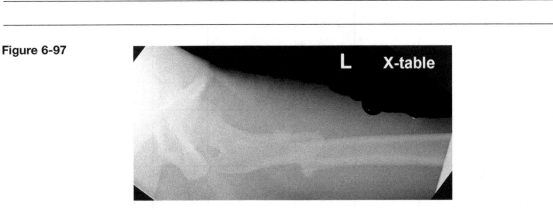

361. (Figure 6-97, trauma proximal femur): _____

_____

_____

_____

Copyright © 2015, 2011, 2006, 1996 by Saunders, an imprint of Elsevier Inc. All rights reserved.

7 | Image Analysis of the Hip and Pelvis

STUDY QUESTIONS

1. Complete Figure 7-1.

   Figure 7-1

Hip and Pelvis Technical Data					
Projection	kV	Grid	AEC	mAs	SID
AP, pelvis					
AP frogleg, pelvis					
AP, hip					
AP frogleg, hip					
Axiolateral (inferosuperior), hip					
AP axial, sacroiliac joints					
AP oblique, sacroiliac joints					
Pediatric					

2. List the four soft tissue structures that are demonstrated on accurately exposed AP hip and pelvis projections and describe their locations.

   A. _____

   B. _____

   C. _____

   D. _____

   Why is it important that these soft tissue structures are visualized?

   E. _____

Copyright © 2015, 2011, 2006, 1996 by Saunders, an imprint of Elsevier Inc. All rights reserved.

Pelvis: AP Projection

3. Identify the labeled anatomy in Figure 7-2.

Figure 7-2

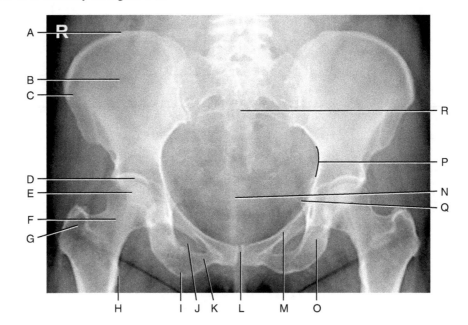

A. _____   J. _____

B. _____   K. _____

C. _____   L. _____

D. _____   M. _____

E. _____   N. _____

F. _____   O. _____

G. _____   P. _____

H. _____   Q. _____

I. _____   R. _____

Copyright © 2015, 2011, 2006, 1996 by Saunders, an imprint of Elsevier Inc. All rights reserved.

4. Complete Figure 7-3.

Figure 7-3

Male and Female Pelvic Differences		
Parameter	Male	Female
Overall Shape		
Ala (iliac wing)		
Pubic arch angle		
Inlet shape		
Obturator foramen		

5. Complete the statements below referring to AP pelvis projection analysis guidelines.

AP Pelvis Projection Analysis Guidelines

■ The ischial spines are aligned with the (A) _pelvic brim_____, the sacrum and coccyx are aligned with the symphysis pubis, and the obturator foramina are open and uniform in size and shape.

■ The femoral necks are demonstrated without foreshortening, the (B) _greater_____ trochanters are in profile laterally, and the (C) _____lesser_____ trochanters are superimposed by the femoral necks.

6. State whether the following pelvis projections are from a female or male patient:

Figure 7-4

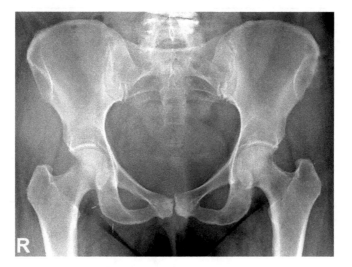

A. (Figure 7-4): _____

Copyright © 2015, 2011, 2006, 1996 by Saunders, an imprint of Elsevier Inc. All rights reserved.

Figure 7-5

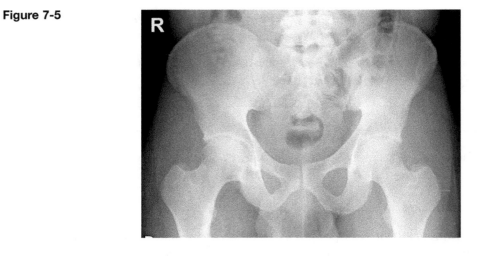

B. (Figure 7-5): _____

7. How can patient positioning be evaluated to ensure that pelvic rotation is not present on an AP pelvic projection?

_____

8. Describe the relationship of the sacrum and coccyx to the symphysis pubis and the symmetry of the iliac wings and obturator foramen on an AP pelvic projection in which the patient's left side was rotated away (RPO) from the IR.

_____

_____

9. Following are descriptions of the femoral neck appearance on different AP pelvic projections. For each description, state the position of the patient's feet and humeral epicondyles that would result in the described projection.

   A. Femoral necks without foreshortening: _____

   _____

   B. Femoral necks on end: _____

   _____

   C. Femoral necks partially foreshortened: _____

   _____

10. How are the patient's feet and femoral epicondyles positioned for an AP pelvic projection with accurate positioning to be obtained?

_____

_____

11. Accurate CR centering on an AP pelvic projection is accomplished by centering a(n) (A) _perp-_ CR to the midsagittal plane at a level halfway between the (B) _symphysis_ and an imaginary line connecting the (C) _ASIS_.

12. What anatomic structures are included on an AP pelvic projection with accurate positioning?
   iliac wings, symphysis, ischia, acetabula, femoral necks, greater & lesser

Copyright © 2015, 2011, 2006, 1996 by Saunders, an imprint of Elsevier Inc. All rights reserved.

For the following descriptions of AP pelvic projections with poor positioning, state how the patient would have been mispositioned for such a projection to be obtained.

13. The right obturator foramen is narrowed, the right ischial spine is demonstrated without pelvic brim superimposition, and the sacrum and coccyx are rotated toward the left hip.

Pelvis rotated to the right

14. The femoral necks are foreshortened, and the lesser trochanters are demonstrated in profile.

For the following AP pelvic projections with poor positioning, state what anatomic structures are misaligned and how the patient should be repositioned for an optimal projection to be obtained.

Figure 7-6

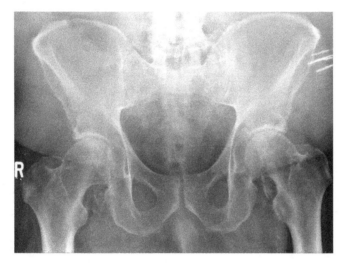

15. (Figure 7-6): _____

Copyright © 2015, 2011, 2006, 1996 by Saunders, an imprint of Elsevier Inc. All rights reserved.

Figure 7-7

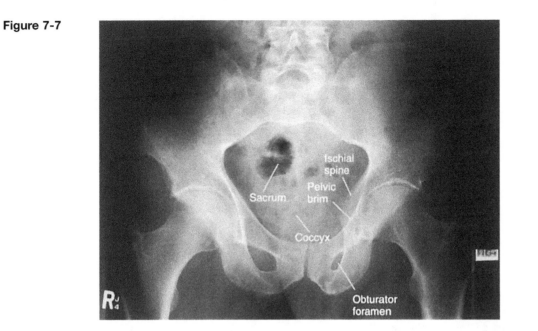

Sacrum
Ischial spine
Pelvic brim
Coccyx
Obturator foramen

16. (Figure 7-7): _____
_____
_____
_____

Figure 7-8

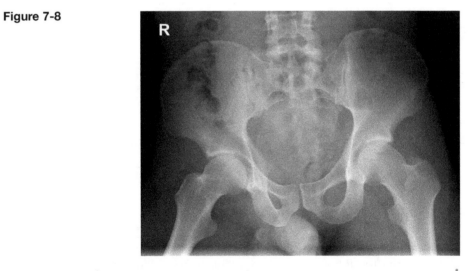

17. (Figure 7-8): right obturator foramen shortened, sacrum & coccyx leaning to left, lessers in profile. Fix: lower left hip, internally rotate legs, & make ASIS equal distant to table top

Copyright © 2015, 2011, 2006, 1996 by Saunders, an imprint of Elsevier Inc. All rights reserved.

Chapter **7 Image Analysis of the Hip and Pelvis**

Pelvis: AP Frogleg Projection (Modified Cleaves Method)

Figure 7-9

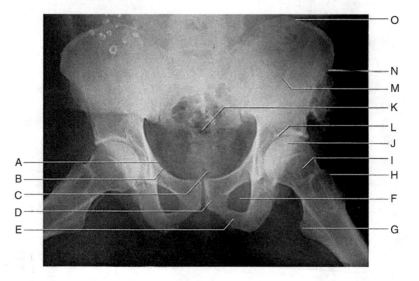

18. Identify the labeled anatomy in Figure 7-9.

A. _____

B. _____

C. _____

D. _____

E. _____

F. _____

G. _____

H. _____

I. _____

J. _____

K. _____

L. _____

M. _____

N. _____

O. _____

19. Complete the statements below referring to AP frogleg pelvis projection analysis guidelines.

AP Frogleg (Modified Cleaves Method) Pelvis Projection Analysis Guidelines

■ The sacrum and coccyx are aligned with the symphysis pubis, the (A) _iliac wings_ are symmetrical, and the obturator foramina are open and uniform in size and shape.

■ The lesser trochanters are in profile (B) _medially_____, and the (C) _femoral necks___ are superimposed over the adjacent greater trochanters.

■ The femoral necks are partially foreshortened, and the (D) _greater trochanters_____ are demonstrated at the same transverse level halfway between the femoral heads and lesser trochanters.

Copyright © 2015, 2011, 2006, 1996 by Saunders, an imprint of Elsevier Inc. All rights reserved.

20. The degree of patient knee and hip flexion determines the position of the greater and lesser trochanters to the

    _____.

21. At what degree with the imaging table are the femurs placed to accurately position the greater and lesser trochanters

    on an AP frogleg pelvic projection? _____

22. The patient's knees and hips were flexed 20 degrees with the imaging table for an AP frogleg pelvic projection. How
    can this positioning error be identified on the resulting projection?

    _____

23. The degree of femoral abduction for an AP frogleg pelvic projection determines what two anatomic relationships?

    A. _____

    B. _____

24. Describe the position of the greater trochanters and the degree of femoral neck foreshortening that are demonstrated
    on an AP frogleg pelvic projection if the femurs are abducted as follows:

    A. Femurs are abducted until placed against the imaging table:

    _____

    B. Femurs are abducted to a 45-degree angle with the imaging table:

    _____

    C. Femurs are abducted only 20 to 30 degrees from vertical:

    _____

25. Accurate CR centering on an AP frogleg pelvic projection is accomplished by centering a (A) _____ CR

    to the (B) _____ plane at a level (C) _____ superior to the (D) _____.

26. What anatomic structures are included on an AP frogleg pelvic projection with accurate positioning?

    _____

**For the following descriptions of AP frogleg pelvic projections with poor positioning, state how the patient would
have been mispositioned for such a projection to be obtained.**

27. The left obturator foramen is narrowed, the left iliac wing is wider than the right, and the sacrum and coccyx are
    rotated toward the right hip.

    _____

28. The femoral necks are demonstrated on end, and the greater trochanters are demonstrated on the same transverse
    level as the femoral heads.

    _____

Copyright © 2015, 2011, 2006, 1996 by Saunders, an imprint of Elsevier Inc. All rights reserved.

For the following AP frogleg pelvic projections with poor positioning, state what anatomic structures are misaligned and how the patient should be repositioned for an optimal projection to be obtained.

Figure 7-10

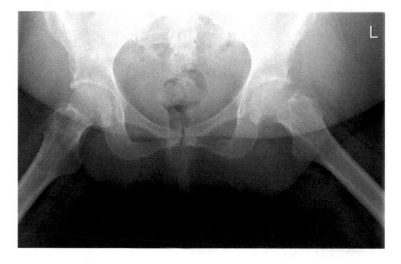

29. (Figure 7-10): _____

_____

_____

_____

Figure 7-11

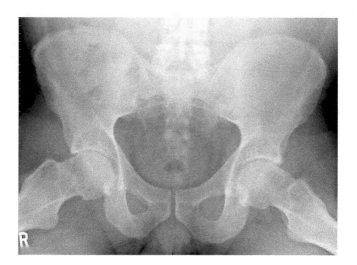

30. (Figure 7-11): _____

_____

_____

_____

Copyright © 2015, 2011, 2006, 1996 by Saunders, an imprint of Elsevier Inc. All rights reserved.

Figure 7-12

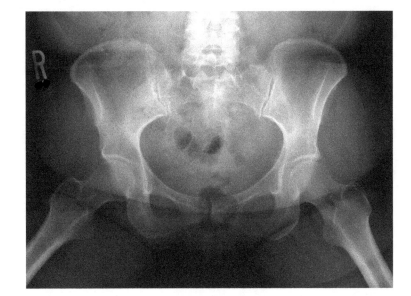

31. (Figure 7-12):_____

_____

_____

_____

Figure 7-13

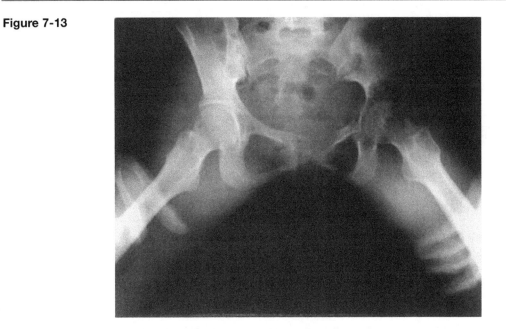

32. (Figure 7-13): _____

_____

_____

_____

Copyright © 2015, 2011, 2006, 1996 by Saunders, an imprint of Elsevier Inc. All rights reserved.

Hip: AP Projection

33. Identify the labeled anatomy in Figure 7-14.

Figure 7-14

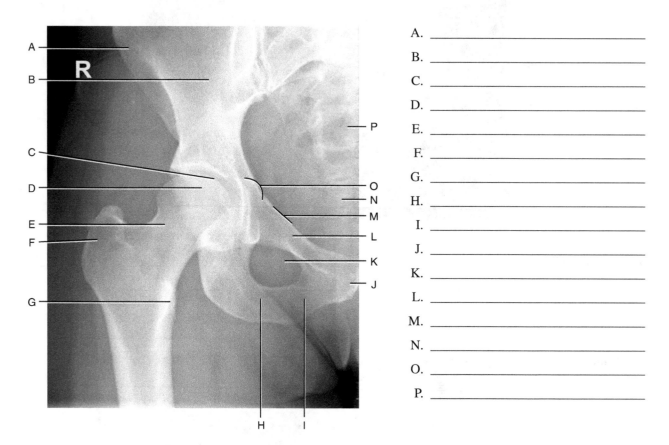

A. _____

B. _____

C. _____

D. _____

E. _____

F. _____

G. _____

H. _____

I. _____

J. _____

K. _____

L. _____

M. _____

N. _____

O. _____

P. _____

34. Complete the statements below referring to AP hip projection analysis guidelines.

AP Hip Projection Analysis Guidelines

- The ischial spine is aligned with the (A) _pelvic brim_, the sacrum and coccyx are aligned with the (B) _symphysis_, and the obturator foramen is open.

- The femoral neck is demonstrated without foreshortening, the greater trochanter is in profile (C) _laterally_, and the lesser trochanter is superimposed by the (D) _femoral neck_.

35. How can patient positioning be evaluated to ensure that pelvic rotation is not present on an AP hip projection?

_____

36. Describe the relationship that would result between the following anatomic structures on an AP hip projection if the affected side was rotated away from the IR.

A. Sacrum and symphysis pubis: _____

B. Iliac spine and pelvic brim: _____

344

Copyright © 2015, 2011, 2006, 1996 by Saunders, an imprint of Elsevier Inc. All rights reserved.

37. If the affected hip is rotated toward the IR for an AP hip projection, how will the obturator foramen appear in comparison with a nonrotated AP hip projection? _____

38. The demonstration of the femoral neck and lesser trochanter on an AP hip projection depends on the position of the femoral epicondyles. For each epicondyle position in the following list, describe how the femoral neck and lesser trochanter are demonstrated on an AP hip projection.

   A. The leg is externally rotated, with the foot at a 45-degree angle and an imaginary line connecting the femoral epicondyles at a 60- to 65-degree angle with the imaging table:

   _____

   B. The leg is internally rotated, with the foot vertical and an imaginary line connecting the femoral epicondyles at a 15- to 20-degree angle with imaging table:

   _____

   C. The leg is internally rotated, with the foot 15 to 20 degrees from vertical and an imaginary line connecting the femoral epicondyles aligned parallel with imaging table:

   _____

39. How are the patient's foot and femoral epicondyles positioned to obtain an AP hip projection with accurate positioning?

   _____

40. Should the technologist attempt to rotate the leg of a patient with a suspected fracture or dislocated hip?

   A. _____ (Yes/No)

   Explain your answer.

   B. _____

41. To center the femoral head in the center of the exposure field, a(n) (A) _____ CR is centered 1½ inches (4 cm) (B) _____ to the midpoint of a line connecting the ASIS and (C) _____.

42. What anatomic structures are included on an AP hip projection with accurate positioning?

   _____

43. How may the positioning procedure require adjusting if the patient has a prosthesis?
   _____Open collimation & may need to center lower_____

44. State whether gonadal shielding should be used for an AP hip projection for the following:

   A. Male: _____

   B. Female: _____

For the following descriptions of AP hip projections with poor positioning, state how the patient would have been mispositioned for such a projection to be obtained.

45. The ischial spine is demonstrated without pelvic brim superimposition, the sacrum and coccyx are not aligned with the symphysis pubis but are rotated away from the affected hip, and the obturator foramen is narrowed.

   _____

   _____

Copyright © 2015, 2011, 2006, 1996 by Saunders, an imprint of Elsevier Inc. All rights reserved.

46. The ischial spine is not aligned with the pelvic brim but is demonstrated closer to the acetabulum, the sacrum and coccyx are not aligned with the symphysis pubis but are rotated toward the affected hip, and the obturator foramen is clearly demonstrated.

_____

_____

47. The femoral neck is completely foreshortened, and the lesser trochanter is demonstrated in profile.

_____

_____

For the following AP hip projections with poor positioning, state what anatomic structures are misaligned and how the patient should be repositioned for an optimal projection to be obtained.

Figure 7-15

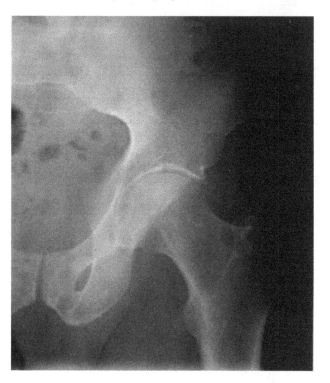

48. (Figure 7-15): _____

_____

_____

_____

 Copyright © 2015, 2011, 2006, 1996 by Saunders, an imprint of Elsevier Inc. All rights reserved.

Figure 7-16

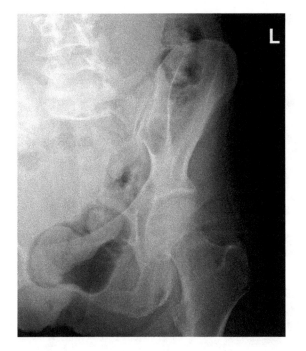

49. (Figure 7-16): _____

_____

_____

_____

Figure 7-17

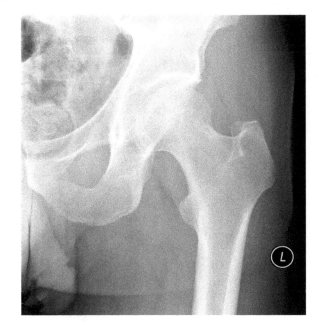

50. (Figure 7-17): _____

_____

_____

_____

_____

Copyright © 2015, 2011, 2006, 1996 by Saunders, an imprint of Elsevier Inc. All rights reserved.   Chapter **7 Image Analysis of the Hip and Pelvis**

Figure 7-18

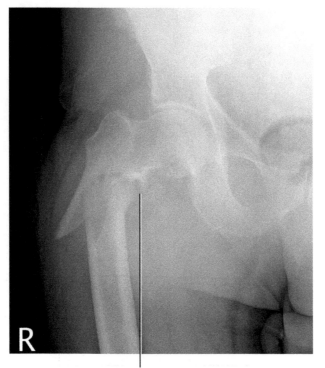

Lesser trochanter

51. (Figure 7-18, fracture): _____

_____

_____

_____

_____

    Copyright © 2015, 2011, 2006, 1996 by Saunders, an imprint of Elsevier Inc. All rights reserved.

Hip: AP Frogleg Projection (Modified Cleaves Method)

52. Identify the labeled anatomy in Figure 7-19.

Figure 7-19

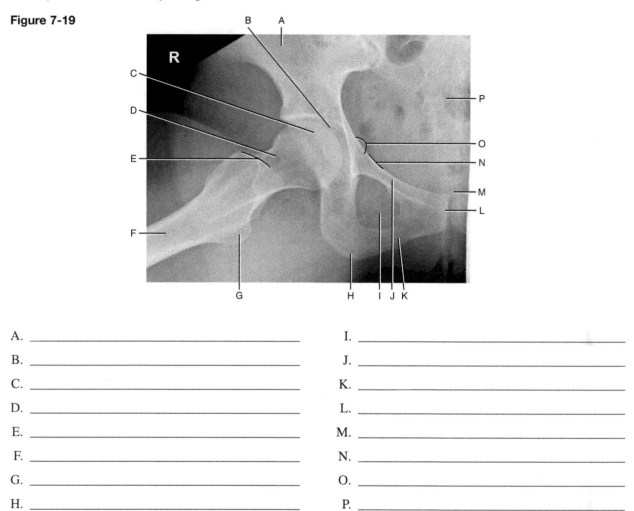

A. _____   I. _____

B. _____   J. _____

C. _____   K. _____

D. _____   L. _____

E. _____   M. _____

F. _____   N. _____

G. _____   O. _____

H. _____   P. _____

53. Complete the statements below referring to the AP frogleg hip projection analysis guidelines.

> **AP Frogleg (Modified Cleaves Method) Hip Projection Analysis Guidelines**
>
> - The (A) _Ischial spine_ is aligned with the pelvic brim, the sacrum and coccyx are aligned with the symphysis pubis, and the obturator foramen is open.
> - The (B) _lesser trochanter_ is in profile medially, and the (C) ___Femoral neck___ is superimposed over the greater trochanter.
> - The (D) ___femoral neck___ is partially foreshortened, and the proximal (E) _greater trochanter_ is demonstrated at a transverse level halfway between the femoral head and the lesser trochanter.

Copyright © 2015, 2011, 2006, 1996 by Saunders, an imprint of Elsevier Inc. All rights reserved.

Chapter **7** **Image Analysis of the Hip and Pelvis**

54. For the Lauenstein and Hickey lateral hip methods, the patient's pelvis is rotated (A) _____ (toward/ away from) the affected hip until the femur is placed (B) _____.

55. The degree of patient knee and hip flexion determines whether or not the greater and lesser trochanter will be in

_____.

56. At what degree with the imaging table is the femur placed to accurately position the greater and lesser trochanters on an AP frogleg hip projection? _____

57. The degree of femoral abduction for an AP frogleg hip projection will determine what two proximal femur anatomic relationships?

A. _____

B. _____

58. Describe the position of the greater trochanter and the degree of femoral neck foreshortening demonstrated on a AP frogleg hip projection if the femur is abducted as stated for each of the following:

A. The femur is abducted until it is placed next to the imaging table:

_____

B. The femur is abducted to a 45-degree angle with the imaging table:

_____

C. The femur is abducted 20 to 30 degrees from vertical:

_____

59. Accurate CR centering on an AP frogleg hip projection is accomplished by centering a(n) (A) _____ CR

(B) _____ inches distal to the midpoint of a line connecting the (C) _____ and symphysis pubis.

60. What anatomic structures are included on an AP frogleg hip projection with accurate positioning?

_____

For the following descriptions of AP frogleg hip projections with poor positioning, state how the patient would have been mispositioned for such a projection to be obtained.

61. The ischial spine is demonstrated without pelvic brim superimposition, the sacrum and coccyx are not aligned with the symphysis pubis but are rotated away from the affected hip, and the obturator foramen is narrowed.

_____

62. The greater trochanter is positioned medially, and the lesser trochanter is obscured.
    Knee flexed more than needed

63. The greater trochanter is positioned laterally.
    Knee not flexed enough

64. The femoral neck is demonstrated on end, and the greater trochanter is demonstrated on the same transverse level as the femoral head.

_____

   Copyright © 2015, 2011, 2006, 1996 by Saunders, an imprint of Elsevier Inc. All rights reserved.

For the following AP frogleg hip projections with poor positioning, state what anatomic structures are misaligned and how the patient should be repositioned for an optimal projection to be obtained.

Figure 7-20

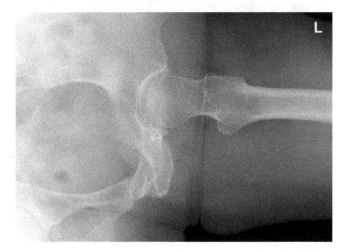

65. (Figure 7-20): *Sacrum & coccyx rotated toward the right hip & left foramen narrowed. Fix: rotate pt. away from affected hip*

Figure 7-21

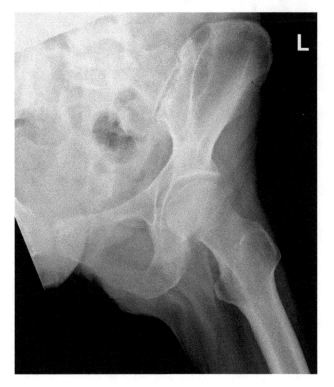

66. (Figure 7-21): _____

_____

_____

_____

Copyright © 2015, 2011, 2006, 1996 by Saunders, an imprint of Elsevier Inc. All rights reserved.

Figure 7-22

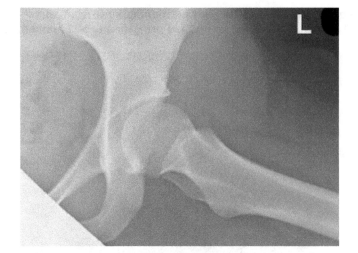

67. (Figure 7-22): _____
_____
_____
_____

Figure 7-23

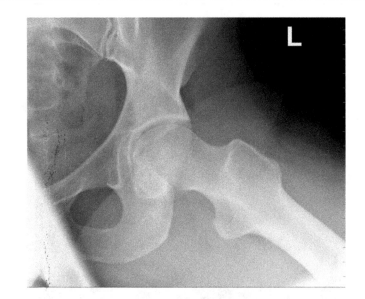

68. (Figure 7-23): _____
_____
_____
_____

Copyright © 2015, 2011, 2006, 1996 by Saunders, an imprint of Elsevier Inc. All rights reserved.

Figure 7-24

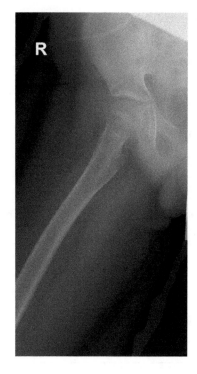

69. (Figure 7-24): _____

_____

_____

_____

Hip: Axiolateral (Inferosuperior) Projection (Danelius-Miller Method)

70. Identify the labeled anatomy in Figure 7-25.

Figure 7-25

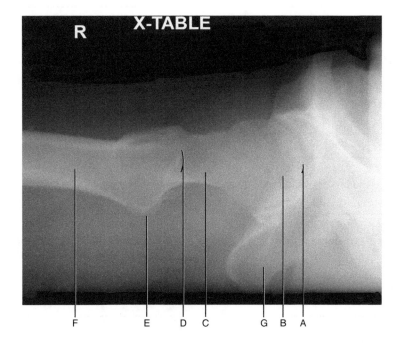

A. _____

B. _____

C. _____

D. _____

E. _____

F. _____

G. _____

Copyright © 2015, 2011, 2006, 1996 by Saunders, an imprint of Elsevier Inc. All rights reserved.

71. Complete the statements below referring to axiolateral hip projection analysis guidelines.

> **Axiolateral Hip Projection Analysis Guidelines**
>
> ■ The femoral neck is demonstrated without foreshortening, and the (A) _greater & lesser_ are demonstrated at approximately the same level.
>
> ■ The lesser trochanter is in profile (B) _posteriorly_, and the greater trochanter is superimposed by the (C) _femoral shaft_.

72. State three ways that the amount of scatter radiation reaching the IR can be reduced on an axiolateral hip projection.

A. _tight collimation_

B. _flat lead strip_

C. _grid_

73. How is the unaffected leg positioned for an axiolateral hip projection to prevent its soft tissue from superimposing the affected hip?

_____

74. Where is the grid-IR placed for an axiolateral hip projection?

A. _____

How is it aligned with the femoral neck?

B. _____

How is the position of the grid-IR changed if the patient has a large amount of lateral soft tissue thickness?

C. _____

How should the CR be positioned with respect to the IR and femoral neck?

D. _____

75. Describe how to localize the femoral neck when positioning for an axiolateral hip projection.

center between ASIS & symphysis, then distally 2.5"

76. Describe the appearance of the femoral neck and greater trochanter if the CR is too large to accurately align it with the femoral neck for an axiolateral hip projection.

A. Femoral neck: _____

B. Greater trochanter: _____

77. How is the leg positioned to accurately place the lesser trochanter on an axiolateral hip projection?

_____

78. On an axiolateral hip projection with accurate positioning, the _____ is centered within the collimated field.

79. What anatomic structures are included on an axiolateral hip projection with accurate positioning?

_____

Copyright © 2015, 2011, 2006, 1996 by Saunders, an imprint of Elsevier Inc. All rights reserved.

For the following descriptions of axiolateral hip projections with poor positioning, state how the patient or CR would have been mispositioned for such a projection to be obtained.

80. The soft tissue from the unaffected thigh is superimposed over the acetabulum and femoral head of the affected hip.

_____

81. The greater trochanter is demonstrated at a transverse level that is proximal to the lesser trochanter, and the femoral neck is partially foreshortened.

_____

82. The greater trochanter is demonstrated posteriorly, and the lesser trochanter is superimposed over the femoral shaft.

_____

For the following axiolateral hip projections with poor positioning, state what anatomic structures are misaligned and how the patient or CR should be repositioned for an optimal projection to be obtained.

Figure 7-26

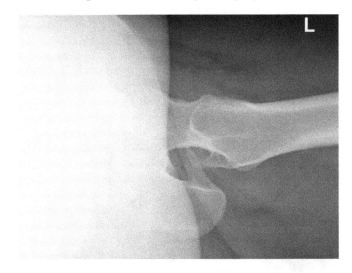

83. (Figure 7-26): _____

_____

_____

_____

_____

Copyright © 2015, 2011, 2006, 1996 by Saunders, an imprint of Elsevier Inc. All rights reserved.

Figure 7-27

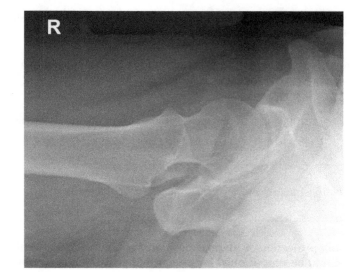

84. (Figure 7-27): _____

_____

_____

_____

Figure 7-28

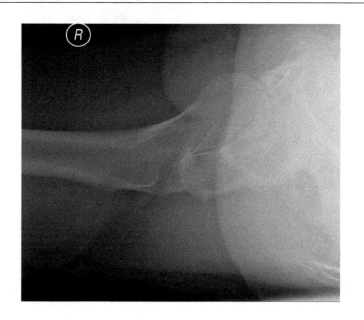

85. (Figure 7-28): _____

_____

_____

_____

              Copyright © 2015, 2011, 2006, 1996 by Saunders, an imprint of Elsevier Inc. All rights reserved.

Figure 7-29

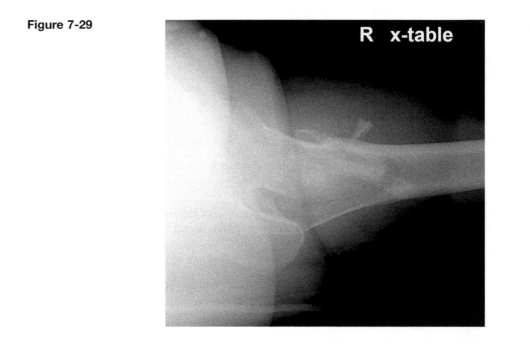

R x-table

86. (Figure 7-29, fracture): _____

_____

_____

_____

Sacroiliac Joints: AP Axial Projection

87. Identify the labeled anatomy in Figure 7-30.

Figure 7-30

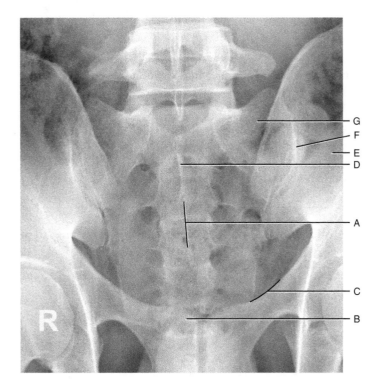

A. _____

B. _____

C. _____

D. _____

E. _____

F. _____

G. _____

Copyright © 2015, 2011, 2006, 1996 by Saunders, an imprint of Elsevier Inc. All rights reserved.

88. Complete the statements below referring to AP axial sacroiliac joints projection analysis guidelines.

AP Axial Sacroiliac Joints Projection Analysis Guidelines

■ The median sacral crest is aligned with the (A) _____, and the sacrum is at equal distance from the lateral wall of the pelvic brim on both sides.

■ The sacroiliac joints are demonstrated without foreshortening, and the sacrum is elongated, with the

(B) _____ superimposed over the inferior sacral segments.

---

89. When a patient is rotated for an AP axial sacroiliac joint projection, the sacrum rotates in the (A) _____ (same/opposite) direction as the symphysis pubis and is positioned next to the lateral wall of the pelvic brim situated

(B) _____ (closer/farther) to/from the IR.

90. How are the patient and CR positioned to demonstrate the sacroiliac joints without foreshortening?

   A. For a male patient: _____

   B. For a female patient: _____

   C. For a patient with greater than average lumbosacral curvature: _____

   D. For a patient with less than average lumbosacral curvature: _____

91. Why is the median sacral crest aligned with the long axis of the collimated field for an AP axial sacroiliac joint projection?

   A. _____

   B. _____

92. Accurate CR centering on an AP axial sacroiliac joint projection is obtained by positioning the CR to the patient's

   (A) _____ plane at a level halfway between an imaginary line connecting the (B) _____

   and (C) _____.

93. What anatomic structures are included on an AP axial sacroiliac joint projection with accurate positioning?

   _____

For the following descriptions of sacroiliac joint projections with poor positioning, state how the patient or CR would have been mispositioned for such a projection to be obtained.

94. The sacrum is situated closer to the right pelvic brim than to the left.

   _____

95. The sacroiliac joints are foreshortened, and the inferior sacrum is demonstrated without symphysis pubis superimposition.

   _____

Copyright © 2015, 2011, 2006, 1996 by Saunders, an imprint of Elsevier Inc. All rights reserved.

For the following sacroiliac joint projections with poor positioning, state what anatomic structures are misaligned and how the patient should be repositioned for an optimal projection to be obtained.

Figure 7-31

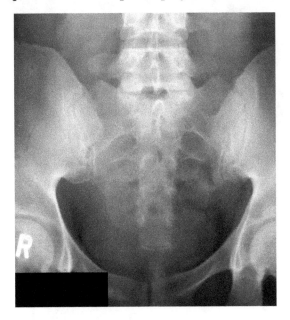

96. (Figure 7-31): _____

_____

_____

_____

Figure 7-32

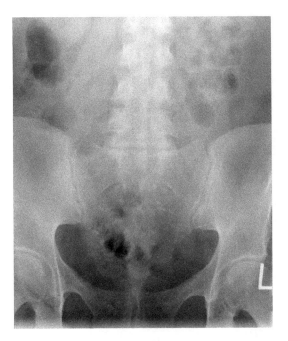

97. (Figure 7-32): _____

_____

_____

_____

Copyright © 2015, 2011, 2006, 1996 by Saunders, an imprint of Elsevier Inc. All rights reserved.

Chapter **7** **Image Analysis of the Hip and Pelvis**

Figure 7-33

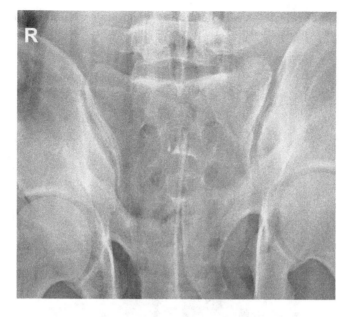

98. (Figure 7-33): _____

_____

_____

Sacroiliac Joints: AP Oblique Projection (LPO and RPO Positions)

99. Identify the labeled anatomy in Figure 7-34.

Figure 7-34

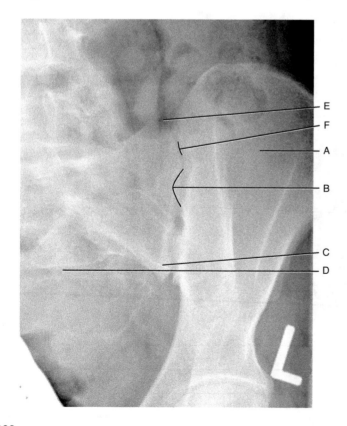

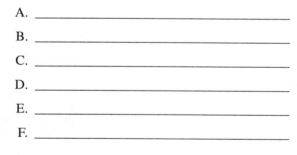

A. _____

B. _____

C. _____

D. _____

E. _____

F. _____

Copyright © 2015, 2011, 2006, 1996 by Saunders, an imprint of Elsevier Inc. All rights reserved.

100. Complete the statements below referring to AP oblique sacroiliac joint projection analysis guidelines.

> **AP Oblique Sacroiliac Joints Projection Analysis Guidelines**
>
> ■ The ilium and (A) _____ are demonstrated without superimposition, and the sacroiliac joint is open.
>
> ■ The long axis of the sacroiliac joint is aligned with the (B) _____ of the exposure field.

101. What two bony structures articulate to form the sacroiliac joints?

    A. _____

    B. _____

102. For an open sacroiliac joint to be obtained on an AP oblique sacroiliac joint projection, the patient is rotated until the (A) _____ plane is at a (B) _____-degree angle with the IR.

103. Which sacroiliac joint is open when the patient is placed in an LPO position?

    _____

104. The affected sacroiliac joint is centered within the collimated field on an AP oblique sacroiliac joint projection with accurate positioning. This centering is obtained by placing the CR 1 inch (A) _____ (medial/lateral) to the elevated (B) _____.

105. What anatomic structures are included on an AP oblique sacroiliac joint projection with accurate positioning?

    _____

    _____

For the following descriptions of AP oblique sacroiliac joint projections with poor positioning, state how the patient would have been mispositioned for such a projection to be obtained.

106. The sacroiliac joint is closed, the superior and inferior sacral ala are demonstrated without iliac superimposition, and the lateral sacral ala is superimposed over the iliac tuberosity.

    _____

107. The sacroiliac joint is closed, and the ilium is superimposed over the lateral sacral ala and inferior sacrum.

    _____

Copyright © 2015, 2011, 2006, 1996 by Saunders, an imprint of Elsevier Inc. All rights reserved.

For the following sacroiliac joint projections with poor positioning, state what anatomic structures are misaligned and how the patient should be repositioned for an optimal projection to be obtained.

Figure 7-35

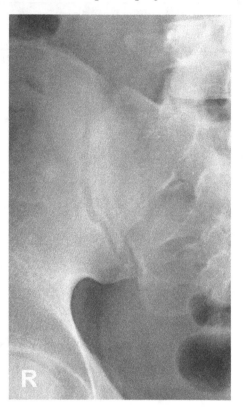

108. (Figure 7-35): _____

_____

_____

_____

_____

Copyright © 2015, 2011, 2006, 1996 by Saunders, an imprint of Elsevier Inc. All rights reserved.

Figure 7-36

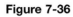

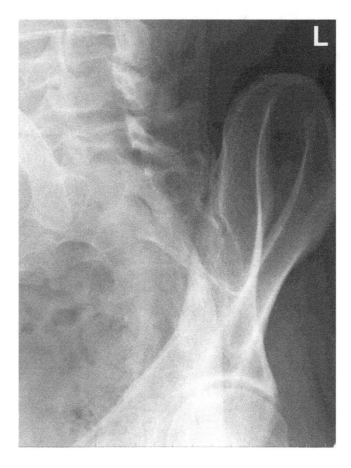

109. (Figure 7-36): _____

_____

_____

_____

Copyright © 2015, 2011, 2006, 1996 by Saunders, an imprint of Elsevier Inc. All rights reserved.

STUDY QUESTIONS

1. Complete Figure 8-1.

   Figure 8-1

Cervical and Thoracic Vertebrae Technical Data					
Projection	kV	Grid	AEC	mAs	SID
AP axial, cervical vertebrae					
AP, open-mouth, C1 and C2					
Lateral, cervical vertebrae					
PA or AP axial oblique, cervical vertebrae					
Lateral (Twining method), cervicothoracic vertebrae					
AP, thoracic vertebrae					
Lateral, thoracic vertebrae					
Pediatric					

Chapter **8** **Image Analysis of the Cervical and Thoracic Vertebrae**   Copyright © 2015, 2011, 2006, 1996 by Saunders, an imprint of Elsevier Inc. All rights reserved.

Cervical Vertebrae: AP Axial Projection

2. Identify the labeled anatomy in Figure 8-2.

Figure 8-2

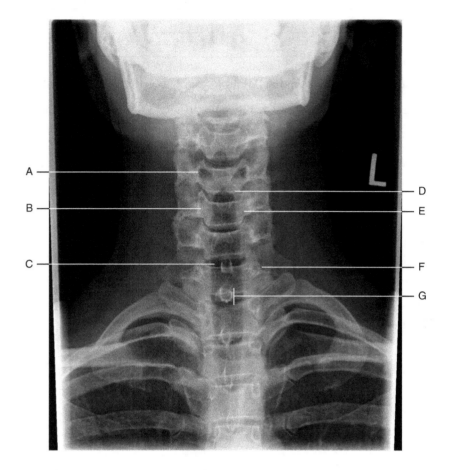

A. _____

B. _____

C. _____

D. _____

E. _____

F. _____

G. _____

3. Complete the statements below referring to AP axial cervical vertebrae projection analysis guidelines.

AP Axial Cervical Vertebrae Projection Analysis Guidelines

- The (A) _____ are aligned with the midline of the cervical bodies, the mandibular angles and mastoid tips are at equal distances from the cervical vertebrae, the articular pillars and pedicles are symmetrically visualized (B) _____ to the cervical bodies, and the distance from the vertebral column to the medial clavicular ends are equal.

- The intervertebral disk spaces are open, the vertebral bodies are demonstrated without distortion, and each vertebra's spinous process is visualized at the level of its (C) _____ intervertebral disk space.

- The third cervical vertebra is demonstrated in its entirety, and the occipital base and mandibular mentum are (D) _____.

Copyright © 2015, 2011, 2006, 1996 by Saunders, an imprint of Elsevier Inc. All rights reserved.

Chapter **8 Image Analysis of the Cervical and Thoracic Vertebrae**

4. How is the patient positioned for an AP cervical projection to prevent rotation of the upper and lower cervical vertebrae?

   A. Upper: *mandibular angles & mastoid tips equal distances from the IR*

   B. Lower: *shoulders equal distances from IR*

   _____

5. When the patient and cervical vertebrae are rotated away from the AP projection, the vertebral bodies will move toward the side positioned (A) _____ (closer to/farther from) the IR, and the spinous processes will move toward the side positioned (B) _____ (closer to/farther from) the IR.

6. Will rotation on an AP cervical projection with poor positioning always be demonstrated throughout the entire cervical column?

   A. _____ (Yes/No)

   Explain your answer.

   B. _____

   _____

7. A patient wearing a collar and on a backboard is taken to the radiography department for a cervical vertebrae series. Should the collar be removed before the radiographs are taken?

   A. _____ (Yes/No)

   The patient's head is rotated. Should it be adjusted?

   B. _____ (Yes/No)

   Explain your answers to parts A and B.

   C. _____

   _____

8. What is the curvature of the cervical vertebral column?

   lordotic

9. How do the intervertebral disk spaces slant on the cervical vertebrae?

   A. _____

   Is the degree of slant higher when the patient is upright or supine?

   B. _____

   What CR angulation is used for an AP cervical projection in a supine patient?

   C. _____

   In an upright patient?

   D. _____

   What causes this difference?

   E. _____

 Copyright © 2015, 2011, 2006, 1996 by Saunders, an imprint of Elsevier Inc. All rights reserved.

10. If the CR angulation is not adequately angled for an AP cervical projection, the intervertebral disk spaces are (A) _____ and each vertebra's spinous process is demonstrated within (B) _____

    _____.

11. Where is each vertebra's spinous process demonstrated if the CR angulation is too cephalad?

    _____

12. Does too much or too little cephalad angulation cause elongation of the uncinate processes on an AP cervical projection? _too much_

13. How is the patient positioned to demonstrate the third cervical vertebra in its entirety on an AP cervical projection with accurate positioning? _lower surface of the upper incisors_ _& tip of mastoid process ⊥ to IR_

14. Accurate CR centering on an AP cervical projection is obtained by placing the CR at the patient's (A) _____ plane at a level halfway between the (B) _____ and (C) _____.

15. What anatomic structures are demonstrated on an AP cervical projection with accurate positioning? _____

    _____

For the following descriptions of AP cervical projections with poor positioning, state how the patient or CR would have been mispositioned for such a projection to be obtained.

16. The spinous processes are not aligned with the midline of the cervical bodies, and the pedicles and articular pillars are not symmetrically demonstrated lateral to the vertebral bodies. The right mandibular angle is visible, the left mandibular angle is superimposed over the cervical vertebrae, and the medial end of the right clavicle is demonstrated without vertebral column superimposition.

    _____

17. The anteroinferior aspects of the cervical bodies are obscuring the intervertebral disk spaces, and each vertebra's spinous process is demonstrated within the vertebral body.

    _____

18. The posteroinferior aspects of the cervical bodies are obscuring the intervertebral disk spaces, the uncinate processes are elongated, and each vertebra's spinous process is demonstrated within the inferior adjoining vertebral body.

    _____

19. A portion of the third cervical vertebra is superimposed over the occipital bone.

    head was tilted too far back

    _____

20. The mandibular mentum is superimposed over a portion of the third cervical vertebra.

    _____

21. The upper cervical vertebra is tilted toward the left side.

    _____

    _____

Copyright © 2015, 2011, 2006, 1996 by Saunders, an imprint of Elsevier Inc. All rights reserved. Chapter **8** **Image Analysis of the Cervical and Thoracic Vertebrae**

For the following AP cervical projections with poor positioning, state what anatomic structures are misaligned and how the patient should be repositioned for an optimal projection to be obtained.

Figure 8-3

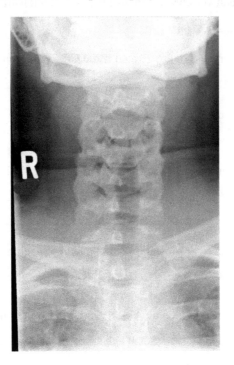

22. (Figure 8-3): _____

_____

_____

_____

Figure 8-4

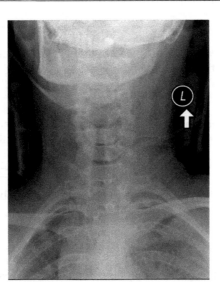

23. (Figure 8-4): <u>pt. rotated (sc. joints not equal), face</u>
<u>towards right.</u>
<u>fix: make shoulders equal distance from IR &</u>
<u>rotate face back straight</u>

Chapter **8 Image Analysis of the Cervical and Thoracic Vertebrae**   Copyright © 2015, 2011, 2006, 1996 by Saunders, an imprint of Elsevier Inc. All rights reserved.

Figure 8-5

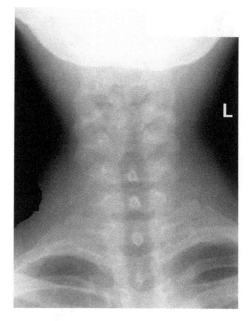

24. (Figure 8-5): _____

_____

_____

_____

Figure 8-6

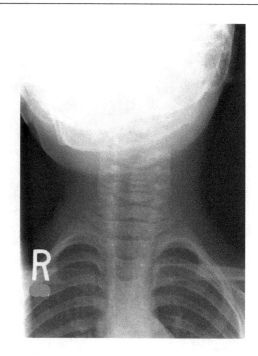

25. (Figure 8-6): _____

_____

_____

_____

Copyright © 2015, 2011, 2006, 1996 by Saunders, an imprint of Elsevier Inc. All rights reserved.   Chapter **8 Image Analysis of the Cervical and Thoracic Vertebrae**

Figure 8-7

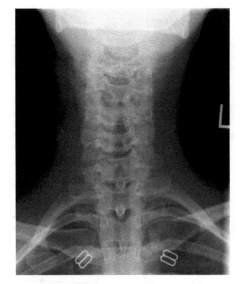

26. (Figure 8-7): _Spinous processes are too low - going into the vertebral body of the one below. Bra clips. fix: decrease amount of cephalic CR angle._

Figure 8-8

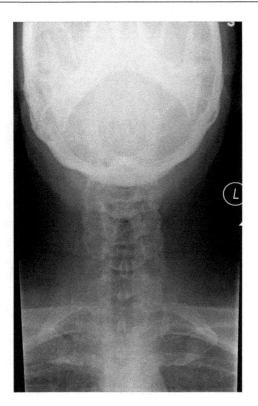

27. (Figure 8-8): _____

_____

_____

_____

Chapter **8 Image Analysis of the Cervical and Thoracic Vertebrae**   Copyright © 2015, 2011, 2006, 1996 by Saunders, an imprint of Elsevier Inc. All rights reserved.

Figure 8-9

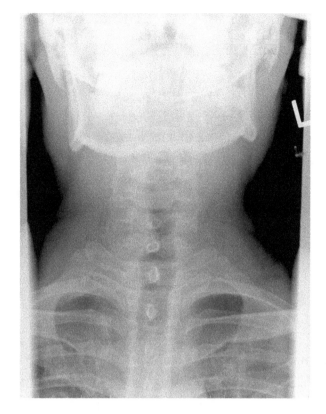

28. (Figure 8-9): _____

_____

_____

_____

Cervical Atlas and Axis: AP Projection (Open Mouth)

29. Identify the labeled anatomy in Figure 8-10.

Figure 8-10

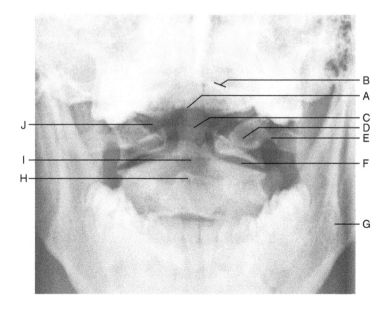

A. _____

B. _____

C. _____

D. _____

E. _____

F. _____

G. _____

H. _____

I. _____

J. _____

371

Copyright © 2015, 2011, 2006, 1996 by Saunders, an imprint of Elsevier Inc. All rights reserved.

30. Complete the statements below referring to AP cervical atlas and axis vertebrae projection analysis guidelines.

AP Cervical Atlas and Axis Projection Analysis Guidelines

- Atlas is symmetrically seated on the (A)_____, with the atlas's lateral masses at equal distances from the (B) _____.

- The spinous processes of the axis is aligned with the midline of the (C) _____ body, and the mandibular rami are visualized at equal distances from the (D) _____.

- The upper incisors and the occipital base are seen (E) _____ to the dens and the atlantoaxial joint.

- The atlantoaxial joint is (F) _____ .

---

31. How is the patient positioned to obtain an AP projection of the atlas and axis without rotation?

_____

_____

32. On head rotation, the atlas pivots around the dens. This results in the lateral mass located on the side toward which the face is turned being displaced (A) _____ (anteriorly/posteriorly), and the side away from which the face is turned being displaced (B) _____ (anteriorly/posteriorly).

33. How is the patient positioned for an AP projection of the atlas and axis to demonstrate the upper incisor and occipital base superior to the dens and atlantoaxial joint?

A. _align lower upper incisors and the tip of_
the mastoid ⊥ to IR

How is a patient without upper teeth positioned?

B. _imagine they have teeth & line up the_
same as if they had teeth

34. Why is it necessary to use a 5-degree cephalic CR angulation on an AP atlas and axis projection? _____

_____

35. Describe how to determine the CR angulation to use for an AP atlas and axis projection on a trauma patient in a collar.

_____

_____

36. How can one determine from an AP atlas or axis projection that the neck was in flexion for the projection?

A. _joint closed + spinous process extremely superior to dens_

That it was in extension for the projection?

B. _joint closed + spinous process extremely inferior to dens_

Copyright © 2015, 2011, 2006, 1996 by Saunders, an imprint of Elsevier Inc. All rights reserved.

37. Accurate CR centering on an AP atlas and axis projection is accomplished by centering the CR through the open mouth to the __MSP__.

38. What anatomic structures are included on an AP atlas and axis projection with accurate positioning?

_____

_____

For the following descriptions of AP atlas and axis cervical projections with poor positioning, state how the patient or CR would have been mispositioned for such a projection to be obtained.

39. The distances from the atlas's lateral masses to the dens and from the mandibular rami to the dens are narrower on the right side of the patient than on the left side, and the axis's spinous process is shifted from the midline.

_____

40. The upper incisors are demonstrated approximately 1 inch (2.5 cm) inferior to the occipital base, obscuring the dens and atlantoaxial joint, and the occipital base is demonstrated directly superior to the dens.

_____

41. The upper incisors are superimposed over the dens, and the occipital base is demonstrated superior to the dens and upper incisors. A 5-degree cephalic angulation was used to obtain this projection.

A. Patient: _____

_____

B. CR: _____

42. The dens is superimposed over the occiput, and the upper incisors are demonstrated approximately 2 inches (5 cm) superior to the occipital base.

A. Patient: _____

_____

B. CR: _____

Copyright © 2015, 2011, 2006, 1996 by Saunders, an imprint of Elsevier Inc. All rights reserved. Chapter **8** **Image Analysis of the Cervical and Thoracic Vertebrae**

For the following AP atlas and axis cervical projections with poor positioning, state what anatomic structures are misaligned and how the patient should be repositioned for an optimal projection to be obtained.

Figure 8-11

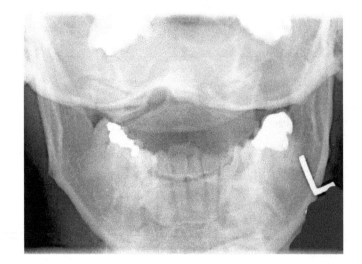

43. (Figure 8-11): _____

_____

_____

_____

Figure 8-12

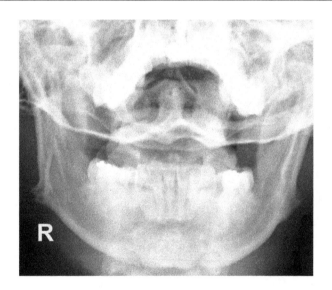

44. (Figure 8-12): _____

_____

_____

_____

Chapter **8 Image Analysis of the Cervical and Thoracic Vertebrae**   Copyright © 2015, 2011, 2006, 1996 by Saunders, an imprint of Elsevier Inc. All rights reserved.

Figure 8-13

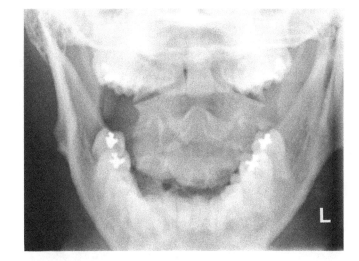

45. (Figure 8-13): _____

_____

_____

_____

Figure 8-14

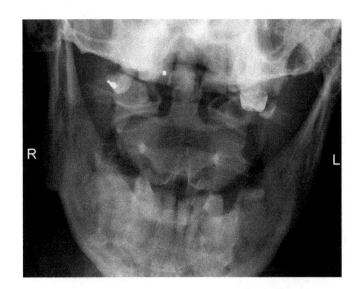

46. (Figure 8-14): _____

_____

_____

_____

Copyright © 2015, 2011, 2006, 1996 by Saunders, an imprint of Elsevier Inc. All rights reserved. Chapter **8 Image Analysis of the Cervical and Thoracic Vertebrae**

Figure 8-15

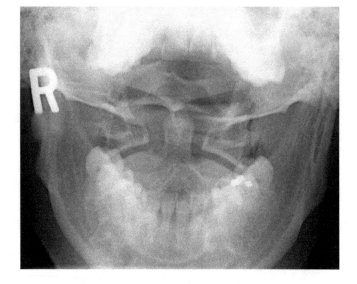

47. Figure 8-15 was taken with the patient in a cervical collar:

    upper incisors too superior to dens, occipital
    bone obsuring dens
    fix: realigned upper incisors w/ base
        of skull

Cervical Vertebrae: Lateral Projection

48. Identify the labeled anatomy in Figure 8-16.

Figure 8-16

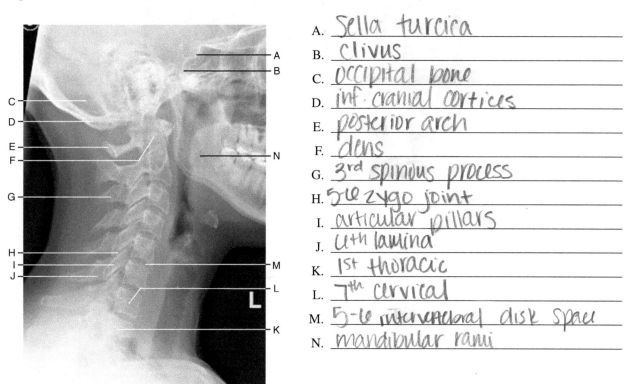

A. Sella turcica
B. clivus
C. occipital bone
D. inf. cranial cortices
E. posterior arch
F. dens
G. 3rd spinous process
H. 5 ½ zygo joint
I. articular pillars
J. 4th lamina
K. 1st thoracic
L. 7th cervical
M. 5-6 intervertebral disk space
N. mandibular rami

Chapter **8** **Image Analysis of the Cervical and Thoracic Vertebrae**   Copyright © 2015, 2011, 2006, 1996 by Saunders, an imprint of Elsevier Inc. All rights reserved.

49. Complete the statements below referring to lateral cervical vertebrae projection analysis guidelines.

Lateral Cervical Vertebrae Projection Analysis Guidelines
■ Contrast resolution is adequate to visualize the (A) _____ fat stripe.
■ The anterior and posterior aspects of the right and left articular pillars and the right and left zygapophyseal joints of each cervical vertebra are (B) _____, and the spinous processes are in (C) _____.
■ The posterior arch of C1 and spinous process of C2 are in profile without (D) _____ superimposition, and their bodies are seen without mandibular superimposition, the cranial cortices and the mandibular rami are (E) _____, the superior and inferior aspects of the right and left articular pillars and the (F) _____ of each cervical vertebra are superimposed, and the intervertebral disk spaces are open.

50. Why is a long SID used for the lateral cervical vertebrae?

_____

51. What body plane is positioned perpendicular to the IR for a lateral cervical projection? *midcoronal*

52. What anatomic structures are aligned with the IR to prevent rotation when positioning the patient for a lateral cervical projection? _____

53. How can rotation be identified on a lateral cervical projection with poor positioning?

_____

54. How must the patient's head be positioned for a lateral cervical projection to demonstrate the posterior arch of C1 and the spinous process of C2 in profile without occiput superimposition, and the bodies of C1 and C2 without mandibular rami superimposition?

AML ‖ to floor, elevate chin
IPL ⊥ to IR

55. How must the patient's head be positioned for a lateral cervical projection to superimpose the superior and inferior aspects of the right and left articular pillars and zygapophyseal joints?

_____

_____

56. What are two advantages of aligning the long axis of the cervical vertebral column with the long axis of the collimated field?

A. _____

B. _____

57. Why are lateral flexion and extension projections of the cervical vertebrae obtained?

_____

Copyright © 2015, 2011, 2006, 1996 by Saunders, an imprint of Elsevier Inc. All rights reserved.

58. How is patient positioning adjusted from a neutral lateral position of the cervical vertebrae to achieve a flexed lateral projection?

tuck chin as tight as they can to their chest

59. How is patient positioning adjusted from a neutral lateral position of the cervical vertebrae to achieve an extended lateral projection? *extend & raise chin as far back as possible*

60. Accurate CR centering on a lateral cervical projection is accomplished by centering the CR to the

(A) _____ plane at a level halfway between the (B) _____ and (C) _____.

61. What anatomic structures are included on a lateral cervical projection with accurate positioning?

_____

_____

62. Why should the clivus be included on all lateral cervical projections?

_____

_____

63. It is often difficult to demonstrate C7 on a routine lateral cervical projection because of shoulder thickness. How should the patient be positioned to improve C7 demonstration?

A. _____

B. _____

C. _____

64. What special projection can be taken to demonstrate C7 when the procedures referred to in the previous question fail? _____

For the following descriptions of lateral cervical projections with poor positioning, state how the patient would have been mispositioned for such a projection to be obtained.

65. The articular pillars and zygapophyseal joints of one side of the patient are situated anterior to the opposite side's pillars and zygapophyseal joints.

_____

66. Neither the posterior nor the anterior cortices of the cranium nor the mandible is superimposed.

_____

67. The inferior cortices of the cranium and mandible are demonstrated without superimposition, and the vertebral foramen of C1 is demonstrated.

head was tilted toward IR

For the following lateral cervical projections with poor positioning, state what anatomic structures are misaligned and how the patient should be repositioned for an optimal projection to be obtained.

Figure 8-17

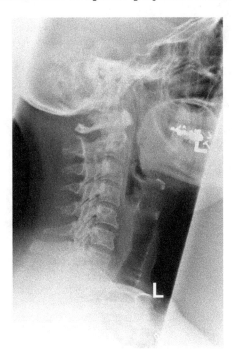

68. (Figure 8-17): ___pt. is rotated___

___fix: rotate back to place midcoronal___
___⊥ to IR___

Figure 8-18

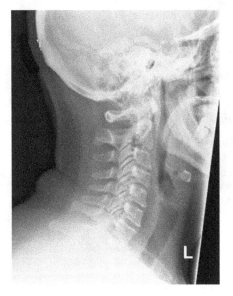

69. (Figure 8-18): _____

_____

_____

_____

Copyright © 2015, 2011, 2006, 1996 by Saunders, an imprint of Elsevier Inc. All rights reserved.
Chapter **8** **Image Analysis of the Cervical and Thoracic Vertebrae**

Figure 8-19

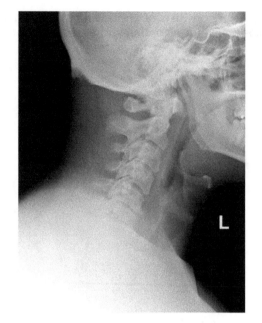

70. (Figure 8-19): _____

_____

_____

_____

Figure 8-20

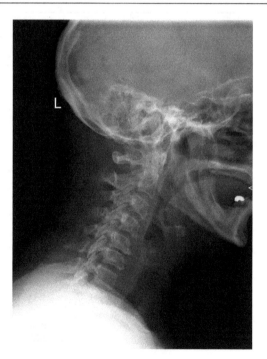

71. (Figure 8-20): _____

_____

_____

_____

Chapter **8 Image Analysis of the Cervical and Thoracic Vertebrae**   Copyright © 2015, 2011, 2006, 1996 by Saunders, an imprint of Elsevier Inc. All rights reserved.

Cervical Vertebrae: PA/AP Axial Oblique Projection (Anterior and Posterior Oblique Positions)

72. Identify the labeled anatomy in Figure 8-21.

Figure 8-21

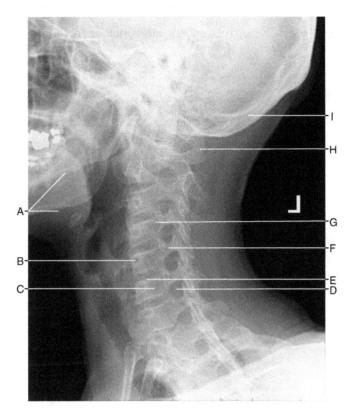

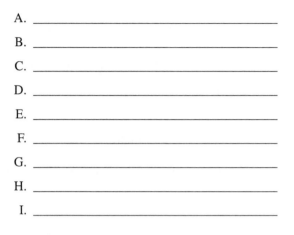

A. _____

B. _____

C. _____

D. _____

E. _____

F. _____

G. _____

H. _____

I. _____

73. Complete the statements below referring to PA/AP axial oblique cervical vertebrae projection analysis guidelines.

PA/AP Axial Oblique Cervical Vertebrae Projection Analysis Guidelines
■ The second through (A) _____ intervertebral foramina are open, demonstrating uniform size and shape, the pedicles of interest are shown in (B) _____, and the opposite pedicles are aligned with the (C) _____ vertebral bodies.
■ The intervertebral disk spaces are open, the cervical bodies are seen as individual structures and are uniform in shape, and the posterior arch of the atlas is seen without foreshortening, demonstrating the (D) _____.

74. Why is a long SID used for AP axial oblique cervical projections?

_____

Copyright © 2015, 2011, 2006, 1996 by Saunders, an imprint of Elsevier Inc. All rights reserved.

Chapter **8 Image Analysis of the Cervical and Thoracic Vertebrae**

75. Why is it not necessary to use a grid even though a high kilovolt-peak (kVp) level is used for AP axial oblique cervical projections?

_____

_____

76. For the following oblique cervical projections, state whether the right or left intervertebral foramina will be demonstrated.

A. Right PA axial oblique (RAO position): __right_____

B. Left AP axial oblique (LPO position): __right_____

C. Left PA axial oblique (LAO position): __left_____

D. Right AP axial oblique (RPO position): __left_____

77. What degree of body rotation is used for oblique cervical projections? _____

78. What body plane is used to set up the degree of obliquity? _____

79. Describe how to position the IR beneath a trauma patient to demonstrate the right intervertebral foramina for an AP axial oblique cervical projection.

A. _____

How is the CR angled and positioned?

B. _____

80. What degree and direction of CR angulation are used for PA axial oblique cervical projections?

A. ____15-20° caudal_____

For AP axial oblique cervical projections?

B. ____15-20° cephalic_____

Why is it necessary to use an angled CR for oblique cervical projections?

C. ____to open up disk spaces_____

81. How should the patient be positioned to demonstrate the alignment of the right and left posterior cranium and mandible cortices and to demonstrate the upper cervical vertebrae without occipital or mandibular superimposition?

_____

_____

82. How should the CR be adjusted from the routinely used angle for a PA axial oblique cervical vertebrae projection in a patient who has severe kyphosis to better demonstrate the lower cervical vertebrae?

_____

_____

83. Which cranial and mandibular cortices will be demonstrated inferiorly on a right PA axial oblique cervical projection?

A. _____

Chapter **8** **Image Analysis of the Cervical and Thoracic Vertebrae**   Copyright © 2015, 2011, 2006, 1996 by Saunders, an imprint of Elsevier Inc. All rights reserved.

On a left AP axial oblique cervical projection?

B. _____

What aspect of the positioning setup causes these cortices to be projected one superior to the other?

C. _____

_____

84. Accurate CR centering on a PA axial oblique cervical projection is accomplished by centering the CR to the

(A) _____ plane at a level halfway between the (B) _____ and

(C)_____.

85. What anatomic structures are included on PA/AP axial oblique cervical projections with accurate positioning?

_____

_____

_____

For the following descriptions of PA/AP axial oblique cervical projections with poor positioning, state how the patient or CR would have been mispositioned for such a projection to be obtained.

86. A left PA axial oblique (LAO) cervical projection, obtained with the patient's head in an oblique position, demonstrates obscured pedicles and intervertebral foramina, and the vertebral column is superimposed over a portion of the left sternoclavicular joint and medial clavicular end.

_____

87. A right PA axial oblique (RAO) cervical projection, obtained with the patient's head in a lateral position, demonstrates the intervertebral foramina, the right pedicles (although they are not in true profile), the left pedicles in the midline of the vertebral bodies, and the right zygapophyseal joints.

_____

88. A left PA axial oblique (LAO) cervical projection, the intervertebral disk spaces are closed, the vertebral bodies are distorted, the posterior tubercles are demonstrated within the vertebral foramina, the C1 vertebral foramen is not demonstrated, and the inferior mandibular rami and the cranial cortices are demonstrated with superimposition.

_____

_____

89. The upper cervical vertebrae are obscured by the patient's cranium and mandible.

_____

90. The atlas and its posterior arch are obscured. The inferior cranial cortices demonstrate more than 1/4 inch (0.6 cm) of distance between them, and the inferior cortices of the mandibular rami demonstrate more than 1/2 inch (1.25 cm) of distance between them.

_____

Copyright © 2015, 2011, 2006, 1996 by Saunders, an imprint of Elsevier Inc. All rights reserved. Chapter **8 Image Analysis of the Cervical and Thoracic Vertebrae**

For the following PA/AP axial oblique cervical projections with poor positioning, state what anatomic structures are misaligned and how the patient should be repositioned for such a projection to be obtained.

Figure 8-22

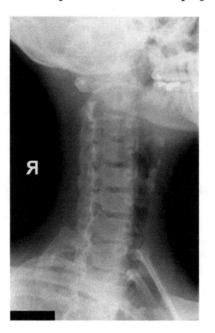

91. (Figure 8-22): _____

_____

_____

_____

_____

_____

Figure 8-23

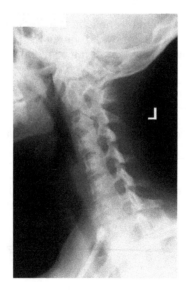

92. (Figure 8-23): _____

_____

_____

Chapter **8** **Image Analysis of the Cervical and Thoracic Vertebrae**   Copyright © 2015, 2011, 2006, 1996 by Saunders, an imprint of Elsevier Inc. All rights reserved.

Figure 8-24

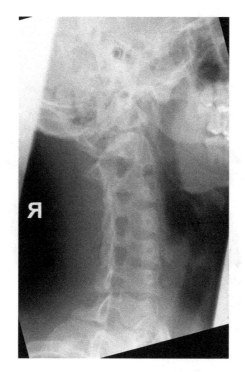

93. (Figure 8-24): _____

_____

_____

Figure 8-25

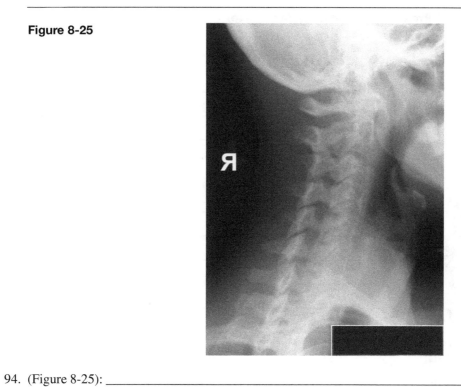

94. (Figure 8-25): _____

_____

_____

Copyright © 2015, 2011, 2006, 1996 by Saunders, an imprint of Elsevier Inc. All rights reserved. Chapter **8 Image Analysis of the Cervical and Thoracic Vertebrae**

Figure 8-26

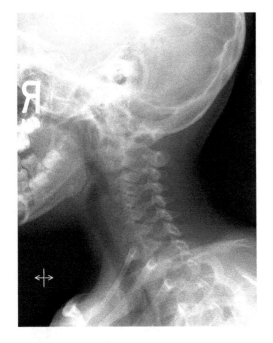

95. (Figure 8-26): _____

_____

_____

_____

Cervicothoracic Vertebrae: Lateral Projection (Swimmer's Technique)

96. Identify the labeled anatomy in Figure 8-27.

Figure 8-27

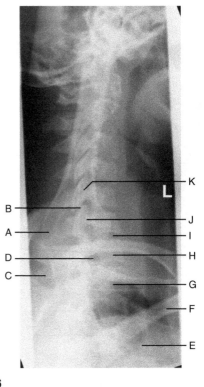

A. _____

B. _____

C. _____

D. _____

E. _____

F. _____

G. _____

H. _____

I. _____

J. _____

K. _____

Chapter **8 Image Analysis of the Cervical and Thoracic Vertebrae**   Copyright © 2015, 2011, 2006, 1996 by Saunders, an imprint of Elsevier Inc. All rights reserved.

97. Complete the statements below referring to lateral cervicothoracic vertebrae projection analysis guidelines.

> **Lateral Cervicothoracic Vertebrae Projection Analysis Guidelines**
>
> ■ The right and left cervical zygapophyseal joints (A) _____, and the posterior ribs are superimposed.
>
> ■ The humerus elevated above the patient's head is aligned with the (B) _____.
>
> ■ The intervertebral disk spaces are (C) _____.

98. List two situations in which a cervicothoracic lateral projection would be indicated.

    A. _____

    B. _____

99. What respiration is used for the cervicothoracic lateral projection? _expiration_

100. To obtain a cervicothoracic lateral projection, how is the arm adjacent to the IR positioned?

    A. _arm elevated above head_

    How is the arm situated farther from the IR positioned?

    B. _arm @ side_

101. How is the patient positioned to prevent rotation on a lateral cervicothoracic projection?

    A. Cervical rotation: _____

    _____

    B. Thoracic rotation: _____

    _____

102. How can rotation be identified on a lateral cervicothoracic projection?

    _____

    _____

103. How is the patient positioned for a lateral cervicothoracic projection to demonstrate open intervertebral disk spaces and undistorted vertebral bodies?

    _____

    _____

104. Accurate CR centering on a lateral cervicothoracic projection is accomplished by centering a perpendicular CR to the (A) _____ plane at a level 1 inch (2.5 cm) superior to the (B) _____ or at the level of the (C) _____.

105. When should a 5-degree caudal CR angulation be used with the cervicothoracic lateral projection?

    _____

Copyright © 2015, 2011, 2006, 1996 by Saunders, an imprint of Elsevier Inc. All rights reserved. Chapter **8 Image Analysis of the Cervical and Thoracic Vertebrae**

106. What anatomic structures are included on a lateral cervicothoracic projection with accurate positioning?

_____

For the following descriptions of lateral cervicothoracic projections with poor positioning, state how the patient would have been mispositioned for such a projection to be obtained.

107. The right and left articular pillars, zygapophyseal joints, and posterior ribs are demonstrated without superimposition. The humerus that was raised and situated closer to the IR is demonstrated posterior to the vertebral column.

_____

108. The right and left articular pillars, zygapophyseal joints, and posterior ribs are demonstrated without superimposition. The humerus demonstrating the lesser amount of magnification is situated anterior to the vertebral column.

_____

109. The intervertebral disk spaces are closed, and the vertebral bodies are distorted.

_____

For the following lateral cervicothoracic projections with poor positioning, state what anatomic structures are misaligned and how the patient should be repositioned for an optimal projection to be obtained.

Figure 8-28

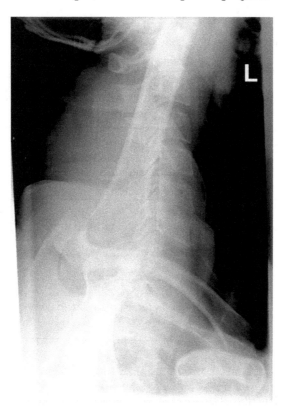

110. (Figure 8-28): _____

_____

_____

Chapter **8** **Image Analysis of the Cervical and Thoracic Vertebrae**   Copyright © 2015, 2011, 2006, 1996 by Saunders, an imprint of Elsevier Inc. All rights reserved.

Figure 8-29

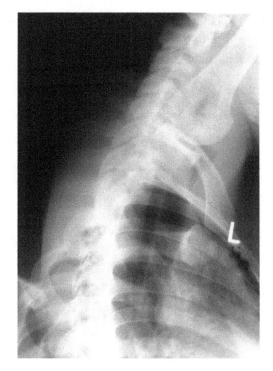

111. (Figure 8-29): _____

_____

_____

Thoracic Vertebrae: AP Projection

112. Identify the labeled anatomy in Figure 8-30.

Figure 8-30

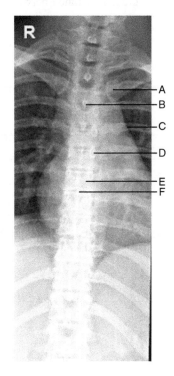

A. _____

B. _____

C. _____

D. _____

E. _____

F. _____

Copyright © 2015, 2011, 2006, 1996 by Saunders, an imprint of Elsevier Inc. All rights reserved.

113. Complete the statements below referring to AP thoracic vertebrae projection analysis guidelines.

AP Thoracic Vertebrae Projection Analysis Guidelines

- The spinous processes are aligned with the midline of the (A) _____, and the distances from the vertebral column to the sternal clavicular ends and from the pedicles to the (B) _____ _____ are equal on the two sides.

- The intervertebral disk spaces are (C) _____, and the vertebral bodies are seen without foreshortening.
---

114. How tightly can one safely collimate transversely on an AP projection of the thoracic vertebrae?

_____

115. How can the patient be positioned with respect to the x-ray tube for an AP thoracic projection to take advantage of the anode-heel effect?

_____

_____

116. What patient respiration is used for an AP thoracic projection to demonstrate the vertebrae and posterior ribs?

_____

117. How is the patient positioned to ensure that rotation will not be demonstrated on an AP thoracic projection?

place shoulders & ASISs equal distance
from the IR

118. When rotation is present on an AP thoracic projection, the side demonstrating the greater distance between the spinous processes and pedicles will be _____ (closer to/farther from) the IR.

119. What patient condition can simulate rotation on an AP thoracic projection?

A. _____

Describe how this condition can be distinguished from rotation.

B. _____

_____

120. What type of curvature does the thoracic vertebral column demonstrate?

A. _kyphotic_

How can the patient be positioned to reduce this curvature and better align the x-ray beams with the intervertebral disk spaces?

B. _head on small pillow & bend knees_
putting feet flat on table

 Copyright © 2015, 2011, 2006, 1996 by Saunders, an imprint of Elsevier Inc. All rights reserved.

121. Accurate CR centering on an AP thoracic projection is accomplished by centering the CR to the (A) _____ plane at a level halfway between the (B) _____ and xiphoid.

122. What anatomic structures are included on an AP thoracic projection with accurate positioning?

_____

For the following descriptions of AP thoracic projections with poor positioning, state how the patient would have been mispositioned for such a projection to be obtained.

123. The lower thoracic intervertebral disk spaces are obscured, and the vertebral bodies are distorted.

_____

124. The distance from the left pedicles to the spinous processes is greater than the distance from the right pedicles to the spinous processes.

_____

125. The upper thoracic vertebrae are overexposed, and the lower thoracic vertebrae demonstrate adequate brightness.

_____

For the following AP thoracic projections with poor positioning, state what anatomic structures are misaligned and how the patient should be repositioned for an optimal projection to be obtained.

Figure 8-31

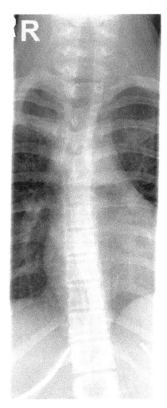

126. (Figure 8-31): _____

_____

_____

Copyright © 2015, 2011, 2006, 1996 by Saunders, an imprint of Elsevier Inc. All rights reserved.   Chapter **8 Image Analysis of the Cervical and Thoracic Vertebrae**

Figure 8-32

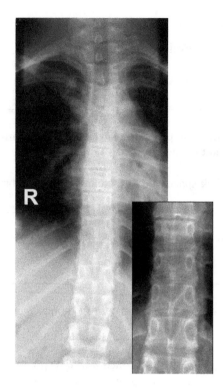

127. (Figure 8-32): _____

_____

Thoracic Vertebrae: Lateral Projection

128. Identify the labeled anatomy in Figure 8-33.

Figure 8-33

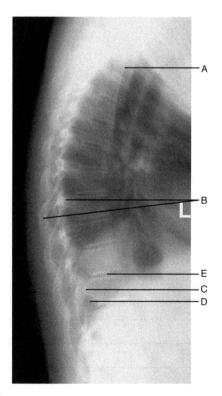

A. _____

B. _____

C. _____

D. _____

E. _____

Chapter **8 Image Analysis of the Cervical and Thoracic Vertebrae**   Copyright © 2015, 2011, 2006, 1996 by Saunders, an imprint of Elsevier Inc. All rights reserved.

129. Complete the statements below referring to lateral thoracic vertebrae projection analysis guidelines.

> **Lateral Thoracic Vertebrae Projection Analysis Guidelines**
>
> ■ The intervertebral foramina are clearly demonstrated, pedicles are in (A) _____, the posterior surfaces of each vertebral body are (B) _____, and no more than (C) _____ inch(es) of space is demonstrated between the posterior ribs.
>
> ■ The intervertebral disk spaces are (D) _____, and the vertebral bodies are demonstrated without distortion.

130. What advantage does using a breathing technique over a nonbreathing technique have when imaging the thoracic vertebrae in the lateral projection?

_____

131. If patient motion cannot be avoided on a lateral thoracic projection when using a breathing technique, what respiration should be used?

_____

132. List two reasons why the patient's arms should be positioned at a 90-degree angle with the body for a lateral thoracic projection.

A. _____

_____

B. _____

_____

133. How is the patient positioned to prevent rotation on a lateral thoracic projection?

_____

_____

134. How can rotation be identified on a lateral thoracic projection?

_____

_____

135. How can scoliosis be distinguished from rotation on a lateral thoracic projection?

_____

136. When the thoracic vertebrae are in a lateral projection, the posterior ribs are positioned on top of each other. Why does the resulting projection demonstrate the posterior ribs without superimposition?

_____

_____

Copyright © 2015, 2011, 2006, 1996 by Saunders, an imprint of Elsevier Inc. All rights reserved. Chapter **8 Image Analysis of the Cervical and Thoracic Vertebrae**

137. How is the patient positioned to obtain open intervertebral disk spaces on a lateral thoracic projection?

_____

138. Describe the patient body forms that demonstrate the greatest thoracic vertebral sagging when the patient is placed in a lateral projection.

A. _____

B. _____

State where the radiolucent sponge is positioned to offset this sagging.

C. _____

State how the CR can be adjusted to offset this sagging.

D. _____

139. Accurate CR centering on a lateral thoracic vertebral projection is accomplished by centering the CR to the

_____ when the patient's arm is positioned at a 90-degree angle with the body.

140. What anatomic structures are included on a lateral thoracic projection with accurate positioning?

_____

141. List two methods of confirming which thoracic vertebra is the twelfth on a lateral thoracic projection.

A. _____

B. _____

_____

142. List two methods of confirming which thoracic vertebra is the first on a lateral thoracic projection.

A. _____

B. _____

143. If the first, second, or third thoracic vertebra is not included on a routine lateral thoracic projection, what supplementary projection is used to demonstrate these vertebrae?

_____

For the following descriptions of lateral thoracic projections with poor positioning, state how the patient would have been mispositioned for such a projection to be obtained.

144. The posterior surfaces of the vertebral bodies are demonstrated without superimposition, and more than 1/2 inch (1.25 cm) of space is demonstrated between the posterior ribs.

_____

145. The posterior surfaces of the vertebral bodies are demonstrated without superimposition, and the posterior ribs are superimposed.

_____

Chapter **8** **Image Analysis of the Cervical and Thoracic Vertebrae**   Copyright © 2015, 2011, 2006, 1996 by Saunders, an imprint of Elsevier Inc. All rights reserved.

146. The eighth through twelfth thoracic intervertebral disk spaces are obscured, and the vertebral bodies are distorted.

_____

For the following lateral thoracic projections with poor positioning, state what anatomic structures are misaligned and how the patient should be repositioned for an optimal projection to be obtained.

Figure 8-34

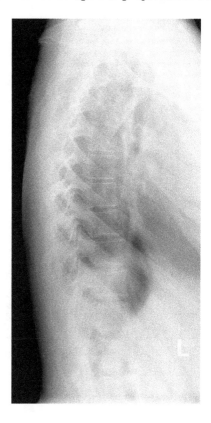

147. (Figure 8-34): _____

_____

_____

Copyright © 2015, 2011, 2006, 1996 by Saunders, an imprint of Elsevier Inc. All rights reserved.   Chapter **8 Image Analysis of the Cervical and Thoracic Vertebrae**

Figure 8-35

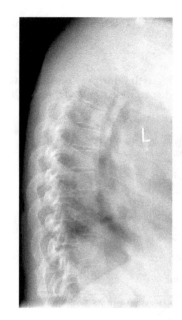

148. (Figure 8-35): _____

_____

_____

_____

_____

Figure 8-36

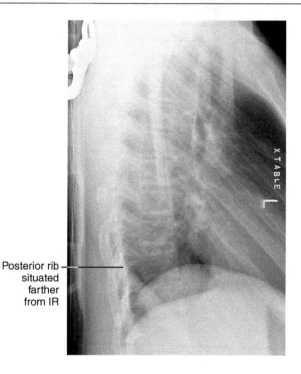

Posterior rib
situated
farther
from IR

149. (Figure 8-36, Cross-table trauma projection): _____

_____

_____

   Copyright © 2015, 2011, 2006, 1996 by Saunders, an imprint of Elsevier Inc. All rights reserved.

9 Image Analysis of the Lumbar Vertebrae, Sacrum, and Coccyx

1. Complete Figure 9-1

   Figure 9-1

Lumbar Vertebrae, Sacrum, and Coccyx Technical Data					
Projection	kV	Grid	AEC	mAs	**SID**
AP, lumber vertebrae					
AP oblique, lumbar vertebrae					
Lateral, lumbar vertebrae					
Lateral, L5-S1 lumbosacral junction					
AP axial, sacrum					
Lateral, sacrum					
AP axial, coccyx					
Lateral, coccyx					
Pediatric					

Copyright © 2015, 2011, 2006, 1996 by Saunders, an imprint of Elsevier Inc. All rights reserved.

Lumbar Vertebrae: AP Projection

2. Identify the labeled anatomy in Figure 9-2.

Figure 9-2

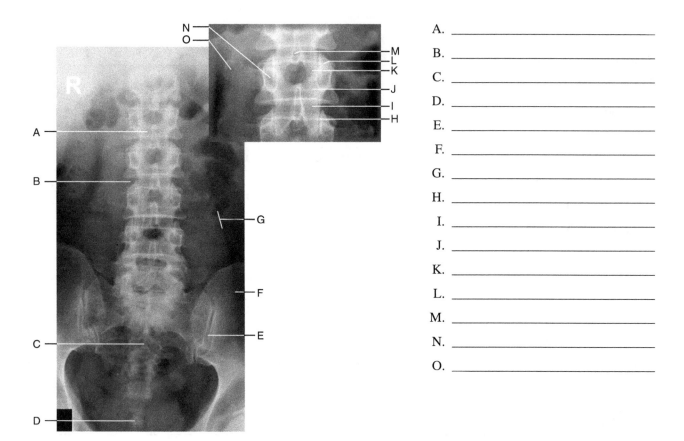

A. _____

B. _____

C. _____

D. _____

E. _____

F. _____

G. _____

H. _____

I. _____

J. _____

K. _____

L. _____

M. _____

N. _____

O. _____

3. Complete the statements below referring to AP lumbar vertebrae projection analysis guidelines.

AP Lumbar Vertebrae Projection Analysis Guidelines

- The distances from the pedicles to the (A) _Spinous process_ and from the sacroiliac joints to the spinous processes are (B) _equal distance_ on both sides. The sacrum and coccyx should be centered within the inlet pelvis and aligned with the symphysis pubis.

- The intervertebral disk spaces are (C) _open_, and the vertebral bodies are seen without distortion.

- The (D) _Spinous process_ are aligned with the midline of the vertebral bodies.

Copyright © 2015, 2011, 2006, 1996 by Saunders, an imprint of Elsevier Inc. All rights reserved.

4. What soft tissue structures are to be included on an AP lumbar projection?

   A. _____

   Where are these structures located?

   B. _____

5. How is rotation identified on an AP lumbar projection?

   _____

   _____

6. How is the patient positioned to ensure that open intervertebral disk spaces and undistorted vertebral bodies are obtained?

   _____

   _____

7. What is the curvature of the lumbar vertebral column?

   _____

8. An AP lumbar projection demonstrates the vertebral column deviating laterally at the level of the second through fourth lumbar vertebrae, the sacrum is centered within the pelvic inlet, and the distances from the pedicles to the spinous processes of the 11th thoracic vertebra and the fifth lumbar vertebra are nearly equal. What has caused the appearance of this projection?

   _____

9. Accurate CR centering on an AP lumbar projection taken using an 8- × 14-inch (20- × 35-cm) field size, is

   accomplished by centering the CR to the (A) _____ plane at a level 1½ inches (4 cm)

   (B) _____ to the (C) _____.

10. What anatomic structures are included on an AP lumbar projection with accurate positioning taken using an 8- × 14-inch (20- × 35-cm) field size?

    _____

11. Accurate CR centering on an AP lumbar projection taken using an 8- ×x 17-inch (20- × 43-cm) field size is

    accomplished by centering the CR to the (A) _____ plane at the level of the (B) _____.

12. What anatomic structures are included on an AP lumbar projection with accurate positioning taken using an 8- × 17-inch (20- × 43-cm) field size?

    _____

13. How tightly can the transversely collimated field be coned and still include all the required anatomic structures?

    _____

For the following descriptions of AP lumbar projections with poor positioning, state how the patient would have been mispositioned for such a projection to be obtained.

14. The distance from the right pedicles to the spinous processes is less than the distance from the left pedicles to the spinous processes, and the sacrum and coccyx are rotated toward the right lateral inlet pelvis.

    _____

Copyright © 2015, 2011, 2006, 1996 by Saunders, an imprint of Elsevier Inc. All rights reserved. Chapter **9 Image Analysis of the Lumbar Vertebrae, Sacrum, and Coccyx**

15. The first through third lumbar vertebrae are demonstrated without rotation, the fourth and fifth vertebrae are rotated, and the sacrum and coccyx are rotated toward the patient's left side.

_____

16. The intervertebral disk spaces between the 12th thoracic vertebra and the third lumbar vertebra are closed, and these lumbar bodies are distorted. The iliac spines are demonstrated without pelvic brim superimposition.

_____

For the following AP lumbar projections with poor positioning, state what anatomic structures are misaligned and how the patient should be repositioned for an optimal projection to be obtained.

Figure 9-3

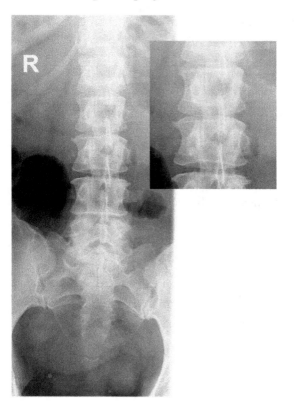

17. (Figure 9-3): _____

_____

_____

Chapter **9 Image Analysis of the Lumbar Vertebrae, Sacrum, and Coccyx**   Copyright © 2015, 2011, 2006, 1996 by Saunders, an imprint of Elsevier Inc. All rights reserved.

Figure 9-4

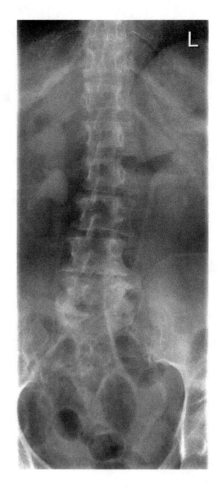

18. (Figure 9-4): _____

_____

_____

_____

_____

_____

Copyright © 2015, 2011, 2006, 1996 by Saunders, an imprint of Elsevier Inc. All rights reserved. Chapter **9 Image Analysis of the Lumbar Vertebrae, Sacrum, and Coccyx**

Figure 9-5

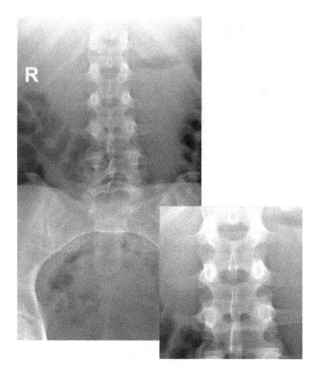

19. (Figure 9-5): _____

_____

Lumbar Vertebrae: AP Oblique Projection (RPO and LPO Positions)

20. Identify the labeled anatomy in Figure 9-6.

Figure 9-6

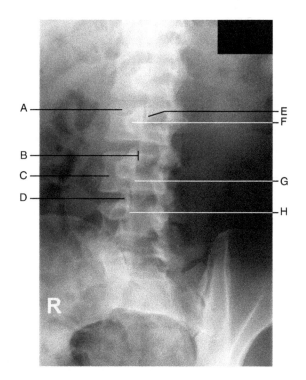

A. 2nd lumbar vertebrae

A. 2ⁿᵈ lumbar vertebrae

B. zygo joint

C. transverse process

D. superior articular process

E. inferior articular process

F. pedicle

G. lamina

H. pars

Chapter **9 Image Analysis of the Lumbar Vertebrae, Sacrum, and Coccyx**   Copyright © 2015, 2011, 2006, 1996 by Saunders, an imprint of Elsevier Inc. All rights reserved.

21. Complete the statements below referring to AP oblique lumbar vertebrae projection analysis guidelines.

AP Oblique Lumbar Vertebrae Projection Analysis Guidelines
■ The superior and inferior (A) _____ are in profile, the (B) _____ joints are demonstrated, and the (C) _____ are seen halfway between the midpoint of the vertebral bodies and the lateral border of the vertebral bodies.

22. For the following positions, state whether the right or left zygapophyseal joints are demonstrated on an AP oblique lumbar projection.

A. RAO: _____

B. LPO: _____

C. RPO: _____

D. LAO: _____

23. What body plane is used to determine patient obliquity for an AP oblique lumbar projection?

A. ___*midcoronal*_____

How much is the patient's torso rotated for an AP oblique lumbar projection?

B. ___*45°*_____

24. Name the anatomic structures of the lumbar vertebrae that correspond with the parts of the "Scottie dog" listed below.

A. Ear: _____

B. Nose: _____

C. Body: _____

D. Eye: _____

E. Front leg: _____

25. Accurate CR centering on an AP oblique lumbar projection is accomplished by centering the CR 2 inches (5 cm)

(A) _____ to the elevated (B) _____ at a level 1½ inches (4 cm) superior to the (C) _____.

26. What anatomic structures are included on an AP oblique lumbar projection with accurate positioning?

___*T12-sacrum & SI joints*_____

_____

For the following descriptions of AP oblique lumbar projections with poor positioning, state how the patient would have been mispositioned for such a projection to be obtained.

27. The vertebrae's superior and inferior articular processes are not demonstrated in profile, their corresponding zygapophyseal joint spaces are closed, and their pedicles are demonstrated adjacent to the vertebrae's lateral vertebral body borders.

_____

_____

Copyright © 2015, 2011, 2006, 1996 by Saunders, an imprint of Elsevier Inc. All rights reserved. Chapter **9** **Image Analysis of the Lumbar Vertebrae, Sacrum, and Coccyx**

28. The vertebrae's superior and inferior articular processes are not demonstrated in profile, their corresponding zygapophyseal joint spaces are closed, their laminae are obscured, and their pedicles are shown at the midpoint of the vertebral bodies.

Vertebrae were rotated more than 45°

For the following oblique lumbar projections with poor positioning, state what anatomic structures are misaligned and how the patient should be repositioned for an optimal projection to be obtained.

Figure 9-7

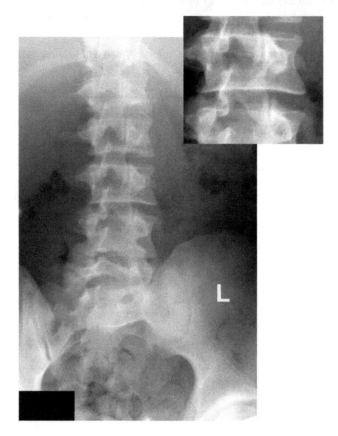

29. (Figure 9-7): _____

_____

_____

Chapter **9** **Image Analysis of the Lumbar Vertebrae, Sacrum, and Coccyx**   Copyright © 2015, 2011, 2006, 1996 by Saunders, an imprint of Elsevier Inc. All rights reserved.

Figure 9-8

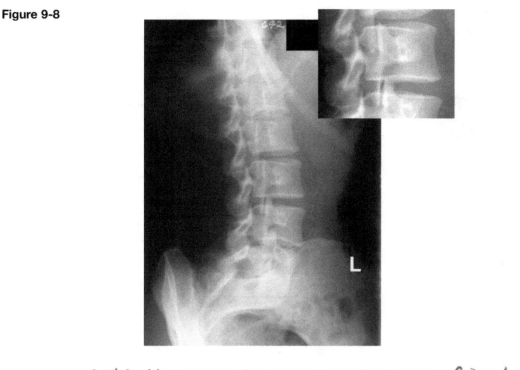

30. (Figure 9-8): _articular processes aren't in profile &_
zygo joints closed
fix. decrease obliquity

Figure 9-9

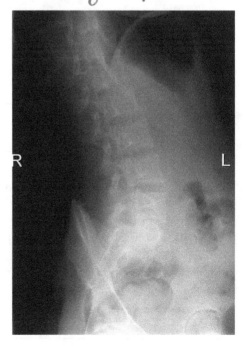

31. (Figure 9-9): _____

_____

_____

Copyright © 2015, 2011, 2006, 1996 by Saunders, an imprint of Elsevier Inc. All rights reserved. Chapter **9 Image Analysis of the Lumbar Vertebrae, Sacrum, and Coccyx**

Lumbar Vertebrae: Lateral Projection

32. Identify the labeled anatomy in Figure 9-10.

Figure 9-10

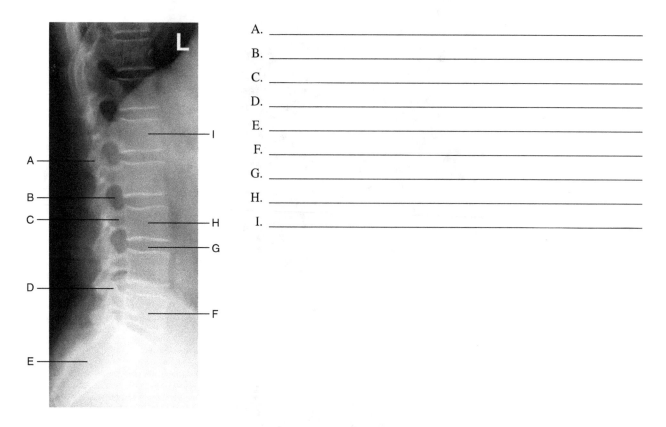

A. _____

B. _____

C. _____

D. _____

E. _____

F. _____

G. _____

H. _____

I. _____

33. Complete the statements below referring to lateral lumbar vertebrae projection analysis guidelines.

Lateral Lumbar Vertebrae Projection Analysis Guidelines
■ The intervertebral foramina are demonstrated, and the (A) _____ are in profile.
■ The right and left pedicles and the posterior surfaces of each vertebral body are (B) _____.
■ The intervertebral disk spaces are (C) _____.
■ The lumbar vertebral column is in a (D) _____ position without anteroposterior flexion or extension.

34. How is the patient positioned to prevent rotation on a lateral lumbar projection?

_____

_____

Chapter **9 Image Analysis of the Lumbar Vertebrae, Sacrum, and Coccyx**   Copyright © 2015, 2011, 2006, 1996 by Saunders, an imprint of Elsevier Inc. All rights reserved.

35. How is the patient positioned to ensure open intervertebral disk spaces and undistorted vertebral bodies on a lateral lumbar projection?

_____

36. Lumbar column lateral flexion or tilt with the IR most often occurs with what patient body types?

    A. _____

    B. _____

37. How can CR be adjusted to obtain open disk spaces and undistorted vertebral bodies on a lateral lumbar projection when the patient's vertebral column is tilted?

_____

38. For a lateral lumbar projection, the patient may be placed on the imaging table in a left or right recumbent position unless the patient has what spinal condition?

    A. ___*Scoliosis*_____

    For this condition, how are the CR and vertebral column positioned?

    B. ___*positioned on table to direct CR to curve*___

39. What is accomplished by placing a pillow or sponge between the patient's legs for a lateral lumbar projection?

_____

40. Will the upper and lower vertebrae on a lateral lumbar projection always demonstrate simultaneous rotation?

    A. _____ (Yes/No)

    Explain your answer.

    B. _____

41. Why is it difficult to determine which side of the body has been rotated anteriorly or posteriorly when a lateral lumbar projection demonstrates rotation?

_____

42. Why are flexion and extension lateral lumbar projections requested?

_____

43. Describe how patient positioning is adjusted from a neutral lateral position to place the patient in maximum flexion for a lateral lumbar projection.

    A. _____

    Describe how patient positioning is adjusted from a neutral lateral position to place the patient in maximum extension for a lateral lumbar projection.

    B. _____

44. The lordotic curvature on a lumbar projection is (A) _____ (increased/decreased) when the patient is positioned in maximum flexion and is (B) _____ (increased/decreased) when the patient is positioned in maximum extension.

Copyright © 2015, 2011, 2006, 1996 by Saunders, an imprint of Elsevier Inc. All rights reserved. Chapter **9** **Image Analysis of the Lumbar Vertebrae, Sacrum, and Coccyx**

45. Accurate CR centering on a lateral lumbar projection when an 8- × 14-inch (20- × 35-cm) field size is used is accomplished by centering the CR to the (A) _____ plane located halfway between the elevated (B) _____ and (C) _____ at a level 1½ inches (4 cm) superior to the (D) _____.

46. What anatomic structures are included on a lateral lumbar projection with accurate positioning taken on an 8- × 14-inch (20- × 35-cm) field size?

_____

47. Accurate CR centering on a lateral lumbar projection when an 8- × 17-inch (20- × 43-cm) field size is used is accomplished by centering the CR to the (A) _____ plane located halfway between the elevated (B) _____ and (C) _____ at the level of the (D) _____.

48. What anatomic structures are included on a lateral lumbar projection with accurate positioning taken on an 8- × 17-inch (20- × 43-cm) field size?

_____

49. Describe two situations in which a tightly collimated lateral view of the L5-S1 lumbar region is indicated after the lateral lumbar projection has been reviewed.

A. _____

B. _____

50. Explain how the shield is positioned for a lateral lumbar projection to protect the patient's gonads.

_____

_____

For the following descriptions of lateral lumbar projections with poor positioning, state how the patient would have been mispositioned for such a projection to be obtained.

51. The posterior surfaces of the first through fourth vertebral bodies and the posterior ribs are demonstrated without superimposition. The most magnified ribs are demonstrated anteriorly.

_____

52. The L4-L5 and L5-S1 intervertebral disk spaces are closed, and the third through fifth vertebral bodies are distorted.

_____

    Copyright © 2015, 2011, 2006, 1996 by Saunders, an imprint of Elsevier Inc. All rights reserved.

53. Explain why the intervertebral joint spaces are closed on the lateral lumbar projection in Figure 9-11 even though the iliac crests and alae are perfectly superimposed.

Figure 9-11

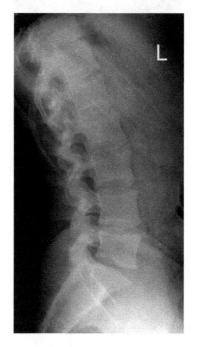

For the following lateral lumbar projections with poor positioning, state what anatomic structures are misaligned and how the patient should be repositioned for an optimal projection to be obtained.

Figure 9-12

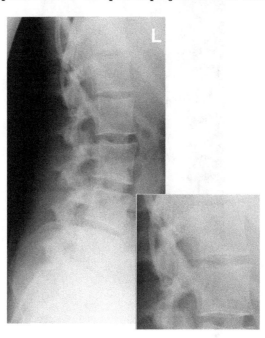

54. (Figure 9-12): _____

_____

_____

_____

_____

Copyright © 2015, 2011, 2006, 1996 by Saunders, an imprint of Elsevier Inc. All rights reserved. Chapter **9** **Image Analysis of the Lumbar Vertebrae, Sacrum, and Coccyx**

Figure 9-13

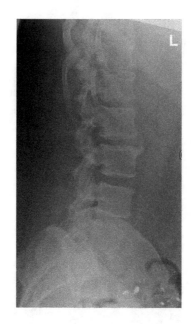

55. (Figure 9-13): _____

_____

_____

Figure 9-14

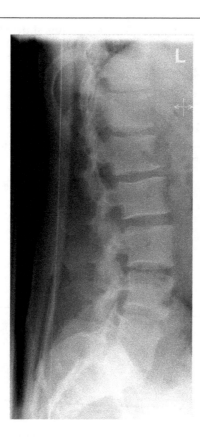

56. (Figure 9-14): _____

_____

_____

Chapter **9 Image Analysis of the Lumbar Vertebrae, Sacrum, and Coccyx**   Copyright © 2015, 2011, 2006, 1996 by Saunders, an imprint of Elsevier Inc. All rights reserved.

Figure 9-15

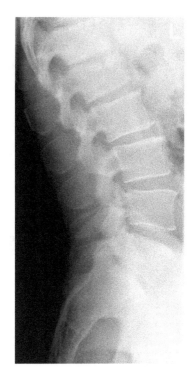

57. (Figure 9-15): _____
_____
_____

L5-S1 Lumbosacral Junction: Lateral Projection

58. Identify the labeled anatomy in Figure 9-16.

Figure 9-16

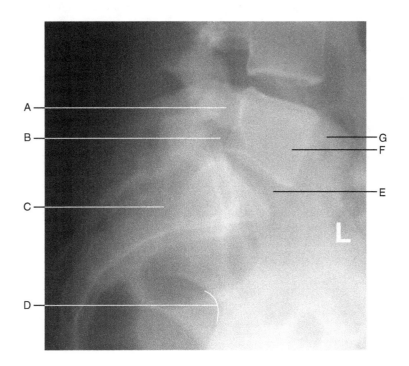

A. _____

B. _____

C. _____

D. _____

E. _____

F. _____

G. _____

Copyright © 2015, 2011, 2006, 1996 by Saunders, an imprint of Elsevier Inc. All rights reserved. Chapter **9 Image Analysis of the Lumbar Vertebrae, Sacrum, and Coccyx**

59. Complete the statements below referring to lateral L5-S1 lumbosacral junction projection analysis guidelines.

Lateral L5-S1 Lumbosacral Junction Projection Analysis Guidelines

■ The L5-S1 intervertebral foramen are demonstrated, the right and left (A) _____ _____ are

superimposed and in profile, and the greater sciatic notches and (B) _____
are nearly superimposed.

■ The L5-S1 intervertebral disk space is (C) _____, the pelvic alae are superimposed, and
the sacrum is seen without foreshortening.

---

60. How tightly can the transverse field be collimated and still include the needed anatomic information on a lateral L5-S1 projection?

_____

61. What is accomplished by placing a pillow or sponge between the patient's legs for a lateral L5-S1 projection?

_____

_____

62. How can rotation be detected on a rotated lateral L5-S1 projection?

_____

_____

63. How is the patient positioned to obtain open intervertebral disk spaces and undistorted vertebral bodies on a lateral L5-S1 projection?

_____

64. How should the CR be adjusted to obtain an open L5-S1 joint space in a patient whose vertebral column curves upwardly?

_____

65. Accurate CR centering on a lateral L5-S1 projection is accomplished by centering the CR to a point 2 inches (5 cm)

(A) _____ to the elevated (B) _____ and 1½ inches (4 cm) (C) _____ to the

(D) _____.

66. What anatomic structures are included on a lateral L5-S1 projection with accurate positioning?

_____

For the following descriptions of lateral L5-S1 lumbar projections with poor positioning, state how the patient would have been mispositioned for such a projection to be obtained.

67. The L5-S1 intervertebral foramen is obscured, and the greater sciatic notches and femoral heads are not superimposed.

_____

 Copyright © 2015, 2011, 2006, 1996 by Saunders, an imprint of Elsevier Inc. All rights reserved.

68. The L5-S1 intervertebral disk space is closed, and the pelvic alae are not superimposed.

_____

For the following lateral L5-S1 lumbar projections with poor positioning, state what anatomic structures are misaligned and how the patient should be repositioned for an optimal projection to be obtained.

Figure 9-17

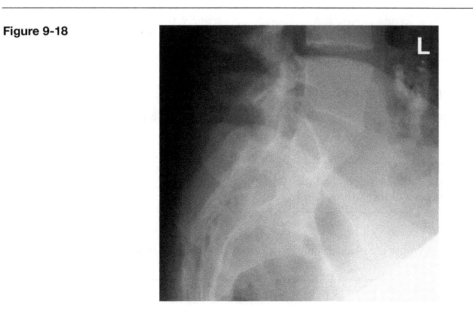

69. (Figure 9-17): _____

_____

_____

Figure 9-18

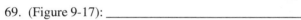

70. (Figure 9-18): _____

_____

_____

Copyright © 2015, 2011, 2006, 1996 by Saunders, an imprint of Elsevier Inc. All rights reserved.
Chapter **9 Image Analysis of the Lumbar Vertebrae, Sacrum, and Coccyx**

Sacrum: AP Axial Projection

71. Identify the labeled anatomy in Figure 9-19.

Figure 9-19

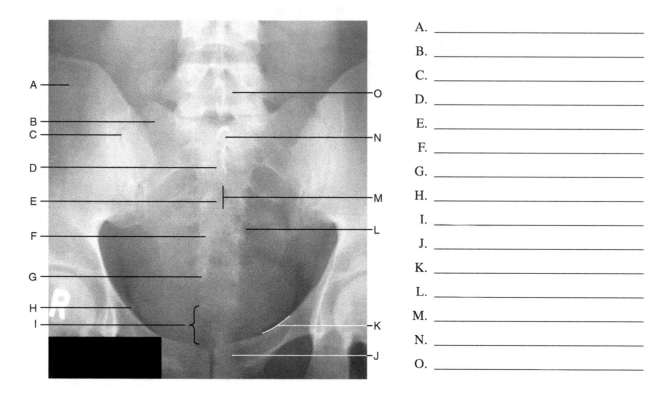

A. _____

B. _____

C. _____

D. _____

E. _____

F. _____

G. _____

H. _____

I. _____

J. _____

K. _____

L. _____

M. _____

N. _____

O. _____

72. Complete the statements below referring to AP axial sacrum projection analysis guidelines.

AP Axial Sacrum Projection Analysis Guidelines
■ The ischial spines are equally demonstrated and are aligned with the (A) _____, and the median sacral crest and (B) _____ are aligned with the symphysis pubis.
■ The first through (C) _____ sacral segments are seen without foreshortening, sacral foramina demonstrate equal spacing, and the (D) _____ is not superimposed over any portion of the sacrum.

73. Why is the patient instructed to empty the bladder and colon before an AP sacral projection is taken?

_____

_____

Chapter **9** **Image Analysis of the Lumbar Vertebrae, Sacrum, and Coccyx**   Copyright © 2015, 2011, 2006, 1996 by Saunders, an imprint of Elsevier Inc. All rights reserved.

74. When a patient is rotated for an AP sacral projection, the sacrum rotates in the (A) _____ (opposite/same) direction as the symphysis pubis and is positioned next to the lateral pelvic brim situated (B) _____ (closer/farther) to/from the IR.

75. What is the curvature of the sacrum? _____

76. How must the patient and CR be positioned to demonstrate the sacrum without foreshortening?

_____

_____

77. Accurate CR centering on an AP sacral projection is accomplished by positioning the CR to the (A) _____ plane at a level halfway between (B) _____ and the (C) _____.

78. What anatomic structures are included on an AP sacral projection with accurate positioning?

_____

For the following descriptions of AP sacral projections with poor positioning, state how the patient or CR would have been mispositioned for such a projection to be obtained.

79. The left ischial spine is demonstrated without pelvic brim superimposition, and the median sacral crest and coccyx are rotated toward the right hip.

_____

80. The first, second, and third sacral segments are foreshortened.

_____

81. The sacrum is elongated, and the symphysis pubis is superimposed over the fifth sacral segment.

_____

Copyright © 2015, 2011, 2006, 1996 by Saunders, an imprint of Elsevier Inc. All rights reserved. Chapter **9 Image Analysis of the Lumbar Vertebrae, Sacrum, and Coccyx**

For the following AP sacral projections with poor positioning, state what anatomic structures are misaligned and how the patient should be repositioned for an optimal projection to be obtained.

Figure 9-20

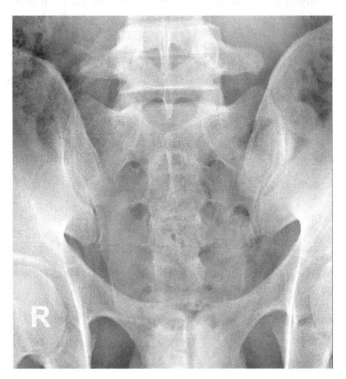

82. (Figure 9-20): _____

_____

_____

Figure 9-21

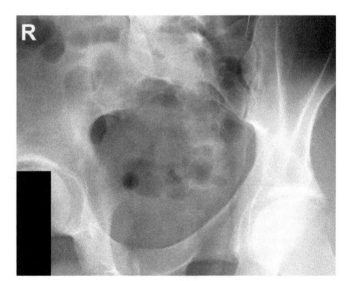

83. (Figure 9-21): _____

_____

_____

_____

Chapter **9 Image Analysis of the Lumbar Vertebrae, Sacrum, and Coccyx**   Copyright © 2015, 2011, 2006, 1996 by Saunders, an imprint of Elsevier Inc. All rights reserved.

Figure 9-22

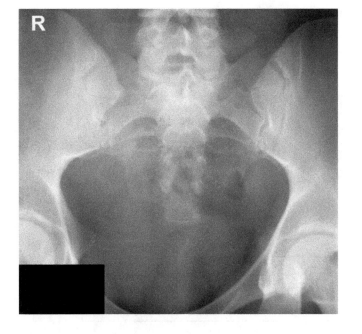

84. (Figure 9-22): Sacrum foreshortened, right ischial spine w/o pelvic brim superimposition
fix: make ASIS₅ equal distance from table top & angle CR 15° cephalic

Figure 9-23

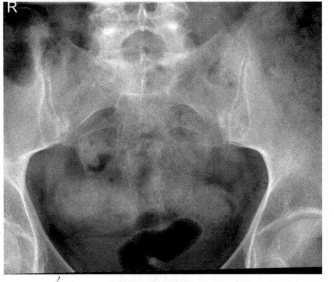

85. (Figure 9-23): Sacrum foreshortened & fecal matter obscuring anatomy
fix: angle CR 15° cephalic & have pt. try to empty colon

Copyright © 2015, 2011, 2006, 1996 by Saunders, an imprint of Elsevier Inc. All rights reserved.
Chapter **9 Image Analysis of the Lumbar Vertebrae, Sacrum, and Coccyx**

Sacrum: Lateral Projection

86. Identify the labeled anatomy in Figure 9-24.

Figure 9-24

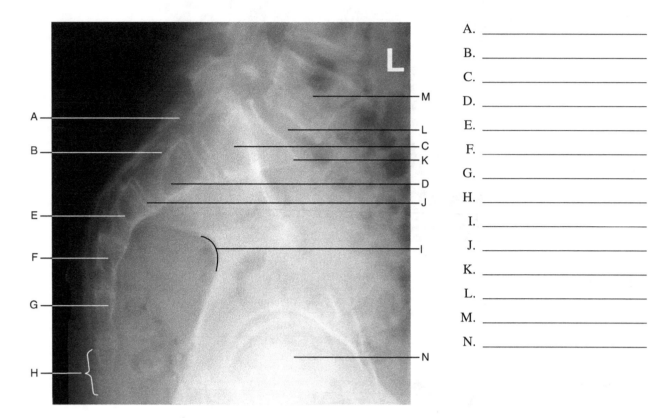

A. _____

B. _____

C. _____

D. _____

E. _____

F. _____

G. _____

H. _____

I. _____

J. _____

K. _____

L. _____

M. _____

N. _____

87. Complete the statements below referring to lateral sacrum projection analysis guidelines.

Lateral Sacrum Projection Analysis Guidelines
■ The median sacral crest is in (A) _____, and the greater sciatic notches and the (B) _____ are nearly superimposed.
■ The L5-S1 intervertebral disk space is open, greater sciatic notches are (C) _____, and the sacrum is seen without foreshortening.

88. How can rotation be detected on a rotated lateral sacral projection?

_____

_____

Chapter **9** **Image Analysis of the Lumbar Vertebrae, Sacrum, and Coccyx**   Copyright © 2015, 2011, 2006, 1996 by Saunders, an imprint of Elsevier Inc. All rights reserved.

89. When a lateral sacral projection demonstrates rotation and the femoral heads are demonstrated on the projection, the hip that is projected inferiorly is situated _____ (closer to/farther away from) the IR.

90. How is the patient positioned to obtain an open L5-S1 disk space and an undistorted fifth lumbar body on a lateral sacral projection?

_____

_____

91. How should the CR be adjusted to obtain an open L5-S1 intervertebral joint space in a patient whose vertebral column curves upwardly?

_____

92. Accurate CR centering on a lateral sacral projection is accomplished by centering the CR to the (A) _____ plane located 3 to 4 inches (7.5 to 10 cm) posterior to the elevated (B) _____.

93. What anatomic structures are included on a lateral sacral projection with accurate positioning?

_____

_____

For the following descriptions of lateral sacral projections with poor positioning, state how the patient would have been mispositioned for such a projection to be obtained.

94. The greater sciatic notches are demonstrated without superimposition, the median sacral crest is not in profile, and the inferiorly located femoral head is rotated posteriorly.

_____

95. The L5-S1 intervertebral disk space is closed, the fifth lumbar vertebra and sacrum are foreshortened, and the greater sciatic notches are demonstrated without superimposition.

_____

Copyright © 2015, 2011, 2006, 1996 by Saunders, an imprint of Elsevier Inc. All rights reserved. Chapter **9 Image Analysis of the Lumbar Vertebrae, Sacrum, and Coccyx**

For the following lateral sacral projections with poor positioning, state what anatomic structures are misaligned and how the patient should be repositioned for an optimal projection to be obtained.

Figure 9-25

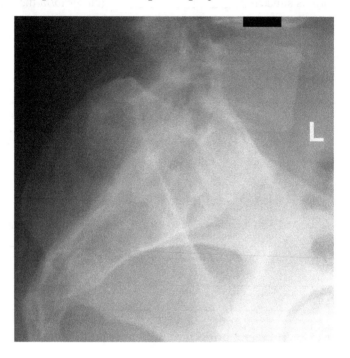

96. (Figure 9-25): _____

_____

_____

Figure 9-26

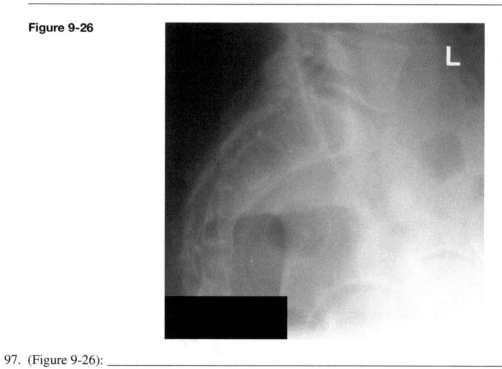

97. (Figure 9-26): _____

_____

_____

Chapter **9 Image Analysis of the Lumbar Vertebrae, Sacrum, and Coccyx**   Copyright © 2015, 2011, 2006, 1996 by Saunders, an imprint of Elsevier Inc. All rights reserved.

Figure 9-27

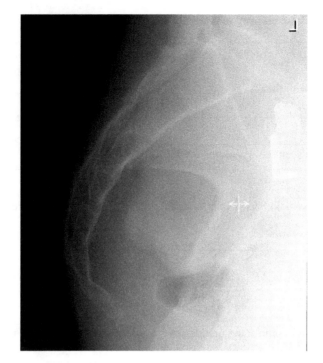

98. (Figure 9-27): _____

_____

_____

Coccyx: AP Axial Projection

99. Identify the labeled anatomy in Figure 9-28.

Figure 9-28

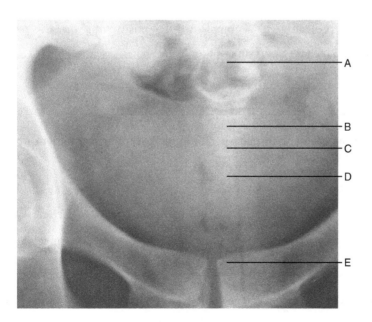

A. _____

B. _____

C. _____

D. _____

E. _____

Copyright © 2015, 2011, 2006, 1996 by Saunders, an imprint of Elsevier Inc. All rights reserved. Chapter **9** **Image Analysis of the Lumbar Vertebrae, Sacrum, and Coccyx**

100. Complete the statements below referring to AP axial coccyx projection analysis guidelines.

AP Axial Coccyx Projection Analysis Guidelines

- The coccyx is aligned with the (A) _____ and is at equal distances from the lateral walls of the (B) _____.

- The first through (C) _____ coccygeal vertebrae are seen without foreshortening and without symphysis pubis superimposition.

---

101. How much can the transverse field be safely collimated and still include the required anatomic structures for an AP coccygeal projection?

_____

102. Where is the marker placed on an AP coccygeal projection that is collimated to a 6-inch (15-cm) field size?

_____

103. Why is the patient instructed to empty the bladder and colon before an AP sacral projection is taken? _____

_____

104. When a patient is rotated for an AP coccygeal projection, the coccyx rotates in the (A) _____ (opposite/same) direction as the symphysis pubis and is positioned next to the lateral pelvic wall situated

(B) _____ (closer/farther) to/from the IR.

105. How must the patient and CR be positioned for an AP coccygeal projection to demonstrate the coccyx without foreshortening?

_____

106. What is the curvature of the coccyx? _____

107. Accurate CR centering on an AP coccygeal projection is accomplished by positioning the CR to the

(A) _____ plane at a level 2 inches (5 cm) superior to the (B) _____.

108. What anatomic structures are included on an AP coccygeal projection with accurate positioning?

_____

For the following descriptions of AP coccygeal projections with poor positioning, state how the patient or CR would have been mispositioned for such a projection to be obtained.

109. The urinary bladder is dense and creating a shadow over the coccyx.

_____

110. The coccyx is not aligned with the symphysis pubis but is situated closer to the left lateral pelvic wall.

_____

111. The symphysis pubis is superimposed over the coccyx, and the second and third coccygeal vertebrae are foreshortened.

_____

Chapter **9** **Image Analysis of the Lumbar Vertebrae, Sacrum, and Coccyx**   Copyright © 2015, 2011, 2006, 1996 by Saunders, an imprint of Elsevier Inc. All rights reserved.

For the following AP coccygeal projections with poor positioning, state what anatomic structures are misaligned and how the patient should be repositioned for an optimal projection to be obtained.

Figure 9-29

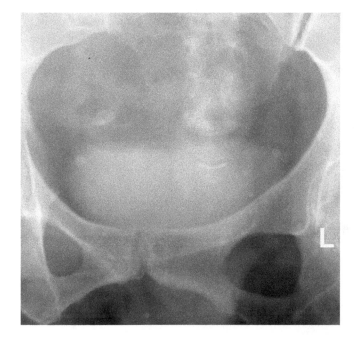

112. (Figure 9-29): _____

_____

_____

Figure 9-30

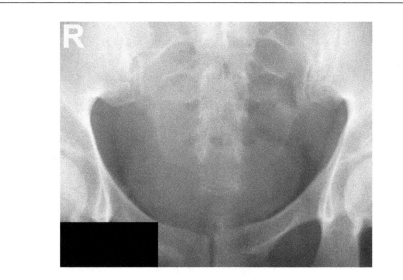

113. (Figure 9-30): _____

_____

_____

Copyright © 2015, 2011, 2006, 1996 by Saunders, an imprint of Elsevier Inc. All rights reserved.   Chapter **9 Image Analysis of the Lumbar Vertebrae, Sacrum, and Coccyx**

114. Identify the labeled anatomy in Figure 9-31.

Figure 9-31

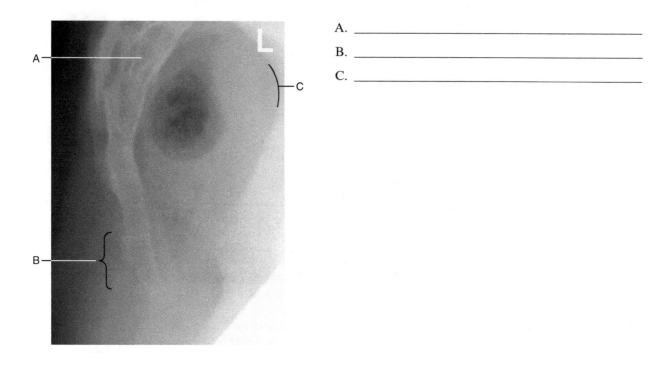

A. _____

B. _____

C. _____

115. Complete the statements below referring to lateral coccyx projection analysis guidelines.

Lateral Coccyx Projection Analysis Guidelines
■ The median sacral crest is in (A) _____, and the greater sciatic notches are superimposed.
■ The coccyx is seen without (B) _____.

116. How can rotation be detected on a rotated lateral coccygeal projection?

_____

117. How is the patient positioned to prevent foreshortening of the coccyx on a lateral coccygeal projection?

_____

_____

118. Accurate CR centering on a lateral coccygeal projection is accomplished by centering a perpendicular central ray approximately 3½ inches (9 cm) (A) _____ and 2 inches (5 cm) (C) _____ to the (B) _____.

Chapter **9 Image Analysis of the Lumbar Vertebrae, Sacrum, and Coccyx**   Copyright © 2015, 2011, 2006, 1996 by Saunders, an imprint of Elsevier Inc. All rights reserved.

119. How tightly can one safely collimate on a lateral coccygeal projection without fear of clipping any portion of the coccyx?

_____

120. What anatomic structures are included on a lateral coccygeal projection with accurate positioning?

_____

For the following description of a lateral coccygeal projection with poor positioning, state how the patient would have been mispositioned for such a projection to be obtained.

121. The greater sciatic notches are demonstrated without superimposition, and the ischium is nearly superimposed over the third coccygeal segment.

_____

For the following lateral coccygeal projection with poor positioning, state what anatomic structures are misaligned and how the patient should be repositioned for an optimal projection to be obtained.

Figure 9-32

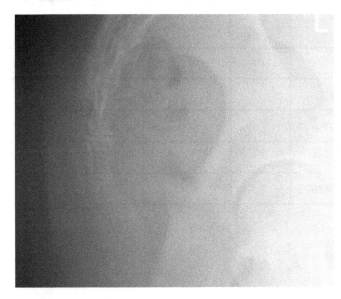

122. (Figure 9-32): _____

_____

_____

Copyright © 2015, 2011, 2006, 1996 by Saunders, an imprint of Elsevier Inc. All rights reserved. Chapter **9 Image Analysis of the Lumbar Vertebrae, Sacrum, and Coccyx**

10 Image Analysis of the Sternum and Ribs

STUDY QUESTIONS

1. Complete Figure 10-1.

   Figure 10-1

Sternum and Ribs Technical Data					
Projection	kV	Grid	AEC	mAs	SID
PA oblique (RAO position), sternum					
Lateral, sternum					
AP or PA, above diaphragm					
AP or PA, below diaphragm					
PA oblique, above diaphragm					
PA oblique, below diaphragm					

Copyright © 2015, 2011, 2006, 1996 by Saunders, an imprint of Elsevier Inc. All rights reserved.

Sternum: PA Oblique Projection (RAO Position)

2. Identify the labeled anatomy in Figure 10-2.

Figure 10-2

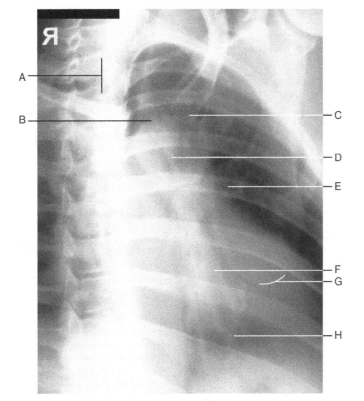

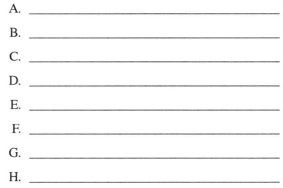

A. _____

B. _____

C. _____

D. _____

E. _____

F. _____

G. _____

H. _____

3. Complete the statements below referring to PA oblique sternum projection analysis guidelines.

> ### PA Oblique Sternum Projection Analysis Guidelines
>
> ■ The ribs and lung markings are (A) _____, and the posterior ribs and (B) _____ are magnified.
>
> ■ The manubrium, SC joints, sternal body, and xiphoid process are demonstrated within the heart shadow without (C) _____ superimposition.

4. Why is a PA oblique projection chosen over a PA oblique (LAO) projection when imaging the sternum?

_____

_____

5. Keeping the entire sternum within the heart shadow for the PA oblique projection provides a sternal projection that demonstrates homogeneous _____ across the entire sternum.

427

Copyright © 2015, 2011, 2006, 1996 by Saunders, an imprint of Elsevier Inc. All rights reserved.

6. List four structures that overlie the sternum in a PA oblique sternal projection.

   A. _____

   B. _____

   C. _____

   D. _____

7. Using a short SID will result in _____ (lower/higher) patient entrance skin dosage.

8. Using a long exposure time and (A) _____ breathing for the PA oblique sternal projection will blur the

   (B) _____ and (C) _____ .

9. The sternum is rotated from beneath the thoracic vertebrae for a PA oblique sternal projection by rotating the patient

   until the (A) _____ plane is aligned (B) _____ degrees with the IR.

10. Any portion of the sternum that is positioned outside the heart shadow on a PA oblique sternal projection demon-

    strates _____ (more/less) brightness than that positioned within the heart shadow.

11. On a PA oblique sternal projection with accurate positioning, the _____ is centered within the collimated
    field.

12. Proper centering for a PA oblique sternal projection is accomplished by centering the CR (A) _____

    inches to the left of the (B) _____ and placing the top of the IR approximately 1½ inches superior

    to the (C) _____ .

13. Because the long axis of the sternum does not align with the long axis of the IR in the PA oblique sternal projection,

    transverse collimation should be limited to the (A) _____ and (B) _____ .

**For the following description of a PA oblique sternal projection with poor positioning, state how the patient would
have been mispositioned for such a projection to be obtained.**

14. The right sternoclavicular (SC) joint and right side of the manubrium are superimposed by the thoracic vertebrae.

    _____

    _____

 Copyright © 2015, 2011, 2006, 1996 by Saunders, an imprint of Elsevier Inc. All rights reserved.

For the following PA oblique sternal projections with poor positioning, state what anatomic structures are misaligned and how the patient should be repositioned for an optimal projection to be obtained.

Figure 10-3

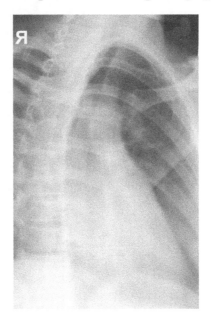

15. (Figure 10-3): _____

_____

_____

_____

Figure 10-4

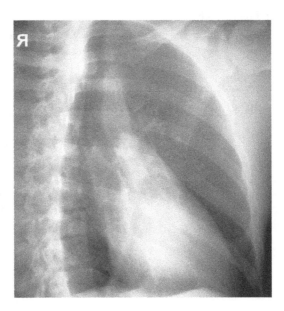

16. (Figure 10-4): _____

_____

_____

_____

Copyright © 2015, 2011, 2006, 1996 by Saunders, an imprint of Elsevier Inc. All rights reserved.   Chapter **10 Image Analysis of the Sternum and Ribs**

Sternum: Lateral Projection

17. Identify the labeled anatomy in Figure 10-5.

Figure 10-5

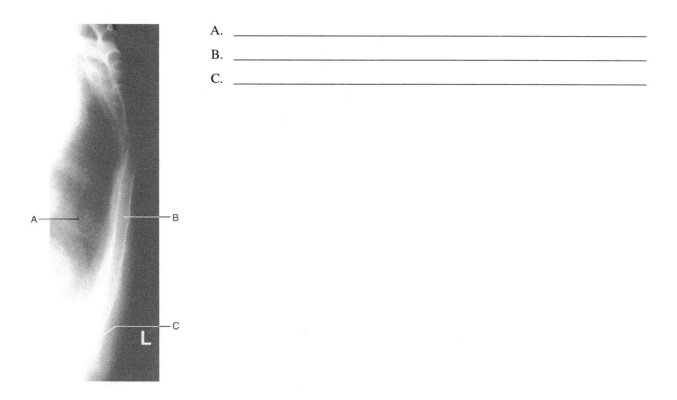

A. _____

B. _____

C. _____

18. Identify the labeled anatomy in Figure 10-6.

Figure 10-6

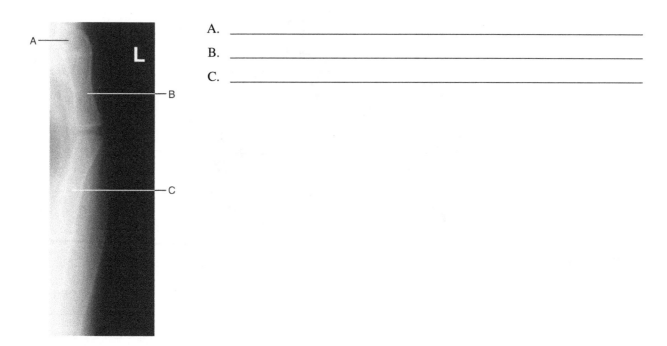

A. _____

B. _____

C. _____

Copyright © 2015, 2011, 2006, 1996 by Saunders, an imprint of Elsevier Inc. All rights reserved.

19. Complete the statements below referring to lateral sternum projection analysis guidelines.

> **Lateral Sternum Projection Analysis Guidelines**
>
> - The manubrium, sternal body, and xiphoid process are in (A) _____, and the anterior ribs are not superimposed over the sternum.
> - No superimposition of (B) _____ soft tissue over the sternum is present.
> - The (C) _____ is at the center of the exposure field.

20. Why is it often difficult to demonstrate the superior and inferior sternum simultaneously on a lateral sternal projection?

   _____

   _____

21. List three methods of controlling the amount of scatter radiation that reaches the IR on a lateral sternal projection.

   A. _____

   B. _____

   C. _____

22. How is rotation avoided when positioning the patient for a lateral sternal projection? _____

   _____

23. Describe how one can determine on a lateral sternal projection with poor positioning that the patient's right thorax is rotated anteriorly.

   _____

24. Deep suspended respiration draws the sternum away from the _____.

25. How is the patient positioned to prevent humeral soft tissue from superimposing the sternum? _____

   _____

26. Accurate CR centering on a lateral sternal projection is accomplished by placing the top edge of the IR

   (A) _____ inches above the (B) _____ and aligning the receptor's long axis and a

   (C) _____ CR to the midsternum.

27. Why is a 72-inch (180-cm) SID used for a lateral sternum projection?

   _____

   _____

28. What anatomic structures are included on a lateral sternal projection with accurate positioning?

   _____

Copyright © 2015, 2011, 2006, 1996 by Saunders, an imprint of Elsevier Inc. All rights reserved.

For the following descriptions of lateral sternal projections with poor positioning, state how the patient would have been mispositioned for such a projection to be obtained.

29. The anterior ribs are demonstrated without superimposition, the sternum is not in profile, and the superior heart shadow extends beyond the sternum and into the anteriorly situated lung.

   _____

30. The anterior ribs are demonstrated without superimposition, the sternum is not in profile, and the superior heart shadow does not extend beyond the sternum.

   _____

For the following lateral sternal projection with poor positioning, state what anatomic structures are misaligned and how the patient should be repositioned for an optimal projection to be obtained.

Figure 10-7

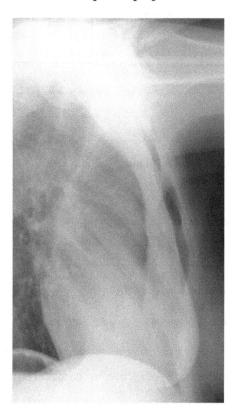

31. (Figure 10-7): _____

   _____

   _____

   _____

   _____

 Copyright © 2015, 2011, 2006, 1996 by Saunders, an imprint of Elsevier Inc. All rights reserved.

Ribs: AP or PA Projection

32. Identify the labeled anatomy in Figure 10-8.

Figure 10-8

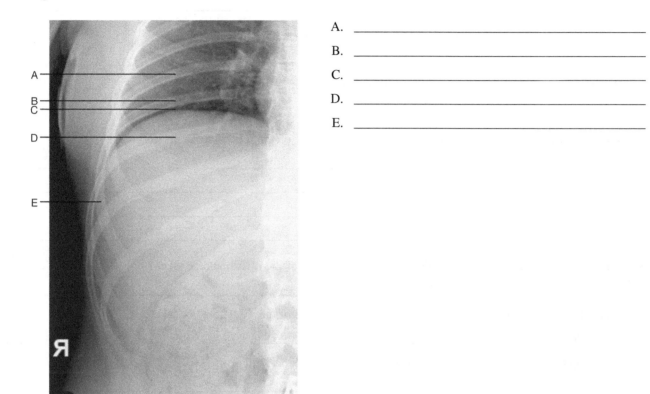

A. _____

B. _____

C. _____

D. _____

E. _____

33. Complete the statements below referring to AP/PA rib projection analysis guidelines.

AP or PA Rib Projection Analysis Guidelines

■ Thoracic vertebrae–rib head articulations are demonstrated, the sternum and (A)_____ are superimposed, and the distances from the (B) _____ to the sternal ends of the clavicles, when seen, are equal.

Above the diaphragm:

■ Scapulae are outside the lung field, and (C) _____ posterior ribs are seen above the diaphragm.

Below the diaphragm:

■ The (D) _____ through 12th posterior ribs are demonstrated below the diaphragm.

Copyright © 2015, 2011, 2006, 1996 by Saunders, an imprint of Elsevier Inc. All rights reserved.

34. Why do some facilities require the technologist to tape a rib marker (lead "BB") on the patient's skin near the area where the ribs are tender?

_____

_____

35. A. What patient respiration is used when imaging ribs located above the diaphragm?

_____

B. What patient respiration is used when imaging ribs located below the diaphragm?

_____

36. What soft tissue structures are evaluated for associated injury on the following rib projections?

A. Upper ribs: _____

_____

B. Lower ribs: _____

_____

37. If the patient complains of anterior rib pain, what projection of the ribs should be taken?

A. (AP/PA) _____

When the patient indicates posterior rib pain, what projection of the ribs should be taken?

B. (AP/PA) _____

If the opposite is taken for these two situations, what difference would result?

C. _____

38. How is spinal scoliosis identified on PA and AP rib projections?

_____

_____

39. Accurate CR centering on an above-diaphragm AP rib projection is accomplished by centering the CR halfway between the (A) _____ and affected lateral rib surface at a level halfway between the (B) _____ and (C) _____. This centering is accomplished on a PA projection by placing the CR halfway between the (D) _____ and lateral rib surface at the level of the (E) _____.

40. What anatomic structures are included on an above-diaphragm AP or PA rib projection with accurate positioning?

_____

_____

41. Accurate CR centering on a below-diaphragm AP or PA rib projection is accomplished by placing the lower border of the IR at the (A) _____, centering a perpendicular CR to the IR, and moving the patient side to side until the longitudinal collimator light line is aligned halfway between the (B) _____ and lateral rib surface.

42. What anatomic structures are included on an AP or PA below-diaphragm rib projection with accurate positioning?

_____

_____

 Copyright © 2015, 2011, 2006, 1996 by Saunders, an imprint of Elsevier Inc. All rights reserved.

For the following descriptions of AP or PA rib projections with poor positioning, state how the patient would have been mispositioned for such a projection to be obtained.

43. The sternum and SC joints are demonstrated to the left of the vertebral column on an AP projection taken because of left rib pain.

_____

_____

44. The left scapula is superimposed over the upper lateral rib field on a PA projection.

_____

_____

45. The 10th through 12th posterior ribs are demonstrated below the diaphragm on a below-diaphragm projection.

_____

_____

For the following AP or PA rib projections with poor positioning, state what anatomic structures are misaligned and how the patient should be repositioned for an optimal projection to be obtained.

Figure 10-9

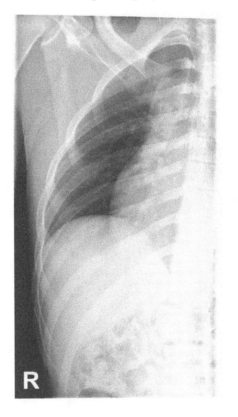

46. (Figure 10-9, AP projection, above-diaphragm ribs):

_____

_____

_____

_____

Copyright © 2015, 2011, 2006, 1996 by Saunders, an imprint of Elsevier Inc. All rights reserved.   Chapter **10 Image Analysis of the Sternum and Ribs**

Figure 10-10

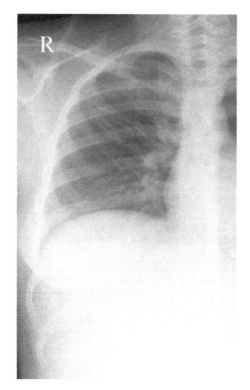

47. (Figure 10-10, AP projection, above-diaphragm ribs):

_____

_____

Figure 10-11

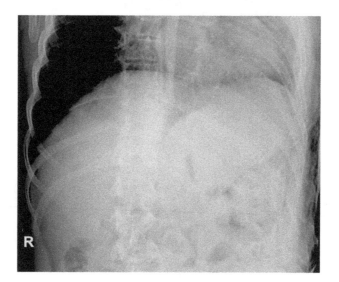

48. (Figure 10-11, AP projection, below-diaphragm ribs):

_____

_____

_____

Copyright © 2015, 2011, 2006, 1996 by Saunders, an imprint of Elsevier Inc. All rights reserved.

Ribs: AP Oblique Projection ((RPO and LPO Positions)

49. Identify the labeled anatomy in Figure 10-12.

Figure 10-12

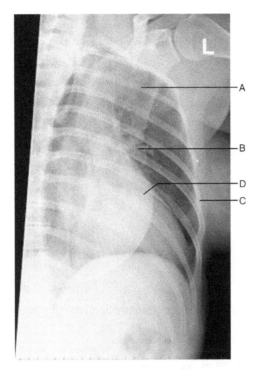

A. _____

B. _____

C. _____

D. _____

50. Identify the labeled anatomy in Figure 10-13.

Figure 10-13

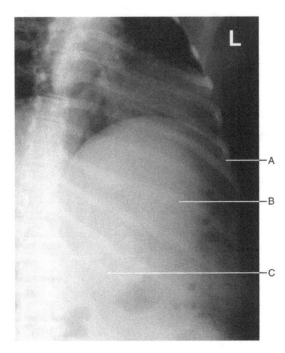

A. _____

B. _____

C. _____

Copyright © 2015, 2011, 2006, 1996 by Saunders, an imprint of Elsevier Inc. All rights reserved.   Chapter **10 Image Analysis of the Sternum and Ribs**

51. Complete the statements below referring to AP oblique ribs projection analysis guidelines.

AP Oblique Rib Projection Analysis Guidelines
■ The (A) _____ is located halfway between the lateral rib surface and the vertebral column, and the axillary ribs are free of superimposition.
■ The (B) _____ are demonstrated without superimposition and are located in the center of the collimated field, and the anterior ribs are located at the lateral edge.
Above the diaphragm:
■ The (C) _____ axillary ribs are demonstrated above the diaphragm.
Below the diaphragm:
■ The (D) _____ through 12th axillary ribs are demonstrated below the diaphragm.

52. What degree of patient rotation is used for AP oblique rib projections?

A. _____

What body plane is used to align this angle?

B. _____

53. State whether the patient is rotated toward or away from the affected side to demonstrate the axillary ribs in the AP

oblique projection. _____

54. How can one determine from an AP oblique rib projection if the patient has been rotated 45 degrees?_____

55. Accurate CR centering on an above-diaphragm AP oblique rib projection is accomplished by centering a

(A) _____ CR halfway between the midsagittal plane and (B) _____ , at a level halfway

between the (C) _____ and (D) _____.

56. What anatomic structures are included on an above-diaphragm AP oblique rib projection with accurate positioning?

_____

_____

57. Accurate CR centering on a below-diaphragm AP oblique rib projection is accomplished by positioning the lower

IR border at the patient's (A) _____ and centering the CR halfway between the (B) _____
and lateral rib surface.

58. What anatomic structures are included on a below-diaphragm AP oblique rib projection?

_____

_____

 Copyright © 2015, 2011, 2006, 1996 by Saunders, an imprint of Elsevier Inc. All rights reserved.

For the following descriptions of AP oblique rib projections with poor positioning, state how the patient would have been mispositioned for such a projection to be obtained.

59. The axillary ribs demonstrate increased foreshortening, and the sternum is rotated toward the patient's left side on a projection taken for right side rib pain.

_____

_____

60. The sternal body is demonstrated adjacent to the vertebral column.

_____

_____

61. An above-diaphragm AP oblique rib projection demonstrates the first through seventh posterior ribs above the diaphragm.

_____

_____

For the following AP and PA oblique rib projections with poor positioning, state what anatomic structures are misaligned and how the patient should be repositioned for an optimal projection to be obtained.

Figure 10-14

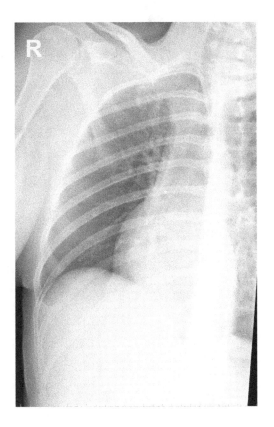

62. (Figure 10-14, AP oblique projection): _____

_____

_____

Copyright © 2015, 2011, 2006, 1996 by Saunders, an imprint of Elsevier Inc. All rights reserved.

Figure 10-15

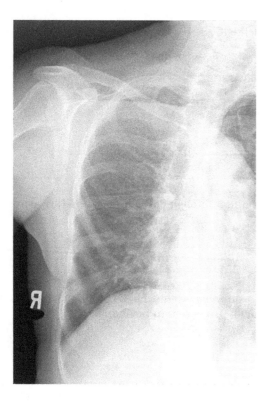

63. (Figure 10-15, PA oblique projection):

_____

_____

_____

Copyright © 2015, 2011, 2006, 1996 by Saunders, an imprint of Elsevier Inc. All rights reserved.

11 Image Analysis of the Cranium

STUDY QUESTIONS

1. Complete Figure 11-1.

   Figure 11-1

Cranium, Facial Bones and Paranasal Sinus Technical Data						
Projection	Structure	kV	Grid	AEC	mAs	SID
AP or PA						
PA axial (Caldwell method)						
AP axial (Towne method)						
Lateral						
Submentovertex (Schueller method)						
Pariet oacanthial (Waters method)						

2. State the cranial positioning lines indicated in Figure 11-2.

   Figure 11-2

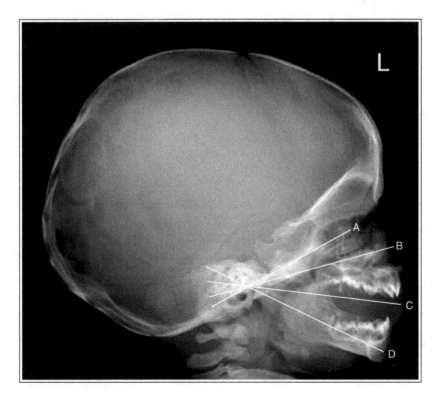

A. _____

B. _____

C. _____

D. _____

Copyright © 2015, 2011, 2006, 1996 by Saunders, an imprint of Elsevier Inc. All rights reserved.

Cranium and Mandible: PA or AP Projection

3. Identify the labeled anatomy in Figure 11-3.

Figure 11-3

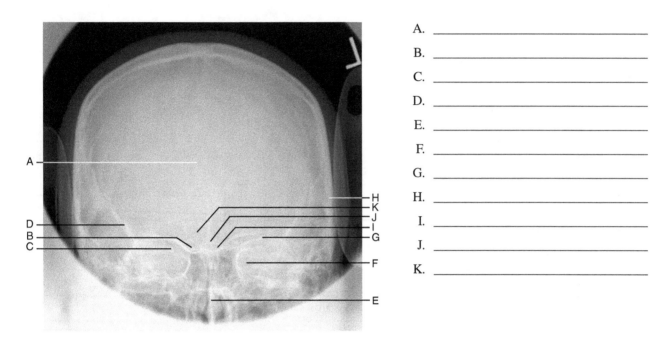

A. _____

B. _____

C. _____

D. _____

E. _____

F. _____

G. _____

H. _____

I. _____

J. _____

K. _____

4. Complete the statements below referring to PA cranial and mandibular projection analysis guidelines.

PA Cranium and Mandible Projection Analysis Guidelines

■ The distances from the lateral margin of orbits to the lateral cranial (A) _____ from the crista galli to the lateral cranial cortices, and from the mandibular rami to the lateral cervical vertebrae on both sides are equal.

■ The anterior clinoids and dorsum sellae are seen superior to the (B) _____.

■ The petrous ridges are superimposed over the (C) _____ and the internal acoustic meatus and visualized horizontally through the center of the orbits.

■ The crista galli and (D) _____ are aligned with the long axis of the exposure field, and the supraorbital margins and the TMJs are demonstrated on the same horizontal plane.

---

5. The midsagittal plane is positioned (A) _____⊥_____ to the IR for a PA cranial projection to prevent rotation.

How is this positioning best accomplished? (B) _place hands on each side of head (parietal) & move accordingly_

6. How is cranial rotation identified on a rotated PA skull projection?

_____

7. How is the patient's head position adjusted to prevent rotation on an AP skull projection taken in a patient with a suspected cervical injury?

_____

   Copyright © 2015, 2011, 2006, 1996 by Saunders, an imprint of Elsevier Inc. All rights reserved.

8. PA and AP skull projections demonstrate different magnified anatomic structures. Which of these projections demonstrates the greater orbital magnification?

A. _____

Which projection demonstrates the greater parietal bone magnification?

B. _____

9. What cranial positioning line is used to obtain an accurate PA projection? (A) _____ How is this line

positioned with respect to the IR? (B) _____

10. If the patient is unable to accurately position the line indicated in the above question to the IR for a PA cranial projection, how is the CR adjusted to compensate?

_____

11. When the patient's chin is tucked for a PA cranial projection, in which direction will the supraorbital margins move

with respect to the petrous ridges? _____ (Inferiorly/Superiorly)

12. If the patient is unable to adjust the degree of chin elevation for an AP trauma cranial projection, how is the CR used to compensate?

_____

13. A PA skull projection with poor positioning demonstrates approximately 1 inch (2.5 cm) of space between the petrous ridges and supraorbital margins. The ridges are inferior. Where are the dorsum sellae and anterior clinoids

demonstrated with respect to the ethmoid sinuses on this projection?_____

14. On a trauma AP cranial projection with poor positioning, the petrous ridges are demonstrated superior to the supraorbital margins. The distance between them is approximately ½ inch (1.25 cm). Will there be an increase or decrease in the amount of dorsum sella and anterior clinoid superimposition above the ethmoid sinuses on this projection?

_____

15. What two anatomic structures are aligned with the long axis on the projection if the patient's midsagittal plane is accurately aligned with the collimated field on a PA or AP cranial projection?

A. _____

B. _____

16. On a PA or AP cranial projection with accurate positioning, the (A) _____ is centered within the

collimated field. This centering is obtained when the CR is centered to the (B) _____.

17. What anatomic structures are included on a PA or AP cranial projection with accurate positioning?

_____

18. On a PA or AP mandible projection with accurate positioning, the (A) _____ is centered within the

exposure field. This centering is obtained when the CR is centered to (B)_____.

19. What anatomic structures are included on a PA or AP mandibular projection with accurate positioning?

_____

Copyright © 2015, 2011, 2006, 1996 by Saunders, an imprint of Elsevier Inc. All rights reserved.

For the following descriptions of PA cranial projections with poor positioning, state how the patient or CR would have been mispositioned for such an image to be obtained.

20. The distance from the lateral orbital margins to the lateral cranial cortex and from the crista galli to the lateral cranial cortex on the left side is greater than on the right side.

   _____

21. The petrous ridges are demonstrated inferior to the supraorbital margins, and the dorsum sellae and anterior clinoids are superimposed over the ethmoid sinuses. How was the patient mispositioned?

   A. ___chin was too far up___

   If this were a trauma AP projection, how would the CR have been mispositioned?

   B. ___CR angled too cephalic___

22. The petrous ridges are demonstrated superior to the supraorbital margins. How was the patient mispositioned?

   A. ___chin was tucked too much___

   If this were a trauma AP projection, how would the CR have been mispositioned?

   B. ___CR angled too caudal___

For the following PA cranial projections with poor positioning, state what anatomic structures are misaligned and how the patient should be repositioned for an optimal image to be obtained.

Figure 11-4

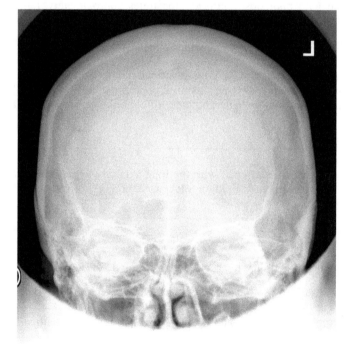

23. (Figure 11-4, PA projection): ___the pt was rotated 3 crista galli not centered fix: rotate face to left 3 place MSP ⊥ to IR___

Copyright © 2015, 2011, 2006, 1996 by Saunders, an imprint of Elsevier Inc. All rights reserved.

Figure 11-5

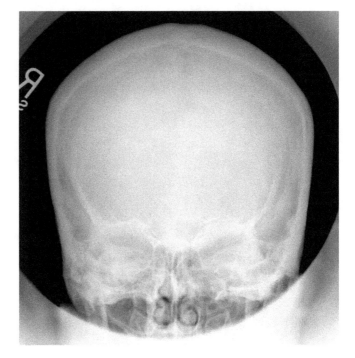

24. (Figure 11-5, PA projection): _____

_____

_____

_____

Figure 11-6

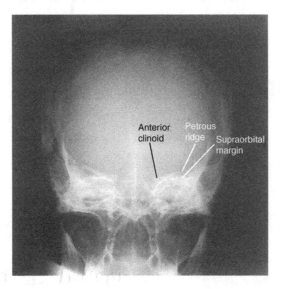

25. (Figure 11-6, PA projection): _____

_____

_____

_____

Copyright © 2015, 2011, 2006, 1996 by Saunders, an imprint of Elsevier Inc. All rights reserved.   Chapter **11 Image Analysis of the Cranium**

Figure 11-7

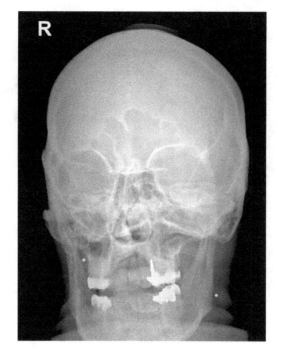

26. (Figure 11-7, AP projection, trauma): _____

_____

_____

_____

Cranium, Facial Bones, and Sinuses: PA Axial Projection (Caldwell Method)

27. Identify the labeled anatomy in Figure 11-8.

Figure 11-8

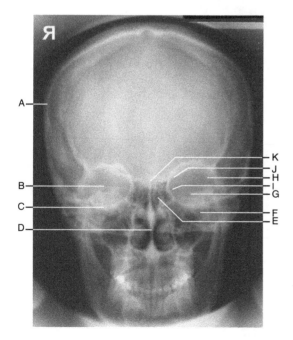

A. lateral cranial cortex

B. greater wing

C. infraorbital margin

D. nasal septum

E. ethmoid sinus

F. petrous pyramid

G. petrous ridge

H. oblique orbital line

I. supraorbital fissure

J. lesser wing

K. crista galli

446

Copyright © 2015, 2011, 2006, 1996 by Saunders, an imprint of Elsevier Inc. All rights reserved.

28. Complete the statements below referring to PA axial cranial, facial bones, and sinuses projection analysis guidelines.

> **PA Axial Cranium, Facial Bones, and Sinuses Projection Analysis Guidelines**
>
> ■ The distances from the lateral orbital margins to the (A) _____ on both sides and from the crista galli to the lateral cranial cortices on both sides are equal.
>
> ■ The petrous ridges are demonstrated horizontally through the lower third of the (B) _____, the petrous pyramids are superimposed over the (C) _____, and the superior orbital fissures are seen within the orbits.
>
> ■ The (D) _____ and nasal septum are aligned with the long axis of the exposure field, and the supraorbital margins are demonstrated on the same horizontal plane.

29. What plane is positioned perpendicular to the IR for a PA axial projection?

_____

30. When rotation is present on a PA axial projection, the patient's face is rotated (A) _____ (toward/away from) the side of the cranium that demonstrates the greater distance. On an AP axial projection, the patient's face is rotated (B) _____ (toward/away from) the side of the cranium that demonstrates the greater distance._____

31. What are the degree and direction of the CR angulation used on a PA axial projection of the cranium?

_____

32. What are the degree and direction of the CR angulation used on an AP axial projection of the cranium when the patient is capable of adequately positioning the head?

_____

33. Accurate positioning for a PA or AP axial cranial projection is obtained when the _____ line is aligned perpendicular to the IR.

34. How is the CR angulation determined for a PA axial cranial projection of a patient who is unable to accurately position the head? _____

_____

35. What is the CR angulation for a PA axial projection of the cranium for a patient who can tuck the chin only enough to place the OML at a 10-degree cephalad angle with the IR?

_____

36. What is the CR angulation for an AP axial projection of the cranium for a patient who can tuck the chin only enough to place the OML at a 5-degree caudal angle with the IR?

_____

37. On a PA and AP axial projection with accurate positioning, the (A) _____ are centered within the exposure field. This is accomplished by centering the CR to (B) _____.

Copyright © 2015, 2011, 2006, 1996 by Saunders, an imprint of Elsevier Inc. All rights reserved.

38. What anatomic structures are included on a PA or AP axial projection of the cranium with accurate positioning?

A. _____

On a projection of facial bones or sinuses?

B. _____

For the following descriptions of PA axial cranial projections with poor positioning, state how the patient or CR would have been mispositioned for such an image to be obtained.

39. The distance from the lateral orbital margin to the lateral cranial cortex on the left side is greater than that on the right side. Will the distance from the left or right side of the crista galli to the lateral cranial cortex demonstrate the smaller distance on this projection?

A. _____

How was the patient mispositioned for this image?

B. _____

40. The petrous ridges are demonstrated inferior to the inferior orbital margins. How was the patient mispositioned for such a projection to be obtained if the CR was accurately angled?

A. _____

How was the CR mispositioned for such a projection to be obtained if the patient was accurately positioned?

B. _____

41. The petrous ridges and pyramids are superior to the supraorbital margins, and the internal auditory canals are distorted. How was the patient mispositioned for such a projection to be obtained if the CR was accurately angled?

A. _____

How was the CR mispositioned for such a projection to be obtained if the patient was accurately positioned?

B. _____

Copyright © 2015, 2011, 2006, 1996 by Saunders, an imprint of Elsevier Inc. All rights reserved.

For the following PA axial cranial projections with poor positioning, state what anatomic structures are misaligned and how the patient should be repositioned for an optimal image to be obtained.

Figure 11-9

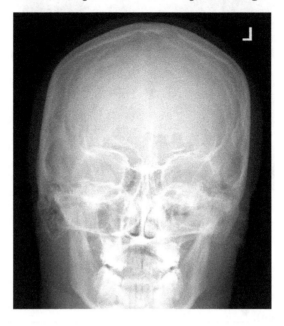

42. (Figure 11-9, PA axial projection): _____

_____

_____

_____

Figure 11-10

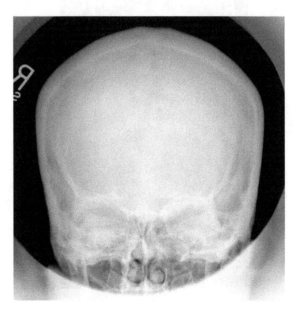

43. (Figure 11-10, PA axial projection): _____

_____

_____

_____

449

Copyright © 2015, 2011, 2006, 1996 by Saunders, an imprint of Elsevier Inc. All rights reserved.

Figure 11-11

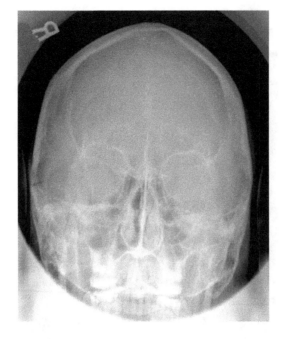

44. (Figure 11-11, PA axial projection): _____

_____

_____

_____

Figure 11-12

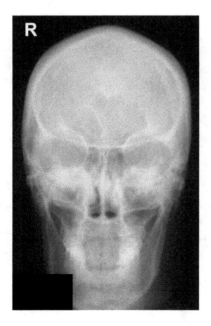

45. (Figure 11-12, AP axial projection, trauma): _____

_____

_____

_____

 Copyright © 2015, 2011, 2006, 1996 by Saunders, an imprint of Elsevier Inc. All rights reserved.

Cranium and Mandible: AP Axial Projection (Towne Method)

46. Identify the labeled anatomy in Figure 11-13.

Figure 11-13

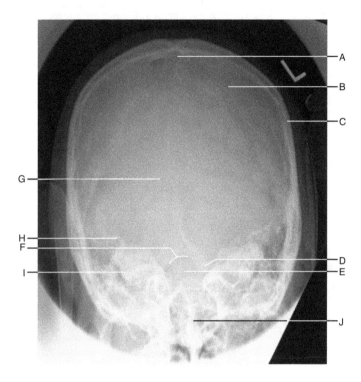

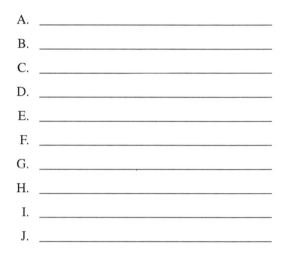

A. _____

B. _____

C. _____

D. _____

E. _____

F. _____

G. _____

H. _____

I. _____

J. _____

47. Identify the labeled anatomy in Figure 11-14.

Figure 11-14

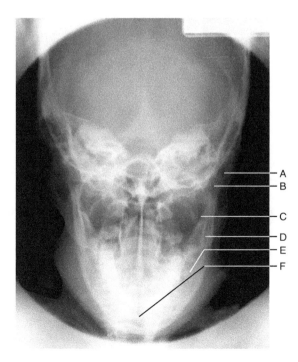

A. _____

B. _____

C. _____

D. _____

E. _____

F. _____

Copyright © 2015, 2011, 2006, 1996 by Saunders, an imprint of Elsevier Inc. All rights reserved.

48. Complete the statements below referring to AP axial cranial and mandibular projection analysis guidelines.

AP Axial Cranium and Mandible Projection Analysis Guidelines

- The distances from the posterior clinoid process to the lateral borders of the (A) _____ on both sides and the mandibular necks to the lateral cervical vertebrae on both sides are equal, the petrous ridges are symmetrical, and the dorsum sellae is centered within the (B) _____.

- Cranium: The dorsum sellae and (C) _____ are seen within the foramen magnum without foreshortening or superimposition of the atlas's posterior arch.

- Mandible: The dorsum sellae and posterior clinoids are at the level of the (D) _____ foramen magnum, and the mandibular condyles and fossae are clearly demonstrated, with minimal mastoid superimposition.

- The (E) _____ and nasal septum are aligned with the long axis of the exposure field.

---

49. The (A) _____ plane is positioned (B) _____ to the IR to prevent rotation on an AP axial projection.

50. When rotation is present on an AP axial projection, the side demonstrating less distance between the posterior clinoid process and the lateral border of the foramen magnum is the side _____ (toward/away from) which the patient's face is rotated.

51. When the correct CR angulation and head position are used on an AP axial projection, the (A) _____ and posterior clinoids are demonstrated within the (B) _____.

52. What are the degree and direction of the CR angulation used on an AP axial projection of the cranium and mandible?
    _____30-40° caudal_____

53. What cranial positioning line is aligned perpendicular to the IR for an AP axial projection of the cranium?
    _____OML_____

54. How is the CR angulation determined for an AP axial projection of the cranial in a patient who is unable to accurately position the head?

    _____

55. What anatomic structures are included on an AP axial projection of the cranium with accurate positioning?

    _____

For the following descriptions of AP axial projections of the cranium with inaccurate positioning, state how the patient or CR would have been mispositioned for such an image to be obtained.

56. The distance from the posterior clinoid process to the lateral foramen magnum on the patient's left side is less than that on the patient's right side.

    _____

   Copyright © 2015, 2011, 2006, 1996 by Saunders, an imprint of Elsevier Inc. All rights reserved.

57. The dorsum sellae and anterior clinoids are demonstrated superior to the foramen magnum. How would the patient have been mispositioned for such a projection to be obtained if the CR was accurately angled?

A. _____

How would the CR have been mispositioned for such a projection to be obtained if the patient was accurately positioned?

B. _____

58. The dorsum sella is foreshortened and superimposed over the atlas's posterior arch. How would the patient have been mispositioned for such a projection to be obtained if the CR was accurately angled?

A. _____

How would the CR have been mispositioned for such a projection to be obtained if the patient was accurately positioned?

B. _____

For the following AP axial projections of the cranium and mandible with poor positioning, state what anatomic structures are misaligned and how the patient should be repositioned for an optimal image to be obtained.

Figure 11-15

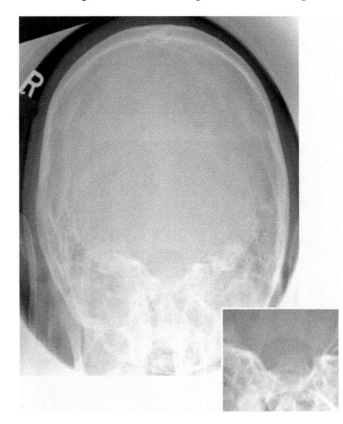

59. (Figure 11-15): _____

_____

_____

_____

Copyright © 2015, 2011, 2006, 1996 by Saunders, an imprint of Elsevier Inc. All rights reserved.

Figure 11-16

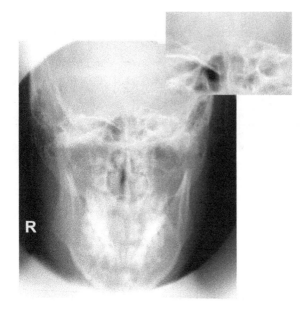

60. (Figure 11-16): _____

_____

_____

_____

Figure 11-17

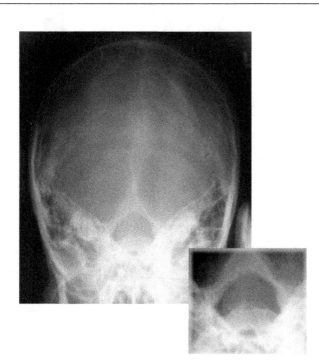

61. (Figure 11-17): _____

_____

_____

Copyright © 2015, 2011, 2006, 1996 by Saunders, an imprint of Elsevier Inc. All rights reserved.

Cranium, Facial Bones, Nasal Bones, and Sinuses: Lateral Projection

62. Identify the labeled anatomy in Figure 11-18.

Figure 11-18

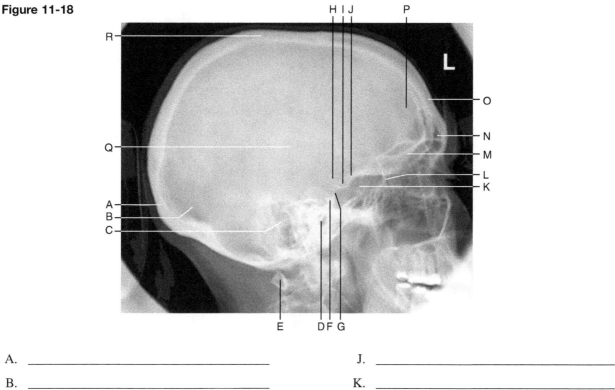

A. _____

B. _____

C. _____

D. _____

E. _____

F. _____

G. _____

H. _____

I. _____

J. _____

K. _____

L. _____

M. _____

N. _____

O. _____

P. _____

Q. _____

R. _____

Copyright © 2015, 2011, 2006, 1996 by Saunders, an imprint of Elsevier Inc. All rights reserved.

63. Identify the labeled anatomy in Figure 11-19.

Figure 11-19

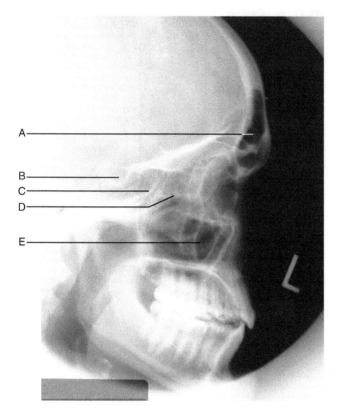

A. _____

B. _____

C. _____

D. _____

E. _____

64. Identify the labeled anatomy in Figure 11-20.

Figure 11-20

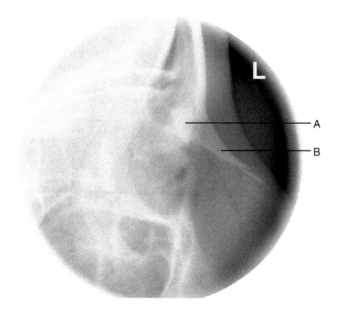

A. _____

B. _____

Copyright © 2015, 2011, 2006, 1996 by Saunders, an imprint of Elsevier Inc. All rights reserved.

65. Complete the statements below referring to lateral cranial, facial and nasal bones, and sinuses projection analysis guidelines.

Lateral Cranium, Facial and Nasal Bones, and Sinuses Projection Analysis Guidelines
■ When visualized, the sella turcica is seen in (A) _____. orbital roofs, mandibular rami, greater wings of the sphenoid, external acoustic canals, zygomatic bones, and cranial cortices are (B) _____.
■ Cranium: The posteroinferior occipital bones and (C) _____ of the atlas are free of superimposition.

66. What sinuses are demonstrated on a lateral projection of the sinuses?

_____ all 4 _____

67. Why is it best to take a lateral sinus projection with the patient in an upright position?

_____ air-fluid levels _____

68. What plane is used to position the patient to prevent rotation and tilting on a lateral cranial projection?

A. _____ MSP _____

How is it aligned with the IR?

B. _____ // _____

How does this positioning align the interpupillary (IP) line with the IR?

C. _____ ⊥ _____

69. How is the patient or IR positioned to include the occipital bone for a lateral cranial projection of a recumbent patient without cervical trauma?

A. _____

Of a recumbent patient with cervical trauma?

B. _____

70. How can cranial tilting be distinguished from rotation on a lateral cranial projection? _____

_____ rotation - throws off anterior/posterior _____

_____ tilt - throws off superior/inferior _____

Copyright © 2015, 2011, 2006, 1996 by Saunders, an imprint of Elsevier Inc. All rights reserved.

71. How is the patient positioned to ensure that the posteroinferior occipital bone and posterior arch of the atlas are free of superimposition?

_____10ML ⊥ to front edge of IR_____

72. On a lateral cranial projection with accurate positioning, the CR is centered 2 inches (5 cm) (A) _____

to the (B) _____.

73. What anatomic structures are included on a lateral cranial projection with accurate positioning?

_____

74. On a lateral sinus projection with accurate positioning, the (A) _Zygoma_ are centered within the exposure field. This is accomplished by centering the CR halfway between the (B) _EAM_ and (C) _outer canthus_.

75. What anatomic structures are included on a lateral sinus projection with accurate positioning?

_____

76. On a lateral nasal projection with accurate positioning, the (A) _____ are centered within the exposure field. This is accomplished by centering the CR ½ inch (1.25 cm) (B) _____ to the nasion.

77. What anatomic structures are included on a lateral nasal bone projection with accurate positioning?

_____nasal bones & surrounding soft tissues_____

For the following descriptions of lateral cranial projections with poor positioning, state how the patient would have been mispositioned for such an image to be obtained.

78. The greater wings of the sphenoid and the anterior cranial cortices are demonstrated without superimposition. One of each corresponding structure is demonstrated anterior to the other.

_____rotation of pts. head_____

79. The orbital roofs, external auditory meatus, and inferior cranial cortices are demonstrated without superimposition. One of each corresponding structure is demonstrated superior to the other, and the posterior arch is seen in profile.

_____

Copyright © 2015, 2011, 2006, 1996 by Saunders, an imprint of Elsevier Inc. All rights reserved.

For the following lateral cranial projections with poor positioning, state what anatomic structures are misaligned and how the patient should be repositioned for an optimal image to be obtained.

Figure 11-21

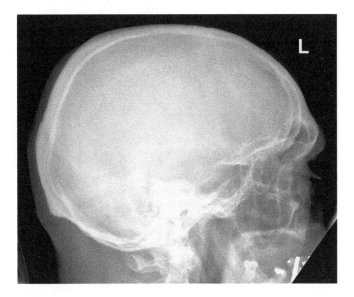

80. (Figure 11-21): _____

_____

_____

_____

Figure 11-22

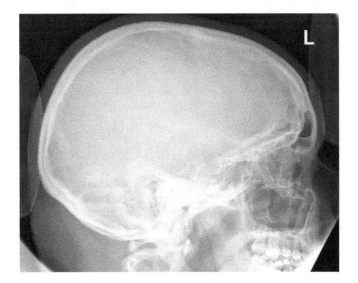

81. (Figure 11-22): _____

_____

_____

_____

Copyright © 2015, 2011, 2006, 1996 by Saunders, an imprint of Elsevier Inc. All rights reserved. Chapter **11 Image Analysis of the Cranium**

Cranium, Mandible, and Sinuses: Submentovertex (SMV) Projection (Schueller Method)

82. Identify the labeled anatomy in Figure 11-23.

Figure 11-23

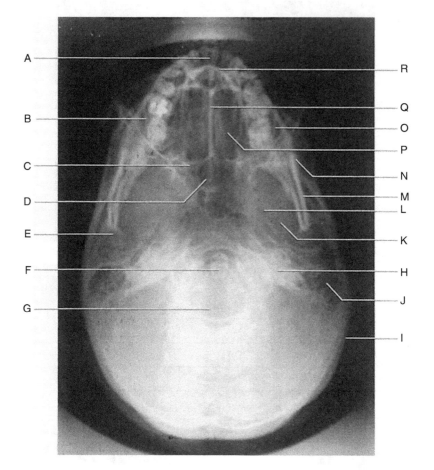

A. _____   J. _____

B. _____   K. _____

C. _____   L. _____

D. _____   M. _____

E. _____   N. _____

F. _____   O. _____

G. _____   P. _____

H. _____   Q. _____

I. _____   R. _____

Copyright © 2015, 2011, 2006, 1996 by Saunders, an imprint of Elsevier Inc. All rights reserved.

83. Complete the statements below referring to SMV cranial, mandibular, and sinuses projection analysis guidelines.

Submentovertex (SMV) Cranium, Mandible, and Sinuses Projection Analysis Guidelines
■ The mandibular mentum and nasal fossae are demonstrated just anterior to the (A) _____.
■ The distances from the mandibular ramus and body to the (B) _____ on both sides are equal.
■ The vomer, bony nasal septum, and (C) _____ are aligned with the long axis of the exposure field.

84. Accurate mandibular mentum and nasal fossae positioning on a SMV cranial projection is obtained when the (A)_____ cranial positioning line is aligned (B) _____ with the IR.

85. What structures are obscured on a SMV cranial projection if the patient's neck is not adequately extended?

    A. _____

    B. _____

    C. _____

    D. _____

86. How is the positioning setup adjusted for a SMV cranial projection in a patient who is unable to extend the neck as far as needed?

    _____

87. How is cranial tilting identified on a tilted SMV cranial projection?

    A. _____

    How is the patient positioned to prevent tilting on a SMV cranial projection?

    B. _____

88. On a SMV cranial projection with accurate positioning, the (A) _____ is centered within the exposure field. This is accomplished when the CR is centered to the (B) _____ plane at a level (C) _____ inch(es) anterior to the level of the (D) _____.

89. What anatomic structures are included on a SMV cranial projection with accurate positioning?

    _____

90. On a SMV sinus and mandible image with accurate positioning, the (A) _Sphenoid sinus_ are centered within the collimated field. This is accomplished by centering the CR to the (B) _MSP_ plane at a level (C) _1.5-2_ inches inferior to the (D) _mandibular symphysis_

91. What anatomic structures are included on a SMV sinus and mandible projection with accurate positioning?

    mandible, mastoids, & lateral cranial cortius

Copyright © 2015, 2011, 2006, 1996 by Saunders, an imprint of Elsevier Inc. All rights reserved.

For the following descriptions of SMV cranial projections with poor positioning, state how the patient or CR would have been mispositioned for such an image to be obtained.

92. The mandibular mentum is demonstrated too far anterior to the ethmoid sinuses.

_____

93. The mandibular mentum is demonstrated posterior to the ethmoid sinuses. How would the patient have been mispositioned?

A. _____

How would the CR have been mispositioned?

B. _____

94. The distance from the left mandibular ramus and body to its corresponding lateral cranial cortex is greater than the distance from the right mandibular ramus and body to its corresponding lateral cranial cortex.

_____

For the following SMV cranial, facial bone, and sinus projections with poor positioning, state what anatomic structures are misaligned and how the patient should be repositioned for an optimal image to be obtained.

Figure 11-24

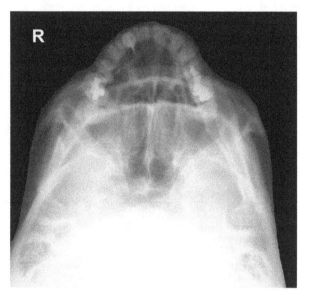

95. (Figure 11-24): _____

_____

_____

_____

Chapter **11 Image Analysis of the Cranium**   Copyright © 2015, 2011, 2006, 1996 by Saunders, an imprint of Elsevier Inc. All rights reserved.

Figure 11-25

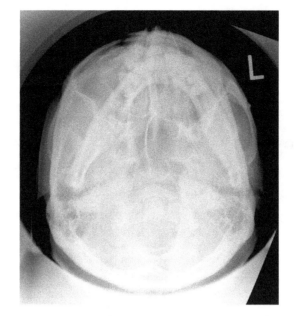

96. (Figure 11-25): _____

_____

_____

_____

_____

_____

Figure 11-26

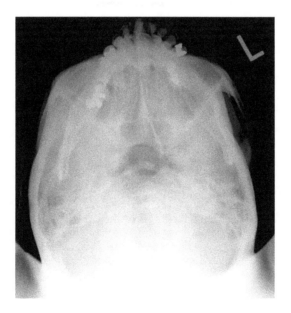

97. (Figure 11-26): _____

_____

_____

_____

Copyright © 2015, 2011, 2006, 1996 by Saunders, an imprint of Elsevier Inc. All rights reserved.

Facial Bones and Sinuses: Parietoacanthial and Acanthioparietal Projection (Waters and Open-Mouth Waters Methods)

98. Identify the labeled anatomy in Figure 11-27.

Figure 11-27

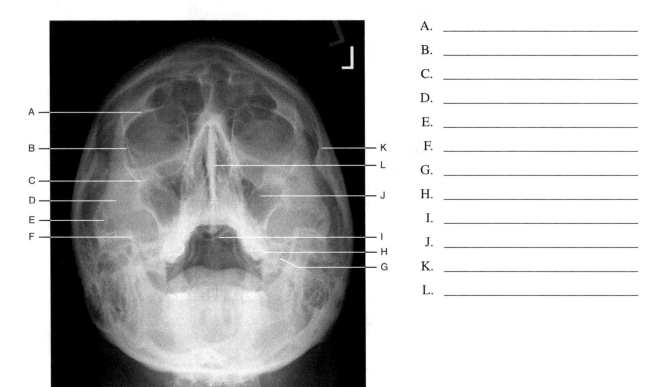

A. _____

B. _____

C. _____

D. _____

E. _____

F. _____

G. _____

H. _____

I. _____

J. _____

K. _____

L. _____

99. Complete the statements below referring to parietoacanthial and acanthioparietal facial bones and sinuses projection analysis guidelines.

Parietoacanthial and Acanthioparietal Facial Bones and Sinuses Projection Analysis Guidelines
■ The distances from the (A) _____ to the lateral cranial cortex and the distance from the bony nasal septum to the lateral cranial cortex on both sides are equal.
■ The petrous ridges are demonstrated (B) _____ to the maxillary sinuses and extend (C) _____ from the posterior maxillary alveolar process.
■ The bony nasal septum is aligned with the long axis of the exposure field, and the (D) _____ are demonstrated on the same horizontal plane.

Copyright © 2015, 2011, 2006, 1996 by Saunders, an imprint of Elsevier Inc. All rights reserved.

100. What sinuses are demonstrated on an open-mouth parietoacanthial projection that are not demonstrated on a closed-mouth parietoacanthial projection? _____

101. When rotation is present on a parietoacanthial projection, the patient's face is rotated (A) _____ (toward/away from) the side of the cranium that demonstrates the greatest distance. If an acanthioparietal projection is taken, the patient's face is rotated (B) _____ (toward/away from) the side of the cranium that demonstrates the greatest distance.

102. How is the patient positioned to accurately demonstrate the petrous ridges inferior to the maxillary sinuses on a parietoacanthial projection? _____

103. On a parietoacanthial projection with accurate positioning, the (A) _____ is centered within the exposure field. This is accomplished by centering the CR to the (B)_____ .

104. What anatomic structures are included on a parietoacanthial projection with accurate positioning?

_____

_____

For the following descriptions of parietoacanthial cranial projections with poor positioning, state how the patient would have been mispositioned for such a projection to be obtained.

105. The distances from the lateral orbital margin to the lateral cranial cortex and from the bony nasal septum to the lateral cranial cortex on the left side of the patient are greater than the distances on the right side.

_____

_____

106. The petrous ridges are demonstrated within the maxillary sinuses and superior to the posterior maxillary alveolar process.

_____

_____

107. The petrous ridges are inferior to the maxillary sinuses and posterior maxillary alveolar process.

_____

_____

Copyright © 2015, 2011, 2006, 1996 by Saunders, an imprint of Elsevier Inc. All rights reserved.   Chapter **11** **Image Analysis of the Cranium**

For the following parietoacanthial projections with poor positioning, state what anatomic structures are misaligned and how the patient should be repositioned for an optimal image to be obtained.

Figure 11-28

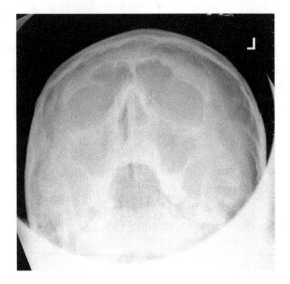

108. (Figure 11-28): _____

_____

_____

_____

Figure 11-29

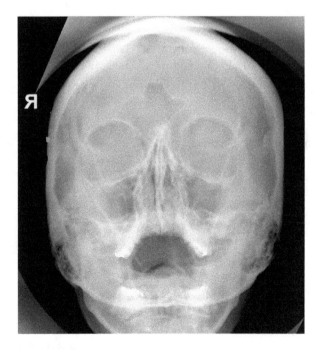

109. (Figure 11-29, parietocanthial):

petrous ridges are in maxillary sinuses
fix: elevate chin so MML ⊥ to IR

_____

Chapter **11** **Image Analysis of the Cranium**   Copyright © 2015, 2011, 2006, 1996 by Saunders, an imprint of Elsevier Inc. All rights reserved.

Figure 11-30

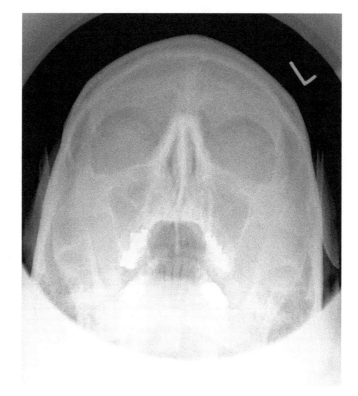

110. (Figure 11-30, parietocanthial): ___petrous ridges below maxillary sinuses___
___fix: depress chin so MML is ⊥ to IR___

Copyright © 2015, 2011, 2006, 1996 by Saunders, an imprint of Elsevier Inc. All rights reserved.

STUDY QUESTIONS

1. List the patient preparation procedure for the following examinations.

    A. Esophagus: _____

    _____

    B. Stomach: _____

    _____

    C. Small intestine: _____

    _____

    D. Large intestine: _____

    _____

2. Why are short exposure times needed when imaging the digestive system?

    involuntary motion & peristaltic activity

    _____

3. Define *peristalsis* and state how it is recognized on stomach and large and small intestine projections.

    _____

    _____

    _____

    _____

Copyright © 2015, 2011, 2006, 1996 by Saunders, an imprint of Elsevier Inc. All rights reserved.

4. Complete Figure 12-1.

Figure 12-1

Digestive System Technical Data					
Projection	kV	Grid	AEC	mAs	SID
Upper Gastrointestinal System					
PA oblique (RAO) position, esophagus					
Lateral, esophagus					
AP or PA, esophagus					
PA oblique (RAO position) stomach					
PA, stomach					
Right lateral, stomach					
AP oblique (LPO position), stomach					
AP, stomach					
Small Intestine					
PA or AP					
Large Intestine					
AP or PA					
Lateral, rectum					
AP or PA (lateral decubitus)					
PA oblique (RAO position)					
PA oblique (LAO position)					
PA axial or PA axial oblique (RAO position)					

Copyright © 2015, 2011, 2006, 1996 by Saunders, an imprint of Elsevier Inc. All rights reserved.

5. State the size, shape, and placement in the abdominal cavity of the stomach for the following habitus.

A. Hypersthenic: _____

_____

_____

B. Asthenic: _____

_____

_____

C. Sthenic: _____

_____

_____

6. State the position of the lower intestine within the abdominal cavity for the following habitus.

A. Hypersthenic: _Stomach: high & transverse_

flexures & transverse high

B. Asthenic: _Stomach: low, verticle, near midline, &_

"J" shaped

intestines: low in abd.

C. Sthenic: _Stomach: somewhat "J" shaped_

intestines: centered to abd.

7. How many posterior ribs are demonstrated superior to the diaphragm dome when an upper or lower gastrointestinal projection is obtained after full expiration, and why is this important?

9 & gives more room, so structures don't overlap

UPPER GASTROINTESTINAL SYSTEM

Esophagram

8. What barium weight or volume suspension is used for esophagus projections? _____

_____

9. When might the patient be asked to swallow cotton balls soaked in barium, barium-filled gelatin capsules, or barium tablets for an esophagram?

_____

470

Copyright © 2015, 2011, 2006, 1996 by Saunders, an imprint of Elsevier Inc. All rights reserved.

Esophagram: PA Oblique Projection (RAO Position)

10. Identify the labeled anatomy in Figure 12-2.

Figure 12-2

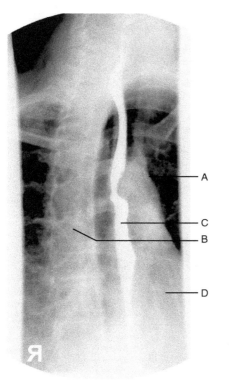

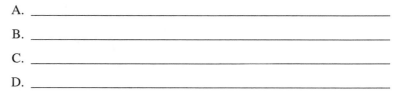

A. _____

B. _____

C. _____

D. _____

11. An adequately rotated PA oblique esophagram projection will demonstrate the esophagus between the

(A) _____ and (B) _____ and approximately (C) _____ inch of the right

sternal clavicular end to the left of the vertebrae and is accomplished by rotating the patient (D) _____ degrees.

12. On a PA oblique esophagram projection with accurate positioning, the (A) _mid-esophagus_ is centered within the collimated field. This centering is obtained when a perpendicular CR is centered 3 inches to the left of

the (B) _spinous processes_ and (C) _2-3_ inches inferior to the jugular notch.

13. What anatomic structures are included on a PA oblique esophagram projection with accurate positioning?

esophagus between spine & heart

For the following descriptions of PA oblique esophagram projections with poor positioning, state how the patient or CR would have been mispositioned for such a projection to be obtained.

14. The superior and inferior ends of the esophagus are not filled with barium.

_____

15. The vertebrae are superimposed over the right sternal clavicular end and a portion of the esophagus.

_____

Copyright © 2015, 2011, 2006, 1996 by Saunders, an imprint of Elsevier Inc. All rights reserved.

For the following PA oblique esophagram projections with poor positioning, state what anatomic structures are misaligned and how the patient should be repositioned for an optimal projection to be obtained.

Figure 12-3

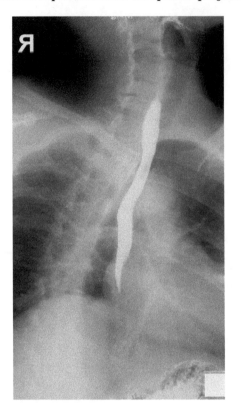

16. (Figure 12-3): _____

_____

_____

_____

Copyright © 2015, 2011, 2006, 1996 by Saunders, an imprint of Elsevier Inc. All rights reserved.

Figure 12-4

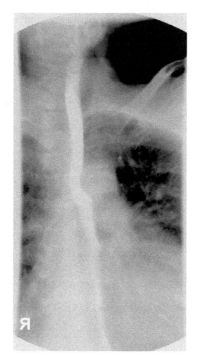

17. (Figure 12-4): _____

_____

_____

_____

Esophagram: Lateral Projection

18. Identify the labeled anatomy in Figure 12-5.

Figure 12-5

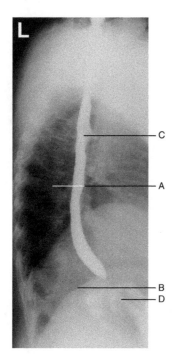

A. _____

B. _____

C. _____

D. _____

Copyright © 2015, 2011, 2006, 1996 by Saunders, an imprint of Elsevier Inc. All rights reserved.

19. A lateral projection of the esophagus is obtained when the esophagus is demonstrated anterior to the thoracic vertebrae, the (A) _____ surfaces of each vertebral body are superimposed, and no more than (B) _____ inch of space is seen between the (C) _____.

20. How should the patient be positioned to prevent rotation on a lateral esophagram projection?

_____

_____

21. How are the patient's shoulders and humeri positioned to place them away from the esophagus on a lateral projection? _____

_____

_____

22. On a lateral esophagram projection with accurate positioning, the (A) _____, at the level of (B) _____, is centered within the collimated field. This centering is obtained when a perpendicular CR is centered 2 to 3 inches inferior to the (C) _____.

23. What anatomic structures are included on a lateral esophagram projection with accurate positioning?

_____

_____

Copyright © 2015, 2011, 2006, 1996 by Saunders, an imprint of Elsevier Inc. All rights reserved.

For the following description of a lateral esophagram projection with poor positioning, state how the patient or CR would have been mispositioned for such a projection to be obtained.

24. The posterior ribs demonstrate more than ½ inch (1.25 cm) of space between them.

_____

Esophagram: PA Projection

25. Identify the labeled anatomy in Figure 12-6.

Figure 12-6

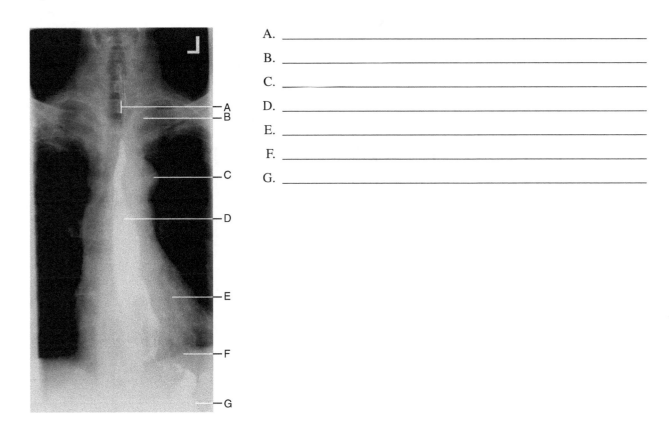

A. _____

B. _____

C. _____

D. _____

E. _____

F. _____

G. _____

26. The distances from the (A) _____ to the (B) _____ are equal, and the vertebrae are superimposed over the esophagus on a nonrotated PA esophagram projection.

27. On a PA esophagram projection with accurate positioning, the (A) _____, at the level of (B) _____, is centered within the collimated field. This centering is obtained when a perpendicular CR is centered 2 to 3 inches superior to the (C) _____.

28. What anatomic structures are included on a lateral esophagram projection with accurate positioning?

_____

Copyright © 2015, 2011, 2006, 1996 by Saunders, an imprint of Elsevier Inc. All rights reserved.

For the following description of a PA esophagram projection with poor positioning, state how the patient or CR would have been mispositioned for such a projection to be obtained.

29. The esophagus is to the right of the vertebrae, and the right sternal clavicular end is demonstrated without vertebral column superimposition.

_____

For the following PA esophagram with poor positioning, state what anatomic structures are misaligned and how the patient should be repositioned for an optimal projection to be obtained.

Figure 12-7

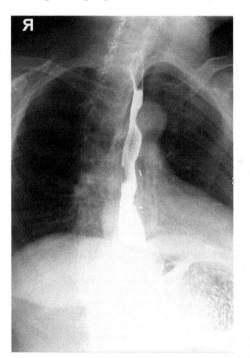

30. (Figure 12-7): _____

_____

_____

_____

STOMACH AND DUODENUM

31. What is the goal of the following upper gastrointestinal studies?

A. Single contrast: _____

_____

B. Double contrast: _____

_____

32. What barium weight or volume suspension is used for single- and double-contrast upper gastrointestinal projections?

A. Single contrast: _____

B. Double contrast: _____

 Copyright © 2015, 2011, 2006, 1996 by Saunders, an imprint of Elsevier Inc. All rights reserved.

33. The negative contrast used in a double-contrast study is mostly commonly (A) _____
and is used to provide (B) _____.

34. The barium in a double-contrast study provides the thin coating that covers the (A) _____.
How is adequate barium coating of the stomach and duodenum achieved? _____

_____

_____

35. List the stomach and duodenum structures that are barium filled and air filled for a double-contrast study when the
patient is placed in the following positions by completing Figure 12-8.

Figure 12-8

Double-Contrast Filling of Upper Gastrointestinal System		
Stomach Projection	Barium-Filled Structures	Air-Filled Structures
PA oblique (RAO position)		
PA		
Right lateral		
AP oblique (LPO position)		
AP		

36. The quality of the mucosal coating depends on:

A. _____

B. _____

C. _____

D. _____

Copyright © 2015, 2011, 2006, 1996 by Saunders, an imprint of Elsevier Inc. All rights reserved. Chapter **12** **Image Analysis of the Digestive System**

Stomach and Duodenum: PA Oblique Projection (RAO Position)

37. Identify the labeled anatomy in Figure 12-9.

Figure 12-9

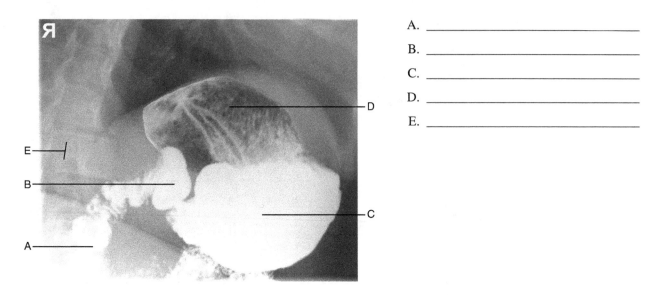

A. _____

B. _____

C. _____

D. _____

E. _____

38. Identify what body type is being represented in the PA oblique stomach and duodenal projections indicated below and state the degree of patient obliquity required to obtain the projection.

A. (Figure 12-9): _hypersthenic_____, 70°_____

Figure 12-10

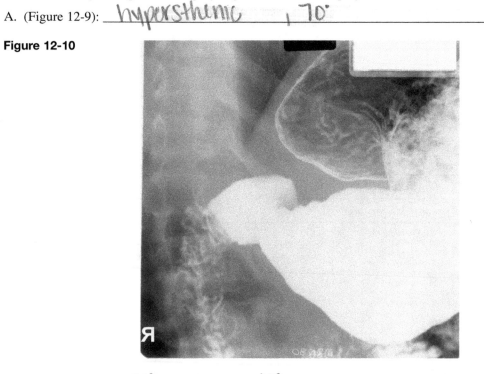

B. (Figure 12-10): _Sthenic_____, 45°_____

Copyright © 2015, 2011, 2006, 1996 by Saunders, an imprint of Elsevier Inc. All rights reserved.

Figure 12-11

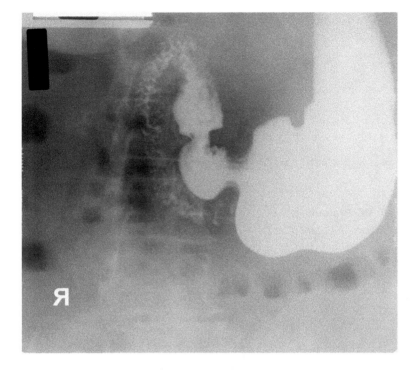

C. (Figure 12-11): ___asthenic___ , ___40°___

39. An adequately rotated hypersthenic PA oblique stomach and duodenal projection will demonstrate the left zygapophyseal joints in the (A) _____ of the vertebral body, the duodenal bulb and

(B) _____ duodenum in profile, and the long axis of the stomach demonstrating foreshortening

with a (C) _____ lesser curvature.

40. An adequately rotated sthenic PA oblique stomach and duodenal projection demonstrates the left zygapophyseal

joints at the (A) ___midline___ of the vertebral body, the duodenal bulb and (B) ___descending___ duodenum in profile, and the long axis of the stomach demonstrating partial foreshortening with a closed

(C) ___lesser curvature___.

41. An adequately rotated asthenic PA oblique stomach and duodenal projection demonstrates the left zygapophyseal

joints in the (A) _____ of the vertebral bodies, the duodenal bulb and (B) _____ duodenum in profile, and the long axis of the stomach demonstrated without foreshortening; the

(C) _____ is open.

42. Explain why it is necessary to rotate the patient differing amounts for a PA oblique stomach and duodenal projection to demonstrate the duodenal bulb and descending duodenum in profile.

___Because structures lie at different positions___
___depending on body habitus___

43. On a sthenic patient for a PA oblique stomach and duodenal projection with accurate positioning, the

(A) _____ is centered within the collimated field. This centering is obtained on the sthenic patient when

a perpendicular CR is centered halfway between the (B) _____ and (C) _____

of the elevated side at a level 1 to 2 inches (2.5 to 5 cm) (D) _____ to the inferior rib margin.

479

Copyright © 2015, 2011, 2006, 1996 by Saunders, an imprint of Elsevier Inc. All rights reserved.

44. State how the CR position is adjusted from the sthenic patient for a PA oblique stomach and duodenal projection for the following habitus.

A. Hypersthenic: _____

_____

B. Asthenic: _____

_____

45. What anatomic structures are included on a PA oblique stomach and duodenal projection with accurate positioning?

_____

Stomach and Duodenum: PA Projection

46. Identify the labeled anatomy in Figure 12-12.

Figure 12-12

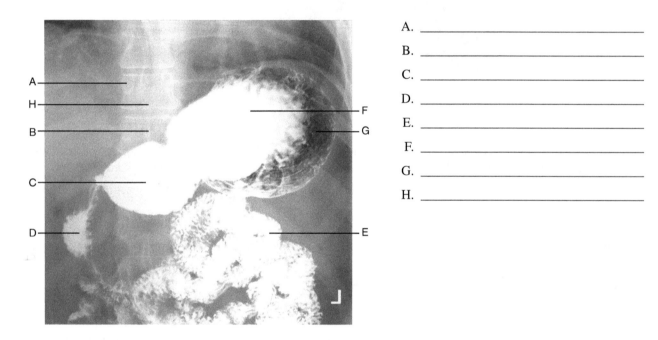

A. _____

B. _____

C. _____

D. _____

E. _____

F. _____

G. _____

H. _____

47. Identify what body type is being represented in the following PA stomach and duodenal projections.

A. (Figure 12-12): ___hypersthenic_____

Copyright © 2015, 2011, 2006, 1996 by Saunders, an imprint of Elsevier Inc. All rights reserved.

Figure 12-13

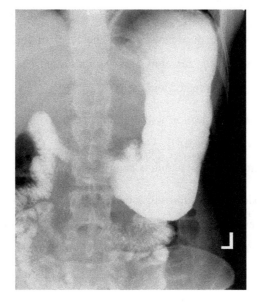

B. (Figure 12-13): _asthenic_

Figure 12-14

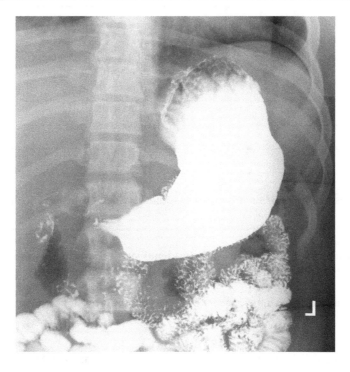

C. (Figure 12-14): _sthenic_

48. An optimal PA stomach and duodenal projection has been obtained when the spinous processes are aligned with the

(A) _____ of the vertebral bodies and the distances from the pedicles to the

(B) _____ are equal on both sides.

Copyright © 2015, 2011, 2006, 1996 by Saunders, an imprint of Elsevier Inc. All rights reserved.   Chapter **12 Image Analysis of the Digestive System**

49. A hypersthenic PA stomach and duodenal projection will demonstrate the stomach aligned nearly (A) _____ with the duodenal bulb at the level of the (B) _____ thoracic vertebrae. The lesser and greater curvatures are demonstrated nearly on end with the greater curvature being more (C) _____ situated and the (D) _____ nearly on end.

50. A sthenic PA stomach and duodenal projection will demonstrate the stomach aligned nearly (A) _vertical_, with the duodenal bulb at the level of the (B) _L1-2_ lumbar vertebrae. The lesser and greater curvature, esophagogastric junction, pylorus, and duodenal bulb are in (C) _partial profile_.

51. An asthenic PA stomach and duodenal projection will demonstrate the stomach aligned (A) _____, with the duodenal bulb at the level of the (B) _____ lumbar vertebrae. The stomach is (C) _____ shaped, and its long axis is demonstrated without foreshortening; the (D) _____, _____, _____, and _____ are in profile.

52. On a sthenic patient for a PA stomach and duodenal projection with accurate positioning, the (A) _____ is centered within the collimated field. For the sthenic patient, this centering is obtained when a perpendicular CR is centered halfway between the (B) _____ and (C) _____ at a point approximately 1 to 2 inches (2.5 to 5 cm) (D) _____ to the lower rib margin.

53. State how the CR position is adjusted from a sthenic patient for a PA stomach and duodenal projection for the following habitus.

    A. Hypersthenic: _____

    _____

    B. Asthenic: _____

    _____

54. What anatomic structures are included on a PA stomach and duodenal projection with accurate positioning?

    _____

For the following descriptions of PA stomach and duodenal projections with poor positioning, state how the patient or CR would have been mispositioned for such a projection to be obtained.

55. The stomach demonstrates a blotchy appearance within the barium. The stomach contains residual food particles.

    _____

56. The distance from the right pedicles to the spinous processes is greater than the distance from the left pedicles to the spinous processes.

    _____

 Copyright © 2015, 2011, 2006, 1996 by Saunders, an imprint of Elsevier Inc. All rights reserved.

Stomach and Duodenum: Lateral Projection (Right Lateral Position)

57. Identify the labeled anatomy in Figure 12-15.

Figure 12-15

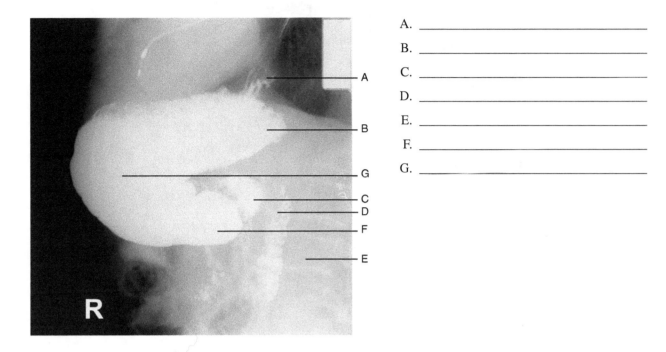

A. _____

B. _____

C. _____

D. _____

E. _____

F. _____

G. _____

58. Identify what body type is being represented in the lateral stomach and duodenal projections indicated below.

A. (Figure 12-15): _____

Figure 12-16

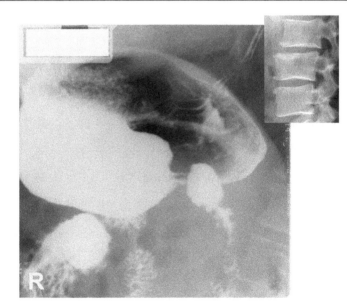

B. (Figure 12-16): _____

Copyright © 2015, 2011, 2006, 1996 by Saunders, an imprint of Elsevier Inc. All rights reserved.

Chapter **12 Image Analysis of the Digestive System**

Figure 12-17

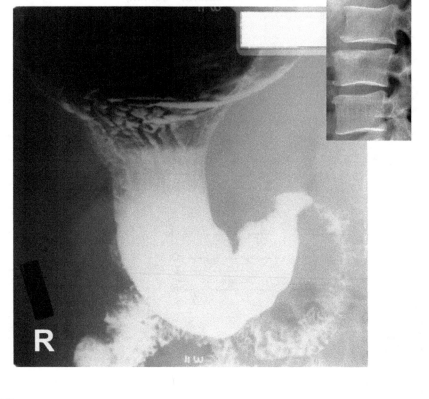

C. (Figure 12-17): _____

59. An optimal right lateral stomach and duodenal projection has been obtained when the (A) _____ surfaces of the vertebral bodies are superimposed and the (B) _____ space is demonstrated.

60. A hypersthenic lateral stomach and duodenal projection demonstrates the (A) _____, (B) _____, and (C) _____ in profile, and the long axis of the stomach demonstrates foreshortening with a (D) _____ lesser curvature.

61. On a sthenic lateral stomach and duodenal projection, the long axis of the stomach is (A) _____ foreshortened, and the lesser curvature is partially (B) _____.

62. On an asthenic lateral stomach and duodenal projection, the long axis of the stomach is demonstrated (A) _____ foreshortening, with a(n) (B) _____ lesser curvature.

63. On a lateral stomach and duodenal projection with accurate positioning, the (A) _____ is centered within the collimated field. For a sthenic patient, this centering is obtained when a perpendicular CR is centered halfway between the (B) _____ and (C) _____ at a level 1 to 2 inches superior to the (D) _____.

Copyright © 2015, 2011, 2006, 1996 by Saunders, an imprint of Elsevier Inc. All rights reserved.

64. State how the CR position is adjusted from the sthenic patient for a lateral stomach and duodenal projection for the following habitus.

A. Hypersthenic: _____

_____

B. Asthenic: _____

_____

65. What anatomic structures are included on a lateral stomach and duodenal projection with accurate positioning?

_____

For the following description of a lateral stomach and duodenal projection with poor positioning, state how the patient or CR would have been mispositioned for such a projection to be obtained.

66. The descending duodenum is partially superimposed over the duodenal bulb and vertebrae, and the posterior surfaces of the thoracic and lumbar vertebrae are not superimposed.

_____

Stomach and Duodenum: AP Oblique Projection (LPO Position)

67. Identify the labeled anatomy in Figure 12-18.

Figure 12-18

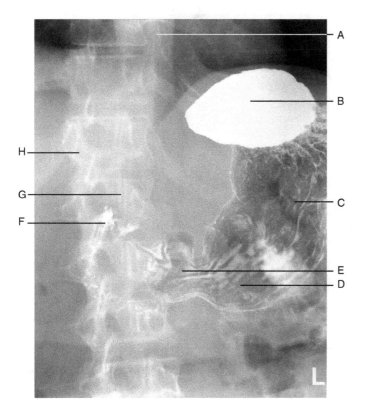

A. _____

B. _____

C. _____

D. _____

E. _____

F. _____

G. _____

H. _____

Copyright © 2015, 2011, 2006, 1996 by Saunders, an imprint of Elsevier Inc. All rights reserved.

68. Identify what body type is being represented in the following AP oblique stomach and duodenal projections, and state the degree of patient obliquity required to obtain the projection.

A. (Figure 12-18): _____

Figure 12-19

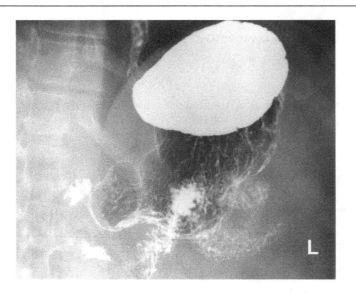

B. (Figure 12-19): _____

Figure 12-20

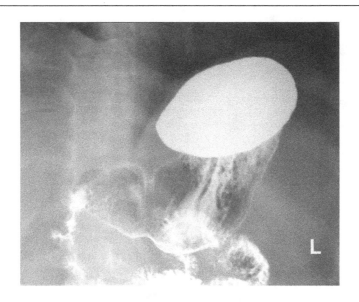

C. (Figure 12-20): _____

69. An adequately rotated hypersthenic AP oblique stomach and duodenal projection demonstrates the left zygapophy-

seal joints in the (A) _____ of the vertebral body and the pylorus superimposed over the

(B) _____.

          Copyright © 2015, 2011, 2006, 1996 by Saunders, an imprint of Elsevier Inc. All rights reserved.

70. An adequately rotated sthenic AP oblique stomach and duodenal projection demonstrates the left zygapophyseal joints at the (A) _____ of the vertebral body and the pylorus with (B) _____ vertebral superimposition.

71. An adequately rotated asthenic AP oblique stomach and duodenal projection demonstrates the left zygapophyseal joints in the (A) _____ of the vertebral bodies and the pylorus with (B) _____ vertebral superimposition.

72. On an AP oblique stomach and duodenal projection with accurate positioning, the (A) _____ is centered within the collimated field. This centering is obtained on the sthenic patient when a perpendicular CR is centered halfway between the (B) _____ and the (C) _____ at a level (D) _____ between the xiphoid process and inferior rib margin.

73. State how the CR position is adjusted from a sthenic patient for an AP oblique stomach and duodenal projection for the following habitus.

    A. Hypersthenic: _____

    _____

    B. Asthenic: _____

    _____

74. What anatomic structures are included on an AP oblique stomach and duodenal projection with accurate positioning?

    _____

Stomach and Duodenum: AP Projection

75. Identify the labeled anatomy in Figure 12-21.

Figure 12-21

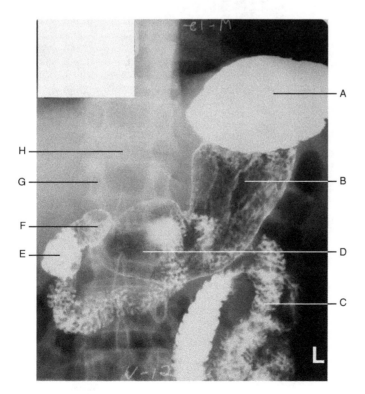

A. _____

B. _____

C. _____

D. _____

E. _____

F. _____

G. _____

H. _____

Copyright © 2015, 2011, 2006, 1996 by Saunders, an imprint of Elsevier Inc. All rights reserved.

76. Identify what body type is being represented in the following AP stomach and duodenal projections.

A. (Figure 12-21): _____

Figure 12-22

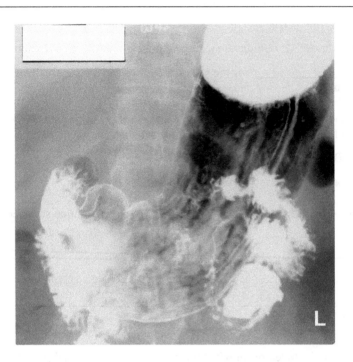

B. (Figure 12-22): _____

Figure 12-23

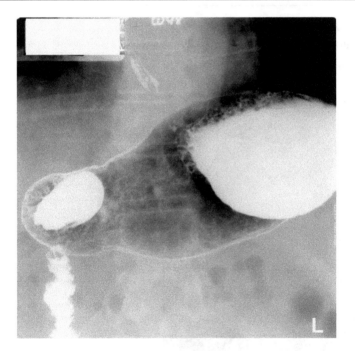

C. (Figure 12-23): _____

488

  Copyright © 2015, 2011, 2006, 1996 by Saunders, an imprint of Elsevier Inc. All rights reserved.

77. An optimal AP stomach and duodenal projection has been obtained when the spinous processes are aligned with the

(A) _____ of the vertebral bodies and the distances from the pedicles to the (B) _____ are equal on each side.

78. A hypersthenic AP stomach and duodenal projection will demonstrate the stomach aligned nearly (A) horizontal

with the duodenal bulb at the level of the (B) T11-12 thoracic vertebrae. The lesser and greater

curvatures are superimposed, with the greater curvature being more (C) anteriorly situated and the

esophagogastric junction nearly (D) on end.

79. A sthenic AP stomach and duodenal projection will demonstrate the stomach aligned nearly (A) _____,

with the duodenal bulb at the level of the (B) _____ lumbar vertebrae. The lesser and greater

curvature, esophagogastric junction, pylorus, and duodenal bulb are in (C) _____.

80. An asthenic AP stomach and duodenal projection will demonstrate the stomach aligned (A) _____,

with the duodenal bulb at the level of the (B) _____ lumbar vertebrae. The stomach is

(C) _____ shaped, and its long axis is demonstrated without foreshortening; the

(D) _____ _____, _____, and _____ are in profile.

81. On an AP stomach and duodenal projection with accurate positioning, the (A) _____ is centered within the collimated field. For a sthenic patient, this centering is obtained when a perpendicular CR is centered halfway

between the (B) _____ and the (C) _____ at a level (D) _____ between the xiphoid process and inferior rib margin.

82. State how the CR position is adjusted from a sthenic patient for an AP stomach and duodenal projection for the following habitus.

A. Hypersthenic: _____

_____

B. Asthenic: _____

_____

83. What anatomic structures are included on an AP stomach and duodenal projection with accurate positioning?

_____

For the following description of an AP stomach and duodenal projection with poor positioning, state how the patient or CR would have been mispositioned for such a projection to be obtained.

84. The distance from the left pedicles to the spinous processes is greater than the distance from the right pedicles to the spinous processes.

_____

_____

Copyright © 2015, 2011, 2006, 1996 by Saunders, an imprint of Elsevier Inc. All rights reserved.

Small Intestine: PA Projection

85. Identify the labeled anatomy in Figure 12-24.

Figure 12-24

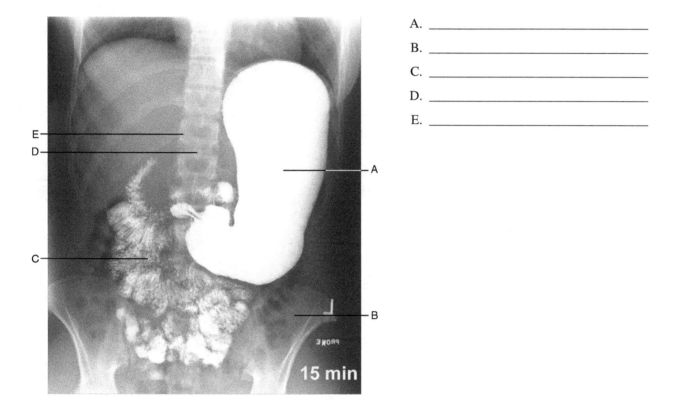

A. _____

B. _____

C. _____

D. _____

E. _____

86. How are PA small intestine projections marked?

_____

_____

87. What is the typical timing sequence for a small intestine series?

_____

 Copyright © 2015, 2011, 2006, 1996 by Saunders, an imprint of Elsevier Inc. All rights reserved.

88. A nonrotated PA small intestine projection demonstrates the spinous processes aligned with the (A) _____ and symmetrical (B) _____.

89. Why is the prone position chosen over the supine position for the small intestine series?

_____

90. Compare Figures 12-25 and 12-26. State which projection was taken earlier in the series and explain how you know this.

Figure 12-25   **Figure 12-26**

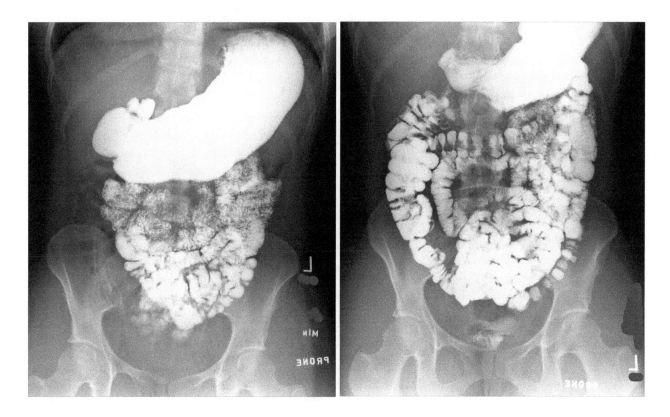

_____
_____
_____
_____

Copyright © 2015, 2011, 2006, 1996 by Saunders, an imprint of Elsevier Inc. All rights reserved.

Chapter **12 Image Analysis of the Digestive System**

91. Figure 12-27 demonstrates the last projection that was taken in a small bowel series. Based on this projection, should the patient wait longer and have another projection obtained? Why or why not?

Figure 12-27

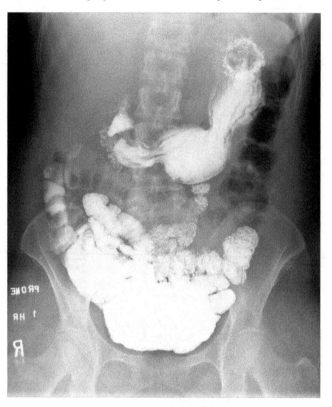

_____

_____

_____

_____

92. On a PA small intestine projection with accurate positioning, the (A) _____ is centered within the

exposure field. Early in the series, a perpendicular CR is centered to the (B) _____ at a level

2 inches (5 cm) (C) _____ to the iliac crest. Later in the series, the CR is centered at the level of the

(D) _____.

93. State why the CR is centered in different locations when a projection is obtained early versus late in the series.

_____

_____

94. What anatomic structures are included on a PA small intestine projection with accurate positioning? _____

Early: Stomach ß prox. Small intestine

later: Small intestine ß cecum

Chapter **12** **Image Analysis of the Digestive System**   Copyright © 2015, 2011, 2006, 1996 by Saunders, an imprint of Elsevier Inc. All rights reserved.

95. Optimal double-contrast coating has been obtained when the lumina are distended, the (A) _____ demonstrates a thin coating of barium, and barium pooling is limited to (B) _____.

96. What is the purpose of the barium pool? _____

    _____

97. State whether air or barium will be within the indicated structure by completing Figure 12-28 for the positions listed.

    Figure 12-28

Double-Contrast Filling of Large Intestinal Structures		
Large Intestine	AP Projection (Supine)	PA Projection (Prone)
Cecum		
Ascending colon		
Ascending limb right colic (hepatic) flexure		
Descending limb right colic (hepatic) flexure		
Transverse colon		
Ascending limb left colic (splenic) flexure		
Descending limb left colic (splenic) flexure		
Descending colon		
Sigmoid colon		
Rectum		

98. How is poor gaseous distension identified on a large intestine projection?

    _____

    _____

99. How is poor barium coating identified on a large intestine projection?

    _____

    _____

Copyright © 2015, 2011, 2006, 1996 by Saunders, an imprint of Elsevier Inc. All rights reserved.

Large Intestine: PA or AP Projection

100. Identify the labeled anatomy in Figure 12-29.

Figure 12-29

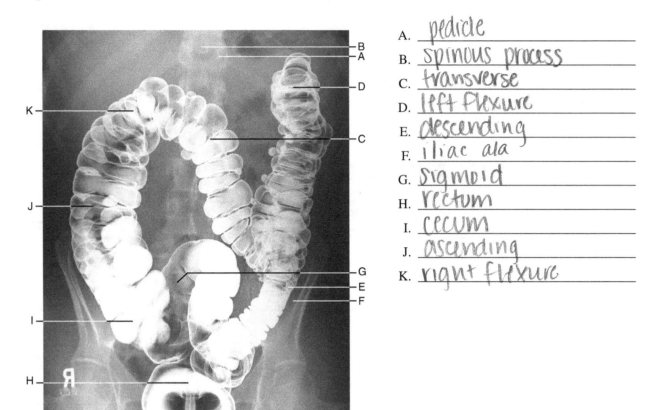

A. pedicle

B. spinous process

C. transverse

D. left flexure

E. descending

F. iliac ala

G. sigmoid

H. rectum

I. cecum

J. ascending

K. right flexure

101. A nonrotated PA or AP large intestine projection is demonstrated when the spinous processes are aligned with the

(A) _____ of the vertebral bodies, the distance from the pedicles to the (B) _____

is the same on both sides, and the iliac ala are (C) _____. The ascending and descending limbs

of the (D) _____ demonstrate some degree of superimposition.

102. To obtain a nonrotated PA or AP large intestine projection, the (A) _____ and (B) _____ are
positioned at equal distances from the imaging table.

103. The side demonstrating the greater distance from the pedicles to the spinous processes, wider iliac ala (wing), and

colic flexure with the greater ascending and descending limb superimposition is the side positioned _farther_
from the IR on a rotated PA large intestine projection.

Copyright © 2015, 2011, 2006, 1996 by Saunders, an imprint of Elsevier Inc. All rights reserved.

104. The iliac wing (ala) on an AP large intestine projection are __wider__ (wider/narrower) than on a PA projection.

105. On an AP or PA large intestine projection with accurate positioning the (A) _____ is centered within the exposure field. This centering is obtained by centering a perpendicular CR with the patient's

(B) _____ plane at the level of the (C) _____ for a PA large intestine projection.

106. For an AP or PA large intestine projection obtained on a hypersthenic patient when two 14- × 17-inch IRs are used, the first projection is obtained with the CR centered to the (A) __MSP__ at a level halfway between the (B) __symphysis__ and (C) __ASIS__ for the lower projection.

107. What anatomic structures are included on an AP or PA large intestine projection with accurate positioning?
    __entire large intestine, left flexure, & rectum__

108. Compare the projections in Figures 12-30 and 12-31. State the projection used to obtain each projection and explain how you know this.

Figure 12-30   **Figure 12-31**

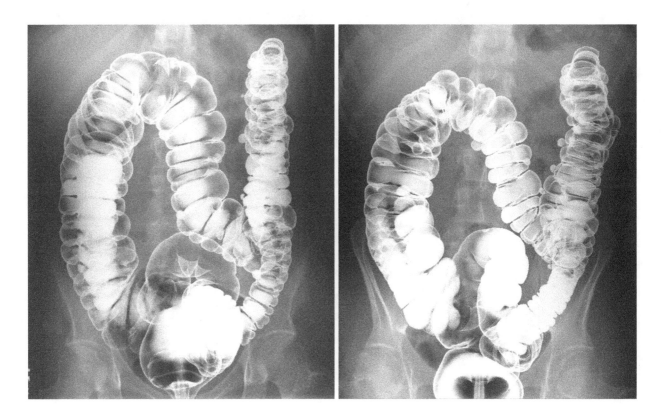

_____

_____

_____

_____

Copyright © 2015, 2011, 2006, 1996 by Saunders, an imprint of Elsevier Inc. All rights reserved.

For the following descriptions of AP or PA large intestine projections with poor positioning, state how the patient or CR would have been mispositioned for such a projection to be obtained.

109. AP projection: The right iliac ala is narrow and the left wide, the distance from the right pedicles to the spinous processes is narrower than the same distance on the left side, and the left colic (splenic) flexure demonstrates greater ascending and descending limb superimposition.

_____

110. PA projection: The left colic (splenic) flexure and part of the transverse colon are not included on the projection.

_____

_____

_____

For the following AP or PA large intestine projections with poor positioning, state what anatomic structures are misaligned and how the patient should be repositioned for an optimal projection to be obtained.

111. (Figure 12-32): _____

Figure 12-32

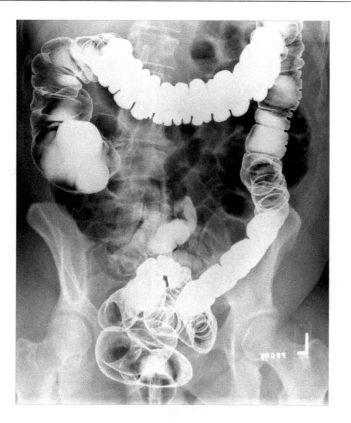

_____

_____

_____

  Copyright © 2015, 2011, 2006, 1996 by Saunders, an imprint of Elsevier Inc. All rights reserved.

Figure 12-33

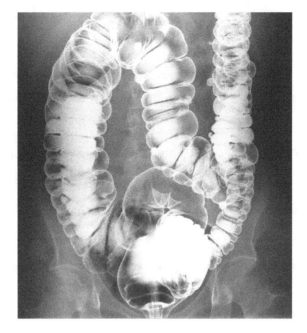

112. (Figure 12-33): _____

_____

_____

_____

Large Intestine (Rectum): Lateral Projection

113. Identify the labeled anatomy in Figure 12-34.

Figure 12-34

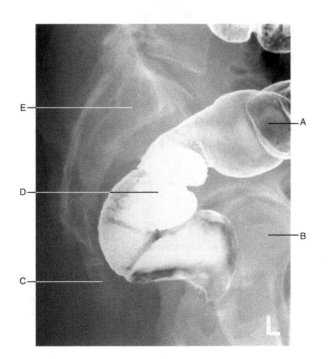

A. _____

B. _____

C. _____

D. _____

E. _____

Copyright © 2015, 2011, 2006, 1996 by Saunders, an imprint of Elsevier Inc. All rights reserved.

114. How is scatter radiation controlled for a lateral large intestine (rectum) projection?

_____

115. A lateral rectum projection with accurate positioning is demonstrated when the sacral medium sacral crest is in

(A) _____ and the (B) _____ are superimposed.

116. On a lateral rectum projection with accurate positioning, the (A) _____ is centered

within the exposure field. This centering is obtained by centering a perpendicular CR with the (B) _____

plane at the level of the (C) _____.

117. What anatomic structures are included on a lateral rectum projection with accurate positioning? _____

_____

For the following description of a lateral rectum projection with poor positioning, state how the patient or CR would have been mispositioned for such a projection to be obtained.

118. The femoral heads are not superimposed; the right femoral head is rotated anterior to the left femoral head.

_____

For the following lateral rectum projections with poor positioning, state what anatomic structures are misaligned and how the patient should be repositioned for an optimal projection to be obtained.

Figure 12-35

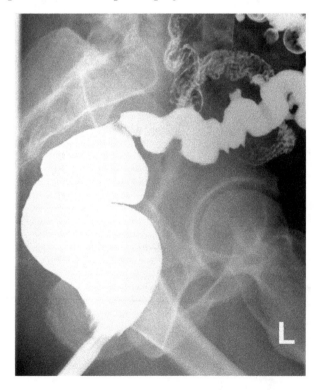

119. (Figure 12-35): _____

_____

_____

_____

Copyright © 2015, 2011, 2006, 1996 by Saunders, an imprint of Elsevier Inc. All rights reserved.

Figure 12-36

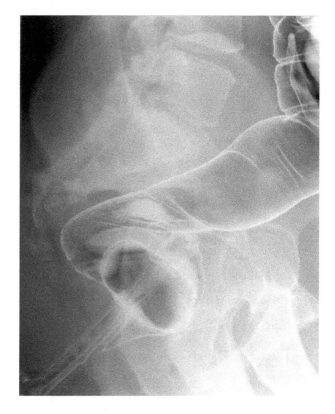

120. (Figure 12-36): _____

_____

_____

_____

Large Intestine: AP or PA Projection (Lateral Decubitus Position)

121. Identify the labeled anatomy in Figure 12-37.

Figure 12-37

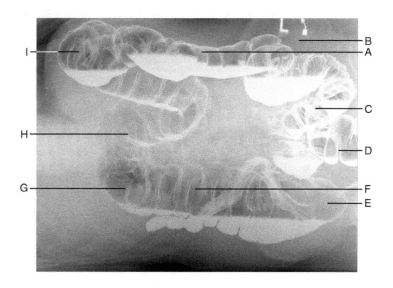

A. _____

B. _____

C. _____

D. _____

E. _____

F. _____

G. _____

H. _____

I. _____

Copyright © 2015, 2011, 2006, 1996 by Saunders, an imprint of Elsevier Inc. All rights reserved.

122. A nonrotated AP (decubitus) projection is obtained when the spinous processes are aligned with the midline of the (A) _____, the distances from the pedicles to the (B) _____ are the same on both sides, and the (C) _____ are symmetrical.

123. The side demonstrating the smaller distance from the pedicles to the spinous processes, narrower iliac wing, and colic flexure with less ascending and descending limb superimposition is the side positioned _____ from the IR on a rotated AP decubitus large intestine projection.

124. The iliac wings on a PA (decubitus) large intestine projection are _narrower_ (wider/narrower) than on an AP (decubitus) projection.

125. Why is the patient elevated on a radiolucent sponge or hard surface for a decubitus large intestine projection?

_____

126. _____ is centered within the exposure field for a PA/AP decubitus large intestine projection. This centering is obtained by centering a perpendicular CR with the (B) _____ plane at the level of the (C) _____.

127. For a PA/AP (decubitus) large intestine projection of a hypersthenic patient in which two projections are taken, the first projection is obtained with the CR centered to the (A) _____ plane at a level halfway between the (B) _____ and (C) _____ for the lower projection.

128. What anatomic structures are included on a decubitus large intestine projection with accurate positioning?

_____

For the following descriptions of AP or PA (decubitus) large intestine projections with poor positioning, state how the patient or CR would have been mispositioned for such a projection to be obtained.

129. Artifact lines are superimposed over the left lateral abdominal region.

_____

130. AP projection: The distances from the right pedicles to the spinous processes are less than the distances from the left pedicles to the spinous processes, the right iliac wing is narrower than the left, and the ascending and descending limbs of the left colic (splenic) flexure demonstrates increased superimposition.

_____

Copyright © 2015, 2011, 2006, 1996 by Saunders, an imprint of Elsevier Inc. All rights reserved.

For the following AP or PA (decubitus) large intestine projections with poor positioning, state what anatomic structures are misaligned and how the patient should be repositioned for an optimal projection to be obtained.

Figure 12-38

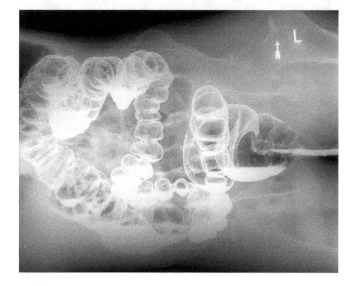

131. (Figure 12-38, AP projection): _____

_____

_____

_____

Figure 12-39

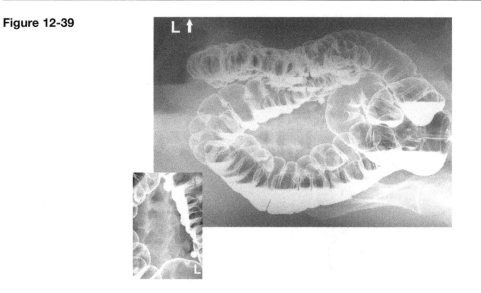

132. (Figure 12-39, AP projection): _____

_____

_____

_____

Copyright © 2015, 2011, 2006, 1996 by Saunders, an imprint of Elsevier Inc. All rights reserved.   Chapter **12 Image Analysis of the Digestive System**

Figure 12-40

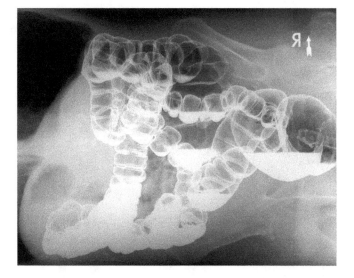

133. (Figure 12- 40, PA projection): _____

_____

_____

_____

Large Intestine: PA Oblique Projection (RAO Position)

134. Identify the labeled anatomy in Figure 12-41.

Figure 12-41

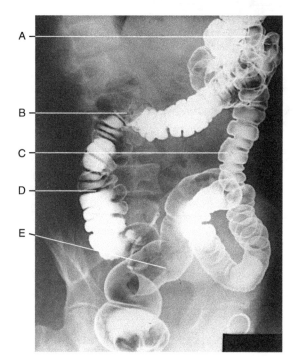

A. _____

B. _____

C. _____

D. _____

E. _____

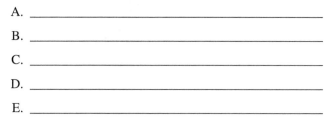

Copyright © 2015, 2011, 2006, 1996 by Saunders, an imprint of Elsevier Inc. All rights reserved.

135. A PA oblique large intestine projection with accurate positioning demonstrates decreased ascending and descending limb superimposition of the (A) _____ compared with the PA projection, and the limbs of the (B) _____ demonstrate increased superimposition. The (C) _____ (right/left) iliac wing is narrower than the opposite wing.

136. To obtain an accurate PA oblique large intestine projection, position the midcoronal plane (A) _____ degrees with the IR. Rotating the patient toward the right side moves the (B) _____ (ascending/descending) right colic (hepatic) flexure from beneath the (C) _____ (ascending/descending) right colic flexure and the distal sigmoid from beneath the (D) _____.

137. On a PA oblique large intestine projection with accurate positioning, the (A) _____ is centered within the exposure field. This centering is obtained by centering a perpendicular CR approximately 1 to 2 inches (2.5 to 5 cm) to the (B) _____ (right/left) of the midsagittal plane at the level of the (C) _____.

138. What anatomic structures are included on a PA oblique large intestine projection with accurate positioning?

_____ *entire large intestine* _____

For the following description of a PA oblique large intestine projection with poor positioning, state how the patient or CR would have been mispositioned for such a projection to be obtained.

139. The ascending and descending limbs of the right colic (hepatic) flexure and the rectum and distal sigmoid, respectively, demonstrate increased superimposition. The iliac wings are uniform in width.

_____ *was not rotated correctly* _____

Large Intestine: PA Oblique Projection (LAO Position)

140. Identify the labeled anatomy in Figure 12-42.

Figure 12-42

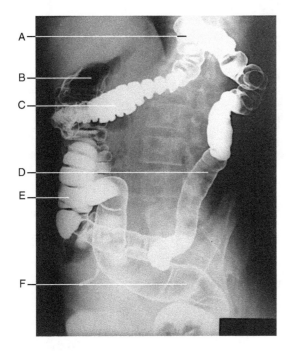

A. _____

B. _____

C. _____

D. _____

E. _____

F. _____

Copyright © 2015, 2011, 2006, 1996 by Saunders, an imprint of Elsevier Inc. All rights reserved.

Chapter **12 Image Analysis of the Digestive System**

141. The ascending and descending limbs of the (A) _____ (right/left) colic flexure are demonstrated with decreased superimposition when compared with the PA projection and the (B) _____ (right/left) iliac wing is narrower on a PA oblique large intestine projection with accurate positioning.

142. To obtain an accurate PA oblique large intestine projection, position the midcoronal plane (A) _____ degrees with the IR. Rotating the patient toward the left side moves the (B) _____ (ascending/descending) left colic (hepatic) flexure from beneath the (C) _____ (ascending/descending) left colic flexure.

143. On a PA oblique large intestine projection with accurate positioning, the (A) _____ is centered within the exposure field. This centering is obtained by centering a perpendicular CR approximately 1 to 2 inches (2.5 to 5 cm) to the (B) _____ (right/left) of the midsagittal plane at the level 1 to 2 inches (2.5 to 5 cm) superior to the (C) _____.

144. What anatomic structures are included on a PA oblique large intestine projection with accurate positioning?

_____

Large Intestine: PA Axial and PA Axial Oblique (RAO Position)

145. Identify the labeled anatomy in Figure 12-43.

Figure 12-43

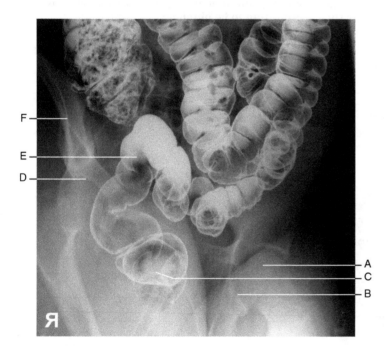

A. _____

B. _____

C. _____

D. _____

E. _____

F. _____

146. (A) _____ are demonstrated without transverse superimposition, the right sacroiliac (SI) joint is shown just (B) _____ to the anterior inferior spine, and the (C) _____ (right/left) obturator foramen is open.

147. To achieve an accurate PA axial oblique large intestine projection, the patient is rotated toward the (A) _____ side until the (B) _____ plane is at a 35- to 45-degree angle with the IR.

 Copyright © 2015, 2011, 2006, 1996 by Saunders, an imprint of Elsevier Inc. All rights reserved.

148. A PA axial large intestine projection with accurate positioning demonstrates _____ iliac wings and obturator foramen.

149. The rectosigmoid segment is demonstrated without (A) _____ superimposition, the pelvis demonstrates elongation, and the left inferior acetabulum is at the level of the (B) _____ when the CR is accurately angled (C) _____ degrees (D) _____ (caudally/cephalically) for a PA axial and PA axial oblique large intestine projection.

150. On a PA axial and PA axial oblique large intestine projection with accurate positioning, the (A) rectosigmoid is centered within the exposure field. This centering is obtained for a PA axial projection by centering so the CR exits at the level of the (B) ASIS and midsagittal plane. This centering is obtained for a PA axial oblique projection by centering the CR to exit at the (C) ASIS and 2 inches (5 cm) to the (D) left (right/left) of the spinous processes.

151. What anatomic structures are included on a PA axial and PA axial oblique large intestine projection with accurate positioning?

_____

For the following descriptions of PA axial oblique large intestine projections with poor positioning, state how the patient or CR would have been mispositioned for such a projection to be obtained.

152. The right SI joint is obscured, and the left obturator foramen is closed.

_____

153. The inferior aspect of the left acetabulum is demonstrated superior to the distal rectum.

_____

Copyright © 2015, 2011, 2006, 1996 by Saunders, an imprint of Elsevier Inc. All rights reserved.

For the following PA axial oblique large intestine projections with poor positioning, state what anatomic structures are misaligned and how the patient should be repositioned for an optimal projection to be obtained.

Figure 12-44

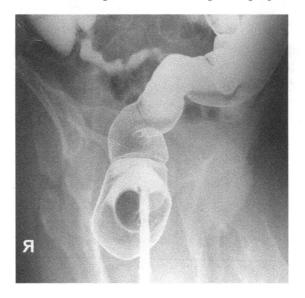

154. (Figure 12-44): _____

_____

_____

_____

Figure 12-45

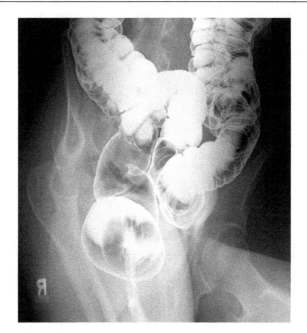

155. (Figure 12-45): _____

_____

_____

_____

  Copyright © 2015, 2011, 2006, 1996 by Saunders, an imprint of Elsevier Inc. All rights reserved.

Study Question Answers

CHAPTER 1   GUIDELINES FOR IMAGE ANALYSIS

1. A. Demographic information (patient and facility name, time, date)
   B. Correct markers in the appropriate position without superimposing the VOI
   C. Desired anatomic structures in accurate alignment with each other
   D. Maximum geometric integrity
   E. Appropriate radiation protection
   F. Best possible contrast resolution, with minimal noise
   G. No preventable artifacts
2. A. Midcoronal
   B. Anterior
   C. Posterior
   D. Superior
   E. Inferior
   F. Anterosuperior
   G. Posteroinferior
3. Anterolateral
4. Posteromedial
5. Anterosuperior
6. Mediolateral
7. A. Midsagittal
   B. Lateral
   C. Medial
   D. Inferolateral
   E. Superolateral
8. A. Proximal
   B. Distal
9. A. Source–object distance
   B. Object–image receptor distance
   C. Source–image receptor distance
10. A. 1 and 3
    B. 2
    C. 1
    D. 1 and 3
    E. 4
    F. 4
    G. 1 and 5
    H. 1 and 5
    I. 1 and 5
    J. 1 and 5
    K. 6
    L. 1
    M. 1
11. A. The AP knee projection is accurately displayed. The marker is correct, and it is accurately displayed as if hanging from the patient's hip.
    B. The marker is reversed, indicating that the projection needs to be flipped horizontally. The image is accurately displayed by the fingertip.
    C. The marker is reversed, indicating that the projection needs to be flipped horizontally. The image is accurately displayed as if the patient were in an upright position.
    D. Forearm projections should be displayed as if hanging by the fingertips and not the elbow. The image is horizontally displayed correctly, as indicated by the correctness of the marker.
    E. Lateral feet projections should be displayed as if hanging from the patient's hip. The projection should be moved 90 degrees counterclockwise. The marker is also reversed and should be correct for a lateral foot projection. The projection should be flipped horizontally.
    F. The marker is reversed and should be correct for AP oblique projections. The projection should be flipped horizontally, with the left marker positioned on the viewer's right side. The projection is accurately displayed as if the patient were in an upright position.
12. Left
13. True
14. False
15. A. Facility's name
    B. Patient's name
    C. Patient's age or birth date
    D. Patient's hospital identification number
    E. Date of examination
    F. Time of examination
16. A. Right
    B. Laterally, adjacent to the patient's right side
17. A. Right
    B. Anteriorly
18. A. The marker is situated too medially, superimposing the VOI. It should remain within the collimated field but be moved as far laterally as possible.
    B. The marker is situated at the midsagittal plane. It should be placed on the left side of the vertebral column as far laterally as possible while staying within the collimated field.
    C. The marker is superimposed on the VOI. Move the marker as far laterally as possible while staying within the collimated field.

Copyright © 2015, 2011, 2006, 1996 by Saunders, an imprint of Elsevier Inc. All rights reserved.

D. The marker is placed to the right of the vertebral column. It should be placed on the left side of the vertebral column as far laterally as possible while staying within the collimated field.

E. The marker is only partially demonstrated. The marker shoulder be placed completely within the collimated field. Annotate an R marker adjacent to the original marker without covering up the original marker.

19. A. Lead
    B. Radiopaque
20. Closer to
21.

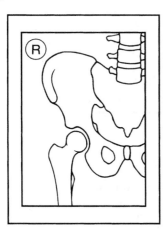

22.

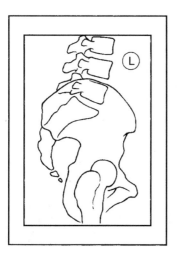

23. Mark the side that is positioned closer to the IR and place a face-up marker laterally adjacent to that side.
24. Annotate the marker next to the original during post-processing for digital systems.
25. CR/collimation
26. True
27. 16 × 16 inches or 17 × 17 inches

28. Needed to prevent the off-centered joint(s) from being projected off the IR because they will move in the direction the diverged x-ray beams that are used to record them on the projection are moving.
29. The ankle joint has been projected off the IR, and more of the distal femur is included than needed. The lower leg was not centered correctly on the IR. Palpate the joints to determine accurate centering.
30. 0.5 to 1 inch
31. A. Decrease
    B. Increase
    C. Decreases
32. Make an imaginary X diagonally connecting the corners of the collimated field. The center of the X indicates where the CR was centered. The CR was centered to the T9-T10 intervertebral disk space.
33. A. Larger
    B. The x-ray beams continue to diverge as they move through the patient to the IR.
34. A. Too much of the patient's abdominal structures have been included, and the lateral collimation borders are not within ½ inch (1.25 cm) of the skin line. The superior aspect of the chest is not included. The CR is centered too inferiorly to collimate tightly.
    B. The posterior and superior collimation borders are within ½ inch (1.25 cm) of the skin line, but the anterior and inferior borders are too wide. The CR is centered too anteroinferiorly to colli-mated tightly.
    C. The CR was centered anterior to the foot instead of on the tarsal bones, and the foot was aligned diagonally instead of with the long axis of the exposure field, preventing the collimation bor-ders from being within ½ inch (1.25 cm) from the skin line.
    D. The CR was centered to the upper cervical verte-brae region instead of to the center of the skull, preventing the shoulder and cervical vertebrae from being collimated off the projection, and the collimation borders are not within ½ inch (1.25 cm) of the skull skin line.
35. A. A
    B. B
    C. The clavicular projection A demonstrates grid cutoff, which occurs when the CR and grid are not properly aligned.
36. A. It would superimpose it.
    B. (1) Proximal
       (2) No
       (3) Because letter A is farther from the IR, it will be projected further proximally than letter B.
    C. (1) Distally
       (2) Letter A would be projected even more distally.
    D. Possibly superimposed over it or positioned only slightly distal or proximal to it depending on the SID used. The placement would vary depending

508

Copyright © 2015, 2011, 2006, 1996 by Saunders, an imprint of Elsevier Inc. All rights reserved.

on the SID because the angle used to record A and B could be perpendicular or proximal if a short SID was used and caudal if a long SIS was used.

37. A.

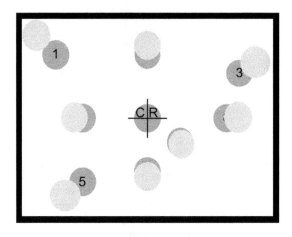

B.

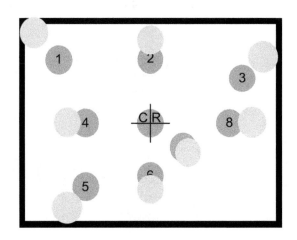

38. A. The SC joints would be projected to the right of the vertebral column.
   B. The SC joints are currently at the level of the third thoracic vertebrae. The 10-degree cephalic angle would project the SC joints superior to this position.
   C. The answers would be the same, although the amount of movement to the right for A and superiorly for B would be less because the x-rays recording the structures would be less diverged.
   D. The answers would be the same, although the amount of movement would be less because the heart shadow is not as far away from the IR as the SC joints are.

39. A. Parallel
   B. Perpendicular
40. A. Foreshortening
   B. Elongation
   C. Elongation
41. A. Magnification: Proportional magnification of the proximal, distal, and midshaft of the humerus
   B. Foreshortening: The proximal humerus was placed farther from the IR as demonstrated by the increased magnification of the proximal humerus when compared with the distal humerus.
   C. Elongation: The distal humerus was placed farther from the IR as demonstrated by the increased magnification of the distal humerus when compared with the proximal humerus.
42. Image 2
43. Image 2
44. A. Use identifiable structures that surround the identical structures.
   B. Use surrounding bony projections.
   C. Identify expected magnification.
45. A. Adjust the patient half the distance demonstrated between the two structures that should be superimposed.
   B. Adjust the patient the entire distance between the structures that should be superimposed.
46. A. 0
   B. 68
   C. 45
   D. 23
   E. 90
47. A. 45
   B. 45
   C. 30
   D. 105
48.

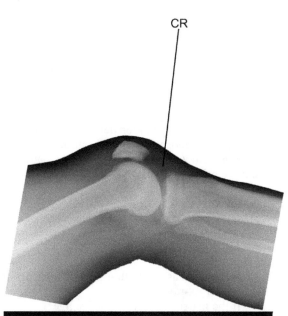

509

Copyright © 2015, 2011, 2006, 1996 by Saunders, an imprint of Elsevier Inc. All rights reserved.

49. A. Fully extend the patient's finger.
    B. Align the CR parallel with the IP joint or perpendicular to the phalange of interest. For this examination the CR would have needed to be angled proximally until it was parallel with the joint of interest.
50. A. Farther from
    B. Closer to
51. A. Internally rotate the hand 0.5 inch (1.25 cm).
    B. Direct the CR anteriorly to move the second metacarpal toward the fifth MC. Because the physical distance between the second and fifth MCs is 2.5 inches (0.6 cm) and a 5-degree angle will move the second MC 0.5 inch (1.25 cm) for this amount of physical separation, and the amount of mispositioning is off by 1 inch (2.5 cm), a 10-degree angle should be placed on the CR.
52. A. Externally rotate the leg 1 inch (2.5 cm).
    B. Direct the CR anteriorly to move the medial condyle toward the lateral condyle. Because the physical distance between the condyles is approximately 2½ inches (6.25 cm), a 5-degree angle will move the medial condyle 0.25 inch (0.6 cm) for this amount of physical separation, and the condyles are mispositioned by 2 inches (5 cm), a 40-degree angle should be placed on the CR.
53. A. Internally rotate the leg 0.125 inch (0.3 cm).
    B. Direct the CR posteriorly to move the medial talar dome toward the lateral dome. Because the physical distance between the talar domes is 1 inch (2.5 cm), a 5-degree angle will move the medial condyle 0.25 inch (0.6 cm) for this amount of physical separation, and the domes are mispositioned by 0.25 inch (0.6 cm), a 5-degree angle should be placed on the CR.
54. A. Small
    B. Smaller
55. Longer/shorter
56. A. Explain the examination to the patient.
    B. Make the patient comfortable.
    C. Keep the exposure time short.
    D. Use positioning devices.
57. Whereas voluntary motion demonstrates blurred gastric patterns and bony cortical outlines, involuntary motion demonstrates blurred gastric patterns and sharp cortical outlines.
58. A. Involuntary
    B. Involuntary
59. Spatial frequency/amount of space (distance)
60. DR system B
61. AP hip projection
62. False
63. A. When gonads are within 2 inches (5 cm) of the primary x-ray beam
    B. If the patient is of reproductive age
    C. If the gonadal shield does not cover the VOI
64. Ovaries, uterine tubes, and uterus

65.

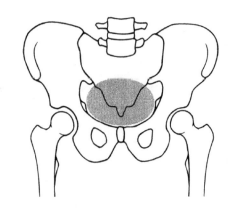

66. Place the narrow end of the shield superior to the palpable symphysis pubis and determine side-to-side centering by placing the shield at equal distances from the anterior superior iliac spines.
67. The shield is placed at a large OID and will greatly magnify, possibly covering the VOI.
68. A. Testes within scrotal pouch
    B. Along midsagittal plane inferior to the symphysis pubis
69. 1 to 1½ inches (2.5 to 4 cm) inferior to the symphysis pubis
70.

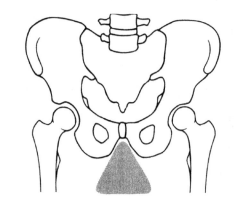

71. This is a male shield used on a female patient. It covers too much of the sacrum and does not cover the required gonadal organs. The shield is situated too superiorly and is not the correct shape.
72. The shield is poorly shaped for a male and does not cover the gonadal organs. The shield should be moved superiorly.
73. The shield is slightly off centered to the left and is smaller than the inlet pelvis.
74. Palpate the patient's coccyx and elevated anterior superior iliac spine (ASIS). Draw an imaginary line connecting the coccyx with a point 1 inch (2.5 cm) posterior to the ASIS. Position the flat contact shield against this imaginary line.

510

Copyright © 2015, 2011, 2006, 1996 by Saunders, an imprint of Elsevier Inc. All rights reserved.

75. A. Breasts
    B. Eyes
    C. Thyroid
    D. Gonads
    E. 2 inches (5 cm)
76. A. Anatomic artifact
    B. Use positioning devices such as sponges and sandbags to aid the patient in holding the position.
77. The technologist must maintain a SSD of at least 12 inches (30 cm) to prevent an unacceptable entrance skin dose. The SID should be elevated at least 2 inches (5 cm).

CHAPTER 2   VISIBILITY OF DETAILS

1. Subject contrast/exposure
2. A. pixel gray shade values
   B. number of pixels with that gray shade value
3. Minimal
4. Air/gas 5
   Bone 2
   Contrast/metal 1
   Fat 4
   Soft tissue 3
5. LUT
6. The displayed projection would have brighter gray shade values and lower contrast.
7. At the midpoint of defined VOI (halfway between S1 and S2)
8. A. wrong body part/projection is selected on workstation
   B. CR not centered to the VOI
   C. insufficient collimation
   D. excessive scatter fogging
   E. wrong technical factors were set for projection
   F. did not cover at least 30% of the IR
   G. multiple projections were not positioned at equal distances from each other
   H. the IP was not erased after days on nonuse
9. Because in DR only the pixels receiving exposure will send signals to the computer for processing.
10. The computer uses the collimated borders. It is best to have four collimated borders shown equal distance from the edges of the IR.
11. 30%
12. A: abdomen; B: chest
13. A. mAs
    B. kV
    C. SID
    D. OID
    E. collimation
    F. grids
14. A. The remnant beam demonstrates the subject contrast in the VOI with a broad range of photon intensities.
    B. Contrast resolution on the displayed projection distinguishes the subject contrast in the VOI with light gray to dark gray shades, and no part of it is completely white or black.
    C. There is no quantum noise or excessive fogging from scatter radiation.
    D. The EI number is within the acceptable exposure range for the digital system.
15. 2
16. Random pattern (grainy)/underexposure
17. A. The IE number indicates the IR received less exposure than needed to put the number within the acceptable exposure range for the digital system when no histogram analysis error has occurred.
    B. The VOI demonstrates a loss of contrast resolution, with some or all of the structures demonstrating a white shade, and postprocessing techniques do not improve their visibility.
    C. Quantum noise is present.
18. A. Determine if a histogram analysis error has occurred.
    B. Determine if all of the structures in the VOI have been adequately penetrated.
    C. Determine how much the exposure needs to be adjusted to move the EI number to the ideal value.
19. A. Atomic density
    B. Atomic number
    C. Part thickness
20. kV
21. False
22. Densest/thickest
23. Pitch black/4 to 5
24. A. The IE number indicates that the IR received more exposure than needed to put the number within the acceptable exposure parameters for the digital system when no histogram analysis error has occurred.
    B. The VOI demonstrates a loss of contrast resolution, with some or all of the structures demonstrating a black shade (saturation), and postprocessing techniques do not improve visibility.
    C. An overall graying is demonstrated because of excessive scatter radiation fogging.
25. Because kV is optimal and the part is penetrated, it should remain the same for the second exposure. To move the EI from 600 to the ideal 200 and reduce quantum noise, the mAs need to be increased by a factor of 3. Use 90 kV at 15 mAs.
26. Because kV is optimal and the part is penetrated, it should remain the same for the second exposure. To move the EI from 4000 to the ideal 1000 and eliminate saturation, the mAs need to be reduced by a factor of 4. Use 80 kV at 2.5 mAs.
27. The EI number indicates that the IE exposure needs to be increased by a factor of 4. Because the hip joints are not fully penetrated and the kV is not at the optimal for a pelvis (80–85), a two times change in kV is needed, and the remainder two times change should be done with mAs. Use 80 kV at 10 mAs.

Copyright © 2015, 2011, 2006, 1996 by Saunders, an imprint of Elsevier Inc. All rights reserved.

28. A. Use a grid.
    B. Use tight collimation.
    C. Place a flat contact shield or edge of an apron along the appropriate collimated border.
29. Place the straight edge of a lead apron along the anterior collimation border.
30. A. 23
    B. 57
    C. 91
    D. 114
31. 125 mAs
32. A. Amount of scatter produced and directed toward the IR.
    B. Degree of OID increase.

33. A. mAs
    B. 10
34. A. Increase by 50%. The new mAs to use is 4.5.
    B. There is no need to increase the mAs for the second projection. The kV is low enough that few of the scatter photons are being diverged at a narrow angle with the IR, so IR exposure is not affected by increasing collimation.
35. A. F
    B. T
    C. F
    D. T
36. Additive

37.

	Technical Adjustment	Additive or Destructive
A. Ascites	+50% mAs	Additive
B. Emphysema	−8% kVp	Destructive
C. Pleural effusion	+35% mAs	Additive
D. Osteoporosis	−8% kVp	Destructive
E. Osteoarthritis	+8% kVp	Additive
F. Pneumothorax	−8% kVp	Destructive
G. Pneumonia	+50% mAs	Additive
H. Bowel obstruction	−8% kVp	Destructive
I. Osteochondroma	+8% kVp	Additive
J. Rheumatoid arthritis	−8% kVp	Destructive
K. Pulmonary edema	+50%	Additive
L. Cardiomegaly	+50%	Additive

38. A. T
    B. F
    C. T
    D. F
    E. T
    F. T
    G. F
    H. T
    I. T
    J. T
    K. F
39. A. The AEC should not have been used when hardware or prosthetic device will be included in the exposure field.

B. The center cell was used on this chest projection. The center cell was positioned beneath a structure that has much greater atomic density than the VOI (lungs).
C. The outside cells were chosen, and the CR was centered too high, positioning part of the cells beneath the lung fields. The lungs have lower atomic density than the abdominal structures.
D. The CR was centered too laterally, so a portion of the AEC chamber was exposed with a part of the x-ray beam that did not go through the patient.
E. The AEC chamber was centered to posterior to the lumbar vertebrae, causing a portion of it to be exposed with a section of the x-ray beam that did not go through the patient.

Copyright © 2015, 2011, 2006, 1996 by Saunders, an imprint of Elsevier Inc. All rights reserved.

40. Brightness/high/greater
41. A. H
    B. H
    C. L
    D. L
    E. L
    F. L
    G. L
42. A. Contrast (length of dynamic range)
    B. Brightness (average gray level)
43. False
44. False
45. A. An anatomic structure within collimated field that could have been removed.
    B. Two exposures are taken on the same IR without processing being done between them.
    C. Patient and hospital belongings that are found outside the patient's body that could have been removed but were not and are demonstrated on a projection.
    D. Objects located within the patient's body that cannot be removed and are demonstrated on the projection.
    E. Artifacts that are caused by the imaging equipment
    F. Artifacts that are caused by the processor or the way the IR was handled or stored
46. A. External artifact
    B. Anatomic artifact
    C. Internal artifact
    D. Equipment-related artifact
    E. Improper film handling or processor artifact
47. A. F
    B. T
    C. F
    D. F
48. Inverted or off-focused grid
49. A. Toward
    B. Increase
    C. Higher
50. A. 3
    B. 2
    C. 4
51. X-ray taken, and the CR was directed toward the basket.
52. An optimal projection is perfect in all aspects, but an acceptable projection does not have to be repeated but has aspects that could be improved.
53. When the artifact can be eliminated and is obscuring a portion of the VOI.
54. The goal of mobile and trauma imaging is to demonstrate accurate relationships between the anatomic structures for the projection without further patient injury and with minimal discomfort.

55. A. Line connecting the MCs
    B. Line connecting the humeral epicondyles
    C. Midsagittal plane
    D. Line connecting the femoral epicondyles
    E. Orbitomeatal line (OML)

56.

	kVp Adjustment	mAs Adjustment
A. Small to medium plaster cast	+5–7	+50%–60%
B. Fiberglass cast	No adjustment	No adjustment
C. Wood backboard	+5	+25%–30%
D. Postmortem imaging of head, thorax, and abdomen	Not recommended	+35%–50%
E. Upper airway obstruction	−15%–20%	Not recommended
F. Wood sliver embedded in soft tissue	−15%–20%	Not recommended

57. A. 20
    B. 30
58. Perpendicular
59. There is a distal ulnar fracture and the wrist is not in a lateral projection. When the patient is unable to place both joints in the true position at the same time, the joint closest to the injury should be in the true position.
60. A. T
    B. T
    C. T
    D. T
    E. T
    F. F
    G. T
    H. F
    I. T
    J. T

Copyright © 2015, 2011, 2006, 1996 by Saunders, an imprint of Elsevier Inc. All rights reserved.

1.

Table 3-1	Adult Chest Technical Data				
Projection	**kV***	**Grid**	**AEC**	**mAs**	**SID**
Adult Chest Technical Data					
PA	110–125	Grid	Both outside		72 inches (183 cm)
Lateral	110–125	Grid	Center		72 inches (183 cm)
AP mobile	110–125			3	50–60 inches (125–150 cm)
AP supine in Bucky	80–100	Grid	Both outside		50–60 inches (125–150 cm)
AP-PA (lateral decubitus)	110–125	Grid	Center	3	72 inches (183 cm)
AP axial (lordotic)	110–125	Grid	Both outside		72 inches (183 cm)
AP-PA oblique	110–125	Grid	Over lung of interest		72 inches (183 cm)
Pediatric Chest Technical Data					
Neonate: AP	70–80			1	50–60 inches (125–150 cm)
Infant: AP	75–85			1.5	50–60 inches (125–150 cm)
Child: AP	75–85			2	50–60 inches (125–150 cm)
Child: PA	75–80	Grid**	Both outside		72 inches (183 cm)
Neonate: Cross-table lateral	75–85			2	50–60 inches (125–150 cm)
Infant: Cross-table lateral	80–90			3	50–60 inches (125–150 cm)
Child: Lateral	85–110	Grid**	Center		72 inches (180 cm)
Neonate: AP (lateral decubitus)	70–80			1	50–60 inches (125–150 cm)
Infant: AP (lateral decubitus)	75–85			1.5	50–60 inches (125–150 cm)
Child: AP (lateral decubitus)	85–110	Grid**	Center		72 inches (183 cm)

2. A. Thoracic vertebra
   B. Mediastinal structures
   C. Vascular lung markings
   D. Fluid-air levels when present
   E. Internal monitoring apparatus when present
3. A. T
   B. T
   C. F
   D. T
   E. T
   F. F
   G. T
   H. T
   I. T
   J. T
   K. F
   L. T
   M. T
   N. F
   O. T
   P. T
   Q. T
4. A. Pleural drainage tube
   B. Central venous catheter
   C. Pulmonary artery catheter (external electrocardiogram leads are also demonstrated)
   D. Automatic implantable cardioverter defibrillator

5. A. 4
   B. 6
   C. 5
   D. 3
   E. 2
   F. 7
   G. 1
6. A. Place in an upright position
   B. Horizontal
7. A. Pleural effusion
   B. Pneumothorax
   C. Pneumectomy
8. A. Hyposthenic
   B. Hypersthenic
   C. Asthenic
   D. Sthenic
9. A. Seventh
   B. Costophrenic angle
   C. Equal
   D. Horizontal
   E. Outside
   F. Fourth thoracic
   G. 10

Copyright © 2015, 2011, 2006, 1996 by Saunders, an imprint of Elsevier Inc. All rights reserved.

10. A. Right lung apex
    B. Clavicle
    C. Fourth thoracic vertebra
    D. Scapula
    E. Fourth anterior rib
    F. Diaphragm
    G. Costophrenic angle
    H. Heart shadow
    I. Lung
    J. Hilum
    K. Seventh posterior rib
    L. Aortic arch
    M. Superior manubrium
    N. Left SC joint
    O. Air-filled trachea
11. A. Transversely
    B. Anteroposteriorly
    C. Vertically
12. Vertical
13. Disease processes, advanced pregnancy, excessive obesity, a slouching patient, or confining clothing
14. A. Hypersthenic
    B. Short and wide
15. A. Asthenic and hyposthenic
    B. Long and narrow
16. Align the shoulders, the posterior ribs, and the ASISs at equal distances from the IR.
17. A. Scoliosis
    B. No
    C. On a rotated patient, the distances will be uniform down the length of the lung field, but with scoliosis, the vertebral column to lateral lung edge distance will vary down the length of the each lung and between each lung.
18. The shoulders are depressed.
19. Place the hands on the hips and rotate the elbows and shoulders anteriorly.
20. A. Midcoronal
    B. Fourth
    C. 1 inch (2.5 cm)
21. A. If the patient's shoulders are not depressed
    B. If the patient's upper midcoronal plane is leaning toward the IR
22. The diaphragm is allowed to move to its lowest position.
23. A. Placing the patient in an upright position
    B. Having the patient perform a deep inspiration
24. It coaxes the patient into a deeper inspiration.
25. A. Pneumothorax
    B. Foreign body
26. A. Higher
    B. 10
    C. Broader
    D. Shorter
27. A. Horizontal
    B. Midsagittal
    C. Vertebral prominens
28. Rotated into an RAO position
29. The shoulders were not depressed.

30. The right elbow and shoulder were not rotated anteriorly.
31. The patient's upper midcoronal plane was tilted toward the IR.
32. Eight posterior ribs are demonstrated above the diaphragm, and the clavicles are not on the same horizontal plane. Expose the projection after coaxing the patient into a deeper inspiration and depress the shoulders.
33. The vertebral column is superimposed over the right sternal clavicular end, and the left inferior posterior ribs are longer than the right. Rotate the patient toward the left side until the shoulders are at equal distances from the IR.
34. The scapulae are demonstrated in the superolateral lung field, the third thoracic vertebra is superimposed over the manubrium, and the inferior tip of the costophrenic angles are not included in the exposure field. Rotate the shoulders and elbows anteriorly, tilt the patient's upper midcoronal plane toward the IR until it is parallel with the IR, and move the CR and IR inferiorly by ½ inch (1.25 cm).
35. Less than 1 inch (2.5 cm) of the lung field is seen above the clavicles and the manubrium is at the level of third thoracic vertebra. Tilt the upper midcoronal plane toward the IR until it is parallel with the IR.
36. The fifth thoracic vertebra is superimposed over the manubrium, only a portion of the 10th posterior rib is seen above the diaphragm, and the right sternal clavicular end is superimposed by the vertebral column. Tilt the upper midcoronal plane away from the IR until it is parallel with the IR, expose the projection after coaxing the patient into a deeper inspiration, and rotate the patient toward the left side until the shoulders are at equal distances from the IR.
37. More than 1 inch (2.5 cm) of the lung field is demonstrated above the clavicles, the manubrium is at the level of the fifth thoracic vertebra, and the scapulae are in the superolateral lung field. Tilt the upper midcoronal plane away from the IR until it is parallel with the IR and rotate the shoulders and elbows anteriorly.
38. A. Lung apex
    B. Scapulae
    C. Thoracic vertebra
    D. Intervertebral foramen
    E. Posterior ribs
    F. Intervertebral disk space
    G. Costophrenic angles
    H. Diaphragm
    I. Heart shadow
    J. Sternum
    K. Hili
    L. Esophagus
    M. Trachea
39. A. Eighth
    B. ½ inch (1 cm)
    C. Hemidiaphragms
    D. Anterior
    E. 11th

515

Copyright © 2015, 2011, 2006, 1996 by Saunders, an imprint of Elsevier Inc. All rights reserved.

40. Align the shoulders, the posterior ribs, and the ASISs in line with each other, with the midcoronal plane aligned perpendicular to the IR.
41. A. Right
    B. It is situated farther from the IR, so diverged x-rays will cause it to magnify.
42. By evaluating the degree of posterior rib superimposition
43. A. Find the gastric air bubble, which is located beneath the left hemidiaphragm.
    B. Look for lung tissue that is anterior to the sternum. When seen, it is the right lung.
    C. Outline the heart shadow, which is located within the left hemidiaphragm.
44. Left
45. Rotate the left side of the patient anteriorly approximately 1 inch (2.5 cm) or rotate the right side of the patient posteriorly approximately 1 inch (2.5 cm).
46. Whereas the anterior ribs will be superimposed, the posterior ribs will demonstrate differing degrees of separation.
47. The midsagittal plane is parallel to the IR.
48. Right
49. A. The heart shadow will be more magnified on the right lateral chest projection.
    B. The left hemidiaphragm will project lower than the right hemidiaphragm on a right lateral chest projection.
50. A. Right lateral
    B. Left lateral
51. Position the humeri vertically.
52. Anteroinferior
53. The 11th thoracic vertebra will be superimposed by the lung field.
54. A. Take exposure after the second full inspiration.
    B. Take exposure with the patient in an upright position.
55. 12th
56. A. Midcoronal
    B. Inferior
57. The lung apices, sternum, posterior ribs, diaphragm, and costophrenic angles
58. The patient's humeri were not positioned vertically.
59. The left thorax was rotated anteriorly.
60. If no medical indication explains this relationship, the patient's lower thorax was situated closer to the IR than the upper thorax (midsagittal plane was not parallel with IR).
61. More than ½ inch (1.25 cm) of separation is present between the posterior ribs. The inferior heart shadow projects into the inferiorly and anteriorly located lung field. Rotate the patient's right side anteriorly approximately ½ inch (1.25 cm).
62. The right and left posterior ribs are separated by more than ½ inch (1.25 cm), indicating that the chest was rotated. The superior heart shadow does not extend beyond the sternum, lung tissue is demonstrated anterior to the sternum, and the gastric air bubble is demonstrated adjacent to the posteriorly situated

lung, verifying that the right lung is situated anterior to the sternum and the left lung posteriorly. Rotate the patient's right side posteriorly approximately ½ inch (1.25 cm).
63. The humeral soft tissue shadows are superimposed over the anterior lung apices. Position the patient's humeri vertically.
64. The hemidiaphragms cover only to the ninth thoracic vertebra. Take the exposure after coaxing the patient into taking a deeper inspiration.
65. A. The manubrium is at the level of the third thoracic vertebra. Tilt the upper midcoronal plane toward the IR until the midcoronal plane is parallel with the IR.
    B. This projection reflects accurate positioning. One might conclude that the left hemidiaphragm is too superior and that the patient's midsagittal plane was tilted, but by evaluating the PA projection, it can be determined that because the left hemidiaphragm is situated higher than the right on this patient, this positioning is accurate.
66 A. Right apex
    B. Right SC joint
    C. Scapula
    D. Fifth posterior rib
    E. Medial scapular border
    F. Diaphragm
    G. Costophrenic angle
    H. Heart shadow
    I. Aortic arch
    J. Manubrium
    K. Third thoracic vertebra
67. A. Seventh
    B. Sternal clavicular ends
    C. Manubrium
    D. Clavicles
    E. Horizontal
    F. Scapulae
    G. 9 to 10
68. So the reviewer knows which projection was taken first if more than one were taken on the same day
69. So the reviewer will know the accuracy of the air-fluid levels demonstrated
70. The fluid is evenly spread throughout the lung field, so no definite air-fluid line is visible.
71. A. The vertical dimension does not fully expand in the recumbent or seated positions.
    B. Because a low SID is used, resulting in increased magnification
72. Align the IR and midcoronal plane parallel with the bed and the front face of the collimator parallel with IR.
73. Rotation is evident when the distances from the sternal clavicular ends to the vertebral column and the lengths of the right and left corresponding posterior ribs are not equal.
74. Clavicles will be on the same horizontal plane.
75. Whereas poor shoulder positioning will demonstrate the manubrium at the level of the fourth thoracic

Study Question Answers
Copyright © 2015, 2011, 2006, 1996 by Saunders, an imprint of Elsevier Inc. All rights reserved.

vertebra, poor CR alignment will demonstrate the manubrium at a level inferior to the fourth thoracic vertebra and increased lung field superior to the clavicles.

76. Place the back of the patient's hands on the hips and rotate the elbows and shoulders anteriorly.

77. A. More than 1 inch (2.5 cm) of apices will be seen above the clavicles, and the posterior ribs will be vertically shaped.
    B. Less than 1 inch (2.5 cm) of the apices will be seen above the clavicles, and the posterior ribs will be horizontal.

78. Angle the CR 5 to 10 degrees cephalically.

79. To offset the upward lift of the manubrium, clavicles, and superior ribs

80. Pressure from the abdominal organs prevents the diaphragm from shifting to an inferior position.

81. Instruct the patient to take two full breaths before the projection is exposed.

82. A. Midsagittal
    B. 4
    C. Jugular notch

83. The lung apices, lateral lungs, and costophrenic angles

84. The patient would have been in a left posterior oblique (LPO) position, or the CR would have been angled toward the left side of the chest.

85. The CR was angled too caudally.

86. The CR was angled too cephalically.

87. The CR was aligned perpendicular to the IR. It would be best to angle 5 to 10 degrees cephalically.

88. Eight posterior ribs are demonstrated superior to the diaphragm, the clavicles are not horizontal, the left SC joint is positioned away from the vertebral column, and the left posterior ribs demonstrate greater length than the right. Expose the projection after coaxing the patient into a greater inspiration, depress the shoulders, and place an elevating device beneath the left IR border to position the IR parallel with the bed or angle the CR toward the right side of the patient until it is aligned perpendicular to the IR.

89. More than 1 inch (2.5 cm) of apical lung field is demonstrated above the clavicles, and the posterior ribs have a vertical contour. Angle the CR cephalically until it is aligned perpendicular to the midcoronal plane.

90. The manubrium is superimposed over the third thoracic vertebra, less than 1 inch (2.5 cm) is demonstrated above the clavicles, and the right sternal clavicular end superimposes the vertebral column. Angle the CR caudally until it is aligned perpendicular to the midcoronal plane and rotate the patient toward the right side until the shoulders are at equal distances from the IR.

91. A. Diaphragm
    B. 10th posterior rib
    C. Heart shadow
    D. Lateral scapular border
    E. Clavicle

92. A. Up and away
    B. Seventh
    C. Vertebral column
    D. Outside the lung field
    E. Fourth thoracic
    F. Clavicle
    G. Diaphragm

93. A. Air
    B. Fluid

94. Within the side of the chest positioned closer to the table or cart

95. A. Left lateral decubitus
    B. Left lateral decubitus

96. A. Posterior ribs
    B. Shoulders
    C. ASISs

97. AP

98. Above the patient's head

99. A. Midcoronal
    B. Parallel

100. Elevate the patient on a radiolucent sponge or cardiac board.

101. The left side of the chest was positioned closer to the IR than the right side.

102. The patient's upper midcoronal plane was tilted toward the IR.

103. The right sternal clavicular end is superimposed over the vertebral column, and the posterior ribs on the left side demonstrate greater length than those on the right. Rotate the left side away from the IR until the midcoronal plane and IR are parallel.

104. The manubrium is superimposed over the fifth thoracic vertebra. Tilt the upper midcoronal plane toward the IR until it and the IR are parallel.

105. A. Lung apex
     B. Posterior fourth rib
     C. Anterior fourth rib
     D. Superior scapular angle
     E. Lateral border scapula
     F. Medial clavicular end
     G. First thoracic vertebra

106. A. Superior
     B. Superior
     C. Horizontally
     D. Lateral
     E. Vertebral column

107. Lung apices

108. A. Have the patient stand 12 inches from IR; then arch the patient's back until the midcoronal plane is at a 45-degree angle to the IR. A horizontal CR is used.
     B. Have the patient remain completely upright and use a 45-degree cephalic CR angle.
     C. The patient's back is arched as much as possible, and the CR is angled cephalically in the amount necessary to equal 45 degrees.

109. A. Increase the degree of patient arch.
     B. Increase the degree of CR angulation.

517

Copyright © 2015, 2011, 2006, 1996 by Saunders, an imprint of Elsevier Inc. All rights reserved.

110. Place the back of the patient's hands on the hips and rotate the elbows and shoulders anteriorly.
111. When the SC joints are not at equal distances from the vertebral column
112. A. Midsagittal
    B. Manubrium
    C. Xiphoid
113. The clavicles, lung apices, and two thirds of the lung field
114. The midcoronal plane was at less than a 45-degree angle to IR, or the CR was angled cephalically less than needed.
115. The elbows and shoulders were not drawn anteriorly.
116. The patient was rotated in an LPO position.
117. The medial clavicular ends are superimposed over the lung apices, and the anterior ribs are demonstrated inferior to their corresponding posterior rib. Cephalically increase the CR angulation or have the patient increase the amount of back arch until the angle of the midcoronal plane and IR is 45 degrees.
118. A. SC joints
    B. Air-filled trachea
    C. Principal bronchi
    D. Heart shadow
    E. Posterior heart shadow
119. A. Principal bronchi
    B. SC joints
    C. Twice
    D. Manubrium
    E. 10
120. Midcoronal
121. 60
122. A. Right
    B. Right
123. LAO
124. Vertebra prominens
125. The apices, costophrenic angles, and lateral chest walls
126. The patient was not rotated enough.
127. The patient was rotated too much.
128. The patient was not rotated enough.
129. Less than two times the lung field is demonstrated on the left side of this thorax than on the right side. Increase the degree of patient obliquity until the midcoronal plane is at a 45-degree angle to the IR.
130. Approximately three times the lung field is demonstrated on the right side of this thorax than on the left side, which indicates that the patient was rotated approximately 60 degrees. An LAO chest position taken to evaluate the lung field should demonstrate only two times the lung field on the right side than the left and would demonstrate the vertebral column superimposed over the heart shadow. Decrease the degree of patient obliquity until the midcoronal plane is at a 45-degree angle to the IR.
131. Neonates and infants have fewer alveoli, causing their lungs to be denser.

132. Head rotation and cervical flexion and extension cause the ET tip to move superiorly and inferiorly, making it difficult for the reviewer to determine exactly where the tube is positioned.
133. A. Clavicle
    B. Right lung apex
    C. Diaphragm
    D. Costophrenic angle
    E. Heart shadow
    F. Anterior rib
    G. Fourth posterior rib
    H. Air-filled airway
134. A. Sixth
    B. Equal
    C. Equal
    D. Downward
    E. Superiorly
    F. 8
    G. 9
    H. Chin
135. A. Midsagittal
    B. Mammary line
    C. Upper airway, lungs, mediastinal structures, and costophrenic angles
136. Shape
137. The dense substances of blood, pus, protein, and cells and the less-dense air
138. A. After neonates take a deep breath as observed by watching chest movements
    B. At any time
139. The patient is rotated toward the right side (RPO position).
140. The CR was centered too inferiorly.
141. The projection was exposed with the ventilator's manometer at a level lower than the highest point.
142. The chin was tucked toward the chest.
143. The left sternal clavicular end is not adjacent to the vertebral column, and the left posterior ribs demonstrate greater length than the right posterior ribs. Rotate the patient toward the right side until the midcoronal plane is parallel with the IR.
144. The anterior ribs are projecting upward, the posterior ribs are horizontal, the sixth thoracic vertebra is in the center of the projection, and the right sternal clavicular end is not adjacent to the vertebral column. Center the CR approximately 1 inch (2.5 cm) superior (at the mammary line) and rotate the patient toward the left side until the midcoronal plane is parallel with the IR.
145. The seventh posterior rib is demonstrated superior to the diaphragm, and the chin is superimposed over the lung apices. If possible, take the exposure after a deeper inhalation and elevate the chin until the cervical vertebrae are in a neutral position.
146. The right sternal clavicular end is not adjacent to the vertebral column, the right posterior ribs demonstrate greater length than the left posterior ribs, and excessive amount of the cervical vertebrae and face are included on projection. Rotate the patient toward the left side until the midcoronal plane is

Copyright © 2015, 2011, 2006, 1996 by Saunders, an imprint of Elsevier Inc. All rights reserved.

parallel with the IR, lift the patient's chin out of collimation field, and increase collimation.

147. A. Second anterior rib
 B. Sixth posterior rib
 C. Lung
 D. Diaphragm
 E. Costophrenic angle
 F. Heart shadow
 G. Hilum
 H. Superior manubrium
 I. Left sternoclavicular joint
 J. Right lung apex
 K. Air-filled trachea

148. The patient's left side is rotated toward the IR (LPO position).

149. The projection was exposed on expiration.

150. The CR was not perpendicular with the midcoronal plane but was angled caudally.

151. The patient's upper midcoronal plane was tilted away from the IR.

152. The shoulders were elevated.

153. The manubrium is at the level of the third thoracic vertebra. Tilt the upper midcoronal plane toward the IR until it is parallel with the IR.

154. The manubrium is at the level of the fifth thoracic vertebra, and the right sternal clavicular end is visualized away from the vertebral column. Tilt the upper midcoronal plane away from the IR until it is parallel with the IR and rotate the patient toward the right side until the IR and midcoronal plane are parallel.

155. Eight posterior ribs are demonstrated above the diaphragm, the right sternal clavicular end is visualized away from the vertebral column, and the right posterior ribs demonstrate greater length than the left. Coax the patient into a deeper inhalation and rotate the patient toward the right side until the IR and midcoronal plane are parallel.

156. The manubrium is at the level of the seventh thoracic vertebra, and the posterior ribs are vertical. Angle the CR cephalically until it is perpendicular to the midcoronal plane.

157. The manubrium is at the level of the second thoracic vertebra, the posterior ribs are horizontal, five posterior ribs are demonstrated above the diaphragm, and the patient is in a slight LPO position. Angle the CR caudally until it is perpendicular to the midcoronal plane, coax the patient into a deeper inhalation, and rotate the patient toward the right side until the IR and midcoronal plane are parallel.

158. A. Intervertebral foramen
 B. Thoracic vertebra
 C. Intervertebral disk space
 D. Costophrenic angle
 E. Diaphragm
 F. Heart shadow
 G. Sternum
 H. Lung apex

159. A. Midcoronal
 B. Mammary line

C. Apices, costophrenic angles, posterior ribs, and airway

160. A. Less disturbance to the sensitive neonate
 B. Will not result in compression of the lung adjacent to the IR and overinflation of the other lung

161. Perpendicular

162. The OID difference between the right and left lungs is minimal.

163. The patient's left side is rotated posteriorly, and the right side is rotated anteriorly.

176. The arms were not elevated to a position near the patient's head.

165. The chin was not tilted upward.

166. The image was taken on expiration.

167. The posterior ribs are demonstrated without superimposition. The right lung is the posterior lung, as indicated by the heart shadow that is demonstrated in the anteriorly and inferiorly located lung. Rotate the right lung anteriorly until the shoulders and the ASISs are perpendicular to the IR.

168. The hemidiaphragms demonstrate an exaggerated cephalic curvature, and the humeral soft tissue is superimposed over the anterior lung apices. Expose the image on full inspiration and raise the arms until the humeri are next to the patient's head.

169. A. Lung apex
 B. Thoracic vertebra
 C. Posterior ribs
 D. Costophrenic angles
 E. Diaphragm
 F. Heart shadow
 G. Sternum
 H. Esophagus
 I. Trachea

170. The patient's left lung was rotated posteriorly.

171. The projection was exposed on expiration.

172. The arms were not elevated.

173. A portion of the right lung is positioned posterior to the left, as indicated by the left side gastric air bubble that is located beneath the superiorly and anteriorly located left lung. Rotate the right side of the patient anteriorly until the shoulders and the ASISs are aligned perpendicular to the IR.

174. The humeral soft tissue is superimposing the apical lung field. Elevate the humeri until they are positioned superior to the lung field.

175. A portion of the right lung is positioned posterior to the left, and the soft tissue of the arms is obscuring the anterior lung apices. Rotate the right side of the patient anteriorly until the shoulder and the ASISs are aligned perpendicular to the IR and elevate the arms.

176. A. Clavicle
 B. Humerus
 C. Third anterior rib
 D. Sixth posterior rib
 E. Chest tube
 F. Heart shadow
 G. Diaphragm

519

Copyright © 2015, 2011, 2006, 1996 by Saunders, an imprint of Elsevier Inc. All rights reserved.

177. A. Sixth
    B. Vertebral column
    C. Clavicles
    D. Above
    E. Eight
    F. Midsagittal
178. Up away from the bed or cart
179. Patient's bottom lip
180. Perpendicular
181. The patient was rotated toward the right side (RPO position).
182. The CR was angled too cephalically.
183. The image was exposed on expiration.
184. The patient was not elevated on a radiolucent sponge.
185. The right arm was not elevated to a position near the patient's head.
186. The left arm is superimposed over the apical lung region, and the right sternal clavicular end is visible away from the vertebral column. Elevate the left arm until it is next to the head, above the lung field, and rotate the right side of the thorax away from the IR until the shoulders and ASISs are at equal distances from the IR.
187. The right arm is superimposed over the apical lung region, and the left arm and upper vertebral column is not on the elevating device, resulting in lateral tilting of the upper vertebral column. Elevate the humeri, positioning them next the head, and elevate the entire thorax on the elevating device, placing the upper vertebral column parallel with the device.
188. The upper vertebral column tilts laterally, the left sternal clavicular end is away from the vertebral column, and the left posterior ribs demonstrate greater length than the right posterior ribs. Elevate the patient's head and upper vertebral column until the midsagittal plane is aligned parallel with the bed and rotate the right side toward the IR until the shoulders and ASISs are at equal distances from the IR.
189. A. Heart shadow
    B. Diaphragm
    C. Eighth posterior rib
    D. Third anterior rib
190. The right side of the patient was positioned closer to the IR than the left side (RAO position).
191. The left side of the patient was positioned closer to the IR than the right side (LPO position).
192. The upper midcoronal plane was tilted posteriorly.
193. The right sternal clavicular end is superimposed over the vertebral column, the posterior ribs on the left side demonstrate the greater length, and the arm is obscuring a small portion of the right lateral lung apex. Rotate the patient's left side away from the IR and elevate the right arm until it is positioned next to the head.
194. The left diaphragm is not included in its entirety. Move the CR and IR inferiorly approximately 2 inches (5 cm).
195. Peristaltic activity
196. A. Involuntary motion; the cortical outlines of the ribs and bony structures are sharp
    B. Voluntary motion; the cortical outlines of the ribs are blurry
197. They are located lateral to the lumbar vertebrae, starting at the first lumbar vertebra and extending to the lesser trochanters.
198. A. They are located lateral to the vertebral column, with the upper poles at approximately the 11th thoracic vertebra and the lower poles at approximately the third lumbar vertebra.
    B. Right
    C. It is located beneath the liver.
199. A. Psoas major muscle
    B. Kidneys
    C. Inferior ribs
    D. Lumbar transverse processes
200. A. 30% to 50% decrease
    B. 5% to 8% decrease
201. A. Obesity
    B. Bowel obstruction
    C. Soft tissue masses
    D. Ascites
202. Diaphragm, bowel gas pattern, and faint outline of bony structures
203. Little intrinsic fat is present to outline the organs.

204.

Adult Abdomen Technical Data					
Projection	kV	Grid	AEC	mAs	SID
AP, supine and upright	70–80	Grid	All three		40–48 inches (100–120 cm)
AP (lateral decubitus)	70–80	Grid	Center		40–48 inches (100–120 cm)
Pediatric Abdomen Technical Data					
Neonate: AP	70–80			3	40–48 inches (100–120 cm)
Infant: AP	70–80			5	40–48 inches (100–120 cm)
Child: AP	70–80	Grid*	All three		40–48 inches (100–120 cm)
Neonate: AP (lateral decubitus)	70–80			3	40–48 inches (100–120 cm)
Infant: AP (lateral decubitus)	70–80			5	40–48 inches (100–120 cm)
Child: AP (lateral decubitus)	70–80	Grid*	Center		40–48 inches (100–120 cm)

Copyright © 2015, 2011, 2006, 1996 by Saunders, an imprint of Elsevier Inc. All rights reserved.

205. A. Kidney
     B. Pedicle
     C. Third lumbar vertebral body
     D. Intestinal gas
     E. Anterior superior iliac spine (ASIS)
     F. Inlet pelvis
     G. Sacrum
     H. Iliac wing
     I. Iliac crest
     J. Spinous process
     K. 11th thoracic vertebra
206. A. Diaphragmatic dome
     B. Pedicle
     C. Inlet pelvis
     D. Sacrum
     E. Spinous process
     F. 12th vertebral body
     G. Gastric bubble
     H. Diaphragmatic dome
     I. Ninth thoracic vertebra
207. A. Vertebral bodies
     B. Symphysis pubis
     C. Ninth
     D. Fourth
     E. Third
208. Intraperitoneal air is located directly beneath each diaphragm dome.
209. A. Hypersthenic
     B. Sthenic
     C. Asthenic
210. Position the patient's shoulders, the posterior ribs, and the ASISs at equal distances from the IR.
211. A. 5 to 20 minutes
     B. It allows time for the air to rise to the level of the diaphragm.
212. A. Inferior
     B. Superior
     C. Eighth or ninth
     D. Ninth
213. A. Expiration
     B. Because less pressure is placed on the abdominal organs
214. A. Ensures that the kidneys, tip of liver, and spleen are included on the projection
     B. Ensures that the inferior border of the peritoneal cavity is included on the projection
215. Because the male patient's pelvis is longer
216. A. The 11th thoracic spinous process, lateral body soft tissue, iliac wings, and symphysis pubis
     B. The diaphragm, lateral body soft tissue, and iliac wings
217. The patient was rotated into an RPO position.
218. The upper abdomen was in an AP projection, and the pelvic area was rotated into an LPO position.
219. The CR and IR were centered too superiorly.
220. The sacrum is not aligned with the symphysis pubis, the distance from the left pedicles to the spinous processes is less than the distance from the right pedicles to the spinous processes, the right

iliac wing is wider than the left, and the lateral soft tissue is not included on the projection. Rotate the patient toward the left side until the shoulders and ASISs are positioned at equal distances from the IR and expose projections of the abdomen using two crosswise computed radiography IRs instead of one lengthwise or for DR open the transverse collimation to ½ inch from the skin line.
221. The symphysis pubis is not included on the projection. Center the CR 1 inch (2.5 cm) superior to the iliac crest and align the IR with the CR.
222. The lateral soft tissue of the abdomen has been clipped on both sides on this obese patient. Use the obese patient protocol to include all soft tissue.
223. The sacrum is not aligned with the symphysis pubis, the distance from the right pedicles to the spinous processes is greater than the distance from the left pedicles to the spinous processes, and the right iliac wing is wider than the left. Rotate the patient toward the left side until the shoulders and ASISs are positioned at equal distances from the IR.
224. The iliac wing is wider than the left, the distance from the right pedicles to the spinous processes is greater than the distance from the left pedicles to the spinous processes, the vertebral column is not aligned with the long axis of the IR, and the symphysis pubis is not included on the projection. Rotate the patient toward the left side until the shoulders and ASISs are positioned at equal distances from the IR, align the midsagittal plane with the long axis of the collimated light field, and move the CR and IR inferior enough to include the symphysis pubis.
225. The domes of the diaphragm are not included on the projection. Center the CR and IR approximately 2 inches (5 cm) superiorly or take an additional AP projection of the upper abdomen only by centering on xiphoid (T9-10) and collimating to a 10-inch longitudinal field size.
226. A. Iliac wing
     B. Intestinal gas
     C. Diaphragmatic dome
     D. Pedicle
     E. Vertebral body
     F. Spinous process
227. A. Vertebral bodies
     B. Spinous processes
     C. Ninth
     D. Third
228. Measure the patient and increase the mAs 30% to 50% or the kVp 5% to 8% from the routine technique that would normally be used for this body measurement.
229. A. Left
     B. This will position the gastric air bubble away from the abdominal area where the intraperitoneal air would be demonstrated.
230. Forward rotation of the side positioned farther from the imaging table

521

Copyright © 2015, 2011, 2006, 1996 by Saunders, an imprint of Elsevier Inc. All rights reserved.

231. A. 5 to 20
    B. To allow time for the air to move away from the soft tissue structures and rise to the level of the right diaphragm
232. A. Right hemidiaphragm
    B. Patient with wide hips and narrow waist and thorax
233. Expiration
234. The right hemidiaphragm, ninth thoracic vertebra, right lateral soft tissue, and right iliac wing
235. The right side of the patient was positioned farther from the IR than the left side.
236. The thorax and upper abdominal region were positioned accurately, and the right side of the pelvis and lower abdomen are closer to the IR than the left side.
237. The IR and CR were positioned too inferiorly.
238. The right iliac wing is narrower than the left iliac wing, and the distance from the right pedicles to the spinous processes is less than the distance from the left pedicles to the spinous processes. Rotate the right side toward the IR until the shoulders and the ASISs are positioned at equal distances from the IR.
239. A. Diaphragm
    B. Iliac wing
    C. Symphysis pubis
    D. Posterior ribs
240. A. Eighth
    B. Fourth lumbar
241. A. Midsagittal
    B. 2
    C. Superior
    D. Iliac crest
242. The CR was centered too inferiorly.
243. The patient's upper thorax is laterally tilted toward the left side.
244. The patient is rotated toward the left side (LPO position).
245. The patient is rotated toward the right side (RPO position).
246. The projection was exposed on inspiration.
247. The CR is centered to the third lumbar vertebra, the symphysis pubis and the lateral soft tissue are not included in the exposure field, the right posterior ribs demonstrate greater length than the left, and the right iliac wing demonstrates greater width than the left. Center the CR 1 inch (2.5 cm) inferiorly, collimate to within ½ inch (1.25 cm) of the lateral skin line, and rotate the patient toward the left side until the shoulders and the ASISs are at equal distances from the IR.
248. The left posterior ribs demonstrate greater length and the left iliac wing greater width than the right side, and the domes of the diaphragm are not included within the collimated field. Rotate the patient toward the right side until the shoulders and

ASISs are at equal distance from the IR and move the CR superiorly as needed to include the diaphragms.
249. A. Intestinal gas
    B. Inlet pelvis
    C. Obturator foramen
    D. Symphysis pubis
    E. Sacrum
    F. Iliac wing
    G. Spinous process
    H. Third lumbar vertebra pedicle
    I. 12th thoracic vertebra
250. The patient was rotated toward the right side (RPO position).
251. The patient was rotated toward the left side (LPO position).
252. Poor radiation protection practices have been followed. The left arm has been included on the projection, transverse and longitudinal collimation is inadequate, and the gonadal shield is positioned too superiorly and slightly too laterally. Move the CR medially until it is positioned at the midsagittal plane, increase transverse collimation to within ½ inch (1.25 cm) of the skin line, longitudinally collimate to the symphysis pubis, and move the gonadal shield slightly inferiorly and medially.
253. The symphysis pubis is not included in the exposure field, the CR is too superior, the right iliac wing is wider than the left, and the right posterior ribs are longer than the left posterior ribs. Center the CR 2 inches (5 cm) inferiorly and rotate the patient toward the left side until the shoulders and the ASISs are at equal distances from the IR.
254. The diaphragm is not included within the exposure field. Move the CR and IR superiorly approximately 2 inches (5 cm) or take an additional AP projection of upper abdomen by centering at the xiphoid (T9-T10) and collimating to a 10-inch longitudinal field size.
255. A. Symphysis pubis
    B. Iliac wing
    C. Posterior rib
    D. Diaphragm
    E. Lumbar vertebra
    F. Intestinal gas
256. To position the gastric bubble away from the elevated diaphragm, where free intraperitoneal air will migrate
257. A. Midsagittal
    B. 2
    C. Superior
    D. Iliac crest
258. The patient was rotated toward the right side (RPO position).
259. The CR was centered too inferiorly.
260. The patient was rotated toward the right side (RPO position).

522

Copyright © 2015, 2011, 2006, 1996 by Saunders, an imprint of Elsevier Inc. All rights reserved.

261. The diaphragm is not included within the exposure field, the posterior ribs on the right side are longer than those on the left, and the right iliac wing is wider than the iliac wing on the left side. Move the CR superiorly enough to include a transverse level 1 inch (2.5 cm) inferior to the mammary line, and rotate the patient away from the IR until the shoulders and the ASISs are at equal distances from the IR.

262. The diaphragm is demonstrated inferior to the ninth posterior rib, and the right pelvic wing is narrower than the left. Expose the patient after exhalation and rotate the right side toward the IR until the shoulders and the ASISs are at equal distances from the IR.

263. A. Right ilium
    B. Spinous process
    C. Pedicle
    D. Second vertebral body
    E. Diaphragm

264. Free interperitoneal air under the right diaphragm

265. The patient was rotated toward the left side (LPO position).

266. The diaphragm is inferior to the ninth posterior rib, indicating that the exposure was taken on inspiration. Center slightly higher and expose the projection after the patient has exhaled. Free intraperitoneal air is demonstrated adjacent to the right hemidiaphragm.

267. The right iliac wing is wider than the left, and the right posterior ribs are longer than the left posterior ribs. Rotate the patient toward the left side until the shoulders and the ASISs are at equal distances from the IR.

CHAPTER 4   IMAGE ANALYSIS OF THE UPPER EXTREMITY

1.

Table 4-1	Upper Extremity Technical Data			
Projection	kV	Grid	mAs	SID
Finger	55–65		1	40–48 inches (100–120 cm)
Thumb	55–65		1	40–48 inches (100–120 cm)
Hand	55–65		1	40–48 inches (100–120 cm)
Wrist	65–70		2	40–48 inches (100–120 cm)
Forearm	70–75		2	40–48 inches (100–120 cm)
Elbow	70–75		2	40–48 inches (100–120 cm)
Humerus	75–85	Grid*	3	40–48 inches (100–120 cm)
Pediatric	60–70		1–2	40–48 inches (100–120 cm)

2. A. Distal phalanx
   B. Middle phalanx
   C. Interphalangeal joints
   D. Proximal phalanx
   E. Metacarpophalangeal joint
   F. Metacarpal head
3. A. Equal
   B. MCP
   C. PIP
   D. MC
4. Shift the ring as far away from the affected area as possible. Note on the orders that the patient was unable to remove the ring.
5. Flat
6. A. Externally into a medial oblique position
   B. The thumb prevents internal rotation.
7. A. Farther
   B. Greater
8. Second
9. Fifth
10. Spread the fingers apart.
11. A. Parallel
    B. Perpendicular
12. A. Closed
    B. Foreshortened
13. A. Supinating
    B. Perpendicular
14. A. Perpendicular
    B. PIP
15. A. Phalanges
    B. MC
16. Within ½ inch (1.25 cm) of the finger skin line
17. The finger was internally rotated into a lateral oblique position.
18. The finger was flexed.
19. Soft tissue width and concavity is increased on the side of the finger facing the thumb. Rotate the hand and finger internally until they are flat against the IR.
20. The phalanges are foreshortened, the IP and MCP joints are closed, and increased concavity is present on the side of the finger facing the third digit. Unflex the finger and internally rotate the hand until the finger and hand are flat against the IR. If patient is unable to fully extend the finger, place it in an AP projection with the joint space of interest perpendicular to IR or phalanges of interest parallel with IR.

Copyright © 2015, 2011, 2006, 1996 by Saunders, an imprint of Elsevier Inc. All rights reserved.

21. A. Distal phalanx
    B. Middle phalanx
    C. Interphalangeal joints
    D. Proximal phalanx
    E. Metacarpophalangeal joint
    F. Metacarpal
22. A. Twice
    B. Concavity
    C. Open spaces
    D. PIP
23. 45
24 A. Externally
    B. Internally or externally
    C. This rotation results in the least amount of OID.
25. A. Extended
    B. Parallel
26. To prevent the finger from tilting toward the IR
27. A. Perpendicular
    B. PIP
28. The distal, middle, and proximal phalanges and half of the MC
29. The finger was not rotated enough and was too close to a PA projection.
30. The finger was rotated closer to a lateral projection than a 45-degree oblique.
31. The finger was flexed or tilted toward the IR.
32. Phalangeal concavity and soft tissue width are equal on each side of the digit. Rotate the hand and finger externally until the finger is at a 45-degree angle to the IR.
33. Whereas the anterior aspects of the middle and proximal phalanges demonstrate midshaft concavity, the posterior aspects of these phalanges demonstrate convexity. Internally rotate the hand until the finger is at a 45-degree angle to the IR. The fourth and fifth digits demonstrate superimposition. Separate the digits.
34. The phalanges are foreshortened, and the IP and MCP joints are closed. The finger was allowed to flex toward the IR. Fully extend the finger until it is parallel with IR.
35. A. Distal phalanx
    B. Distal interphalangeal joint
    C. Middle phalanx
    D. Proximal interphalangeal joint
    E. Proximal phalanx
    F. Metacarpophalangeal joint
    G. Metacarpals
36 A. Anterior
    B. Posterior
    C. IP joints
    D. PIP joint
37. 90
38. A. Internally
    B. Internally
    C. Externally
    D. Externally
39. The hand is rotated to obtain the least amount of OID.

40. Flex the hand into a tight fist with the affected finger extended.
41. The distal, middle, and proximal phalanges and the metacarpal head
42. A device to extend the finger and move the proximal phalanx away from the other phalanges should not be used distal to a fracture, or displacement of the fracture may occur.
43. The hand was not flexed into a tight fist.
44. The finger was not in a lateral projection but was in an oblique position.
45. The affected finger was allowed to tilt toward the IR.
46. Twice as much soft tissue and more phalangeal concavity are present on one side of the digit as on the other, there is soft tissue overlap of fourth and fifth fingers, and the DIP and PIP joints are closed. Flex the unaffected fingers into a fist and increase the degree of external hand obliquity until the finger is in a lateral projection. Position the long axis of the finger parallel with the IR.
47. The unaffected fingers are superimposed over the proximal phalanx. Flex the unaffected fingers into a fist while the finger of interest remains extended. Use a positioning device if needed to help extend the finger if no proximal phalanx injury is suspected.
48. A. Distal phalanx
    B. Interphalangeal joint
    C. Proximal phalanx
    D. Metacarpophalangeal joint
    E. Metacarpal
    F. Carpometacarpal joint
    G. Trapezium
49 A. Concavity
    B. Soft tissue
    C. Thumb
    D. Open spaces
    E. Medial palm
    F. MCP joint
50. A. Internally
    B. Directly
51. Closer
52. Extended
53. Draw the medial palm surface away from the thumb by using the opposite hand or an immobilization device.
54. A. Perpendicular
    B. MCP
55. The phalanges, MC, and CM joint
56. The hand was internally rotated more than needed to place the thumb in an AP projection.
57. The thumb was flexed.
58. The medial palm soft tissue was not drawn away from the proximal first MC.
59. The medial palm soft tissue is superimposed over the proximal MC and CM joint. Using the opposite hand, draw the medial palm away from the proximal MC.
60. More soft tissue width and phalanx concavity are present on the side adjacent to the other digits, and

524

Copyright © 2015, 2011, 2006, 1996 by Saunders, an imprint of Elsevier Inc. All rights reserved.

the thumbnail is facing away from the second through fifth digits. Decrease the amount of internal rotation until the fingernail is flat against the IR.
61. A. Distal phalanx
    B. Interphalangeal joint
    C. Proximal phalanx
    D. Metacarpophalangeal joint
    E. First metacarpal
    F. Second metacarpal
    G. Carpometacarpal joint
62. A. Anterior
    B. Posterior
    C. Open spaces
    D. Second
    E. MP joint
63. Flexed
64. Second proximal MC
65 A. Perpendicular
    B. MP
    C. To the thumb
66. The distal and proximal phalanges, MC, and CM joint
67. The hand was overflexed, and possibly the thumb was not in maximum abduction.
68. The hand was not flexed enough, resulting in under-rotation.
69. The proximal second and third MCs are superimposed over the proximal first MC. Abduct the thumb and slightly decrease the amount of hand flexion while maintaining a lateral thumb projection.
70. Twice as much soft tissue and more phalangeal and MC midshaft concavity are present on the side of the thumb facing the fingers. Increase the amount of hand flexion until the thumb is in a lateral projection.
71. A. Distal phalanx
    B. Interphalangeal joint
    C. Proximal phalanx
    D. Metacarpophalangeal joint
    E. First metacarpal
    F. Carpometacarpal joint
72. A. Twice
    B. Phalanges
    C. First MCP joint
73. 45
74. A. Extended
    B. Flat
75. The phalanges, MC, and CM joint
76. The hand was not flat against the IR, causing the thumb to be rotated closer to a lateral projection.
77. Whereas the anterior aspect of the proximal phalanx and MC demonstrates midshaft concavity, the posterior aspect of the phalanx and MC demonstrates slight convexity. Decrease the degree of hand flexion, positioning the hand flat against the IR.
78. The IP joint is closed and the distal phalanx is foreshortened. Extend the thumb until it is parallel with the IR.
79. A. Distal phalanx
    B. Interphalangeal joint

C. Proximal phalanx
D. Metacarpophalangeal joint
E. First metacarpal
F. Carpometacarpal joint
G. Radius
H. Ulna
I. Carpals
J. Carpometacarpal joint
K. Fifth metacarpal
L. Metacarpophalangeal joint
M. Proximal phalanx
N. Proximal interphalangeal joint
O. Middle phalanx
P. Distal interphalangeal joint
Q. Distal phalanx
80. A. MC heads
    B. Phalanges
    C. IP, MCP, and CM
    D. Third MCP
81. A. Pronate
    B. Flat
82. The joint spaces would be closed, and the phalanges and MCs would be foreshortened.
83. The thumb would move into a lateral projection.
84. The distal, middle, and proximal phalanges, MCs, and carpals and 1 inch (2.5 cm) of the forearm
85. The hand was externally rotated into a medial oblique position.
86. The second through fifth MC midshafts are more concave on one side than on the other, and the third through fifth MC heads demonstrate slight superimposition. The IP joint spaces are closed, and the proximal and middle phalanges are foreshortened. Extend and internally rotate the hand, placing it flat against the IR.
87. The second through fifth phalanges are foreshortened, and the IP joint spaces are closed. Extend the hand and place it flat against the IR.
88. Angle the CR laterally until it is aligned perpendicular to the MCs. Prop the IR on an angled sponge until it is perpendicular to the CR.
89. A. Interphalangeal joints
    B. Metacarpophalangeal joint
    C. Second metacarpal
    D. Radius
    E. Ulna
    F. Carpals
    G. Fifth metacarpal
    H. Phalanges
90. A. First and second
    B. Third through fifth
    C. Fourth and fifth
    D. Third MCP joint
91. A. 45
    B. Externally
92. Because the wrist will demonstrate more obliquity than the hand when they are rotated
93. They must be extended so they are aligned parallel with the IR.

525

Copyright © 2015, 2011, 2006, 1996 by Saunders, an imprint of Elsevier Inc. All rights reserved.

94. The phalanges, MCs, and carpals and 1 inch (2.5 cm) of the forearm
95. The hand was not rotated 45 degrees but was closer to a PA projection.
96. The hand was rotated more than 45 degrees.
97. The third through fifth MC heads are demonstrated without superimposition, the phalanges are foreshortened, and the IP joints are closed. Externally rotate the hand until it forms a 45-degree angle with the IR and elevate the distal fingers until they are aligned parallel with the IR.
98. The midshafts of the third through fifth MCs are superimposed. The phalanges are foreshortened, and the IP and MCP joints are closed. Internally rotate the hand until it forms a 45-degree angle with the IR and elevate the distal fingers until they are aligned parallel with the IR.
99. Angle the CR perpendicular to the MCs and then adjust it 45-degrees medially. Prop the IR until it is aligned perpendicular to the CR.
100. Angle the CR perpendicular to the MCs and then adjust it 45-degrees medially. Prop the IR until it is aligned perpendicular to the CR.
101. A. Distal phalanx
    B. Distal interphalangeal joint
    C. Middle phalanx
    D. Proximal interphalangeal joint
    E. Proximal phalanx
    F. Metacarpophalangeal joint
    G. First metacarpal
    H. Radius
    I. Ulna
    J. Carpals
    K. Metacarpals
    L. Metacarpophalangeal joint
102. A. Fifth
    B. Fifth
    C. MCP joints
103. The thicknesses of the fingers and the MCs are so different in this position that uniform image brightness is difficult to obtain.
104. A. Anteriorly
    B. Posteriorly
105. PA projection to a slight oblique position
106. Depress the thumb until it is parallel with the IR.
107. The phalanges, MCs, and carpals and 1 inch (2.5 cm) of the forearm
108. The hand was externally rotated or supinated.
109. The hand was internally rotated or pronated.
110. The fingers were not fanned.
111. The second through fifth MC midshafts are not all superimposed. The fifth MC is demonstrated anteriorly. Internally rotate the hand until the MCs are superimposed.
112. The second through fifth MC midshafts are demonstrated without superimposition. The second MC is demonstrated anteriorly. Externally rotate the hand until the MCs are superimposed.

113. The second through fifth digits are extended and superimposed, and the fifth MC is slightly anterior to other MCs. Fan or spread the fingers as far apart as possible without superimposing the thumb and internally rotate the hand until the second through fifth MCs are superimposed.
114. A. Trapezoid
    B. Trapezium
    C. Capitate
    D. Scaphoid
    E. Radial styloid
    F. Radius
    G. Ulna
    H. Ulnar styloid
    I. Lunate
    J. Triquetrum
    K. Pisiform
    L. Hamate
    M. Metacarpals
115. A. Scaphoid
    B. Radioulnar
    C. ¼ inch
    D. Second through fifth
    E. Forearm
    F. Carpal bones
116. Convex in shape and located lateral to the scaphoid
117. A change in the convexity of this stripe may indicate joint effusion or fracture.
118. A. Lateral
    B. Parallel
119. A. Posterior
    B. Anterior
120. Slightly depress the proximal forearm.
121. Allow the proximal forearm to hang off the IR and table enough to slightly depress the proximal forearm.
122. Flex the hand until MCs form a 10- to 15-degree angle with the IR.
123. Flexed
124. A. Anteriorly
    B. Foreshortened
    C. Medially
125. Posteriorly
126. Perpendicular
127. The carpal bones, one fourth of the distal ulna and radius, and half of the proximal MCs
128. The CR centering should be the same, but the longitudinally collimated field should be opened to include the needed amount of forearm.
129. The elbow was not in a lateral projection, and the humerus was not parallel with the IR.
130. The wrist was externally rotated (in a medial oblique position).
131. The wrist was internally rotated (in a lateral oblique position).
132. The proximal forearm was elevated.
133. The hand was extended, causing wrist flexion.
134. The hand was overflexed, causing wrist extension.

Study Question Answers   Copyright © 2015, 2011, 2006, 1996 by Saunders, an imprint of Elsevier Inc. All rights reserved.

135. The wrist was in radial flexion.
136. The wrist was in ulnar flexion.
137. The laterally located carpals and MCs are superimposed, and the radioulnar articulation is closed. Externally rotate the hand and wrist into a PA projection.
138. The medially located carpals and MCs are superimposed, and the radioulnar articulation is closed. Internally rotate the hand and wrist into a PA projection. The carpals are not centered in the exposure field. Move the CR proximally 1 inch (2.5 cm).
139. The scaphoid is slightly elongated, and the second through fourth CM joints are closed. Decrease hand flexion until the second through fifth MCs are at a 10- to 15-degree angle with the IR.
140. The scaphoid is foreshortened, and the third MC and midforearm are not aligned. Ulnar-deviate the wrist until the third MC and midforearm are aligned.
141. A. Capitate
    B. Hamate
    C. Pisiform
    D. Triquetrum
    E. Lunate
    F. Ulnar styloid
    G. Ulna
    H. Radius
    I. Radial styloid
    J. Scaphoid
    K. Trapezoid
    L. Trapezium
    M. Carpometacarpal joint
    N. First metacarpal
    O. Trapeziotrapezoidal joint
142. A. Scaphoid fat
    B. Trapezoid
    C. Trapezium
    D. Second
    E. Ulnar styloid
    F. Carpal bones
143. A. 45
    B. Externally
144. Trapezium
145. A. Third MC
    B. Midforearm
146. The posterior margin will be projected distal to the anterior margin.
147. Posterior
148. Perpendicular
149. The carpal bones, one fourth of the distal forearm, and half of the proximal MCs
150. The wrist was in less than a 45-degree external PA oblique projection.
151. The wrist was in radial deviation.
152. The proximal forearm was depressed.
153. The trapezoid and trapezium are superimposed, the trapeziotrapezoidal joint space is obscured, and the trapezoid demonstrates minimal capitate superimposition. Increase the degree of obliquity until the wrist forms a 45-degree angle with the IR.

154. The scaphoid demonstrates foreshortening, and the long axis of the third MC is not aligned with the midforearm. Ulnar-deviate the wrist until the third MC and midforearm are aligned.
155. The trapezium demonstrates minimal trapezoidal superimposition, the trapeziotrapezoidal joint space is obscured, and more than one-fourth of the trapezoid superimposes the capitate. Decrease the degree of obliquity until the wrist forms a 45-degree angle with the IR.
156. The scaphoid is demonstrated with decreased foreshortening, the second CM and scaphotrapezium joints are obscured, and more than ¼-inch (0.6 cm) of the radial articulating surface is demonstrated. Radial-deviate the wrist until the long axis of the third MC and midforearm are aligned, decrease the amount of hand flexion until the MCs are at a 10- to 15-degree angle with the IR, and depress the proximal forearm until the forearm is parallel.
157. A. Capitate
    B. Lunate
    C. Ulnar styloid
    D. Radius
    E. Pisiform
    F. Distal scaphoid
    G. Trapezium
    H. First metacarpal
158. A. Pronator
    B. Anterior
    C. Distal
    D. 10 to 15
    E. Forearm
    F. Posteriorly
    G. Trapezium
159. It is convex in shape and is located next to the anterior surface of the distal radius.
160. Changes in the shape and visualization of this stripe may indicate a fracture.
161. A. Ulnar
    B. Lateromedial
    C. Pisiform
162. Align the long axes of the third MC and the midforearm parallel with the IR.
163. A. Distal
    B. Proximal
164. Radial
165. Flex the hand until the second to fifth MCs are placed at a 10- to 15-degree angle with the anterior plane of the wrist.
166. Position the humerus parallel with the IR and the elbow in a lateral projection.
167. Do not abduct the humerus. Position the humeral epicondyles parallel with the IR in an AP projection.
168. The position described in the second question, when the elbow is in an AP projection and the humerus is not abducted
169. Depress the distal first MC until it is at the same level as the second MC.

Copyright © 2015, 2011, 2006, 1996 by Saunders, an imprint of Elsevier Inc. All rights reserved.

170. Perpendicular
171. The carpal bones, one-fourth of the distal ulna and radius, and half of the proximal MCs
172. A. AP projection
    B. Lateral projection
173. The wrist was externally rotated (or supinated).
174. The wrist was in ulnar deviation.
175. The humerus was not abducted but was placed against the patient, and the elbow was in an AP projection.
176. The distal first metacarpal was elevated.
177. The distal scaphoid is demonstrated anterior to the pisiform. Externally rotate the wrist until it is in a lateral projection. The ulnar styloid is in profile.
178. The distal scaphoid is demonstrated posterior to the pisiform. Internally rotate the wrist until it is in a lateral projection. The ulnar styloid is in profile.
179. The wrist is in extension. Align the long axis of the third MC with the midforearm. The ulnar styloid is in profile.
180. The trapezium is superimposed by the proximal first MC. Depress the first MC until it is at the same level as the second MC. The ulnar styloid is in profile.
181. The pisiform is proximal to the distal scaphoid. Ulnar deviate the wrist until the long axis of the third MC and midforearm are aligned. The wrist is flexed. Flex the hand until the second through fifth MCs are placed at a 10- to 15-degree angle with the anterior plane of the wrist. The ulnar styloid is in profile.
182. Angle the CR posteriorly.
183. A. Capitate
    B. Hamate
    C. Scaphocapitate joint
    D. Ulnar styloid
    E. Radioulnar articulation
    F. Scapholunate joint
    G. Radioscaphoid joint
    H. Scaphoid
    I. Scaphotrapezoidal joint
    J. Scaphotrapezium joint
    K. Trapezium
    L. Trapezoid
    M. CM joint
    N. First metacarpal
184. A. Scaphoid
    B. Scaphotrapezium
    C. First MC
    D. Scaphocapitate
    E. Medially
    F. Scaphoid
185. A. First MC
    B. Radius
    C. Radius
186. In ulnar deviation, the scaphoid has the space it needs to move posteriorly and will demonstrate a decrease in foreshortening.

187. Ulnar deviate the wrist until the long axis of the first MC and radius are aligned and the wrist is externally rotated 25 degrees with the IR.
188. 15 degrees proximally
189. A. 20 degrees proximally
    B. Without ulnar deviation, the distal scaphoid is positioned anteriorly, and the scaphoid demonstrates increased foreshortening.
190. Waist
191. A. Increase 5 to 10 degrees
    B. Decrease 5 to 10 degrees
192. No
193. Elevate (5–6 degrees) the proximal forearm.
194. The carpal bones, radioulnar joint, and proximal first through fourth MCs
195. A. Distal fracture. The first MC is not aligned with the ulna, so the starting CR angulation should be 20 degrees. This amount should then be increased by 5 to 10 degrees to a maximum angle of 25 degrees. A 25-degree angle should be used.
    B. Proximal fracture. The first MC and ulna are aligned, so the starting CR angulation should be 15 degrees. This amount should then be decreased by 5 degrees because the fracture is close to the waist. A 10-degree angle should be used.
    C. Waist fracture. The first MC is aligned with the ulna. A 15-degree CR angulation should be used.
196. The wrist was medially (externally) rotated more than needed.
197. The hand and fingers were flexed.
198. The scapholunate joint is closed, and the capitate and hamate demonstrate a small degree of superimposition. Decrease the degree of medial wrist obliquity.
199. The scaphocapitate joint space is closed, the capitate and hamate are demonstrated without superimposition, and the first MC is not aligned with the radius. Increase the degree of medial obliquity until the wrist forms a 25-degree angle with the IR and if the patient is capable, ulnar deviate the wrist until the first MC and radius are aligned.
200. The scaphotrapezium, scaphotrapezoid, and CM joints are closed. Extend the fingers and place the hand flat against the IR.
201. A. First metacarpal
    B. Trapezium
    C. Scaphoid
    D. Capitate
    E. Carpal canal
    F. Hamulus of hamate
    G. Triquetrum
    H. Pisiform
202. Pisiform
    B. Carpal
    C. Carpal canal
203. A. Narrowing
    B. Fractures

Copyright © 2015, 2011, 2006, 1996 by Saunders, an imprint of Elsevier Inc. All rights reserved.

204. Rotate the hand 10 degrees internally or until the fifth MC is perpendicular to the IR.
205. A. Vertical
    B. 25 to 30 degrees
206. A. Increased
    B. 35 degrees
    C. Acute angle between the CR and IR
207. The patient's wrist and distal forearm were either in a PA projection or in slight external rotation.
208. The angle between the CR and MCs was too great.
209. The angle between the CR and MCs was too small.
210. The pisiform is superimposed over the hamulus of the hamate. Internally (toward the radius) rotate the hand until the fifth MC is vertical.
211. The metacarpal bases obscure the bases of the hamate's hamulus process, pisiform, and scaphoid. Increase the CR angle until it is within 15 degrees of the MCs or increase the amount of wrist hyperextension by pulling the fingers posteriorly until the MCs are close to vertical.
212. The carpal canal is not demonstrated in its entirety, and the carpal bones are foreshortened. Decrease the CR angle until it is within 15 degrees of the MCs.
213. A. Radioscaphoid joint
    B. Radial styloid
    C. Radius
    D. Radial tuberosity
    E. Radial head
    F. Capitulum–radial (elbow) joint
    G. Lateral epicondyle
    H. Olecranon fossa
    I. Medial epicondyle
    J. Olecranon
    K. Ulna
    L. Radioulnar articulation
    M. Ulnar head
    N. Ulnar styloid
    O. Fifth metacarpal base
214. Position the wrist at the anode end and the elbow at the cathode end of the tube.
215. It is located ¾ inch (2 cm) distal to the medial epicondyle.
216. A. Forearm midpoint
    B. Perpendicular
    C. Midforearm
217. The wrist and elbow joints and the forearm soft tissue
218. A. Medially
    B. Ulna
219. The joint that is closer to the area of interest or near the fracture site should be positioned into an AP projection, but the other joint is positioned as close to an AP projection as possible.
220. Because the diverged x-ray beams, used to record this joint, do not align parallel with the joint space
221. Parallel
222. Supinate the hand and wrist, placing them in an AP projection.

223. The elbow was accurately positioned, but the hand and wrist were internally rotated.
224. The wrist and hand were accurately positioned, but the elbow was externally rotated.
225. The elbow is accurately positioned, but the hand was pronated.
226. The wrist was internally rotated and the elbow was externally rotated.
227. The lateral and PA projections of the forearm reflect accurate positioning. When forearm projections are obtained in a patient with a fracture where the patient is unable to position the distal and proximal forearm in a true position simultaneously, the joint closer to the fracture site should be placed in the true position. For these projections, the wrist joint demonstrates accurate positioning.
228. The radial head is demonstrated without ulna superimposition. Internally rotate the elbow until the humeral epicondyles are aligned parallel with the IR. Maintain the same wrist positioning.
229. The radial head is demonstrated without ulnar superimposition. Align the CR perpendicular to the humeral epicondyles (this will require the CR to be adjusted toward the medial surface). Prop the IR as needed to align it perpendicular to the CR.
230. A. Ulnar styloid
    B. Ulna
    C. Coronoid
    D. Olecranon
    E. Humerus
    F. Elbow joint
    G. Radial head
    H. Radius
    I. Pisiform
    J. Distal scaphoid
231. Forearm midpoint
232. The wrist and elbow joints and the forearm soft tissue
233. A. Pisiform
    B. Superimposed
234. The distal scaphoid will be anterior to the pisiform.
235. A. It will be demonstrated in profile posteriorly.
    B. Place the elbow in a lateral position and abduct the humerus, positioning it parallel with the IR.
236. A. No
    B. Supinate the hand to place the tuberosity in profile anteriorly and pronate the hand to place the tuberosity in profile posteriorly.
237. Thick or muscular proximal forearm
238. Radial head will be too posterior to the coronoid.
239. Place the elbow and proximal forearm in a lateral projection and allow the distal forearm to rotate as close to a lateral projection as the patient will allow.
240. The arm could have been externally rotated a slight amount to superimpose the distal radius and ulna or angle the CR posteriorly. The elbow is accurately positioned if the fracture is preventing it from being in a lateral projection.
241. The hand and wrist were externally rotated.

529

Copyright © 2015, 2011, 2006, 1996 by Saunders, an imprint of Elsevier Inc. All rights reserved.

Study Question Answers

242. The hand and wrist were internally rotated, and the proximal humerus was depressed more than the distal humerus.
243. The elbow was not in a lateral projection but was closer to an AP projection.
244. The wrist and hand were in external rotation.
245. The proximal humerus was elevated.
246. The radial head is posterior to the coronoid, and the distal scaphoid is anterior to the pisiform. Depress the proximal humerus until the humerus is parallel with the IR and externally rotate the wrist until it is in a lateral projection.
247. Adjust the CR posteriorly until it is aligned with an imaginary line connecting the distal radius and ulna. Prop the IR as needed to align it perpendicular to the CR.
248. A. Olecranon
   B. Lateral epicondyle
   C. Capitulum–radial joint
   D. Radial head
   E. Radial neck
   F. Radius
   G. Ulna
   H. Radial tuberosity
   I. Coronoid
   J. Medial trochlea
   K. Medial epicondyle
   L. Olecranon fossa
   M. Humerus
249. A. Profile
   B. Radial head
   C. Medially
   D. Open
   E. Elbow joint
250. The wrist and hand position
251. A. CR accurately centered to joint
   B. Forearm aligned parallel with the IR
252. Find where the CR was positioned by diagonally connecting the corners of the exposure field on the elbow projection. The two lines connect where the CR was located and discern whether the olecranon is within the olecranon fossa.
253. Do two AP views—one with the humerus parallel with the IR and one with the forearm parallel with the IR.
254. A. Perpendicular
   B. ¾ inch (2 cm)
   C. Distal
255. The elbow joint, one fourth of the proximal forearm and distal humerus, and the lateral soft tissue
256. Dislocated elbow. Note that the radial head and capitulum do not articulate.
257. The arm was internally (medially) rotated.
258. The hand was pronated.
259. The distal forearm was elevated.
260. The humeral epicondyles are not in profile, and more than ⅛th of the radial head superimposes the ulna. Externally rotate the elbow until the humeral epicondyles are at equal distances to the IR.

261. The humeral epicondyles are not in profile, and the radial head demonstrates less than ¼ inch (0.6 cm) of superimposition. Internally rotate the elbow until the humeral epicondyles are at equal distances from the IR.
262. The capitulum–radial joint is closed, and the radial articulating surface is demonstrated. If the patient's condition allows, fully extend the elbow. If the patient is unable to extend the elbow, take a second AP projection that is positioned with the forearm aligned parallel with the IR. Both projections should be sent to PACS.
263. Angle the CR laterally until it is aligned perpendicular to the humeral epicondyles. Prop the IR as needed to align it perpendicular to the CR.
264. Angle the CR medially until it is aligned perpendicular to the humeral epicondyles. Prop the IR as needed to align it perpendicular to the CR. If the elbow is of interest, center the CR on the elbow joint.
265. A. Medial epicondyle
   B. Medial trochlea
   C. Coronoid
   D. Radial tuberosity
   E. Radial head
266. A. Radial tuberosity
   B. Ulna
   C. Radial head
   D. Capitulum
267. A. Medial trochlea
   B. Trochlear–coronoid process
   C. Radial head
   D. Capitulum
   E. Ulna
   F. Elbow joint
268. A. The forearm was not positioned parallel with the IR.
   B. The CR was not centered to the elbow joint.
269. A. Forearm
   B. Forearm
   C. Humerus
   D. Humerus
   E. Forearm
270. 45 degrees
271. A. Perpendicular
   B. ¾ inch (2 cm)
   C. Medial epicondyle
272. The elbow joint, one-fourth of the distal humerus and proximal forearm, and the lateral soft tissue
273. The distal forearm was elevated.
274. The patient's arm was rotated less than 45 degrees.
275. The patient's arm was rotated more than 45 degrees.
276. The patient's arm was rotated less than 45 degrees.
277. The patient's arm was rotated more than 45 degrees.
278. A small portion of the radial head and tuberosity is superimposed over the ulna. Increase the degree of external obliquity until the humeral epicondyles are at a 45-degree angle to the IR.

Study Question Answers   Copyright © 2015, 2011, 2006, 1996 by Saunders, an imprint of Elsevier Inc. All rights reserved.

279. The capitulum–radial head joint is closed, and a small portion of the radial head is superimposed over the ulna. If the patient's condition allows, fully extend the arm, and if the patient is unable to fully extend the arm, position the forearm parallel with the IR. Increase the degree of external obliquity until the humeral epicondyles are at a 45-degree angle to the IR.

280. The radial head is demonstrated lateral to the coronoid process without complete superimposition of the ulna. Increase the degree of internal obliquity until the humeral epicondyles are at a 45-degree angle to the IR.

281. The radial head is demonstrated lateral to the coronoid process without complete superimposition of the ulna, the capitulum–radial joint is closed, and the articulating surface of the radial head is demonstrated. Increase the degree of internal obliquity until the humeral epicondyles are at a 45-degree angle with the IR. If the patient's condition allows, fully extend the arm, and if the patient is unable to fully extend the arm, position the forearm parallel with the IR.

282. A. Medial trochlea
   B. Coronoid
   C. Radial head
   D. Radius
   E. Ulna
   F. Trochlear notch
   G. Olecranon process
   H. Capitulum
   I. Trochlear sulcus
   J. Humerus

283. A. Trochlear sulcus
   B. Anterior
   C. Profile
   D. Elbow joint

284. A. Anterior fat pad anterior to the distal humerus
   B. Posterior fat pad within the olecranon fossa
   C. Supinator fat stripe, seen parallel to the anterior aspect of the distal radius
   D. Joint effusion and elbow injury

285. The posterior fat pad can be used as a diagnosing tool only when the elbow is flexed 90 degrees and the olecranon is out of the fossa.

286. A. Capitulum
   B. Trochlear sulcus
   C. Medial trochlea
   D. Trochlear sulcus
   E. Medial trochlea
   F. It will close it.

287. The capitulum would be distal to the medial trochlea.

288. The radial head would be distal to the coronoid, and the capitulum would be anterior to the medial trochlea.

289. The radial head will be proximal to the coronoid.

290. The radial head will be anterior to the coronoid, and the capitulum will be proximal to the medial trochlea.

291. A. Superimposed by the radius
   B. In profile, anteriorly
   C. In profile, posteriorly
   D. Superimposed by the radius

292. A. Perpendicular
   B. ¾ inch (2 cm)
   C. Distal

293. The elbow joint, one-fourth of the proximal forearm and distal humerus, and the surrounding soft tissue

294. The patient's arm was in extension.

295. The patient's hand and wrist were supinated.

296. The patient's proximal humerus was elevated.

297. The patient's proximal humerus was depressed.

298. The patient's distal forearm was not adequately elevated.

299. The patient's distal forearm was elevated more than needed.

300. The radial head is proximal to the coronoid (capitulum is posterior to the medial trochlea), and the radial tuberosity is seen anteriorly. Depress the distal forearm until the humeral epicondyles are aligned perpendicular to the IR, and internally rotate the distal forearm until the wrist is in a lateral projection.

301. The radial head is distal to the coronoid (capitulum is anterior to the medial trochlea). Elevate the distal forearm until the humeral epicondyles are aligned perpendicular to the IR.

302. The radial head is distal and posterior to the coronoid (capitulum is distal and anterior to the medial trochlea), the radial tuberosity is demonstrated anteriorly, and the elbow is not flexed to 90 degrees. Elevate the distal forearm and depress the proximal humerus until the humeral epicondyles are aligned perpendicular to the IR, externally rotate the distal forearm until the wrist is in a lateral position, and flex the elbow to 90 degrees.

303. The radial head is proximal and anterior to the coronoid (capitulum is posterior and proximal to the medial trochlea), and the radial tuberosity is visible posteriorly. Depress the distal forearm and elevate the proximal humerus until the humeral epicondyles are aligned perpendicular to the IR and externally rotate the distal forearm until the wrist is in a lateral projection.

304. The radial head is distal and anterior to the coronoid (capitulum is anterior and proximal to the medial trochlea). Elevate the distal forearm and proximal humerus until the humeral epicondyles are aligned perpendicular to the IR.

305. Adjust the CR angle posteriorly with the humerus (proximally on the forearm) until it is aligned parallel with the humeral epicondyles. Prop the IR as needed to align it perpendicular to the CR.

306. Adjust the angle anteriorly on the humerus (distally on the forearm) until it is aligned parallel with the humeral epicondyles. Prop the IR as needed to align it perpendicular to the CR.

Copyright © 2015, 2011, 2006, 1996 by Saunders, an imprint of Elsevier Inc. All rights reserved.

307. A. Capitulum
    B. Elbow joint
    C. Anterior aspect radial head
    D. Radial tuberosity
    E. Posterior aspect radial head
    F. Medial trochlea
308. A. Medial trochlea
    B. Open
    C. Radial head
309. Lateral
310. Radial head and coronoid and the capitulum and medial trochlea
311. The radial head will be proximal to the coronoid, and the capitulum will be posterior to the medial trochlea.
312. The capitulum will be anterior to the medial trochlea.
313. A. Perpendicular
    B. 45
    C. Proximally
    D. Radial head
    E. Capitulum
314. Radial tuberosity
315. A. The radial tuberosity will be in profile posteriorly, the lateral surface of the radial head will be in profile anteriorly, and the medial surface will be in profile posteriorly.
    B. The radial tuberosity will not be in profile but will be superimposed by the radius. The anterior surface of the radial head will appear in profile anteriorly, and the posterior surface will appear in profile posteriorly.
316. A. Lateral
    B. Medial
317. Radial head, located ¾ inch (2 cm) distal to the lateral epicondyle
318. The proximal forearm, distal humerus, and surrounding soft tissue
319. The distal forearm was positioned too far away from the IR.
320. The capitulum–radial joint space is closed, the radial head is demonstrated distal to the coronoid process, and the capitulum is demonstrated too far anterior to the medial trochlea. Elevate the distal forearm until the humeral epicondyles are aligned perpendicular to the IR.
321. The capitulum–radial joint space is closed, and the radial head is too distal to the coronoid process (the capitulum is too anterior to the medial trochlea). The radial head is not anterior enough to the coronoid (the capitulum is not proximal enough to the medial trochlea). Elevate the distal forearm and proximal humerus until the humeral epicondyles are perpendicular to the IR. Place a 45-degree proximal angle on the CR.
322. First align the CR parallel with an imaginary line connecting the humeral epicondyles; then adjust the CR 45 degrees proximally (toward the humerus).

The resulting angle will be more than 45 degrees. Prop the IR as needed to align it perpendicular to the humeral epicondyles.
323. The CR was aligned at an angle halfway between the humerus and forearm, which moved the radial head distal to the coronoid and the capitulum anterior to the medial trochlea.
324. A. Greater tubercle
    B. Lesser tubercle
    C. Humeral midshaft
    D. Medial epicondyle
    E. Lateral epicondyle
    F. Radial head
    G. Ulna
325. ⅛th
326. A. Greater
    B. Humeral head
    C. Lesser tubercle
327. A. Forced external rotation may result in an increased risk of radial nerve damage.
    B. Rotate the patient 35 to 40 degrees toward the affected side for the proximal humerus and rotate the patient toward the affected side until the humeral epicondyles are parallel with the IR when the distal humerus is of interest.
328. Abduct the humerus and place it diagonally on the IR.
329. To ensure that the joints will be included after the beam's divergence projects the elbow joint distally and the shoulder joint proximally
330. A. Locate at the same level as the coracoid
    B. Locate ¾ inch (2 cm) distal to the epicondyles
331. Humeral midpoint
332. The humerus, shoulder and elbow joints, and lateral humeral soft tissue
333. The arm was externally rotated.
334. The greater tubercle and the humeral epicondyles are not in profile, and the radial head is superimposed over more than ¼ inch (0.6 cm) of the ulna. Externally rotate the arm until the humeral epicondyles are at equal distances to the IR.
335. The greater and lesser tubercles are nearly superimposed, and the ulna is demonstrated without radial superimposition. Internally rotate the arm until the humeral epicondyles are at equal distances from the IR.
336. Lateromedial
337. A. Lesser tubercle
    B. Humeral shaft
    C. Medial trochlea
    D. Coronoid
    E. Radial tuberosity
    F. Radial head
    G. Capitulum
338. A. Lesser tubercle
    B. Humeral shaft
    C. Capitulum

Copyright © 2015, 2011, 2006, 1996 by Saunders, an imprint of Elsevier Inc. All rights reserved.

D. Radial head
E. Radial tuberosity
F. Capitulum–radial joint
G. Medial trochlea

339. A. Lesser
B. Medially
340. A. Arm
B. Humeral epicondyles
341. A. PA oblique (scapular Y) projection
B. Transthoracic lateral projection
342. Humeral midpoint
343. The humerus, elbow and shoulder joints, and lateral soft tissue
344. The greater tubercle is in profile, and the humeral epicondyles are not superimposed. Internally rotate the arm until the humeral epicondyles are perpendicular to the IR.
345. The image demonstrates a lateral projection, as indicated by the optimal distal humerus positioning. The brightness is higher at the proximal humerus than at the distal humerus, preventing proximal humerus visualization. Rotate the torso away from the proximal humerus into a PA projection.

CHAPTER 5   IMAGE ANALYSIS OF THE SHOULDER

1. A. 75 to 85
   B. 40 to 48 inches
2. When the part thickness measurement is more than 4 inches (10 cm)
3. A. Superior scapular angle
   B. Clavicle
   C. Acromion process
   D. Humeral head
   E. Greater tubercle
   F. Glenoid cavity
   G. Superolateral border of the scapula
   H. Thorax
   I. Coracoid process
4. A. Half
   B. Lateral edge of the vertebral column
   C. Midclavicle
   D. Greater
   E. Medially
   F. Laterally
   G. Medially
   H. Lesser
5. Position the shoulders at equal distances from the IR, aligning the midcoronal plane parallel with the IR.
6. A. 35 to 45 degrees
   B. Lateral
7. Glenoid cavity
8. Anterior
9. The upper midcoronal plane is straightened and positioned parallel with the IR.

10. Midclavicle
11. Angle the CR cephalically until it is perpendicular to the scapular body or lean the upper thoracic vertebrae posteriorly until the scapular body is parallel with IR and use a horizontal CR.
12. A. Greater
    B. Head
13. A. Position the humeral epicondyles at a 45-degree angle with the IR.
    B. Position the humeral epicondyles perpendicular to the IR.
    C. Position the humeral epicondyles parallel with the IR.
    D. Position the humeral epicondyles parallel with the IR.
14. Do not move the patient's arm. The projection is taken with the arm positioned as is.
15. A. Perpendicular
    B. Inferior
16. The glenohumeral joint, clavicle, proximal one-third of the humerus, and superior scapula
17. The patient was rotated toward the affected shoulder.
18. The patient was rotated toward the unaffected shoulder.
19. The patient's upper midcoronal plane was tilted away from the IR.
20. The patient's humerus was externally rotated until the humeral epicondyles were positioned parallel with the IR.
21. The patient's humerus was rotated internally until the humeral epicondyles were aligned perpendicular to the IR.
22. The superior scapular angle is demonstrated superior to the clavicle, and the lesser tubercle is demonstrated in profile medially. Tilt the upper midcoronal plane posteriorly until it is aligned parallel with the IR, and if a neutral shoulder is indicated, externally rotate the arm until the humeral epicondyles are at a 45-degree angle to the IR.
23. The superior scapular angle is demonstrated inferior to the clavicle. Tilt the upper midcoronal plane anteriorly until it is aligned parallel with the IR.
24. The medial clavicular end is superimposed over the vertebral column, the superior scapular angle is demonstrated superior to the clavicle, and the lesser tubercle is demonstrated in profile medially. Rotate the patient toward the left shoulder until the shoulders are at equal distances from the IR and tilt the upper midcoronal plane posteriorly until it is aligned parallel with the IR. If a neutral shoulder is indicated, externally rotate the arm until the humeral epicondyles are at a 45-degree angle to the IR.
25. A. Greater tubercle
    B. Acromion process
    C. Scapular spine
    D. Glenohumeral joint
    E. Clavicle
    F. Coracoid process
    G. Humeral head
    H. Lesser tubercle

Copyright © 2015, 2011, 2006, 1996 by Saunders, an imprint of Elsevier Inc. All rights reserved.

26. A. Glenoid cavity
    B. Inferior
    C. Lesser tubercle
    D. Lesser tubercle
    F. Posteriorly
    E. Humeral head
27. A. Glenohumeral joint
    B. Scapula
28. 30- to 35-degree
29. A. The angle should be decreased to approximately 20 degrees.
    B. Because the humerus has not been abducted enough to move the glenoid cavity superiorly until it is abducted more than 60 degrees
30. Position the IR vertically at the top of the affected shoulder so it is aligned perpendicular to the CR.
31. A. The lesser tubercle is in partial profile anteriorly, and the posterolateral aspect of the humeral head is in profile posteriorly.
    B. The humeral head and neck is in profile anteriorly, and the greater tubercle is in profile posteriorly.
    C. The humeral head and neck are in profile posteriorly, and the lesser tubercle is in profile anteriorly.
32. A. Horizontal
    B. Coracoid process
33. The glenoid cavity, coracoid process, acromion process, scapular spine, and one-third of the proximal humerus
34. Posterior
35. Medial aspect of the coracoid
36. A. The humeral epicondyles were at a 45-degree angle with the floor.
    B. The humeral epicondyles were perpendicular to the floor.
37. The angle formed between the lateral body surface and the CR was smaller than needed to align the CR parallel with the glenohumeral joint space.
38. The angle formed between the lateral body surface and the CR was larger than needed to align the CR parallel with the glenohumeral joint.
39. The humerus was externally rotated enough to position the humeral epicondyles perpendicular to the floor.
40. The patient's shoulder was not adequately elevated with a sponge or washcloth.
41. The glenoid fossa is demonstrated lateral to the base of the coracoid process. Increase the angle formed by the lateral body and the CR.
42. The inferior margin of the glenoid fossa is demonstrated medial to the coracoid process base. Decrease the angle formed by the lateral body and the CR.
43. The coracoid is not included in the projection. Laterally flex the neck toward the right shoulder and position the IR more medially.
44. A. Clavicle
    B. Scapular neck
    C. Coracoid process

D. Humeral head
    E. Glenohumeral joint
45. A. In profile
    B. Open
    C. ¼ inch (0.6 cm)
    D. Coracoid process
    E. Glenoid cavity
    F. Glenohumeral joint
46. A. Sternoclavicular
    B. Acromioclavicular
47. A. Coracoid process
    B. Acromion angle
48. A. The patient has kyphosis.
    B. The patient is imaged in a recumbent position.
    C. The patient leans against the IR while in an upright position.
49. Vertically
50. A. Horizontal
    B. Coracoid process
51. The glenoid cavity, humeral head, coracoid process, acromion process, and lateral clavicle
52. The patient was rotated more than needed to obtain an open glenohumeral joint space.
53. The patient was rotated less than needed to obtain an open glenohumeral joint space.
54. The patient was rotated more than needed to obtain an open glenohumeral joint space.
55. The upper midcoronal plane is tilted posteriorly.
56. The glenohumeral joint space is closed, more than ¼ inch (0.6 cm) of the lateral tip of the coracoid process is superimposed over the humeral head, and the clavicle demonstrates excessive transverse foreshortening. Decrease the degree of patient obliquity.
57. The glenohumeral joint space is closed, the lateral tip of the coracoid process is not superimposed over the humeral head, and the clavicle demonstrates little foreshortening. Increase the degree of patient obliquity.
58. A. Humeral head
    B. Coracoid process
    C. Clavicle
    D. Superior scapular angle
    E. Acromion process
    F. Glenoid cavity
    G. Scapular body
59. A. Superimposed
    B. Acromion process
    C. Coracoid process
    D. Superior scapular angle
    E. Midscapular body
60. A. Acromion angle
    B. Coracoid process
61. A. Shoulder dislocation
    B. Proximal humeral fracture
62. A. Affected
    B. Unaffected
63. The cortical outline of the lateral border is thicker than the cortical outline of the vertebral border.

Copyright © 2015, 2011, 2006, 1996 by Saunders, an imprint of Elsevier Inc. All rights reserved.

64. The humeral head should be superimposed over the glenoid cavity, and the humeral shaft should be superimposed over the scapular body.
65. Yes
66. A. Anteriorly and beneath the coracoid process
    B. Posteriorly and beneath the acromion process
67. Straighten the upper thoracic vertebrae, positioning the midcoronal plane parallel with the IR.
68. A. Kyphosis
    B. Angle the CR caudally until it is perpendicular to the scapular body.
69. A. Horizontal
    B. Vertebral (medial)
    C. Inferior scapular angle
    D. Acromial angle
70. The entire scapula and the proximal humerus
71. The patient was rotated more than needed to superimpose the scapular body.
72. The patient was rotated less than needed to superimpose the scapular body.
73. The patient's upper midcoronal plane was leaning toward the IR.
74. The lateral and vertebral borders of the scapula are demonstrated without superimposition. The vertebral scapular border is demonstrated next to the ribs, and the lateral border is demonstrated laterally. Increase the degree of patient obliquity.
75. The lateral and vertebral borders of the scapula are demonstrated without superimposition. The lateral border is demonstrated next to the ribs, and the vertebral border is demonstrated laterally. Decrease the degree of patient rotation.
76. The superior scapular angle is demonstrated superior to the clavicle. Tilt the upper midcoronal plane posteriorly until it is parallel with the IR.
77. The lateral and vertebral borders of the scapula are demonstrated without superimposition. The vertebral scapular border is demonstrated next to the ribs, and the lateral border appears laterally. Increase the degree of patient obliquity.
78. A. Greater tubercle
    B. Posterolateral humeral head
    C. Conoid tubercle
    D. Coracoid process
    E. Clavicle
    F. Lesser tubercle
79. A. Conoid tubercle
    B. Posterolateral
    C. Coracoid process
    D. Coracoid process
80. A. Hill-Sachs
    B. Posterolateral
81. A. Vertical
    B. On top of the patient's head
82. Coracoid process
83. Humeral head, coracoid process, lateral clavicle, glenoid cavity, and the upper one-third of scapular body.

84. The upper thoracic vertebrae were arched upward or the CR was angled less than the required 10-degree cephalic angle.
85. The distal humerus is tilted laterally.
86. The humerus was elevated to less than a vertical position.
87. The coracoid process is seen inferior to the clavicle, and the humeral shaft demonstrates increased foreshortening. Place a 10-degree cephalic angulation on the CR.
88. The posterolateral humeral head is obscured, and the humeral shaft demonstrates increased foreshortening and a decrease in density. Elevate the humerus until it is placed at a 90-degree position with the patient's torso.
89. The posterolateral humeral head and lesser tubercle are obscured. The greater tubercle is in profile laterally. Tilt the distal humerus laterally until it is parallel with midsagittal plane.
90. A. Scapular body
    B. Glenoid cavity
    C. Humeral head
    D. Acromion process
    E. Clavicle
    F. Superior scapular angle
    G. Coracoid process
    H. Thorax
91. A. Superimposed
    B. Scapular body
    C. Acromion
    D. Coracoid process
    E. Coracoid process
    F. Clavicle
    G. AC joint
92. PA oblique projection
93. Less
94. Inferior
95. A. 10 to 15 degrees caudally
    B. Superior aspect of the humeral head
96. Acromion and coracoid processes, lateral clavicle, superior scapular spine, and half of the scapular body
97. The patient was rotated more than needed to superimpose the scapular body.
98. The upper midcoronal plane was tilted toward the IR or the CR was not angled 10 to 15 degrees caudally.
99. The lateral and vertebral borders of the scapula are demonstrated without superimposition, and the glenoid cavity is not demonstrated on end but is seen medially. The lateral scapular border is demonstrated next to the ribs, and the vertebral border is demonstrated laterally. Decrease patient obliquity until the scapular borders are superimposed.
100. The outlet is not open, the lateral clavicle and acromion process do not from a smooth arch, and the superior scapular angle is superior to the coracoid process. Straighten the upper midcoronal plane, aligning it vertically, and angle the CR 10 to 15 degrees caudally.

535

Copyright © 2015, 2011, 2006, 1996 by Saunders, an imprint of Elsevier Inc. All rights reserved.

101. A. Acromion process
    B. Lateral clavicle
    C. Coracoid process
    D. Superior scapular angle
    E. Vertebral border of scapula
    F. Medial clavicle
    G. Vertebral column
102. A. Lateral edge
    B. Superior scapular angle
    C. Transverse
    D. Midclavicle
103. Position the shoulders at equal distances from the table or IR.
104. A. Perpendicular
    B. Midclavicle
105. The clavicle and acromion process
106. The patient was rotated away from the affected shoulder.
107. The patient was rotated toward the affected shoulder.
108. The patient's upper midcoronal plane was leaning away from the IR.
109. The superior scapular angle is demonstrated superior to the clavicle. Tilt the upper midcoronal plane posteriorly until it is aligned parallel with the IR.
110. The medial clavicular end is superimposed over the vertebral column, and the vertebral border of the scapula is positioned away from the thoracic cavity. Rotate the patient toward the affected shoulder.
111. A. Acromion process
    B. Lateral clavicle
    C. Middle clavicle
    D. Superior scapular angle
    E. Medial clavicle
112. A. Clavicular
    B. Inferior
    C. First, second, or third
    D. Acromion process
    E. Midclavicle
113. A 15- to 30-degree cephalic angle
114. Middle third of the clavicle
115. A. Clavicle
    B. Acromion process
116. The patient was rotated toward the affected shoulder.
117. The CR was not angled enough cephalically.
118. The lateral and medial thirds of the clavicle are superimposed over the scapula, and the medial clavicular end is superimposed over the vertebral column. Increase the degree of cephalic CR angulation and rotate the patient toward the right shoulder until the shoulders are at equal distances from the IR.
119. A. Superior scapular angle
    B. Scapular spine
    C. Lateral clavicle
    D. AC joint
    E. Acromial apex

120. A. With the patient holding weights
    B. Horizontal
    C. Acromion process
    D. AC joint
121. To compare the projections so the AC joint can be evaluated for possible ligament injury
122. Separation between the acromion process and clavicle will be increased when one compares the weight-bearing with the non–weight-bearing projections.
123. 5 to 8 lb
124. The AC joint, lateral clavicle, acromion, and superior scapular angle
125. To ensure that the same centering is obtained and the x-ray beam's divergence does not result in a false reading
126. The patient is rotated toward the affected AC joint.
127. The superior scapular angle is demonstrated superior to the clavicle. Tilt the upper midcoronal plane posteriorly until it is parallel with the IR.
128. A. Acromion process
    B. Lesser tubercle
    C. Glenoid cavity
    D. Glenoid neck
    E. Lateral border
    F. Inferior angle
    G. Vertebral border
    H. Scapular body
    I. Supraspinous fossa
    J. Scapular spine
    K. Coracoid process
    L. Superior angle
    M. Clavicle
129. A. Glenoid cavity
    B. Clavicle
    C. Thoracic cavity
    D. Vertebral border
    E. Midscapular body
130. Because the thorax, which is filled with air, has less density than the shoulder soft tissue
131. Expiration
132. A. 35 to 45 degrees
    B. Transverse
133. A. The arm is abducted to a 90-degree angle with the body, the elbow is flexed, and the hand is supinated by externally rotating the arm.
    B. It forces it to retract.
    C. When the arm is positioned to cause retraction, the glenoid cavity is positioned closer to profile.
134. Longitudinal
135. A. Perpendicular
    B. 2
    C. Inferior
136. The entire scapula, which includes the inferior and superior angles, coracoid and acromion processes, body, and glenoid cavity

Study Question Answers   Copyright © 2015, 2011, 2006, 1996 by Saunders, an imprint of Elsevier Inc. All rights reserved.

137. Place the patient supine to maximize shoulder retraction. If the glenoid cavity area is of interest, roll the patient onto the affected shoulder.
138. Make sure that the arm is abducted to 90 degrees and externally rotate by flexing the elbow and supinating the hand.
139. A portion of the inferolateral border of the scapula is superimposed by the thoracic cavity, and the superior angle is superimposed by the clavicle. Abduct the humerus to a full 90-degree angle with the body.
140. The inferolateral border of the scapula is superimposed by the thoracic cavity, and the superior angle is superimposed by the clavicle. Abduct the humerus to a 90-degree angle with the body.
141. A. Clavicle
    B. Coracoid process
    C. Thorax
    D. Inferior angle
    E. Scapular body
    F. Acromion process
    G. Glenoid cavity
142. A. Clavicle
    B. Superimposed
    C. Midscapular body
143. A. Away from
    B. Toward
144. The elevation of the humerus
145. The borders of the scapula will not be superimposed.
146. A. Body
    B. Neck
147. Placing the humerus at a 90-degree angle with the body
148. Elevating the humerus higher than a 90-degree angle with the body
149. A. Less
    B. Because the scapula is drawn laterally around the thorax as the humerus is abducted
150. The entire scapula, which includes the inferior and superior angles, coracoid and acromion processes, and scapular body
151. The patient was rotated more than needed to superimpose the scapular borders.
152. The patient was rotated less than needed to superimpose the scapular borders.
153. The lateral and vertebral borders of the scapula are demonstrated without superimposition. The vertebral border is visible next to the ribs. Increase the degree of patient rotation.
154. The lateral and vertebral borders of the scapula are demonstrated without superimposition. The lateral border is next to the ribs, and the vertebral border is demonstrated laterally. The patient's arm was not elevated, positioning the vertebral border of the scapula parallel with the IR. Decrease the degree of patient obliquity and elevate the arm to 90 degrees with the torso.

CHAPTER 6   IMAGE ANALYSIS OF THE LOWER EXTREMITY

1. A. 65 to 75 kV
   B. 75 to 85 kV
   C. 75 to 85 kV
2. A. 3
   B. 9
   C. 7
   D. 10
   E. 2
   F. 4
   G. 1
   H. 6
   I. 5
   J. 8
3. A. Distal phalanx
   B. Distal IP joint
   C. Middle phalanx
   D. Proximal IP joint
   E. Proximal phalanx
   F. MTP joint
   G. Metatarsal
4. A. Soft tissue
   B. Concavity
   C. IP
   D. MTP
   E. MTP
   F. Third
5. A. Lateral
   B. Lateral
6. A. Parallel
   B. Perpendicular
7. The phalanges and half of the MT
8. The foot and toe were laterally rotated.
9. The toe was flexed.
10. The proximal phalanx demonstrates greater soft tissue width and midshaft concavity on the medial surface. Medially rotate the foot and toe until they are placed flat against the IR. The IP joint space is closed, and the distal phalanx is foreshortened. Angle the CR proximally until it is aligned perpendicular to the distal phalanx or elevate the toe on a radiolucent sponge, bringing the distal phalanx parallel with the IR.
11. A. Distal phalanx
    B. IP joint
    C. Proximal phalanx
    D. MTP joint
    E. Metatarsal
12. A. Twice
    B. Away from
    C. IP
    D. MTP
    E. MTP
13. A. 45 degrees
    B. Twice as much soft tissue width is present on the side of the digit rotated away from the IR when accurate.

Copyright © 2015, 2011, 2006, 1996 by Saunders, an imprint of Elsevier Inc. All rights reserved.

14. A. Medially
    B. Laterally
    C. To obtain an oblique using the least amount of OID
15. Closed joint spaces and foreshortened phalanges
16. The phalanges and half of the metatarsal
17. Connecting tissue between the toes
18. The toe and foot were close to an AP projection.
19. The toe was close to a lateral projection.
20. The toe was flexed, and the CR was not aligned perpendicular to the phalanges or parallel with the joint spaces.
21. Nearly equal soft tissue width and midshaft concavity are demonstrated on each side of the phalanges. Increase the degree of toe and foot obliquity until the affected toe is at a 45-degree angle with the IR.
22. Soft tissue and bony overlap of the adjacent digit onto the affected digit is present. Draw the unaffected toes away from the affected toe.
23. The proximal phalanx demonstrates more concavity on the lateral aspect of the toe than the medial aspect, and more than twice as much soft tissue is shown on one side of the toe as on the other. Decrease the degree of toe and foot obliquity until the toe is at a 45-degree angle with the IR.
24. A. Distal phalanx
    B. Distal IP joint
    C. Middle phalanx
    D. Proximal IP joint
    E. Proximal phalanx
    F. MTP joint
    G. Metatarsal
25. A. Posterior
    B. Anterior
    C. PIP
26. A. Medially
    B. Laterally
27. The phalanges and the MTP joint space
28. The foot and toe were not rotated enough to place the toe in a lateral projection.
29. The foot and toe were rotated too much to place the toe in a lateral projection.
30. The adjacent unaffected digits were not drawn away from the affected digit.
31. The proximal and distal phalanges demonstrate nearly equal midshaft concavity, the condyles of the proximal phalanx are demonstrated without superimposition, and the first and second MT heads are not superimposed. Increase the degree of toe and foot obliquity until the affected toe is in a lateral projection.
32. The proximal phalange's condyles are not superimposed, and the MT heads demonstrate slight superimposition. Increase the degree of toe and foot obliquity until the affected toe is in a lateral projection.
33. A. Phalanges
    B. Metatarsals
    C. Medial cuneiform

    D. Medial-intermediate cuneiform joint
    E. Intermediate cuneiform
    F. Navicular–cuneiform joint
    G. Navicular bone
    H. Talus
    I. Calcaneus
    J. Cuboid
    K. Lateral cuneiform
    L. Fifth metatarsal tuberosity
    M. Fourth tarsometatarsal joint
    N. Fifth metatarsal base
34. A. Medial (first)
    B. Intermediate (second)
    C. One-third
    D. TMT
    E. Third
35. A. Plantar
    B. Lower leg
    C. Ankle
    D. Foot
36. Medial
37. Lateral
38. A. 5 to 15
    B. High arch requires more CR angulation.
39. Proximal calcaneus, talar neck, tarsals, MTs, phalanges, and surrounding soft tissue
40. The foot was laterally rotated.
41. The foot was medially rotated.
42. The CR was not angled enough proximally.
43. The joint space between the medial and intermediate cuneiforms is closed, and one-third of the talus superimposes the calcaneus. Rotate the foot medially until the pressure is equal over the entire plantar surface.
44. The joint space between the medial and intermediate cuneiforms is closed, the distal calcaneus is demonstrated without talar superimposition, and the MT bases demonstrate decreased superimposition. Rotate the foot laterally until the pressure is equal over the entire plantar surface.
45. A. Phalanges
    B. Metatarsals
    C. Medial cuneiform
    D. Lateral cuneiform
    E. Intermediate cuneiform
    F. Navicular
    G. Talus
    H. Tarsal sinus
    I. Calcaneus
    J. Cuboid
    K. Cuboid-cuneiform joint
    L. Fifth metatarsal tuberosity
    M. Intermetatarsal joint
    N. Fifth metatarsal base
46. A. Cuboid-cuneiform
    B. Second through fifth
    C. Fifth
    D. Third MT
47. Medially

Study Question Answers   Copyright © 2015, 2011, 2006, 1996 by Saunders, an imprint of Elsevier Inc. All rights reserved.

48. A. 60 degrees
    B. 30 degrees
    C. 45 degrees
49. A. High
    B. The first MT base is superimposed by the second and part of the third MT bases.
50. A. Figure 6-15
    B. More of the cuboid is demonstrated posterior to the navicular in Figure 6-15 than in Figure 6-17.
51. A. Beneath
    B. Second
    C. Closer to
52. A. Fourth MT tubercle
    B. The fifth MT will be superimposed over the fourth MT tubercle.
53. The phalanges, MTs, tarsals, calcaneus, and surrounding soft tissue
54. The foot was underrotated.
55. The foot was overrotated.
56. The lateral cuneiform-cuboid, navicular-cuboid, and third through fifth intermetatarsal joint spaces are closed. The fifth MT is not superimposed over the fourth MT tubercle. Increase the degree of medial foot obliquity.
57. A. Fibula
    B. Calcaneus
    C. Cuboid
    D. Metatarsals
    E. Phalanges
    F. Cuneiforms
    G. Navicular
    H. Talus
    I. Tibiotalar joint
    J. Tibia
58. A. Anterior patellar
    B. Posterior pericapsular
    C. Tibiotalar
    D. 90-degree angle
    E. Distal tarsals
59. Lateral
60. A. The posterior pericapsular located within indention formed by the articulation of the posterior tibia and talar bone.
    B. Anterior pretalar located anterior to the ankle joint, next to the talus.
61. Position the lower leg parallel with the imaging table.
62. A. Position the long axis of the foot at a 90-degree angle with the lower leg.
    B. Position the lateral foot surface parallel with the IR.
63. A. The medial talar dome would be demonstrated distal to the lateral talar dome.
    B. Elevate the distal lower leg and ankle until the lower leg is parallel with the imaging table.
64. A. Posterior
    B. Navicular
65. ½ (1.25 cm)

66. A. Less
    B. More
67. Talar domes
68. A. Leg
    B. Foot
69. This question can be answered two different ways:
    A. Medial   A. Lateral
    B. Proximal   B. Distal
    C. Lateral   C. Medial
    D. Higher   D. Higher
70. This question can be answered two different ways:
    A. Medial   A. Lateral
    B. Distal   B. Proximal
    C. Lateral   C. Medial
    D. Lower   D. Lower
71. Lateral
72. This question can be answered two different ways:
    A. Medial   A. Lateral
    B. Posterior   B. Anterior
    C. Lateral   C. Medial
    D. Anterior   D. Anterior
73. This question can be answered two different ways:
    A. Medial   A. Lateral
    B. Anterior   B. Posterior
    C. Lateral   C. Medial
    D. Posterior   D. Posterior
74. A. It demonstrates the anterior pretalar fat pad without forced flattening.
    B. It places the tibiotalar joint in a neutral position.
    C. It prevents anterior foot rotation.
75. A. Medial
    B. Lateral
76. Move the patient's heel away from the IR.
77. A. Perpendicular
    B. Fifth MT base
78. The phalanges, MTs, tarsals, talus, calcaneus, 1 inch (2.5 cm) of the distal lower leg, and the surrounding foot soft tissue
79. The proximal lower leg was elevated higher than the distal lower leg.
80. The distal lower leg was elevated higher than the proximal lower leg.
81. The heel was elevated, and the forefoot was depressed.
82. The heel was depressed, and the forefoot was elevated.
83. The lower leg and long axis of the foot do not form a 90-degree angle. The foot was in plantarflexion. Dorsiflex the foot until the lower leg and long axis of the foot form a 90-degree angle.
84. The medial talar dome is positioned posterior to the lateral dome, and the distal fibula is anterior on the tibia. Depress the forefoot and elevate the heel (external leg rotation) until the lateral foot surface is parallel with the IR.
85. The lateral talar dome is proximal to the medial talar dome and less than ½ of the cuboid is seen posterior to the navicular. Depress the proximal lower leg or elevate the distal lower leg.

Copyright © 2015, 2011, 2006, 1996 by Saunders, an imprint of Elsevier Inc. All rights reserved.

86. The lateral talar dome is posterior to the medial talar dome and the fibula is too posterior on the tibia. Move the heel away from the IR (internal leg rotation).
87. A. Talus
    B. Talocalcaneal joint
    C. Sustentaculum tali
    D. Tuberosity
    E. Fifth metatarsal base
88. A. Talocalcaneal
    B. Medial
    C. Lateral
    D. Proximal calcaneal tuberosity
89. A. Vertical
    B. 40
    C. Plantar
90. A. Parallel
    B. Perpendicular
91. A. Increase the degree of CR angulation.
    B. Decrease the degree of CR angulation.
92. Base of the fifth MT and distal point of the fibula
93. A. Place the ankle in an AP projection without medial or lateral rotation.
    B. The first MT will be demonstrated medially, or the fourth and fifth MTs will be demonstrated laterally.
94. Fifth MT base
95. The calcaneal tuberosity and talocalcaneal joint
96. The foot was in plantarflexion.
97. The leg and ankle were medially rotated.
98. The leg and ankle were laterally rotated.
99. The second through fifth MTs are demonstrated laterally. Internally rotate the leg until the ankle is in an AP projection.
100. The talocalcaneal joint space is obscured, and the calcaneal tuberosity is foreshortened. If the patient's condition allows, dorsiflex the foot to a vertical, neutral position. If the patient cannot dorsiflex the foot, increase the CR angulation, aligning the CR with the fifth MT base and the distal point of the fibula.
101. The talocalcaneal joint space is obscured, and the calcaneal tuberosity is elongated. The foot was dorsiflexed beyond the vertical position, and a 40-degree central angulation was used. Plantar flex the foot to a vertical position and use a 40-degree angulation.
102. A. Tibiotalar joint
    B. Talar domes
    C. Calcaneus
    D. Tuberosity
    E. Talocalcaneal joint
    F. Cuboid
    G. Navicular
    H. Talus
    I. Tibia
103. A. Posterior
    B. Lower leg
    C. Midcalcaneus

104. Parallel with the imaging table
105. A. Position the long axis of the foot at a 90-degree angle with the lower leg.
    B. Position the lateral foot surface parallel with the IR.
106. The medial talar dome would be demonstrated distal to the lateral talar dome.
107. A. Posterior
    B. Navicular
108. ½ (1.25 cm)
109. This question can be answered two different ways:
    A. Medial   A. Lateral
    B. Proximal   B. Distal
    C. Lateral   C. Medial
    D. Higher   D. Higher
110. This question can be answered two different ways:
    A. Medial   A. Lateral
    B. Posterior   B. Anterior
    C. Lateral   C. Medial
    D. Anterior   D. Anterior
111. A. Perpendicular
    B. Distal
    C. Medial malleolus
112. The tibiotalar joint, talus, calcaneus, and calcaneal articulating tarsal bones
113. The proximal tibia was elevated.
114. The forefoot was depressed, and the heel was elevated (leg externally rotated).
115. The medial talar dome is anterior to the lateral talar dome, and the fibula is too posterior on the tibia. Elevate the forefoot and depress the heel until the lateral foot surface is parallel with the IR.
116. The foot is plantarflexed, the medial talar dome is posterior and distal to the lateral talar dome, the fibula is too anterior on the tibia, and less than ½ inch (1.25 cm) of the cuboid is demonstrated posterior to the navicular. Dorsiflex the foot to a 90-degree angle with the lower leg, depress the forefoot and elevate the heel (externally rotate leg) until the lateral foot surface is parallel with the IR, and depress the proximal lower leg until it is parallel with the imaging table.
117. The lateral talar dome is posterior and proximal to the medial talar dome, the fibula is too far posterior on the tibia, and more than ½ inch (1.25 cm) of the cuboid is demonstrated posterior to the navicular. Internally rotate the leg until the lateral foot surface is parallel with the IR and elevate the proximal lower leg until it is parallel with the IR.
118. A. Tibia
    B. Medial malleolus
    C. Medial mortise
    D. Talus
    E. Lateral malleolus
    F. Tibiotalar joint
    G. Fibula
119. A. Half
    B. Open
    C. Tibiotalar joint

Copyright © 2015, 2011, 2006, 1996 by Saunders, an imprint of Elsevier Inc. All rights reserved.

120. Medial malleolus
121. The tibia is superimposed over the fibula.
122. 15 to 20 degrees
123. The tibia and talus will demonstrate increased superimposition of the fibula, and the medial mortise will be closed.
124. The lower leg should be positioned parallel with the IR and CR centered to ankle joint.
125. The tibiotalar joint space will be closed or narrowed, and the anterior tibial margin will be projected distally.
126. A. Perpendicular
    B. Medial malleolus
127. The distal one-fourth of the tibia and fibula, talus, and surrounding ankle soft tissue
128. The ankle was laterally rotated.
129. The proximal tibia was elevated, or the CR was centered too proximally.
130. The medial mortise is obscured, the tibia and talus demonstrate increased superimposition of the fibula, and the posterior aspect of the medial malleolus is situated medial to the anterior aspect. Rotate the leg internally, placing the long axis of the foot in a vertical position.
131. The talus is demonstrated without fibular superimposition. Externally rotate the leg until the long axis of the foot is vertical.
132. A. Fibula
    B. Lateral malleolus
    C. Lateral mortise
    D. Calcaneus
    E. Talus
    F. Medial mortise
    G. Medial malleolus
    H. Tibiotalar joint
    I. Tibia
133. A. Talar
    B. Lateral
    C. Fibula
    D. Tibial
    E. Distal
    F. Tibiotalar joint
134. A. 15 to 20 degrees
    B. Medially (internally)
135. Position the lower leg parallel with the imaging table and center CR to ankle joint.
136. Dorsiflex the foot to a 90-degree angle with the lower leg.
137. A. Perpendicular
    B. Medial malleolus
138. The distal one fourth of the fibula and tibia, talus, and surrounding ankle soft tissue
139. The leg and ankle were overrotated.
140. The leg and ankle were internally rotated more than 45 degrees.
141. The distal tibia was elevated, or the CR was positioned distal to the joint space.
142. The foot was in plantarflexion.

143. The calcaneus is obscuring the distal aspect of the lateral mortise and the distal fibula. Dorsiflex the foot until its long axis forms a 90-degree angle with the lower leg.
144. The lateral mortise is closed, the medial mortise is open, and the tarsal sinus is not demonstrated. Increase the degree of internal (medial) leg rotation until the most prominent aspects of the malleoli are positioned at equal distances from the IR.
145. The medial mortise is partially closed, the fibula is demonstrated without tibial superimposition, and the tarsal sinus is partially shown. Decrease the degree of internal (medial) leg rotation until the malleoli are positioned at equal distances from the IR.
146. The lateral and medial mortises are closed, and the tarsal sinus is demonstrated. Rotate the leg laterally until the long axis of the foot is at a 45-degree angle with the IR.
147. The lateral and medial mortises are closed, and the tarsal sinus is demonstrated. Rotate the leg laterally until the long axis of the foot is at a 45-degree angle with the IR.
148. The tibia superimposes the fibula by ½ inch. Angle the CR medially.
149. A. Fibula
    B. Tibiotalar joint
    C. Talar domes
    D. Calcaneus
    E. Talocalcaneal joint
    F. Cuboid
    G. Fifth metatarsal tuberosity
    H. Navicular bone
    I. Talus
    J. Tibia
150. A. Open
    B. Distal tibia
    C. Lower leg
    D. Tibiotalar joint
151. A. Parallel
    B. Lateral
152. Proximal
153. This question can be answered two different ways:
    A. Medial   A. Lateral
    B. Distal   B. Proximal
    C. Lateral   C. Medial
    D. Lower   D. Lower
154. A. Anterior
    B. Posterior
155. This question can be answered two different ways:
    A. Medial   A. Lateral
    B. Anterior   B. Posterior
    C. Lateral   C. Medial
    D. Posterior   D. Posterior
156. A. Perpendicular
    B. Medial malleolus
157. The talus, 1 inch (2.5 cm) of the fifth MT base, surrounding ankle soft tissue, and distal one-fourth of the fibula and tibia

541

Copyright © 2015, 2011, 2006, 1996 by Saunders, an imprint of Elsevier Inc. All rights reserved.

158. A fracture of the fifth MT base that results from inversion of the foot
159. So a Jones fracture can be ruled out
160. The distal lower leg was elevated.
161. The heel was depressed, and the forefoot was elevated.
162. The foot is plantarflexed. Dorsiflex the foot until the long axis of the foot forms a 90-degree angle with the lower leg.
163. The lateral talar dome is demonstrated distal to the medial dome, more than ½ inch (1.25 cm) of the cuboid is demonstrated posterior to the navicular, and the talocalcaneal joint is widened. Depress the distal lower leg until the lower leg is aligned parallel with the IR.
164. The lateral talar dome is proximal to the medial dome. Less than ¾ inch (2 cm) of the cuboid is demonstrated posterior to the navicular, and the talocalcaneal joint is narrowed. Elevate the distal lower leg until the lower leg is parallel with the IR.
165. The lateral talar dome is demonstrated anterior and proximal to the medial dome, and the fibula is too far anterior on the tibia. Move the calcaneus away from the IR (externally rotate leg) until the lateral surface of the foot is aligned parallel with the IR and depress the proximal tibia.
166. The lateral talar dome is posterior to the medial dome, and the fibula is posterior on the tibia. Adjust the CR anteriorly until it is aligned perpendicular to the lateral aspect of the foot or 10 degrees (the domes are physically approximately 1 inch (2.5 cm) apart and are off by ¼ inch (0.6 cm) on projection, with a needed 5-degree angulation adjustment for every ⅛ inch (0.3 cm) that the domes are off).
167. The lateral talar dome is proximal and anterior to the medial talar dome.
    Patient: Adjust the distal lower leg ⅛ inch (0.3 cm) toward the IR (need to move half the distance the talar domes are off) and externally rotate the ankle and leg ⅛ inch (0.3 cm) or until the lateral foot surface is parallel with the IR.
    CR: Adjust the CR distally and posteriorly 5 degrees for every ⅛ inch (0.3 cm) the domes are off anterior-posteriorly and proximal-distally, respectively (10 degrees proximally and anteriorly).
168. The foot is plantarflexed, the fibula is too posterior on the tibia, and the lateral talar dome is posterior to the medial talar dome. Dorsiflex the foot if the patient is able and angle the CR anteriorly.
169. A. Intercondylar fossa
    B. Lateral femoral condyle
    C. Fibular head
    D. Fibula
    E. Tibia
    F. Intercondylar eminence
    G. Medial femoral condyle

170. A. One-fourth
    B. Half
    C. Free
    D. Closed
    E. Tibial midshaft
171. Position the ankle toward the anode end of the tube and the knee toward the cathode end.
172. A. The fibula will be demonstrated with reduced or without tibial superimposition.
    B. The fibula will be demonstrated with reduced or without tibial and talar superimposition.
173. Place the knee in an AP projection and allow the ankle to be positioned as is.
174. A. Yes
    B. The proximal tibia slopes in the opposite direction as the diverged x-rays, and the distal tibia does not slope at the same degree as the diverged x-rays. If the x-ray divergence and joints are not parallel, the joints will be closed.
175. To ensure that the diverged beams used to record the ankle and knee will be included on the projection
176. A. Medial malleolus
    B. Distal
    C. Medial epicondyle
177. Tibial midshaft
178. The tibia, fibula, ankle and knee joints, and surrounding lower leg soft tissue
179. The leg was externally rotated.
180. The leg was internally rotated.
181. The distal lower leg has been clipped and the distal and proximal fibula are free of talar superimposition. Move the CR and IR 1 inch (2.5 cm) distally and laterally rotate the patient's leg until the femoral epicondyles are close to being positioned at equal distances from the IR.
182. A. Medial femoral condyle
    B. Fibula
    C. Talar domes
    D. Tibia
183. A. Half
    B. Posterior
    C. Midshaft
    D. Tibial midshaft
184. A. The tibia is partially superimposed over the fibular head.
    B. The tibia and fibula are free of superimposition.
    C. The distal fibula is superimposed by the posterior half of the distal tibia.
185. A. The fibula will be demonstrated with reduced or without tibial superimposition.
    B. The fibula will be demonstrated with reduced or without tibial superimposition.
186. At least 1 inch
187. Tibial midshaft
188. The tibia, fibula, ankle and knee joints, and surrounding lower leg soft tissue
189. The leg was rotated too far posteriorly.
190. The fibula is fully superimposed by the tibia. Rotate the leg externally.

542

Copyright © 2015, 2011, 2006, 1996 by Saunders, an imprint of Elsevier Inc. All rights reserved.

191. The fibular head is demonstrated without tibia superimposition, and the fibula is demonstrated too posterior on the tibia. Rotate the leg internally.
192. A. Patella
    B. Lateral epicondyle
    C. Lateral condyle
    D. Intercondylar eminence
    E. Fibular head
    F. Tibia
    G. Femorotibial joint
    H. Medial epicondyles
    I. Femur
193. A. Profile
    B. Half
    C. Tibial plateau
    D. Proximal
    E. Lateral
    F. Knee joint
194. 10
195. A. Extended
    B. Internally
    C. Equal distances (parallel)
196. The proximal tibia is superimposed over the proximal fibula.
197. Farther away
198. The medial condyle will appear larger than the lateral condyle, and the head, neck, and possibly the shaft of the fibula will be superimposed by the tibia.
199. Parallel with it
200. The tibial plateau slopes approximately 5 degrees anterior to posterior.
201. The thicker the upper thigh, the more the leg slopes down toward the IR, causing the tibial plateau to be at a different angle with the IR.
202. No
203. A. 5 degrees cephalic
    B. 5 degrees caudal
204. A. The fibular head will be foreshortened and demonstrated more than ½ inch (1.25 cm) distal to the tibial plateau.
    B. The fibular head will be elongated and demonstrated less than ½ inch (1.25 cm) distal to the tibial plateau.
205. A. Lateral compartment
    B. Medial compartment
206. Valgus
207. Decrease the angulation approximately 5 degrees to align it with the tibial plateau.
208. A. Distally
    B. Medially
    C. Laterally
209. A. 2
    B. 3
    C. 1
210. A. 1 (2.5 cm)
    B. Distal
    C. Medial epicondyle
211. One-fourth of the distal femur and proximal lower leg and surrounding knee soft tissue

212. The leg was externally (laterally) rotated.
213. The leg was internally (medially) rotated.
214. The CR was angled too cephalically.
215. The CR was angled too caudally.
216. The femorotibial joint space is obscured, the fibular head is more than ½ inch (1.25 cm) distal to the tibial plateau, and the fibular head is foreshortened. Adjust the CR angulation 5 degrees caudally.
217. The femorotibial joint space is obscured, the fibular head is less than ½ inch (1.25 cm) distal to the tibial plateau, and the fibular head is elongated. Adjust the CR angulation 5 degrees cephalically.
218. The medial femoral condyle appears larger than the lateral condyle, and the tibia superimposes more than half of the fibula head. Internally rotate the leg until the femoral epicondyles are at equal distances from the IR. The femorotibial joint space is obscured, and the fibular head is less than ½ inch (1.25 cm) distal to the tibial plateau. Adjust the CR angulation 5 degrees cephalically.
219. The lateral femoral condyle appears larger than the medial condyle, and the tibia superimposes less than half of the fibular head. Externally rotate the patient's leg until the femoral epicondyles are at equal distances from the IR.
220. Angle the CR until it is perpendicular to the anterior surface of the lower leg and then adjust the angle 5 degrees distally, aligning the CR with the tibial plateau.
221. The medial femoral condyle appears larger than the lateral condyle, and the tibia superimposes more than half of the fibular head. Angle the CR medially until it is perpendicular to a line connecting the femoral epicondyles.
222. The lateral femoral condyle appears larger than the medial condyle, the tibia superimposes less than half of the fibular head, the femorotibial joint space is obscured, and the fibular head is more than ½ inch (1.25 cm) distal to the tibial plateau. Angle the CR laterally until it is perpendicular with an imaginary line connecting the femoral epicondyles and rotate the imaging tube until the CR is aligned perpendicular to the anterior surface of the lower leg and then adjust the angle 5 degrees distally, aligning the CR with the tibial plateau.
223. A. Femur
    B. Patella
    C. Medial condyle
    D. Tibia
    E. Fibular head
    F. Tibiofibular joint
    G. Femorotibial joint
    H. Lateral condyle
224. A. Femur
    B. Medial condyle
    C. Tibia
    D. Fibula

543

Copyright © 2015, 2011, 2006, 1996 by Saunders, an imprint of Elsevier Inc. All rights reserved.

E. Femorotibial joint
F. Lateral condyle
G. Patella
225. A. Distal
B. Tibial plateau
C. Tibial
D. Anterior
E. Knee joint
226. 45
227. The femoral condyles will be nearly superimposed.
228. The fibular head will be aligned with the anterior edge of the tibia but will be positioned posterior to this placement.
229. A. Angle 5 degrees caudally
B. The hip is often elevated to accomplish the degree of needed internal obliquity.
C. The hip is placed closer to the imaging table to obtain the needed external obliquity.
230. A. Midline of the knee
B. Knee joint
231. One-fourth of the distal femur and proximal lower leg and surrounding knee soft tissue
232. The knee was rotated less than 45 degrees.
233. The knee was rotated more than 45 degrees.
234. The knee was rotated less than 45 degrees.
235. The CR was angled too cephalically.
236. The tibia is partially superimposed over the fibular head. Increase the degree of internal knee obliquity until an imaginary line connecting the femoral epicondyles is aligned at a 45-degree angle with the IR.
237. The fibular head, neck, and shaft are not entirely superimposed by the tibia. Increase the degree of external knee obliquity until an imaginary line connecting the femoral epicondyles is aligned at a 45-degree angle with the IR.
238. The fibular head is not aligned with the anterior edge of the tibia but is situated posterior to this placement. Decrease the degree of external knee rotation until the femoral epicondyles are aligned at a 45-degree angle with the IR.
239. A. Femur
B. Femoral condyles
C. Intercondylar eminence
D. Fibular head
E. Fibular neck
F. Tibia
G. Femorotibial joint
H. Patellofemoral joint
I. Patella
240. A. Suprapatellar
B. Proximal
C. Femoral condyles
D. Fibular head
E. Knee joint
241. When the knee is flexed more than 20 degrees, the muscles and tendons tighten, forcing the patella to come in contact with the patellar surface of the femur and obscuring the fat pads.

242. A. Parallel
B. Medially
C. 10 to 15
D. Wide
E. Short
243. A. Medial
B. Distal
C. Lateral
244. A. 5 to 7
B. Medial
C. Reduced
245. A. Locate the adductor tubercle on the posterior aspect of the medial condyle.
B. Locate the distal articulating surface that is the flattest. It is the lateral condyle.
246. When the leg is laterally abducted
247. A. The tibia will be partially superimposed over the fibular head.
B. The fibula will be demonstrated free of tibial superimposition.
248. Because it is situated farthest from the IR
249. The fibula will be demonstrated with decreased or without tibial superimposition.
250. The fibula will be demonstrated with increased or complete tibial superimposition.
251. A. 1 (2.5 cm)
B. Distal
C. Medial epicondyle
252. One-fourth of the distal femur and proximal lower leg and surrounding knee soft tissue
253. The knee was overflexed.
254. The CR was angled too caudally.
255. The CR was angled too cephalically.
256. The patella was situated too far away from the IR (leg internally rotated).
257. The patella was situated too close to the IR (leg externally rotated).
258. The knee is overflexed; the patella is in contact with the patellar surface of the femur. The marker is superimposed over the soft tissue structures. Decrease the degree of knee flexion to meet your facility's requirements. Move the marker off of the soft tissue structures.
259. The medial femoral condyle is anterior to the lateral condyle. Rotate the patella farther away from the IR (internal leg rotation).
260. The medial femoral condyle is posterior to the lateral condyle. Rotate the patella closer to the IR (external leg rotation).
261. The medial femoral condyle is proximal to the lateral condyle and the tibiofibular joint is visualized. Adjust the CR angle 5 to 7 degrees caudally.
262. The knee is overflexed; the patella demonstrates a fracture. If a patellar or other knee fracture is suspected, the knee should remain extended to prevent displacement of bony fragments or vascular injury.
263. The medial femoral condyle is anterior to the lateral condyle. Rotate the knee internally until the femoral epicondyles are parallel with the imaging table

Study Question Answers Copyright © 2015, 2011, 2006, 1996 by Saunders, an imprint of Elsevier Inc. All rights reserved.

or the cart on which the patient is lying or adjust the CR anteriorly until it is aligned parallel with the femoral epicondyles.

264. The medial femoral condyle is distal to the lateral condyle. Adduct the patient's leg until the epicondyles are perpendicular to the IR or rotate the x-ray tube toward the patient's feet, adjusting the CR caudally (moves the lateral condyle toward the medial condyle).

265. The lateral femoral condyle is proximal and posterior to the medial condyle. Rotate the imaging tube to direct CR distally and angle the CR anteriorly.

266. A. Lateral fossa surfaces
    B. Lateral epicondyle
    C. Lateral condyle
    D. Tibial condylar margin
    E. Fibular head
    F. Intercondylar eminence
    G. Femorotibial joint
    H. Medial condyle
    I. Medial epicondyle
    J. Medial fossa surfaces
    K. Intercondylar fossa
    L. Proximal fossa surfaces

267. A. Half
    B. Profile
    C. Proximal
    D. Open
    E. Distal
    F. Intercondylar fossa

268. A. Allow the femur to incline medially approximately 10 to 15 degrees.
    B. Position the long axis of the foot perpendicular to the imaging table.

269. A. The patella rotates laterally.
    B. The patella rotates medially.

270. A. 20 to 30
    B. 60 to 70

271. Distally

272. A. The posterior tibial margin is distal to the anterior tibial margin.
    B. Dorsiflex the foot until its long axis is aligned perpendicular to the imaging table.
    C. Femorotibial
    D. Intercondylar eminence
    E. Tubercles

273. A. Perpendicular
    B. 1
    C. Medial femoral epicondyle

274. The distal femur, proximal tibia and intercondylar fossa, eminence, and tubercles

275. The femur was too vertical, or the heel was rotated medially.

276. The heel was laterally rotated.

277. The knee was overflexed; the femur was too close to vertical.

278. The knee was underflexed; the femur was more than 20 to 30 degrees from vertical.

279. The foot was in plantarflexion.

280. The proximal surface of the intercondylar fossa is demonstrated without superimposition, and the patellar apex is positioned at the intercondylar fossa. Unflex the knee, positioning the proximal femur closer to the imaging table. The femorotibial joint is closed, and the fibular head is slightly more than ½ inch (1.25 cm) from the tibial plateau. Increase the degree of foot dorsiflexion, elevating the distal lower leg.

281. The femorotibial joint is obscured, the tibial plateau is demonstrated, and the fibular head is less than ½ inch (1.25 cm) from the tibial plateau. Plantarflex the foot, lowering the distal lower leg.

282. The medial and the lateral aspects of the intercondylar fossa are not superimposed, the patella is situated medially, and the tibia is demonstrated without fibular head superimposition. The knee joint is obscured, the tibial plateau is demonstrated, and the fibula is positioned closer than ½ inch (1.25 cm) closer to the tibial plateau. Rotate the heel medially until the foot's long axis is aligned perpendicular to the imaging table and depress the distal lower leg by decreasing the amount of foot dorsiflexion.

283. A. Medial epicondyle
    B. Proximal intercondylar fossa surfaces
    C. Intercondylar fossa
    D. Medial intercondylar fossa surfaces
    E. Medial femoral condyle
    F. Femorotibial joint space
    G. Intercondylar eminence
    H. Fibular head
    I. Lateral condyle
    J. Lateral intercondylar fossa surfaces
    K. Lateral epicondyle

284. A. Femoral epicondyles
    B. Fibular head
    C. Proximal
    D. ½ inch
    E. Intercondylar fossa

285. Internally rotated to AP projection, with femoral epicondyles parallel with the imaging table

286. A. CR aligned parallel with tibial plateau
    B. Femur position at a 60-degree angle with the imaging table

287. A. CR
    B. Tibial plateau

288. A. Perpendicular
    B. Decreasing
    C. Medial femoral condyle

289. Distal femur, proximal tibia, and intercondylar fossa, eminences, and tubercles

290. The patient's leg was internally rotated.

291. The patient's leg was externally rotated.

292. The femur was angled more than 60 degrees with the imaging table.

293. The femur was angled less than 60 degrees with the imaging table.

294. The distal lower leg was depressed, or the CR was angled too caudally.

545

Copyright © 2015, 2011, 2006, 1996 by Saunders, an imprint of Elsevier Inc. All rights reserved.

295. The distal lower leg was elevated too high, or the CR was angled too cephalically.
296. The medial and the lateral aspects of the intercondylar fossa are not superimposed, the medial femoral condyle is wider than the lateral condyle, and the fibular head demonstrates increased tibial superimposition. Internally rotate the leg until an imaginary line connecting the femoral epicondyles is aligned parallel with the imaging table.
297. The proximal surfaces of the intercondylar fossa are not superimposed, and the patellar apex is demonstrated within the intercondylar fossa. Decrease the degree of hip and knee flexion until the long axis of the femur is aligned 60 degrees with the imaging table. The femorotibial joint is closed, and the fibular head is demonstrated less than ½ inch (1.25 cm) distal to the tibial plateau. Elevate the distal lower leg until the knee is flexed 45 degrees or adjust the CR cephalically.
298. A. Patella
    B. Patellofemoral joint
    C. Anterolateral femoral condyle
    D. Intercondylar sulcus
    E. Anteromedial femoral condyle
299. A. Lateral
    B. Medial
    C. Open
    D. Patellofemoral joint space
300. Because a long OID is used
301. Internally rotate the legs and secure them by wrapping the Velcro straps of the axial viewer around the patient's calves.
302. A. They will be situated laterally.
    B. The condyles will demonstrate equal heights, or the medial condyle will demonstrate more height than the lateral condyle.
303. A. Patellar subluxation
    B. The patella will be demonstrated laterally.
    C. The intercondylar sulci will remain facing superiorly on a subluxed patella but not on a rotated one.
304. Because tightening of the quadriceps muscles will prevent patella subluxation from being demonstrated
305. Parallel with the imaging table.
306. Directly above the bend of the axial viewer until the knees are flexed 45 degrees
307. A. Decrease the angulation set on the axial viewer, or increase the CR angulation 5 to 10 degrees.
    B. The tibial tuberosities will be demonstrated within the patellofemoral joint spaces.
308. 60 degrees caudally
309. 105 degrees
310. To offset the magnification caused by the large OID
311. The patellae, anterior femoral condyles, and intercondylar sulci
312. The legs were externally rotated.
313. The height of the axial viewer was not set high enough to position the long axes of the femurs parallel with the imaging table.

314. The posterior knee curve was positioned at or below the bend of the axial viewer.
315. The posterior knee curve was positioned too far above the bend of the axial viewer.
316. The patellae are demonstrated directly above the intercondylar sulci and rotated laterally, and the heights of the lateral and medial condyles are nearly equal. Internally rotate the legs until the patellae are situated superiorly and restrain the legs with the Velcro straps of the axial viewer.
317. The patellae are resting against the intercondylar sulci, obscuring the patellofemoral joint spaces. Slide the knees away from the axial viewer until the posterior knee curvatures are positioned just superior to the bend of the axial viewer.
318. The tibial tuberosities are demonstrated within the patellofemoral joint spaces. Slide the knees toward the axial viewer until the posterior knee curvatures are just superior to the bend of the axial viewer.
319. The patellae, anterior femoral condyles, and intercondylar sulci are demonstrated superiorly; the lateral femoral condyle demonstrates more height than the medial condyle; the patellofemoral joint space is open; and the patellae are laterally located. Positioning is accurate; the patient's patellae are subluxed.
320. A. Femoral shaft
    B. Lateral epicondyle
    C. Lateral condyle
    D. Femorotibial joint
    E. Fibular head
    F. Medial condyle
    G. Medial epicondyle
321. A. Pelvic brim
    B. Obturator foramen
    C. Lesser trochanter
    D. Femoral shaft
    E. Greater trochanter
    F. Femoral neck
    G. Femoral head
    H. Acetabulum
322. A. Profile
    B. Fibular head
    C. Distal femoral shaft
323. A. Pelvic brim
    B. Greater
    C. Lesser
    D. Proximal femoral shaft
324. Position the knee toward the anode end of the tube and the hip toward the cathode end.
325. It can be used to detect subcutaneous air or hematomas.
326. A. Supine
    B. Extended
    C. Internally
327. A. No
    B. Forced internal rotation of a fractured femur may cause injury to the blood supply and nerves that surround the injured area.

546

Copyright © 2015, 2011, 2006, 1996 by Saunders, an imprint of Elsevier Inc. All rights reserved.

328. A. 2
    B. Knee
329. The distal femoral shaft, surrounding femoral soft tissue, femorotibial joint, and 1 inch (2.5 cm) of the lower leg
330. Position the ASISs at equal distances from the imaging table.
331. A. Parallel with the imaging table
    B. It will demonstrate the femoral neck without foreshortening and the greater trochanter in profile.
332. A. Proximal femoral shaft
    B. Affected ASIS
333. The proximal femoral shaft, hip joint, and surrounding femoral soft tissue
334. The leg was externally rotated.
335. The pelvis was rotated toward the affected femur.
336. The patient was rotated away from the affected femur.
337. The patient's leg was externally rotated.
338. The femoral epicondyles are not in profile, the medial condyle appears larger than the lateral condyle, and the tibia superimposes more than half of the fibular head. Internally rotate the leg until the femoral epicondyles are at equal distances from the IR.
339. The femoral neck is partially foreshortened, and the lesser trochanter is demonstrated in profile medially. Internally rotate the leg until the femoral epicondyles are positioned at equal distances from the imaging table.
340. A. Femoral shaft
    B. Fibula
    C. Tibia
    D. Medial femoral condyle
    E. Patella
    F. Lateral femoral condyle
341. A. Femoral head
    B. Femoral neck
    C. Femoral shaft
    D. Lesser trochanter
    E. Greater trochanter
342. A. Femoral shaft
    B. Femoral neck
    C. Femoral head
    D. Lesser trochanter
    E. Greater trochanter
343. A. Lateral
    B. Medial
    C. Distal femoral shaft
344. A. Medially
    B. Greater trochanter
    C. Greater
    D. Proximal femoral shaft
345. A. Lateral
    B. Perpendicular

346. The femur should not be moved or the patient rotated. The projection is obtained using a cross-table (horizontal) beam.
347. A. 2
    B. Knee joint
348. The distal femoral shaft, surrounding femoral soft tissue, femorotibial joint, and 1 inch (2.5 cm) of the lower leg
349. The pelvis is rotated until the femoral epicondyles are aligned perpendicular to the imaging table.
350. Lateral surface of femur is placed next to the imaging table.
351. Axiolateral projection
352. A. Proximal femoral shaft
    B. ASIS
353. The proximal femoral shaft, hip joint, and surrounding femoral soft tissue
354. The patella was positioned too far away from the IR.
355. The pelvis is overrotated, and the femoral epicondyles are not aligned perpendicular to the imaging table; the medial epicondyle is anterior to the lateral epicondyle.
356. The pelvis is underrotated, and the femoral epicondyles are not aligned perpendicular to the imaging table; the medial epicondyle is posterior to the lateral epicondyle.
357. The medial femoral condyle is anterior to the lateral epicondyle. Internally rotate the leg (moving the patella away from the IR).
358. The medial femoral condyle is anterior to the lateral epicondyle. Internally rotate the femur until the femoral epicondyles are aligned perpendicular to the IR or angle the CR anteriorly until it is aligned parallel with the femoral epicondyles.
359. The greater trochanter is positioned laterally, the femoral neck is demonstrated with only partial foreshortening, and the femoral shaft is foreshortened. Rotate the pelvis, increase the degree of external leg rotation, and abduct the leg as needed to place the femur against the imaging table, with the femoral epicondyles aligned perpendicular to the IR.
360. The soft tissue from the unaffected thigh is superimposed over the acetabulum and femoral head of the affected femur. Flex and abduct the unaffected leg, drawing it away from the affected acetabulum and femoral head.
361. The greater trochanter is demonstrated posteriorly, and the lesser trochanter is superimposed over the femoral shaft. A proximal femoral shaft fracture is present. The patient's affected leg was in external rotation. Do not attempt to adjust the patient's leg position if a fracture of the proximal femur is suspected. No corrective movement is needed.

Copyright © 2015, 2011, 2006, 1996 by Saunders, an imprint of Elsevier Inc. All rights reserved.

1.

Hip and Pelvis Technical Data					
Projection	kV	Grid	AEC	mAs	SID
AP, pelvis	80–85	Grid	Both outside		40–48 inches (100–120 cm)
AP frogleg, pelvis	80–85	Grid	Both outside		40–48 inches (100–120 cm)
AP, hip	80–85	Grid	Center		40–48 inches (100–120 cm)
AP frogleg, hip	80–85	Grid	Center		40–48 inches (100–120 cm)
Axiolateral (inferosuperior), hip	80–85	Grid		60	40–48 inches (100–120 cm)
AP axial, sacroiliac joints	80–85	Grid	Center		40–48 inches (100–120 cm)
AP oblique, sacroiliac joints	80–85	Grid	Center		40–48 inches (100–120 cm)
Pediatric	65–75	Grid		3–5	40–48 inches (100–120 cm)

2. A. The obturator internus fat plane lies within the pelvic inlet next to the pelvic brim.
   B. The iliopsoas fat plane lies medial to the lesser trochanter.
   C. The pericapsular fat plane is found superior to the femoral neck.
   D. The gluteal fat plane lies superior to the pericapsular fat plane.
   E. They will aid in the detection of intraarticular and periarticular disease.
3. A. Iliac crest
   B. Iliac ala
   C. ASIS
   D. Acetabulum
   E. Femoral head
   F. Femoral neck
   G. Greater trochanter
   H. Lesser trochanter
   I. Ischial tuberosity
   J. Obturator foramen
   K. Inferior ramus of ischium
   L. Symphysis pubis
   M. Superior ramus of pubis
   N. Coccyx
   O. Superior ramus of ischium
   P. Pelvic brim
   Q. Ischial spine
   R. Sacrum

7. Make sure that the ASISs are positioned at equal distances from the IR.
8. The sacrum and coccyx would not be aligned with the symphysis pubis but would be rotated toward the left hip; the right iliac is wider than the left, and the right obturator foramen is narrower than the left.
9. A. The patient's legs were internally rotated with the feet at 15 to 20 degrees from vertical and the femoral epicondyles placed parallel with the imaging table.
   B. The patient's legs were externally rotated with the feet at a 45-degree angle from vertical and the femoral epicondyles positioned at a 60- to 65-degree angle with the imaging table.
   C. The patient's legs were externally rotated with the feet vertical and the femoral epicondyles at a 15- to 20-degree angle with the imaging table.
10. The feet are tilted internally 15 to 20 degrees from vertical, and the line connecting the femoral epicondyles is aligned parallel with the imaging table.
11. A. Perpendicular
    B. Symphysis pubis
    C. ASISs
12. The ilia, pubis, ischia, acetabula, femoral necks and heads, and greater and lesser trochanters
13. The pelvis was rotated onto the right side (RPO).

4.

Sternum and Ribs Technical Data					
Projection	kV	Grid	AEC	mAs	SID
PA oblique (RAO position), sternum	70-80	Grid	Center		30-40 inches (75-100 cm)
Lateral, sternum	75-80	Grid		50	72 inches (180 cm)
AP or PA, above diaphragm	75-85	Grid	Center		40-48 inches (100-120 cm)
AP or PA, below diaphragm	80-90	Grid	Center		40-48 inches (100-120 cm)
PA oblique, above diaphragm	75-85	Grid	Center		40-48 inches (100-120 cm)
PA oblique, below diaphragm	80-90	Grid	Center		40-48 inches (100-120 cm)

5. A. Pelvic brim
   B. Greater
   C. Lesser
6. A. Female
   B. Male

14. The legs were externally rotated, with the feet and an imaginary line connecting the femoral epicondyles positioned at a 45-degree angle with the table.
15. The femoral necks are completely foreshortened, and the lesser trochanters are demonstrated in profile. The legs were externally rotated, with the feet

                                   Copyright © 2015, 2011, 2006, 1996 by Saunders, an imprint of Elsevier Inc. All rights reserved.

at a 45-degree angle and the femoral epicondyles positioned at a 60- to 65-degree angle with the imaging table. Internally rotate the legs until the feet are angled 15 to 20 degrees from vertical and the femoral epicondyles are positioned parallel with the imaging table.

16. The left obturator foramen is narrower than the right foramen, the left iliac wing is wider than the right, and the sacrum and coccyx are rotated toward the right hip. Rotate the patient toward the right hip until the ASISs are positioned at equal distances from the IR.

17. The femoral necks are foreshortened, and the lesser trochanters are demonstrated in profile. The right obturator foramen is narrower, the right iliac wing is wider than the left, and the sacrum and coccyx is rotated toward the left hip. Internally rotate the legs until the femoral epicondyles are positioned parallel with the imaging table and rotate the patient toward the left hip until the ASISs are positioned at equal distances from the IR.

18. A. Ischial spine
    B. Pelvic brim
    C. Coccyx
    D. Symphysis pubis
    E. Ischial tuberosity
    F. Obturator foramen
    G. Lesser trochanter
    H. Greater trochanter
    I. Femoral neck
    J. Femoral head
    K. Sacrum
    L. Acetabulum
    M. Iliac ala
    N. ASIS
    O. Iliac crest

19. A. Iliac wings
    B. Medially
    C. Femoral necks
    D. Proximal greater trochanters

20. Proximal femurs

21. 60 to 70 degrees

22. The greater trochanters will be demonstrated lateral to the proximal femur.

23. A. The amount of femoral neck foreshortening
    B. The transverse level at which the greater trochanters will be demonstrated between the femoral heads and lesser trochanters

24. A. The femoral necks would be demonstrated on end, and the greater trochanters would be demonstrated at the same transverse level as the femoral heads.
    B. The femoral necks would be partially foreshortened, and the greater trochanters would be positioned at a transverse level halfway between the femoral heads and lesser trochanters.
    C. The femoral necks would be demonstrated without foreshortening, and the greater trochanters would be positioned at the same transverse level as the lesser trochanters.

25. A. Perpendicular
    B. Midsagittal
    C. 1 inch (2.5 cm)
    D. Symphysis pubis

26. The ilia, pubis, ischia, acetabula, femoral necks and heads, and greater and lesser trochanters

27. The left side of the patient's pelvis was rotated closer to the IR than the right (LPO).

28. The patient's femurs were abducted beyond 45 degrees.

29. The femoral necks are demonstrated "on end." The greater trochanters are demonstrated on the same transverse level as the femoral heads. Consult with reviewers in your facility to determine whether this is an acceptable image. Because the femoral necks cannot be evaluated because of foreshortening, it may be necessary to have the patient position the femurs at a 45-degree angle with the imaging table. The iliac crest has been clipped. The CR and IR were positioned too inferiorly.

30. The femoral necks are demonstrated "on end." The greater trochanters are demonstrated on the same transverse level as the femoral heads. Consult with reviewers in your facility to determine whether this is an acceptable image. Because the femoral necks cannot be evaluated because of foreshortening, it may be necessary to have the patient position the femurs at a 45-degree angle with the imaging table.

31. The greater trochanters are partially demonstrated laterally. Increase the degree of knee and hip flexion until the femurs are placed at a 60- to 70-degree angle with the imaging table.

32. The sacrum is rotated toward the right hip, the patient's hands are demonstrated within the exposure field, the right femur is abducted more than the left, and the inferior sacrum is not in the center of the projection. Rotate the patient toward the right hip, move the patient's hands away from the collimated field, and abduct both femurs equally and accurately center the CR.

33. A. ASIS
    B. Iliac wing (ala)
    C. Acetabulum
    D. Femoral head
    E. Femoral neck
    F. Greater trochanter
    G. Lesser trochanter
    H. Ischial tuberosity
    I. Inferior ramus of pubis
    J. Symphysis pubis
    K. Obturator foramen
    L. Superior ramus of pubis
    M. Pelvis brim
    N. Coccyx
    O. Ischial spine
    P. Sacrum

34. A. Pelvic brim
    B. Symphysis pubis
    C. Laterally
    D. Femoral neck

549

Copyright © 2015, 2011, 2006, 1996 by Saunders, an imprint of Elsevier Inc. All rights reserved.

35. Make sure that the ASISs are at equal distances from the imaging table.
36. A. The sacrum would not be aligned with the symphysis pubis but would be rotated toward the affected hip.
    B. The iliac spine would be closer to the acetabulum than the pelvic brim.
37. It will be narrower.
38. A. The femoral neck will be demonstrated on end, and the lesser trochanter will be demonstrated in profile medially.
    B. The lesser trochanter is in partial profile medially, and the femoral neck is only partially foreshortened.
    C. The femoral neck is demonstrated without foreshortening, the greater trochanter is demonstrated in profile laterally, and the lesser trochanter is obscured.
39. The foot should be tilted internally 15 to 20 degrees from vertical, and an imaginary line connecting the epicondyles should be positioned parallel with the imaging table.
40. A. No
    B. Forced internal rotation of a fractured or dislocated hip may result in injury to the blood supply and nerves that surround the injured area.
41. A. Perpendicular
    B. Distal
    C. Symphysis pubis
42. The acetabulum; greater and lesser trochanters; femoral head and neck; and half of the sacrum, coccyx, and symphysis pubis
43. A larger IR and lower CR centering may be required.
44. A. Yes, no anatomic structures will be covered.
    B. Yes but use a shield that is small enough and is shaped for the female pelvis to avoid covering any pelvic structures.
45. The patient was rotated toward the affected hip.
46. The patient was rotated away from the affected hip.
47. The patient's leg was in external rotation, with the foot and femoral epicondyles positioned at a 45-degree angle with the imaging table.
48. The ischial spine is demonstrated without pelvic brim superimposition, the sacrum and coccyx are not aligned with the symphysis pubis but are rotated away from the affected hip, and the obturator foramen is narrowed. Rotate the patient away from the affected hip. The lesser trochanter is demonstrated in profile. Internally rotate the leg until the femoral epicondyles are aligned parallel with the imaging table.
49. The ischial spine is not aligned with the pelvic brim but is demonstrated closer to the acetabulum, the sacrum and coccyx are not aligned with the symphysis pubis but are rotated toward the affected hip, and the iliac wing is narrowed. Rotate the patient toward the affected hip. The lesser trochanter is demonstrated in profile. Internally rotate the leg until the femoral epicondyles are aligned parallel with the imaging table.

50. The femoral neck is partially foreshortened, and the lesser trochanter is demonstrated in profile. The leg was externally rotated, bringing the foot vertical and the femoral epicondyles positioned at approximately a 15- to 20-degree angle with the imaging table. Internally rotate the leg until the foot is angled 15 to 20 degrees from vertical and the femoral epicondyles are positioned parallel with the imaging table.
51. The lesser trochanter is in profile, and there is a proximal femur fracture. The leg should not be internally rotated when a femoral or hip fracture is suspected. Adequate positioning is demonstrated.
52. A. Iliac (ala) wing
    B. Acetabulum
    C. Femoral head
    D. Femoral neck
    E. Greater trochanter
    F. Femoral shaft
    G. Lesser trochanter
    H. Ischial tuberosity
    I. Obturator foramen
    J. Superior ramus
    K. Inferior ramus
    L. Symphysis pubis
    M. Coccyx
    N. Pelvic brim
    O. Ischial spine
    P. Sacrum
53. A. Ischial spine
    B. Lesser trochanter
    C. Femoral neck
    D. Femoral neck
    E. Greater trochanter
54. A. Toward
    B. Against the imaging table
55. Profile
56. 60 to 70 degrees
57. A. The amount of femoral neck foreshortening
    B. The transverse level at which the greater trochanter will be demonstrated between the femoral head and lesser trochanter
58. A. Demonstrates the femoral neck on end and the greater trochanter at the same transverse level as the femoral head
    B. Demonstrates the femoral neck with only partial foreshortening and positions the greater trochanter at a transverse level halfway between the femoral neck and lesser trochanter
    C. Demonstrates the femoral neck without foreshortening and the greater trochanter at the same transverse level as the lesser trochanter
59. A. Perpendicular
    B. 2½ (6.25 cm)
    C. ASIS
60. The acetabulum; greater and lesser trochanters; femoral head and neck; and half of the sacrum, coccyx, and symphysis pubis
61. The patient was rotated toward the affected hip.

Copyright © 2015, 2011, 2006, 1996 by Saunders, an imprint of Elsevier Inc. All rights reserved.

62. The patient's knee was flexed more than needed, placing the femur at an angle greater than 60 to 70 degrees with the imaging table.
63. The patient's knee was not flexed enough to align the femur at a 60- to 70-degree angle with the imaging table, or the affected leg's foot and ankle were resting on top of the unaffected leg, elevating it off the imaging table.
64. The patient's femur was abducted until it was positioned next to the imaging table.
65. The ischial spine is demonstrated without pelvic brim superimposition, the sacrum and coccyx are rotated toward the right hip, and the left obturator foramen is narrowed. Rotate the patient away from the affected hip until the ASISs are at equal distances from the imaging table.
66. The ischial spine is not aligned with the pelvic brim but is demonstrated closer to the acetabulum; the sacrum and coccyx are not aligned with the symphysis pubis but are rotated toward the affected hip; and the iliac ala is narrowed and the obturator foramen widened. Rotate the patient toward the affected hip.
67. The femoral neck is foreshortened, and the greater trochanter is demonstrated at the same transverse level as the femoral head. Adduct the patient's femur until it is aligned at a 45-degree angle with the imaging table.
68. The greater trochanter is positioned laterally. The patient's knee was not flexed enough to align the femur at a 60- to 70-degree angle with the imaging table (20 to 30 degrees from vertical). Increase the knee flexion until the femur is aligned at a 60- to 70-degree angle with the imaging table.
69. The greater trochanter is positioned medially. Decrease knee flexion until the femur is at a 60- to 70-degree angle with the imaging table (20 to 30 degrees from vertical).
70. A. Acetabulum
    B. Femoral head
    C. Femoral neck
    D. Greater trochanter
    E. Lesser trochanter
    F. Femoral shaft
    G. Ischial tuberosity
71. A. Lesser and greater trochanters
    B. Posteriorly
    C. Femoral shaft
72. A. Use tight collimation.
    B. Place a flat lead contact strip over the top of the unused half of the IR.
    C. Use a grid.
73. Place the unaffected leg in maximum flexion and abduction.
74. A. Against the patient's affected side at the level of the iliac crest
    B. Parallel
    C. It should be positioned superior to the iliac crest.
    D. Perpendicular to both

75. Find the center of an imaginary line drawn between the symphysis pubis and the ASIS. Bisect that line and draw a perpendicular line distally. This imaginary line parallels the long axis of the femoral neck.
76. A. The femoral neck will be foreshortened.
    B. The greater trochanter will be demonstrated proximal or distal to the lesser trochanter depending on the angle.
77. Internally rotate the leg until an imaginary line connecting the femoral epicondyles is positioned parallel with the imaging table.
78. Femoral neck
79. The acetabulum, femoral head and neck, greater and lesser trochanters, and ischial tuberosity
80. The unaffected leg was not adequately flexed and abducted.
81. The angle of the CR to the femur was too great.
82. The patient's leg was in external rotation.
83. Soft tissue from the unaffected thigh is superimposed over the acetabulum and femoral head of the affected hip. Flex and abduct the unaffected leg, drawing it away from the affected acetabulum and femoral head. If the patient is unable to further adjust the unaffected leg, the kVp and mAs can be increased to demonstrate this area.
84. The greater trochanter is demonstrated at a transverse level proximal to the lesser trochanter, and the femoral neck is partially foreshortened. Localize the femoral neck. Position the IR parallel with the femoral neck and the CR perpendicular to the IR and femoral neck.
85. The greater trochanter is demonstrated posteriorly, the lesser trochanter is superimposed over the femoral shaft, the greater trochanter is demonstrated at a transverse level that is proximal to the lesser trochanter, and the femoral neck is foreshortened. Internally rotate the leg and decrease the angle of the CR to the femur.
86. A fracture of the femoral neck is present. The greater trochanter is demonstrated posteriorly, and the lesser trochanter is superimposed over the femoral shaft. Do not attempt to adjust the position if a fracture of the proximal femur is suspected. No corrective movement is needed.
87. A. Median sacral crest
    B. Symphysis pubis
    C. Pelvic brim
    D. Second sacral segment
    E. Ilium
    F. Sacroiliac joint
    G. Sacral ala
88. A. Symphysis pubis
    B. Symphysis pubis
89. A. Opposite
    B. Farther
90. A. 30 degrees cephalic
    B. 35 degrees cephalic
    C. Increase the angle over the routine amount used until the CR and sacroiliac joints are aligned.
    D. Decrease the angle over the routine amount used until the CR and sacroiliac joints are aligned.

551

Copyright © 2015, 2011, 2006, 1996 by Saunders, an imprint of Elsevier Inc. All rights reserved.

91. A. To obtain tight collimation
    B. To ensure that the CR is accurately aligned with the sacroiliac joints
92. A. Midsagittal
    B. ASISs
    C. Symphysis pubis
93. The sacroiliac joints and first through fourth sacral segments
94. The right side of the patient's pelvis was situated farther away from the IR than the left side (LPO).
95. The CR was inadequately angled.
96. The sacroiliac joints are foreshortened, and the inferior sacrum is demonstrated without symphysis pubis superimposition. Increase the degree of cephalic CR angulation.
97. The CR is centered to the L5-S1 joint disk space, causing less diverged beams to record the sacroiliac joints than required to demonstrate them without foreshortening. Move the CR inferiorly, centering to the second sacral segment (1.5 inches superior to the symphysis pubis).
98. The sacroiliac joints and sacrum are elongated, and the symphysis pubis is superimposed over the inferior aspects of the sacrum and sacroiliac joints. Angle the CR 30 to 35 degrees cephalad.

99. A. Ilium
    B. Iliac tuberosity
    C. Inferior sacral ala
    D. Sacrum
    E. Superior sacral ala
    F. Sacroiliac joint
100. A. Sacrum
     B. Longitudinal axis
101. A. Ilium
     B. Sacrum
102. A. Midcoronal
     B. 25 to 30
103. Right
104. A. Medial
     B. ASIS
105. The sacroiliac joint, sacral ala, and ilium
106. The patient was underrotated.
107. The patient was overrotated.
108. The sacroiliac joint is closed. The superior and inferior sacral alae are demonstrated without iliac superimposition, and the lateral sacral ala is superimposed over the iliac tuberosity. Increase the pelvic obliquity.
109. The sacroiliac joint is closed, and the ileum is superimposed over the lateral sacral ala and the inferior sacrum. Decrease the degree of pelvic obliquity.

CHAPTER 8 IMAGE ANALYSIS OF THE CERVICAL AND THORACIC VERTEBRAE

1.

Cervical and Thoracic Vertebrae Technical Data					
Projection	kV	Grid	AEC	mAs	SID
AP axial, cervical vertebrae	75–85	Grid	Center		40–48 inches (100–120 cm)
AP, open-mouth, C1 and C2	75–85	Grid		5	40–48 inches (100–120 cm)
Lateral, cervical vertebrae	75–85	Grid*	Center		72 inches (150–180 cm)
PA or AP axial oblique, cervical vertebrae	75–85	Grid*	Center		72 inches (150–180 cm)
Lateral (Twining method), cervicothoracic vertebrae	80–95	Grid	Center		40–48 inches (100–120 cm)
AP, thoracic vertebrae	80–90	Grid	Center		40–48 inches (100–120 cm)
Lateral, thoracic vertebrae	80–90	Grid	Center		40–48 inches (100–120 cm)
Pediatric	65–75	Grid**		2–3	40–48 inches (100–120 cm)

2. A. Articular pillar
   B. Pedicle
   C. Sixth to seventh intervertebral disk space
   D. Fourth spinous process
   E. Fifth vertebral body
   F. Seventh uncinate process
   G. Air-filled trachea
3. A. Spinous processes
   B. Lateral
   C. Inferior
   D. Superimposed
4. A. Position the mastoid tips and mandibular angles at equal distances from the imaging table.
   B. Position the shoulders at equal distances from the imaging table.

5. A. Closer to
   B. Farther from
6. A. No
   B. The upper and lower cervical vertebrae can move independently of each other.
7. A. No
   B. No
   C. Spinal cord injury may be caused by moving the patient when a fracture is suspected.
8. Lordotic
9. A. Upwardly, anteriorly to posteriorly
   B. Higher when upright
   C. 15 degrees cephalad
   D. 20 degrees cephalad
   E. The gravitational pull on the vertebrae that results when the patient is supine

Study Question Answers   Copyright © 2015, 2011, 2006, 1996 by Saunders, an imprint of Elsevier Inc. All rights reserved.

10. A. Closed
    B. Its vertebral body
11. Within the inferior adjoining vertebral body
12. Too much
13. Align the lower surface of the upper incisors and the tip of the mastoid process perpendicular to the IR.
14. A. Midsagittal
    B. External auditory meatus (EAM)
    C. Jugular notch
15. The second through seventh cervical vertebrae, first thoracic vertebra, and surrounding soft tissue
16. The head was turned, and the torso was rotated toward the right side.
17. The CR was not angled cephalically enough.
18. The CR was angled too cephalically.
19. The chin was not adequately tucked. Position the lower surface of the upper incisors and the mastoid tip.
20. The chin was overtucked. Position the lower surface of the upper incisors with the mastoid tip.
21. The head and upper cervical vertebrae's midsagittal plane was not aligned with the lower cervical vertebrae.
22. The spinous processes are not aligned with the midline of the cervical bodies but are closer to the right side, and the medial end of the right clavicle is superimposed over the vertebral column and the anteroinferior aspects of the cervical bodies are obscuring the intervertebral disk spaces, and each vertebra's spinous process is demonstrated within its vertebral body. Rotate the patient toward the right side until the shoulders are at equal distances from the IR and increase the amount of cephalic CR angulation.
23. The spinous processes are closer to the left side, the medial end of the left clavicle superimposes the vertebral column, and the patient's face is turned toward the right side. Rotate the body and face toward the left side until the shoulders are at equal distances from the IR and the face is looking forward.
24. The anteroinferior aspects of the cervical bodies are obscuring the intervertebral disk spaces, and each vertebra's spinous process is demonstrated within its vertebral body. Increase the amount of cephalic CR angulation.
25. The anteroinferior aspects of the cervical bodies are obscuring the intervertebral disk spaces, and each vertebra's spinous process is demonstrated within its vertebral body. The head and upper cervical vertebrae are tilting toward the right side. Increase the amount of cephalic CR angulation and align the midsagittal planes of the head and cervical vertebrae.
26. The posteroinferior aspects of the cervical bodies are obscuring the intervertebral disk spaces, the uncinate processes are elongated, and each vertebra's spinous process is demonstrated within the inferior adjoining vertebral body. Decrease the amount of cephalic CR angulation.
27. A portion of the third cervical vertebra is superimposed over the occiput, preventing clear visualization of the third cervical vertebra. Tuck the chin half the distance demonstrated between the base of the skull and the mandibular mentum or until an imaginary line connecting the upper occlusal plane and the base of the skull is aligned perpendicular to the imaging table or upright grid holder.
28. The mandible is superimposed over a portion of the third cervical vertebra, the anteroinferior aspects of the cervical bodies are obscuring the intervertebral disk spaces, and each vertebra's spinous process is demonstrated within its vertebra body. Raise the chin half the distance demonstrated between the occipital base and the mandibular mentum or until the lower surface of the upper incisors and the tip of the mastoid process is aligned perpendicular to the IR, and increase the degree of cephalic CR angulation.
29. A. Upper incisors
    B. Occiput
    C. Dens
    D. C1 lateral mass
    E. Transverse process
    F. Atlantoaxial joint
    G. Mandibular ramus
    H. C2 spinous process
    I. C2 body
    J. Occipitoatlantal joint
30. A. Axis
    B. Dens
    C. Axis's
    D. Lateral masses
    E. Superior
    F. Open
31. Position the patient's shoulders, mandibular angles, and mastoid tips at equal distances from the imaging table.
32. A. Posteriorly
    B. Anteriorly
33. A. Tuck the patient's chin until the lower surface of the upper incisors and mastoid tip are aligned perpendicular to the IR and have the patient open the mouth.
    B. Imagine where the teeth would be if the patient had them and position the patient in the same manner.
34. To offset the magnification of the upper incisors that is caused by the long OID.
35. Angle the CR until it is aligned parallel with the IOML.
36. A. The atlantoaxial joint will be closed, and the axis's spinous process will demonstrate an increased superior location to the dens.
    B. The atlantoaxial joint will be closed, and the axis's spinous process will demonstrate an increased inferior location to the dens.
37. Midsagittal plane
38. The atlantoaxial and occipitoatlantal joints, atlas's lateral masses and transverse processes, and axis's dens and body
39. The patient's face was rotated toward the left side.
40. The CR was not angled 5 degrees cephalad.
41. A. The chin was tucked more than needed.
    B. The CR was angled too caudally.

553

Copyright © 2015, 2011, 2006, 1996 by Saunders, an imprint of Elsevier Inc. All rights reserved.

42. A. The patient's chin was not tucked enough to position the acanthiomeatal line perpendicular to the imaging table.
    B. The CR was angled too cephalically.
43. The distances from the atlas's lateral masses to the dens and from the mandibular rami to the dens are narrower on the left side than on the right side, and the dens is superimposed over the occiput. Rotate the face toward the left side until the mandibular angles and mastoid tips are positioned at equal distances from the imaging table or upright grid holder and tuck the chin toward the chest until the lower edge of the upper incisors and the mastoid tip are aligned perpendicular to the IR.
44. The dens is superimposed over the occiput. The upper incisors are demonstrated directly superior to the dens. Tuck the chin toward the chest until the lower edge of the upper incisors and the mastoid tip are aligned perpendicular to the IR. A 5-degree cephalad angulation should be used.
45. The upper incisors are demonstrated inferior to the occipital base, superimposing the dens and atlanto-axial articulation. The occipital base is demonstrated directly superior to the dens. If the lower edge of the upper incisors and the occipital base were aligned perpendicular to the IR and a perpendicular CR was used for this projection, do not adjust patient positioning; simply direct the CR 5 degrees cephalad. If a 5-degree cephalad angulation was used for this projection, do not adjust patient positioning; simply increase the cephalad angulation by 5 degrees.
46. The atlantoaxial joint space is closed, and the axis's spinous process is demonstrated too inferior to the dens. The neck was in extension. Place a small sponge under the head to reduce neck extension and then realign the lower edge of the upper incisors and the occipital base.
47. The upper incisors are demonstrated superior to the dens and the occipital base, and the dens is superimposed over the occiput. Adjust the CR angulation caudally until it is aligned parallel with the IOML.
48. A. Sella turcica
    B. Clivus
    C. Occiput
    D. Inferior cranial cortices
    E. Posterior arch
    F. Dens
    G. Third spinous process
    H. Fifth through sixth zygapophyseal joints
    I. Articular pillars
    J. Sixth lamina
    K. First thoracic vertebra
    L. Seventh cervical vertebra
    M. Intervertebral disk space
    N. Mandibular rami
49. A. Prevertebral
    B. Superimposed
    C. Profile
    D. Posterior occiput

E. Superimposed
F. Zygapophyseal joints
50. Using a long SID will decrease the cervical magnification that results from the long OID that is created between the cervical vertebrae and IR.
51. Midcoronal
52. Align the shoulders, mastoid tips, and mandibular rami.
53. The articular right or left pillars and zygapophyseal joints will be demonstrated one anterior to the other.
54. Position the AML parallel with the floor and align the IPL perpendicular to the IR.
55. Position the AML parallel with the floor and align the IPL perpendicular to the IR.
56. A. Places the cervical vertebrae in a neutral position
    B. Allows for tight transverse collimation
57. To demonstrate AP vertebral mobility
58. Instruct the patient to tuck the chin against the chest as tightly as possible.
59. Instruct the patient to extend the chin up and backward as far as possible.
60. A. Midcoronal
    B. EAM
    C. Jugular notch
61. The sella turcica, clivus, first through seventh cervical vertebrae, superior half of the first thoracic vertebra, and surrounding soft tissue
62. The clivus with the dens can be used to evaluate cervical injury.
63. A. Take the projection with the patient in an upright position.
    B. Have the patient hold weights on each arm to depress the shoulders.
    C. Take the exposure on suspended expiration.
64. Lateral cervicothoracic (Twining method)
65. The cervical vertebrae were rotated.
66. The head was rotated.
67. The head and upper cervical vertebrae were tilted toward the IR.
68. The articular pillars and zygapophyseal joints on one side of the patient are situated anterior to those on the other side. Rotate the patient until the midcoronal plane is aligned perpendicular to the IR.
69. Neither the inferior nor the posterior cortices of the cranium nor the mandible is superimposed, the posterior arch of C1 is demonstrated in profile, and the right and left articular pillars and zygapophyseal joints demonstrate a superoinferior separation. Rotate the head until the midsagittal plane is aligned parallel with the IR and then tilt the head toward the IR until the interpupillary line is perpendicular to the IR.
70. The vertebral body of C7 is not demonstrated in its entirety, and the superior body of T1 is not demonstrated. Have the patient hold 5- to 10-lb weights on each arm to depress the shoulders. If the patient cannot hold weights or if the weights do not sufficiently drop the shoulders, a special projection known as the cervicothoracic lateral (Twining method) should be taken to demonstrate this area.

Copyright © 2015, 2011, 2006, 1996 by Saunders, an imprint of Elsevier Inc. All rights reserved.

71. The posterior cortices of the mandible are not super-imposed, causing C1 and C2 to superimpose the left mandibular ramus, the left articular pillars and zygapophyseal joints demonstrate a superoinferior separation, and the long axis of the cervical vertebral column is not aligned with the long axis of the exposure field. Rotate the face away from the IR until the midsagittal plane is parallel with the IR, tilt the head toward the IR until the interpupillary line is perpendicular to the IR, and elevate the chin until the eyes are facing forward and the long axis of the neck is aligned with the long axis of the collimated field.

72. A. Inferior mandibular cortices
    B. Pedicle
    C. Sixth vertebral body
    D. Intervertebral foramen
    E. Intervertebral disk space
    F. Pedicle
    G. Fourth uncinate process
    H. Posterior arch
    I. Inferior cranial cortices

73. A. Seventh
    B. Profile
    C. Anterior
    D. Vertebral foramen

74. To offset the magnification that would result because of the long OID used for the examination

75. When a long OID is used, causing scatter radiation to be diverged away from the IR and decreasing the amount of scatter radiation that reaches the IR

76. A. Right
    B. Right
    C. Left
    D. Left

77. 45 degrees

78. Midcoronal

79. A. Align the left mastoid tip with the longitudinal axis of the IR and the right gonion with the transverse axis of the IR.
    B. Direct it 45 degrees medially and 15 degrees cephalically. Center it to the right side of the patient's neck halfway between the AP surfaces of the neck at the level of the thyroid cartilage.

80. A. 15 to 20 degrees caudally
    B. 15 to 20 degrees cephalically
    C. To open the intervertebral disk spaces and demonstrate undistorted vertebral bodies

81. Turn the face away from the side of interest and until the head's midsagittal plane is aligned parallel with the IR.

82. Increase the degree of CR angulation.

83. A. Left
    B. Left
    C. The angulation of the CR projects the mandible situated farther from the IR inferiorly on PA oblique projections and superiorly on AP oblique projections.

84. A. Midsagittal plane
    B. EAM
    C. Jugular notch

85. The first through seventh cervical vertebrae, first thoracic vertebra, and surrounding soft tissue

86. The patient was rotated less than 45 degrees.

87. The patient was rotated more than 45 degrees.

88. The CR was not angled enough caudally.

89. The head was not turned to a lateral position.

90. The head and upper cervical vertebrae were tilted away from the IR.

91. This patient was in a right PA axial oblique projection (RAO), with the head in an oblique position. The right pedicles and intervertebral foramina are obscured. Increase patient obliquity until the midcoronal plane is placed at a 45-degree angle with the IR.

92. This patient was in a left PA axial oblique projection (LAO), with the head in a lateral position. The intervertebral foramina are demonstrated, the left pedicles are visible (although they are not in true profile), the right pedicles are demonstrated in the midline of the vertebral bodies, and the left zygapophyseal joints are demonstrated. Decrease patient rotation until the midcoronal plane is placed at a 45-degree angle with the IR.

93. This patient was in a right PA axial oblique projection (RAO), with the head in a lateral position. The atlas and its posterior arch are obscured. The inferior cranial cortices demonstrate more than ¼ inch (0.6 cm) between them, and the inferior cortices of the mandibular rami demonstrate more than ½ inch (1.25 cm) between them. The first thoracic vertebra is not included in its entirety. Tilt the patient's head toward the IR until the interpupillary line is aligned perpendicular to the IR and move the CR and IR inferiorly.

94. This patient was in a right PA axial oblique projection (RAO), with the head in a lateral position. The intervertebral disk spaces are closed, the cervical bodies are distorted, the posterior tubercles are demonstrated within the intervertebral foramina, the C1 vertebral foramen is not demonstrated, and the inferior mandibular rami and the cranial cortices are demonstrated with superimposition. The CR was directed perpendicular to the IR. Angle the CR 15 to 20 degrees caudally for anterior oblique images.

95. This patient was in a right PA axial oblique projection (RAO), with the head in a lateral position. The intervertebral foramina are demonstrated, the left pedicles are shown although they are not in true profile, the right pedicles are demonstrated in the midline of the vertebral bodies, and the left zygapophyseal joints are demonstrated. Decrease the degree of patient rotation to 45 degrees with the IR.

96. A. Humeral head
    B. Zygapophyseal joints
    C. C7 spinous process
    D. Intervertebral foramen
    E. Humeral head
    F. Clavicle
    G. T1 vertebra
    H. C7 vertebral body
    I. Intervertebral disk space

555

Copyright © 2015, 2011, 2006, 1996 by Saunders, an imprint of Elsevier Inc. All rights reserved.

J. Pedicles
K. Articular pillars
97. A. Articular pillars
    B. Vertebral column
    C. Open
98. A. When the routine lateral cervical projection does not demonstrate the seventh cervical vertebra
    B. When the routine lateral thoracic projection does not demonstrate the first through third thoracic vertebrae
99. Expiration
100. A. The arm is elevated above the patient's head as high as possible.
    B. The arm is against the patient's side and should be depressed.
101. A. Position the patient's head in a lateral position.
    B. Position the shoulders, posterior ribs, and ASISs on top of each other, aligning the midcoronal plane perpendicular to the IR.
102. The right and left articular pillars, posterior ribs, and zygapophyseal joints will be demonstrated without superimposition.
103. Place the head in a lateral projection with the IPL perpendicular to and midsagittal plane parallel with the IR.
104. A. Midcoronal
    B. Jugular notch
    C. Vertebral prominens
105. When the patient is unable to depress the shoulder positioned farther from the IR
106. The fifth through seventh cervical vertebrae and first through fourth thoracic vertebrae
107. The shoulder that was depressed and positioned farther from the IR was rotated anteriorly.
118. The shoulder that was depressed and positioned farther from the IR was rotated posteriorly.
109. The vertebral column was not positioned parallel with the IR.
110. The intervertebral disk spaces are closed, and the vertebral bodies are distorted. The cervical vertebral column was not positioned parallel with the IR. Position the midsagittal plane parallel with the IR. It may be necessary to prop the head on a sponge to help the patient maintain the position.
111. The right and left articular pillars, zygapophyseal joints, and posterior ribs are demonstrated without superimposition. The patient's thorax was rotated. The humerus that was raised and situated closer to the IR is demonstrated anterior to the vertebral column. Rotate the shoulder positioned farther from the IR anteriorly until your flat palms placed against the shoulders and the posterior ribs, respectively, are aligned perpendicular to the IR.
112. A. Medial clavicular end
    B. Spinous process
    C. Posterior rib
    D. Pedicle
    E. Vertebral body
    F. Intervertebral disk space

113. A. Vertebral bodies
    B. Spinous processes
    C. Open
114. To an 8-inch field size
115. Position the patient's head and upper thoracic vertebrae at the anode end of the tube and the lower thoracic vertebrae at the cathode end of the tube.
116. Suspended expiration
117. Position the shoulders, posterior ribs and ASISs at equal distances from the IR, aligning the midcoronal plane parallel with the IR.
118. Closer to
119. A. Scoliosis
    B. Whereas a rotated lateral thoracic projection will demonstrate rotation of the thoracolumbar vertebrae and either the upper thoracic or lower lumbar vertebrae, scoliosis will demonstrate rotation of the thoracolumbar vertebrae without corresponding rotation of the upper thoracic or lower lumbar vertebrae.
120. A. Kyphotic
    B. Position the patient's head on a thin pillow and bend his or her knees, placing the feet flat against the imaging table.
121. A. Midsagittal
    B. Jugular notch
122. The seventh cervical vertebra, first through 12th thoracic vertebrae, first lumbar vertebra, and 2½ inches (6.25 cm) of the posterior ribs and mediastinum on each side of the vertebral column
123. The legs were extended.
124. The left side of the patient was positioned closer to the IR than was the right side (LPO).
125. The patient's head was positioned at the cathode end of the tube.
126. The upper thoracic vertebrae demonstrate uneven distance from the left pedicle to the spinous process than from the right pedicle to the spinous process, and the left medial clavicle is demonstrated away from the vertebral column. Discern whether the patient has scoliosis. If not, rotate the patient toward the right side until the shoulders are at equal distances from the imaging table.
127. The eighth through 12th intervertebral disk spaces are obscured, and the vertebral bodies distorted. Flex the patient's hips and knees, placing the feet and back firmly against the imaging table.
128. A. First thoracic vertebra
    B. Posterior ribs
    C. Pedicles
    D. Intervertebral foramen
    E. Intervertebral disk space
129. A. Profile
    B. Superimposed
    C. ½
    D. Open
130. It will blur the ribs and lung markings.
131. Suspended expiration

 Copyright © 2015, 2011, 2006, 1996 by Saunders, an imprint of Elsevier Inc. All rights reserved.

Let's Practice Key Words

Directions: Fill in each blank with a Key A (main idea) word or a Key B (detail) word.

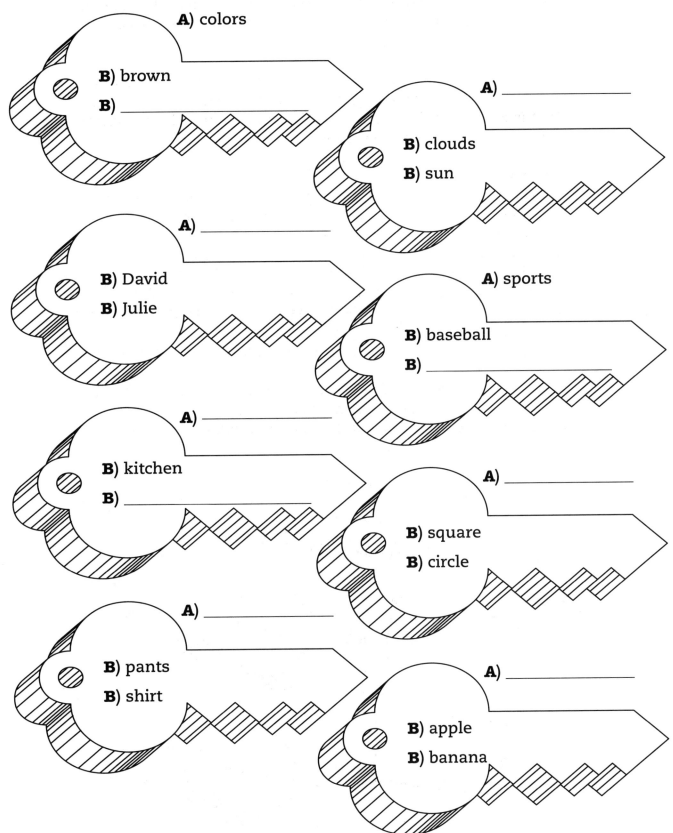

A) colors

B) brown

B) _____

A) _____

B) clouds

B) sun

A) _____

B) David

B) Julie

A) sports

B) baseball

B) _____

A) _____

B) kitchen

B) _____

A) _____

B) square

B) circle

A) _____

B) pants

B) shirt

A) _____

B) apple

B) banana

Key Paragraphs © 2002 Creative Teaching Press

Let's Practice More Key Words

Directions: Fill in each blank with a Key A (main idea) word or a Key B (detail) word.

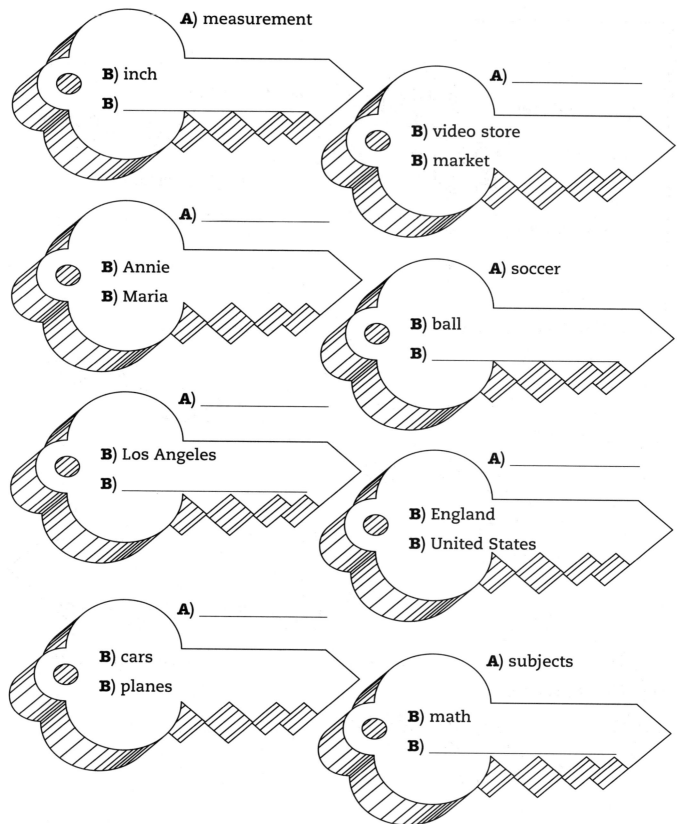

A) measurement

B) inch

B) _____

A) _____

B) video store

B) market

A) _____

B) Annie

B) Maria

A) soccer

B) ball

B) _____

A) _____

B) Los Angeles

B) _____

A) _____

B) England

B) United States

A) _____

B) cars

B) planes

A) subjects

B) math

B) _____

Key Paragraphs © 2002 Creative Teaching Press

Unlock the Door Practice

Directions: Fill in each blank with a Key B (detail) word from the door.

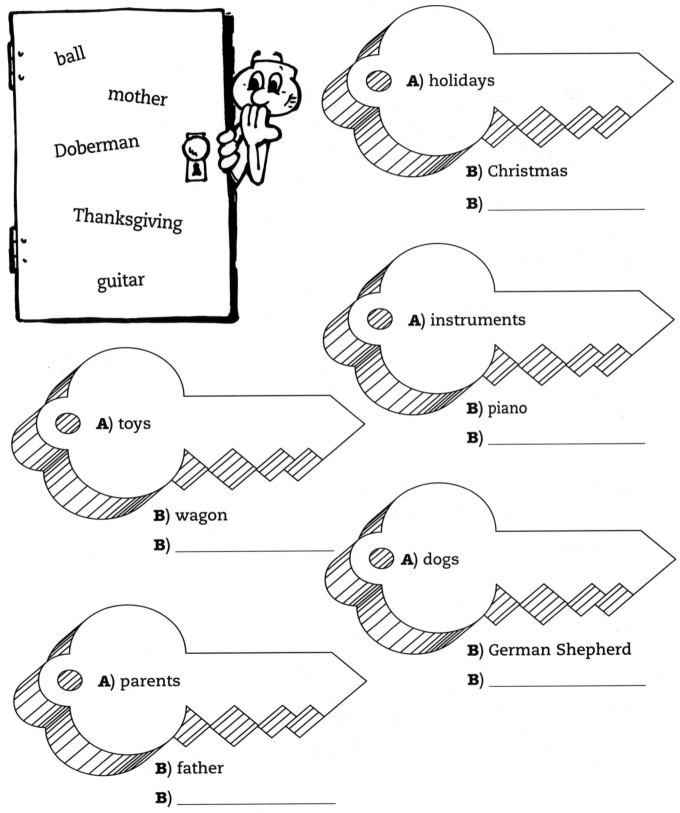

ball

mother

Doberman

Thanksgiving

guitar

A) holidays

B) Christmas

B) _____

A) instruments

B) piano

B) _____

A) toys

B) wagon

B) _____

A) dogs

B) German Shepherd

B) _____

A) parents

B) father

B) _____

Key Paragraphs © 2002 Creative Teaching Press

More Unlock the Door Practice

Directions: Fill in each blank with a Key B (detail) word from the door.

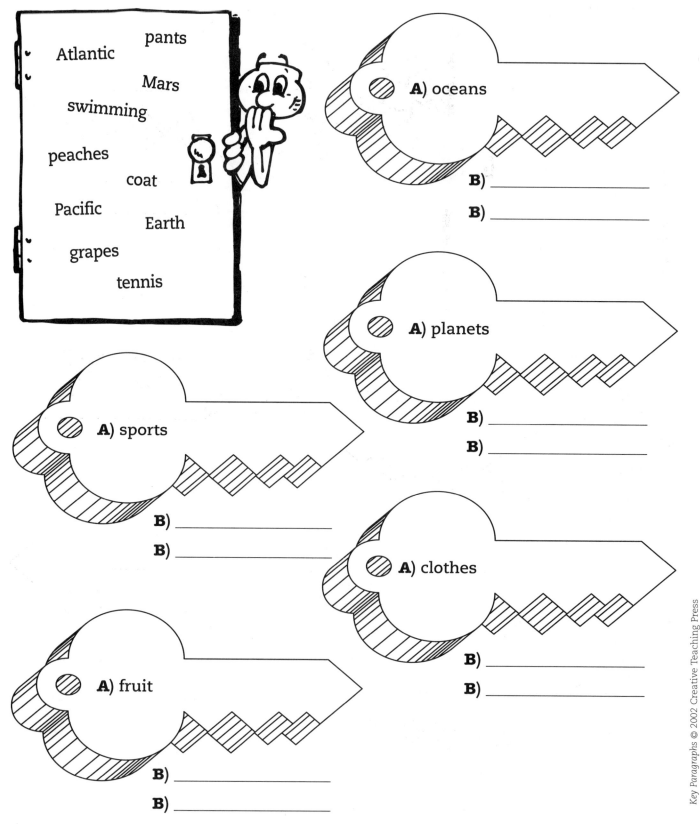

pants
Atlantic
Mars
swimming
peaches
coat
Pacific
Earth
grapes
tennis

A) oceans

B) _____

B) _____

A) planets

B) _____

B) _____

A) sports

B) _____

B) _____

A) clothes

B) _____

B) _____

A) fruit

B) _____

B) _____

Key Paragraphs © 2002 Creative Teaching Press

Unlock the Door

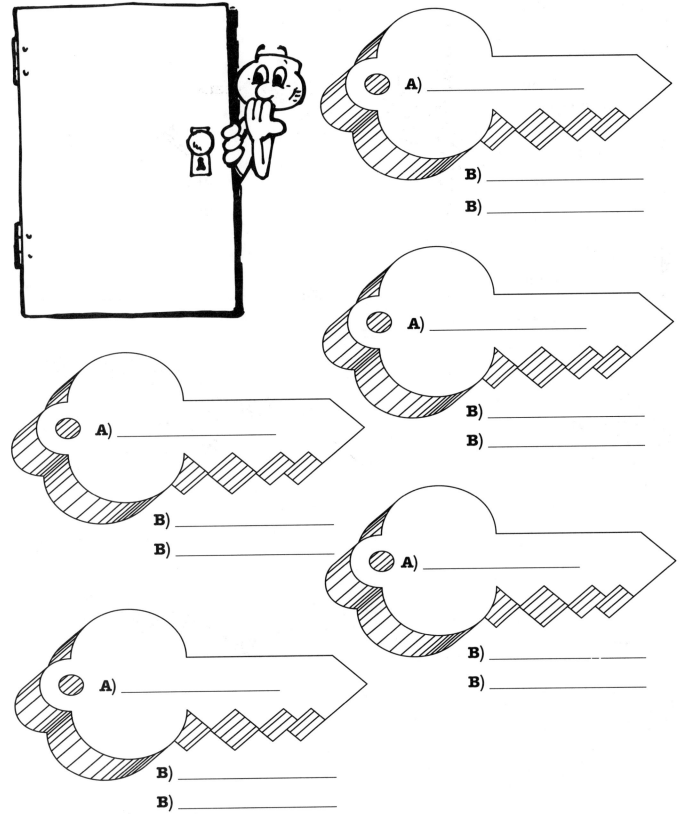

Key Paragraphs © 2002 Creative Teaching Press

Extending Key Words to Key Phrases

Introduce key phrases to help students transition from key words to key sentences. A key phrase is merely a simple extension from one word to a few words. The additional word(s) can be an adjective, a prepositional phrase, or any words that further describe the key word. The goal is to have students think "bigger." Explain to students that key phrases are extensions of key words and that a key phrase is not a sentence. Give students opportunities to practice the A B B method with phrases. Students do not need to spend a great deal of time on the key phrase stage. However, this stage is a necessity because it is a bridge between writing key words and key sentences.

Key word = lion

Key phrase = lion and tigers
or ferocious lion

Have students complete the following activities for key phrase practice:

◉ Have each student complete the Let's Practice Key Phrases reproducibles (pages 19 and 20). Explain to students that the Key A phrases on the reproducibles are indented as a reminder that each time they write a new paragraph they will need to indent.

◉ Find a paragraph from a published source, or write your own. Ask students to color-code the sentences. Have them use a red crayon or marker to underline the main idea sentence (Key A) and a blue crayon or marker to underline the details (Key B). Ask them to use a pencil to circle the key phrase in each sentence.

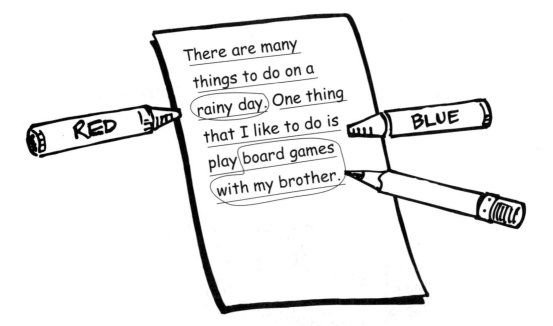

Let's Practice Key Phrases

Directions: Fill in each blank with a Key A (main idea) phrase or Key B (detail) phrase.

A) my favorite foods

B) cheese pizza

B) _____

A) yummy desserts

B) _____

B) chocolate chip cookies

A) toy balls

B) yellow tetherball

B) _____

A) _____

B) shiny penny

B) silver dime

A) bikes to ride

B) two-wheeler

B) _____

A) _____

B) handball with friends

B) jump rope

A) different shapes

B) big triangle

B) _____

A) nice house pets

B) _____

B) green turtle

Key Paragraphs © 2002 Creative Teaching Press

Let's Practice More Key Phrases

Directions: Fill in each blank with a Key A (main idea) phrase or Key B (detail) phrase.

A) _____

B) my friend, David

B) my cousin, Jerry

A) stores in my community

B) Von's Supermarket

B) _____

A) things that go fast

B) sports cars

B) _____

A) items found in school

B) lined paper

B) _____

A) my favorite foods

B) spaghetti with sauce

B) _____

A) _____

B) math book

B) language book

A) _____

B) tetherball

B) hopscotch

A) _____

B) animals with fur

B) animals with feathers

Key Paragraphs © 2002 Creative Teaching Press

Transitioning to Key Sentences and Paragraphs

When students fully understand the concept of key phrases, it is time to have them create A B B paragraphs. First, ask students to complete an Unlock the Door reproducible (page 17). Then, have them turn each Key A word into a main idea sentence and write each sentence on a separate piece of paper. (Remind them to indent.) Ask students to use the Key B words from their reproducible to write detail sentences for each main idea sentence. Have students complete the Key Sentences reproducibles (pages 23 and 24) for more sentence-writing practice.

There are many kinds of cars. One kind of car is Ford. Another kind of car is Honda.

There are many kinds of drinks. One kind is soda.

Repetitive Pattern

The easiest way to introduce students to the A B B concept is to use the repetitive pattern. In this pattern, the Key A sentence states that two ideas (Key B sentences) will be presented (e.g., *I like school for* **two reasons** or *I have* **two favorite** *books*). Have students complete the Key Sentences Practice reproducible (page 23) to give them practice creating A B B paragraphs using the repetitive pattern.

I like school for two reasons. One reason that I like school is that I want to learn many things. Another reason is that I like helping my teacher.

A
B

B

Using the Word "Many"

When you feel the class is ready to move on from the repetitive pattern, have students complete the "Many" Key Sentences Practice reproducible (page 24). The sentences on this reproducible reinforce the use of "many" in the Key A (main idea) sentence. The word "many" is considered to be the "magic" word for a Key A sentence because it so easily reinforces the bigger, main idea concept.

At home, I help in many ways. **A**
One way I help in my house **B**
is by cleaning my room.
Another way I help is by **B**
helping my mom sweep
the kitchen.

Checklist

Give each student a Key Paragraph Checklist (page 25). Ask students to use the checklist as a reminder of things to do each time they write a key paragraph.

Checking Work

After students have completed the Key Sentences reproducibles (pages 23 and 24), divide the class in pairs. Ask partners to exchange papers. Have each student check his or her partner's work. Ask students to label each sentence with an A or B. This activity provides students with additional practice identifying A B B sentences and saves you time from grading papers.

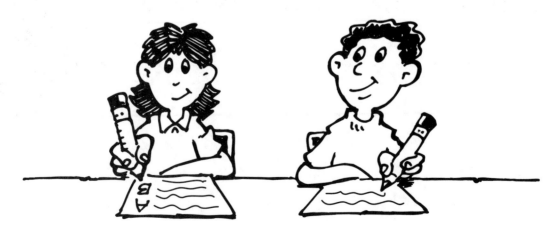

Key Sentences Practice

Directions: Complete an A B B paragraph for each sentence. Copy a Key A sentence on a separate piece of paper. Then, add two Key B sentences to form an A B B paragraph. Remember to indent when you begin your paragraph.

1. I like school for two reasons.

2. I enjoy holidays for two reasons.

3. There are two kinds of pies that I love.

4. I do two things every morning.

5. There are two fruits I like to eat.

6. Last weekend, I did two things that made me happy.

7. I like my friend for two reasons.

8. I have two favorite books.

9. At Thanksgiving, I am grateful for two things.

10. There are two special people in my life.

Key Paragraphs © 2002 Creative Teaching Press

"Many" Key Sentences Practice

Directions: Complete an A B B paragraph for each sentence. Copy a Key A sentence on a separate piece of paper. Then, add two Key B sentences to form an A B B paragraph. Remember to indent when you begin your paragraph.

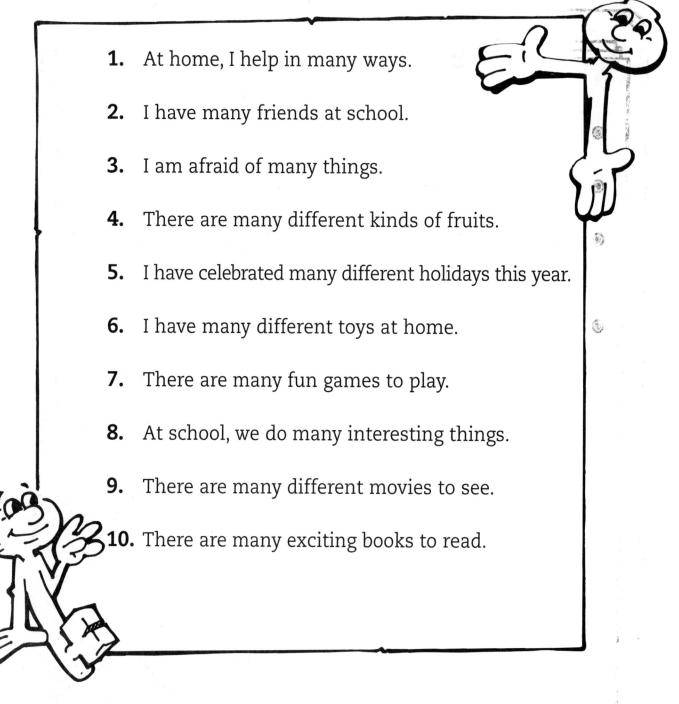

1. At home, I help in many ways.

2. I have many friends at school.

3. I am afraid of many things.

4. There are many different kinds of fruits.

5. I have celebrated many different holidays this year.

6. I have many different toys at home.

7. There are many fun games to play.

8. At school, we do many interesting things.

9. There are many different movies to see.

10. There are many exciting books to read.

Key Paragraphs © 2002 Creative Teaching Press

Key Paragraph Checklist

⊙ _____ I copied the Key A sentence correctly.

⊙ _____ I added two complete Key B sentences.

⊙ _____ I used capital letters and punctuation marks where needed.

⊙ _____ I indented when I began my paragraph.

⊙ _____ I reread my Key A B B paragraph and made any necessary changes.

Key Paragraphs © 2002 Creative Teaching Press

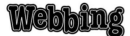

Webbing

Webbing (a form of a graphic organizer) is a method of prewriting that enables the writer to map out all his or her thoughts on a subject and then choose which ones to use. These are the main benefits of webbing:

◉ helps writing seem more like taking a picture, which is less intimidating

◉ helps students generate ideas and relate to something and write about it

◉ creates motivation and imaginative thinking

◉ frees the thoughts, allowing for the opportunity to focus on sentence and paragraph structure

◉ can be used with nonwriters by employing pictures and symbols for a feeling of success

◉ allows students to be uninhibited in expressing their thoughts and ideas

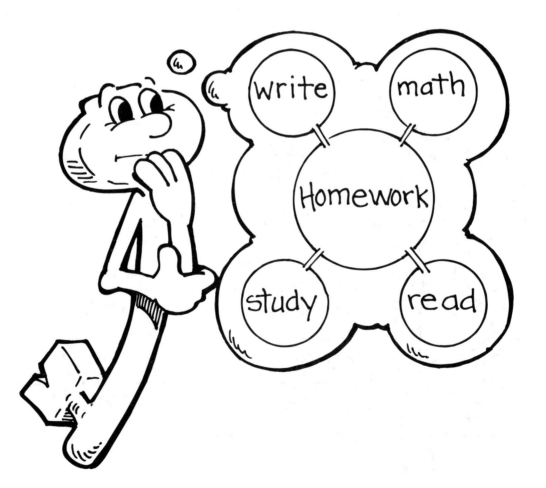

Planning a Key Paragraph Using a Web

Use this easy, one-step web to introduce the use of webs as a method of planning. Make a transparency of the Web reproducible (page 28), or draw it on the chalkboard. Explain that the center of the circle always stands for the main idea (Key A) and the circles branching out represent the details (Key B). Use the following directions to model and explain the steps for completing the reproducible:

1. Have the class choose a subject, and write it in the main circle of the web. Remind them that this is the main idea (Key A) of the paragraph.
2. Brainstorm with the class words or phrases that relate to the main idea. Write them in the other circles of the web, and explain that these ideas are details (Key B).
3. Discuss how to turn the Key A word or phrase into a sentence. Encourage students to use the word *many* in their Key A sentence to reinforce the bigger concept of a main idea.
4. Write a sample Key A sentence on the transparency or board. Choose two Key B words or phrases, and use them to develop sentences that support Key A.
5. Give each student a Web reproducible, and invite students to use it to generate their own ideas and paragraphs.

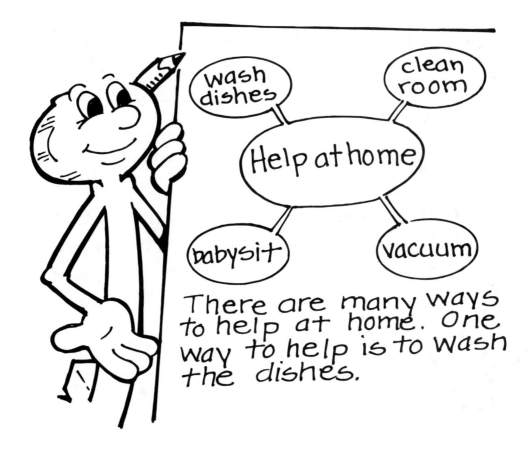

Name _____   Date _____

Web

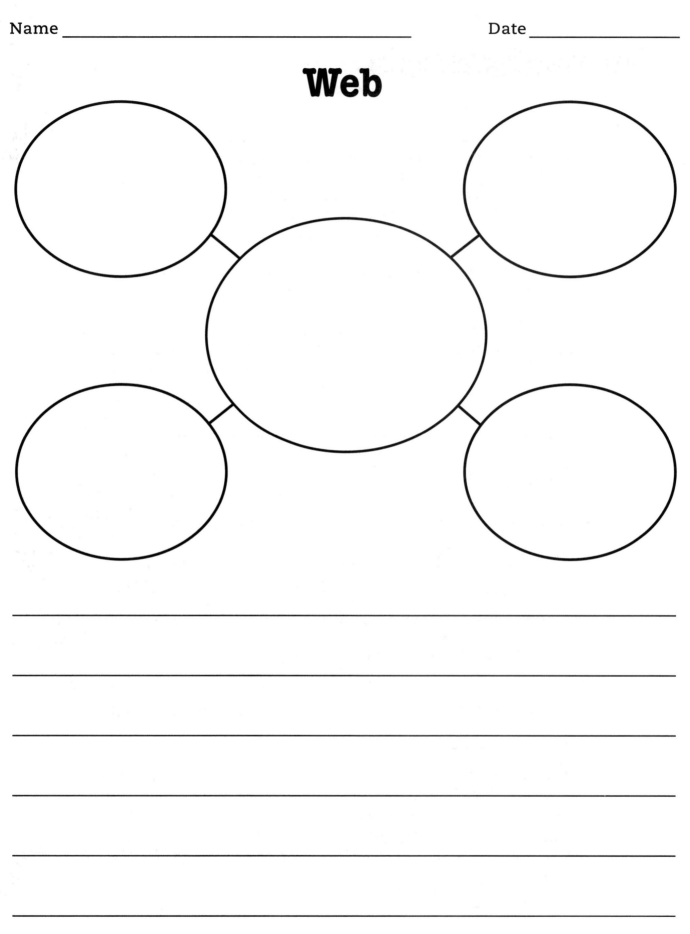

_____

_____

_____

_____

_____

Key Paragraphs © 2002 Creative Teaching Press

Complex Paragraphs

When students have mastered the concept of the A B B format, they are extremely motivated and ready to make their paragraphs grow into bigger and better ones! After much practice and reinforcement with journal writing (see pages 67–70), students can add "C" to their paragraphs. Tell students that they can add a Key C sentence (another detail that tells more about the Key B sentence) to the A B B format to create an A B C B C paragraph.

Brainstorm a list of Key A words, and write them on the chalkboard. Model how to create a complex paragraph. Choose a word from the list (e.g., recess), and write a topic sentence using that word (e.g., *There are many things to do during recess*). Then, write a B sentence that provides details about the A sentence (e.g., *One of my favorite games is handball*). Ask students to brainstorm C sentences to tell more about the B sentence. Write one of their responses (e.g., *I am usually a winner when I play handball*) on the chalkboard.

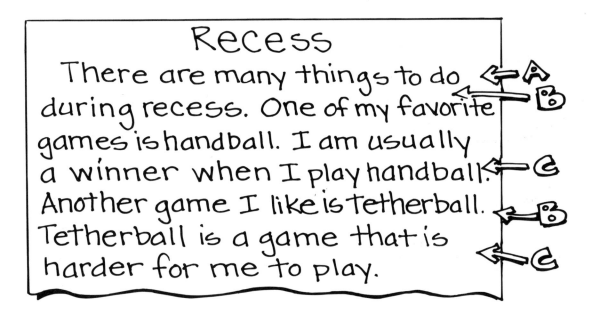

Have students practice writing A B C B C paragraphs in their journals, or have them complete the activities on the following pages. Give each student a Key Signals reproducible (page 30). Explain that the key signal words are found at the beginning of a sentence and help ideas flow from sentence to sentence. Invite students to refer to the reproducible to help them develop Key B and Key C sentences.

Key Signals

Key signals are words and phrases found at the beginning of a sentence that help ideas flow from sentence to sentence. Introduce the key signal words shown below to help students develop Key B and Key C sentences.

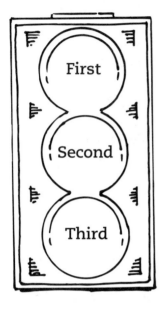

Key B Signals

First	Then
Second	To begin with
Third	As well as
More	In addition to
Even more	Lastly
Moreover	Finally
More than that	Some
Besides	Others
Furthermore	Still others
Also	Above all
Likewise	One
Again	Another
Next	Equally important

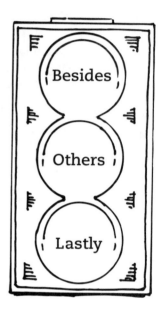

Key C Signals

Namely	For example
As	In the same manner
Just as	To be specific
This can be made clearer	Such as
To be sure	In other words
In such cases	This can be explained
It is necessary to	Because of this

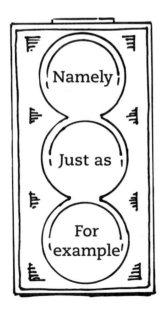

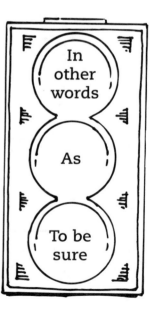

Key Paragraphs © 2002 Creative Teaching Press

Publishing

Have students use the self-edited version of their work or feedback from a completed response sheet to write their final draft. Writers are now ready to present their final product in its finished form. When students are ready to share their work with an audience, the writing process is complete! Allow students to present their work in many different forms. Students can present a typed or handwritten copy of their work, create illustrations for the text, or submit their work for inclusion in a class-made book. Writers will feel proud when others read their work. This is a wonderful time to display students' final drafts and share them with other classes.

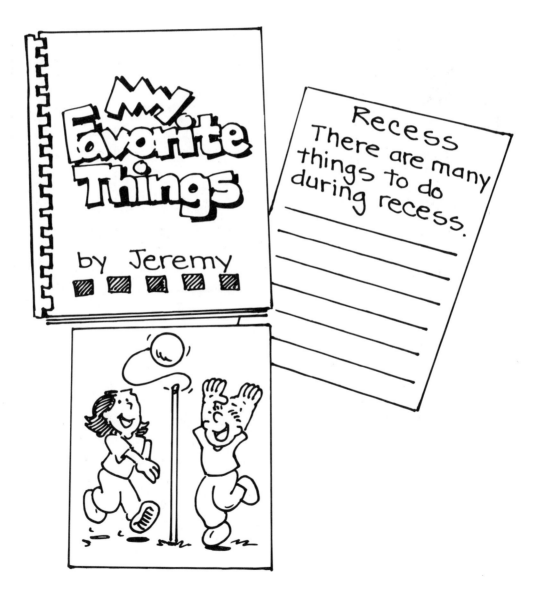

Key Web

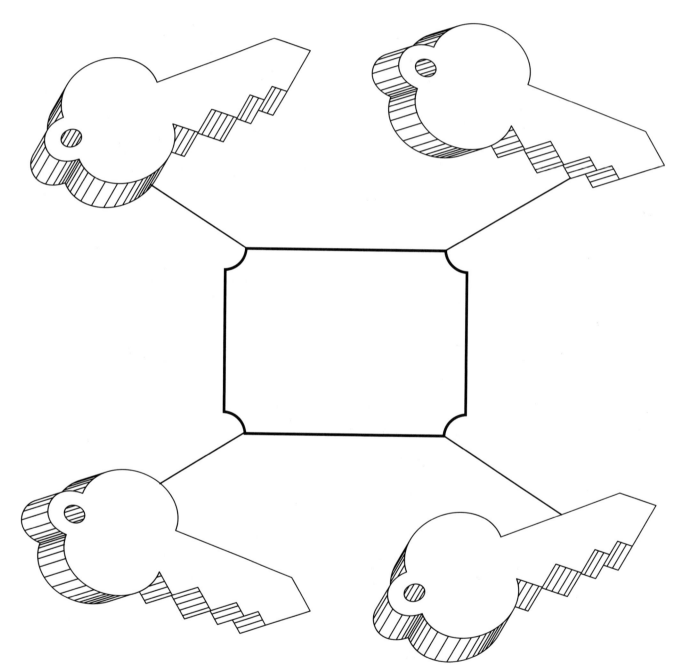

Key Paragraphs © 2002 Creative Teaching Press

Star Web

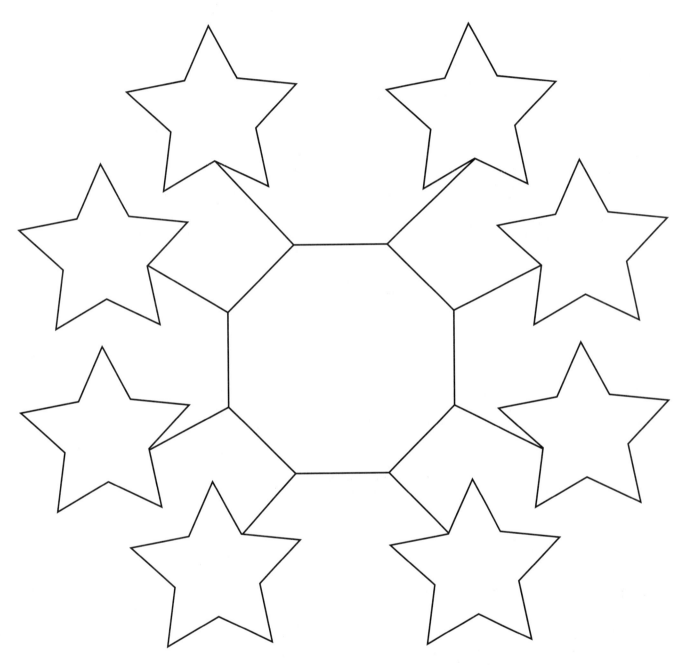

Key Paragraphs © 2002 Creative Teaching Press

Use Your Senses Web

Directions: Think about a specific place or event. Write words that describe what you heard, saw, tasted, smelled, and touched.

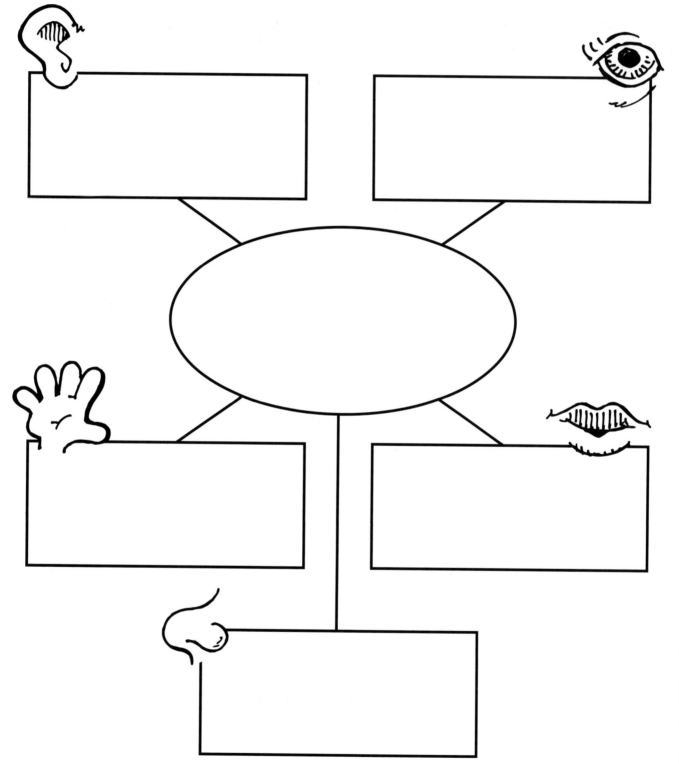

Key Paragraphs © 2002 Creative Teaching Press

Response Sheet

Your name: _____

Partner's name: _____

Directions: Read your partner's paper. When you finish, carefully fill out this sheet. Remember that you are helping your partner improve his or her writing.

1. One thing I remember best about this writing is _____

_____

_____

2. I would like the author to tell more about _____

_____

_____

3. This made sense to me because _____

_____

_____

4. I was confused because _____

_____

_____

Key Paragraphs © 2002 Creative Teaching Press

Editing Marks

delete line *e* remove letters, words, or sentences	We have too many ~~many~~ things. We have too many things.
caret ∧ add words	We went to ∧ store. the We went to the store.
rubber band ○→ move words	We ⟨every day⟩ do our homework. We do our homework every day.
three lines ≡ change a lowercase letter to a capital letter	On saturday we will go to the park. On Saturday we will go to the park.
slash / change a capital letter to a lowercase letter	We went to the M̸ovies this week. We went to the movies this week.
circle and *sp* for spelling ○ **sp** shows a spelling error	We are learning ⟨wekly⟩ words. sp We are learning weekly words.
paragraph symbol ¶ indent to start a new paragraph	¶ There are many new things to study in school. There are many new things to study in school.

Key Paragraphs © 2002 Creative Teaching Press

Peer Editing Form

Your name: _____

Partner's name: _____

Put an **X** in each box after you have checked your partner's paper. Make sure you use the correct editing marks when you are proofreading.

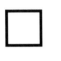 All sentences begin with a capital letter.

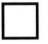 All sentences end with the proper punctuation.

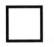 I checked all words for spelling.

 No words are missing.

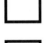 The writing is easy to read and it makes sense.

Paragraphs are indented.

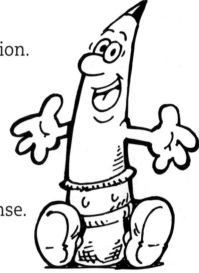

Comments _____

_____

_____

_____

_____

_____

_____

Key Paragraphs © 2002 Creative Teaching Press

Spelling Practice

Have students memorize the spellings of frequently used words to reduce the time they spend on editing spelling errors on their first drafts. Each week, present the class with a given number of high-frequency words from one of the lists on pages 57–60. Give students 10–25 words per week. Teach students the following memorization technique to help them minimize spelling mistakes when they are writing:

Step 1: Read each word, and have students repeat it after you. Have students write the words on a piece of paper.

Step 2: Define any words that are unclear, and talk about any "tricky" words.
Example: *their, they're* and *they're* or other homonyms
Example: *w* vs. *wh* words
Example: *them—then*

Step 3: Demonstrate the Say—Spell—Say memorization technique. Choose a word, and write it on the chalkboard. Say the word aloud, then spell it aloud, and then say it again. Repeat this two more times. Then, repeat the process three times with your eyes closed and again three more times as you look at the board.

Step 4: Have students practice saying, spelling, and saying each word nine times. The first three times, have them look at the word. The next three times, have them close their eyes and visualize the word in their mind. The last three times, ask them to look at the word again.

Step 5: Ask students to silently practice the technique with all the words for approximately 3 minutes.

Step 6: Ask students to copy the words in their homework folder.

Step 7: Have students practice spelling the words at home.

Step 8: Give a spelling test at the end of the week. Dictate each word, a sentence using the word, and the word again.

(Note: Include a 3–5 minute time frame during every writing period for students to practice high-frequency word memorization.)

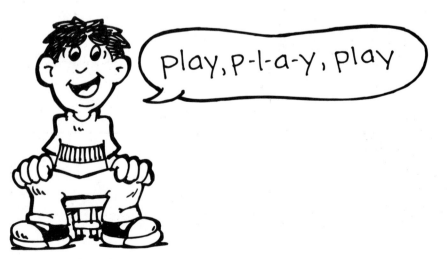

Primer Word List
1–50

1–10	11–20	21–30	31–40	41–50
a	are	as	at	away
and	be	big	blue	his
for	can	come	find	little
I	from	down	go	on
in	he	funny	have	play
is	look	help	here	that
it	my	jump	me	three
the	run	make	of	up
to	they	not	said	was
you	two	see	this	where

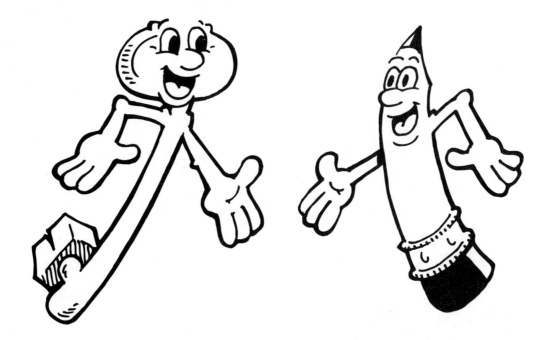

Key Paragraphs © 2002 Creative Teaching Press

High-Frequency Words
1–100

1–25	26–50	51–75	76–100
all	about	after	also
an	again	always	back
but	before	been	children
by	came	call	didn't
do	does	could	end
each	don't	day	fast
had	every	did	four
how	fun	ever	friend
if	get	first	goes
kind	give	good	him
last	happy	house	just
more	has	its	most
off	her	know	much
or	into	long	must
red	keep	made	never
she	let	may	next
stop	like	now	often
their	many	over	own
there	other	people	ready
use	out	say	saw
we	so	than	these
were	them	us	those
what	then	very	thought
which	told	way	want
your	will	who	when

Key Paragraphs © 2002 Creative Teaching Press

High-Frequency Words
101–200

101–125	126–150	151–175	176–200
another	any	around	ate
because	ask	beautiful	book
best	both	chair	boy
better	dear	eye	bring
clean	few	father	cold
done	glad	found	grow
enough	home	got	hand
gave	large	green	head
girl	myself	heard	left
hope	name	laugh	letter
live	nice	none	man
mother	open	one	men
night	sister	pass	new
only	soon	past	nobody
pretty	sure	read	once
put	teacher	some	party
right	too	something	place
school	try	take	shall
thank	went	talk	should
thing	why	together	small
think	work	until	time
used	would	wash	through
while	year	week	under
with	yellow	well	wish
write	yes	zoo	yard

Key Paragraphs © 2002 Creative Teaching Press

High-Frequency Words
201–300

201–225	226–250	251–275	276–300
asked	add	across	above
buy	along	almost	against
carry	began	begin	better
cut	between	below	body
draw	city	car	book
drink	close	country	color
eight	earth	example	eat
five	food	feet	face
fly	group	grow	family
full	head	hard	far
going	important	hear	himself
hold	it's	I'll	idea
hurt	life	list	Indian
light	might	mile	knew
old	near	music	late
pick	paper	night	leave
pull	plant	question	listen
road	run	remember	miss
round	sea	river	mountain
sit	seem	side	real
sleep	story	song	second
start	tree	state	several
today	usually	whole	slowly
took	walk	without	sometimes
warm	white	young	watch

Key Paragraphs © 2002 Creative Teaching Press

Writing Folders

Writing folders are an absolute necessity for a successful writing program because they
- ◎ provide a place to store all ongoing work related to the writing program.
- ◎ are a resource center for students.
- ◎ contain crucial writer's information (e.g., writing process, editing symbols, vocabulary).
- ◎ document each student's work in progress.

Organizing the Folders

1. For each student, glue a copy of the Draft Checklist (page 63) on the back of a two-pocket folder.
2. Give each student a folder.
3. Have students place a copy of the following reproducibles in their folder: Editing Marks (page 54), High-Frequency Word Lists (pages 57–60), Your Writing Process (page 62), Word Substitution (page 64), and Words for Feelings (page 65).
4. Give each student a journal (simple ruled composition book or any ruled paper stapled together) to place in one pocket.
5. Ask students to write their name on the cover of their folder.

Have students keep their prewriting, drafts, completed response sheets, and final drafts in these folders. Explain to students that they will take out their folder each time they use the writing process to work on a piece of writing. Have students keep their folders at their desks or store them in one location (e.g., a decorated box). Set aside time each month to have a conference with each student to review his or her writing folder.

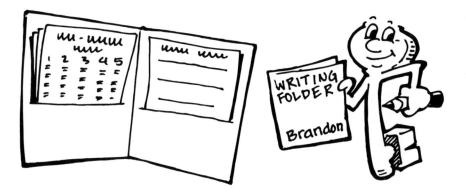

Your Writing Process

Prewriting
◉ Choose a topic
◉ Brainstorm ideas—jot down key words and phrases
◉ Plan your writing
◉ Talk to others

Think First!

Drafting
◉ Turn your key words and phrases into sentences
◉ Form some A B C B C paragraphs
◉ Write a first draft

Writing!

Revising
◉ Read what you wrote
◉ Change words or ideas
◉ Write more

Improving!

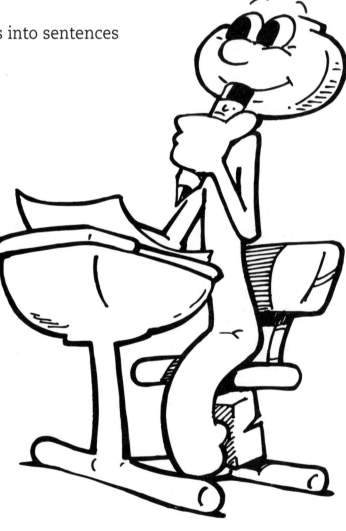

Editing
◉ Use complete sentences
◉ Have someone check your work
◉ Use proofreading marks

Correcting!

Publishing
◉ Think of a good title
◉ Make a clean copy
◉ Display it for others to see

Final Draft!

Key Paragraphs © 2002 Creative Teaching Press

Draft Checklist

Check your
paper after each
draft!

Did you indent your paragraphs?

Did you check your spelling?

Did you use capital letters and
punctuation marks?

Did you use the A B B or A B C B C
format for your paragraphs?

Key Paragraphs © 2002 Creative Teaching Press

Word Substitution

every   common, frequent, regular, routine, usual

fun   enjoyable, exciting, fantastic, incredible, marvelous, pleasure, terrific, wonderful

go   advance, continue, depart, leave, move, pass, proceed, travel

good   acceptable, all right, appropriate, decent, fine, nice, right

got   acquired, earned, gathered, obtained, received, won

great   important, large, mighty, notable, outstanding, remarkable, sensational

happy   cheerful, content, fulfilled, glad, joyful, pleased, satisfied

like   admire, appreciate, enjoy, prefer

lots   abundant, countless, many, numerous, various

mad   angry, annoyed, exasperated, furious, irritated, upset

make   assemble, build, compose, create, form, invent, originate, produce

nice   agreeable, courteous, fine, friendly, good, kind, pleasant

sad   blue, depressed, forlorn, gloomy, unhappy

said   announced, asked, claimed, declared, explained, hollered, mentioned, remarked, replied, spoke, stated, told, whispered, yelled

see   detect, discover, note, notice, observe, picture, spot

then   after, finally, later, next

very   extremely, incredibly, quite, wonderfully

want   crave, desire, long for, need, wish for

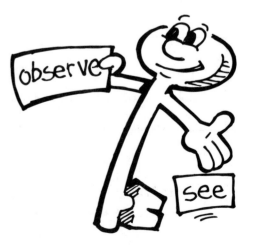

Key Paragraphs © 2002 Creative Teaching Press

Words for Feelings

HAPPINESS	amused	delighted	joyful
	calm	eager	peaceful
	cheerful	ecstatic	proud
	content	excited	satisfied
	curious	glad	

SADNESS	afraid	fearful	miserable
or	angry	frightened	nervous
WORRY	anxious	gloomy	serious
	disappointed	hopeless	sorrowful
	discouraged	lonely	tearful
			upset

LOVING	calm	gentle	kind
or	caring	glad	pleasant
FRIENDLY	generous	helpful	true

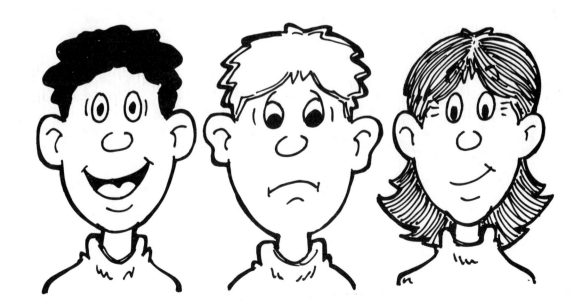

Key Paragraphs © 2002 Creative Teaching Press

Making the Connection

Once students are comfortable with writing key paragraphs and the writing process, give them opportunities to practice throughout their school day. Invite students to practice their paragraph writing in their journals. See the journal ideas on pages 67–70.

Incorporate paragraph writing into other curriculum areas. Key Paragraphs across the Curriculum on page 71 provides some suggested topic ideas.

An awareness of different genres and writing domains helps students become more discriminating writers. Share with the class the explanation of the domains and the different modes of writing from pages 72–73.

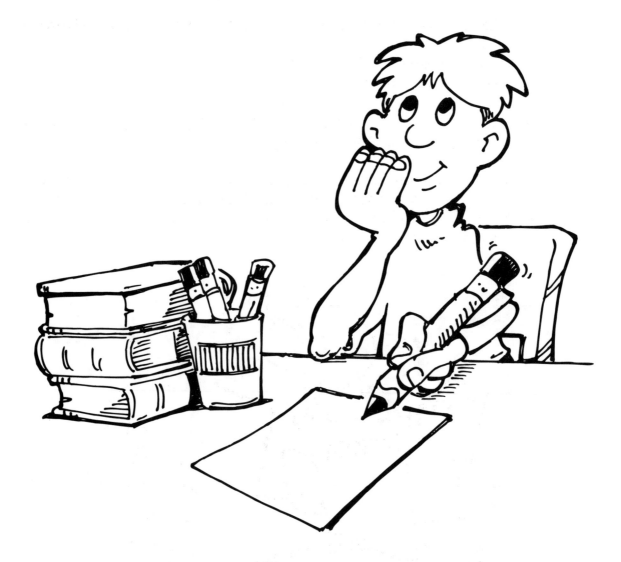

Journals

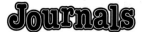

There are various reasons why teachers do not use journals in the classroom. Many teachers have their own quandaries about journaling and, therefore, end up not dealing with it at all. Do any of these statements or questions sound familiar?

I can't add one more thing to the daily schedule.
Should I check or not check? How can you ignore obvious mistakes?
When will I have time to respond?
My kids won't sit still long enough to write.
What about the nonwriters? What do I do with them?
Most kids are stuck and don't feel comfortable.
I don't have enough time.

Keep the following in mind when implementing journal writing into your classroom:

- Keep a simple system for responding.
- Make it easy on yourself.
- Make it a comfortable experience for students.
- Use it as a tool to reinforce your lessons, especially the key paragraphs!
- Do not grade, correct, or collect the journals.

Remember that the experience is meant to encourage more writing because, as in reading, the more you do the better you will be. As students practice their writing skills, they will also develop a love of writing. Students feel empowered as their journals begin to fill with their own writing.

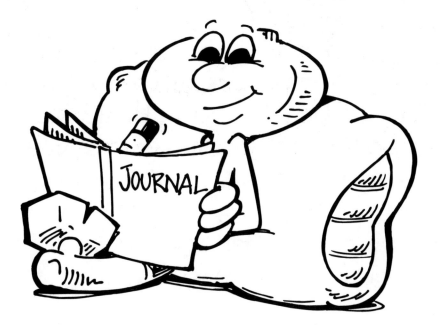

Practicing through Journals

Give students daily practice with writing key paragraphs in their journal. Use the following directions to explain to students how to use the journal prompts to write A B B paragraphs:

1. Write a topic on the chalkboard. Use topics that are relevant to what is happening at school or in general (e.g., holidays), or choose journal prompts from pages 69–70.
2. Brainstorm ideas with the class. Draw a web, and use student ideas to complete it.
3. Change the topic into a Key A sentence.
4. Discuss how to turn the details from the web into Key B sentences.
5. Have students date the entry and begin writing. Encourage them to write on the topic for 5 minutes.
6. At the end of 5 minutes, have students stop.
7. Invite several students to read aloud their writing. Do not make sharing mandatory, but provide a wonderful experience for those who are comfortable with sharing. It is very helpful to those reluctant writers who need to hear ideas.

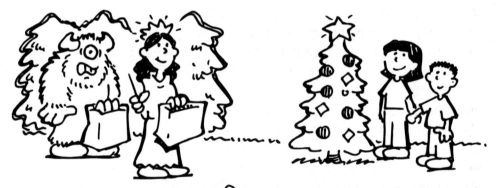

I have two favorite holidays. Ⓐ One is Halloween. Halloween Ⓑ is so cool because we wear Ⓒ costumes, like a monster or a princess. Another is Ⓑ Christmas because I gather with my family.

Journal Prompts

The following Key A sentences reinforce the simple key paragraph A B B:

- There are two things I like to do at recess.
- I have two favorite sports.
- There are two things I learned in school this week.
- I remember kindergarten for two reasons.
- I have two favorite holidays.
- I feel good about _____ for two reasons.
- I feel good about (school). (two reasons)
- There are two TV shows I like to watch.
- I have two best friends.
- I have been to two different cities.
- My two favorite subjects in school are _____.

The following Key A sentences reinforce the key paragraph concept of using "many" in the Key A sentence:

- I am thankful for many things.
- I celebrated many holidays during my vacation.
- I enjoy school for many reasons.
- I enjoy being with my friends for many reasons.
- There are many things that make me feel good.
- There are many things that don't make me feel good.
- There are many things I like about (favorite TV show).
- There are many fun things to do at parties.
- There are many fun holidays to celebrate.
- There are many things I find boring.
- I did (did not do) many great things on the weekend.
- There are many things to do before I finish ____ grade.
- I have had many different teachers in school.
- I worry about many things.

Encourage the use of the A B C B C paragraph format and variations of it (e.g., A B B C B, A B C C B C).

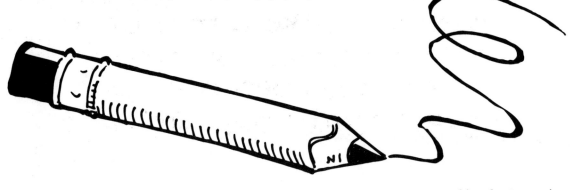

The following are more advanced Key A sentences. These sentences move away from "two" and "many."

◉ I am learning how to write.
◉ I have learned a new (word, fact, idea) this week.
◉ I remember when I went to . . .
◉ I had a (adjective) vacation.
◉ Christmas is a fun holiday.
◉ I have had a _____ vacation from school. I did (not do) many things.
◉ I feel _____ about my parents seeing my report card.
◉ Every student in (state) is taking a test.
◉ I feel _____ about taking tests.
◉ Writing can sometimes be difficult for me.
◉ I feel _____ about going to _____ grade.
◉ There are four seasons in a year.
◉ I enjoyed celebrating (holiday) with my family.

Key Paragraphs across the Curriculum

Have students write key paragraphs throughout the school day to incorporate writing across your curriculum. Choose one of these topics, or create your own.

Math
◉ Explain how you solved a math problem.
◉ Describe the differences between two shapes.
◉ Write about the value of a coin and its characteristics.

Social Studies
◉ Compare two historic people.
◉ Retell a historical event.
◉ Describe how you would feel if you lived during a historical event (e.g., war, Great Depression).

Science
◉ Explain an experiment you completed.
◉ Compare two animals.
◉ Explain what a scientist does.
◉ Describe a science-related observation.

Reading
◉ Compare two characters in a story.
◉ Describe an event in a story.
◉ Describe how you felt about a story.
◉ Describe the main character.

Fine Arts
◉ Describe a work of art.
◉ Describe your feelings about a work of art.
◉ Describe what materials you would use to create a work of art and explain why you would use them.

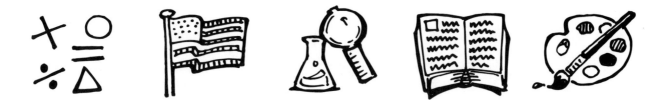

Writing Domains

The domains of writing classify the different types of writing and distinguish a writing selection by its purpose and audience. Although there are various ways of grouping the different domains, the most common fall into four groups:

◉ Sensory/Descriptive

◉ Imaginative/Narrative

◉ Practical/Informative

◉ Analytical/Expository

An awareness of different genres and writing domains helps students become more discriminating writers. Introduce them to the four domains, and discuss all the different modes of writing as follows:

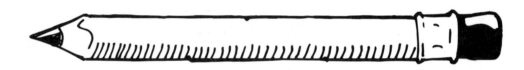

1. Sensory/Descriptive—Be able to describe in detail and to express individual feelings.

Modes	Student Uses	Genre
✓ Journal/Diary entry ✓ Autobiography ✓ Personal letter ✓ Poem	✓ Descriptive language to tell about experiences ✓ Use of five senses ✓ Descriptive words for sounds, people, animals and their actions	✓ Nonfiction: autobiography ✓ Fiction: realistic

2. Imaginative/Narrative—Be able to tell what happens in a sequence of time. The events can be real or imaginary.

Modes	Student Uses	Genre
✓ Short story	✓ Write own stories	✓ Nonfiction: autobiography
✓ Poem	✓ Describe imaginary	✓ Fiction: realistic, fantasy,
✓ Myth	characters	traditional
✓ Dialogue	✓ Create simple rhymes	

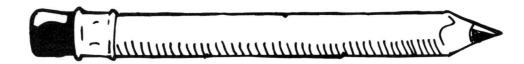

3. Practical/Informative—Be able to relate information clearly.

Modes	Student Uses	Genre
✓ Letter	✓ Facts about an event	✓ Nonfiction: biography,
✓ Summary	✓ Greetings	autobiography,
✓ Notes	✓ Information	information
✓ Report		

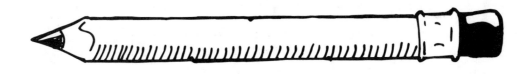

4. Analytical/Expository—Be able to explain, analyze, and persuade.

Modes	Student Uses	Genre
✓ Paragraph	✓ Gathers information	✓ Nonfiction: information
✓ Research paper	✓ Points of view	
✓ Speech	✓ Supporting details	
✓ Report	✓ Persuasive language	

Assessment

Assessment is an ongoing process throughout the year. Use assessment and evaluation to guide your classroom instruction to meet the needs of your students as well as track students' progress.

After students have written their paragraphs and practiced the writing process, it is time for you to assess their writing. This section explains two methods of assessment: writing rubrics and portfolios.

Rubrics are a method of informal assessment. Use rubrics to assess and analyze students' writing skills. This section includes two sample rubrics.

Writing portfolios provide a way for collecting student writing samples. See pages 78–79 for more information about writing portfolios.

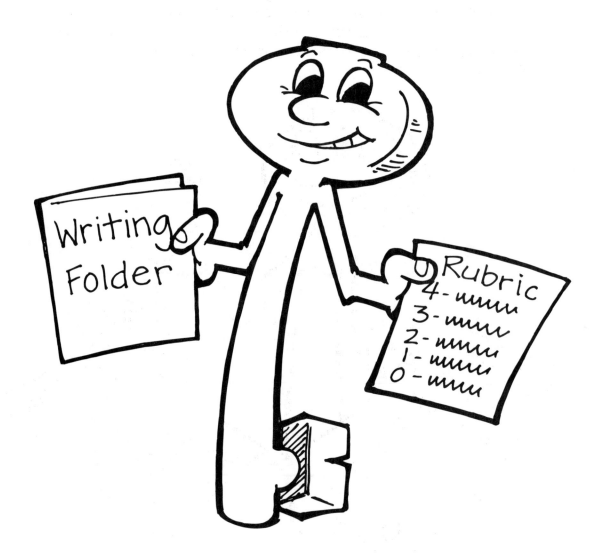

Rubrics

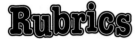

A rubric is a scoring guide designed to evaluate a student's performance. In the writing curriculum, a rubric could measure the following components of a student's writing:

- Ideas
- Organization
- Word choice
- Sentence structure
- Mechanics—punctuation, capitalization, spelling

Use the Writing Rubric 0–5 on page 76 to score students' writing. Determine which number best describes the student's writing, and write that number on his or her paper. The Primary Writing Rubric on page 77 can be used to evaluate emergent writers. Or, create a customized rubric for a specific writing assignment. When designing your own rubric, design it to have guidelines for observation, assessment, and evaluation. Make sure the rubric values the students' process as well as the final product.

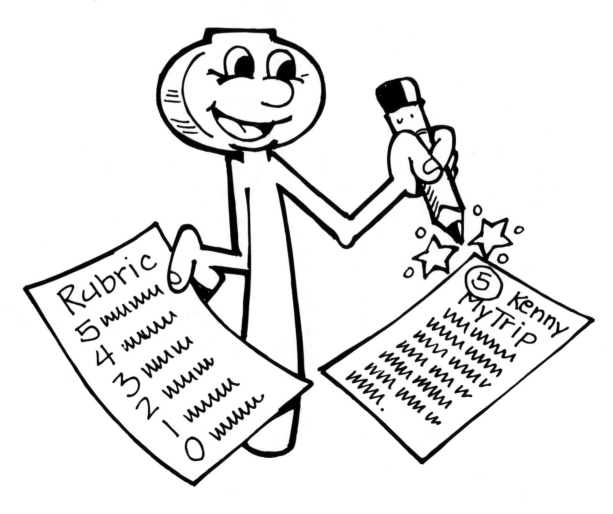

Safety First _____

Heed the warnings in these boxes so your soap-making experience is a safe one!

Soap Stats _____

These boxes offer a little more information and fun facts.

Acknowledgments

Zonella and I both would like to say a special thank you to Ken Bower for creating SoapCalc. You opened a whole new world for soap-makers!

I would like to dedicate my part of this book to my family, for all their support and help. My mother, Iris Wyman, thank you for being such a great mom. My husband, Mark Trew; my children, Doug, Carissa, and Alicia; my son-in-law Keith; and my grandchildren, Hunter, Trenten, Shawn, Trinity, Sydney, and Pacey, I love you all. A special thanks to Sandra Morrow and all our list mates on the Apple! Your support and encouragement have meant the world to me! And lastly, K. C. Massey, thanks for all your help with my computer and for always being willing to test my formulations.

—Sally Trew

I would like to dedicate my part of this book to my family, for all their support and help. From Darrell and Dan and their families to sisters and brother and all the local people that have given nothing but encouragement.

—Zonella Gould

Trademarks

All terms mentioned in this book that are known to be or are suspected of being trademarks or service marks have been appropriately capitalized. Alpha Books and Penguin Group (USA) Inc. cannot attest to the accuracy of this information. Use of a term in this book should not be regarded as affecting the validity of any trademark or service mark.

Part 1

The Basics of Natural Soap-Making

Taking the first step to making homemade soap is a start to an adventure. But as with anything you want to do, and do well, you need a good foundation. In Part 1, you begin building that strong foundation and take the first steps on the path to becoming a great soap-maker. You learn all about the oils and butters used to make soap and how to use SoapCalc to formulate your soap batch recipe. We also look at the fragrances and essential oils you can use and then cover the molds you pour all your delicious-smelling concoctions into.

By the time you've finished Part 1, you'll be ready to make your very first batch of soap!

Introduction to Soap-Making

In This Chapter

- ◆ The basics of making soap
- ◆ What ingredients you need to make soap
- ◆ Soap-making safety and other equipment

If the soap-making bug hasn't bitten you yet, it's about to! As you'll learn in the following pages and chapters, natural, homemade soaps have many wonderful benefits. They're nonirritating to your skin—in fact, we've seen facial and other skin blemishes clear up after using natural soap. Properly made soap not only cleanses but is gentle and moisturizing and never leaves your skin feeling dry or itchy. The soap is such a pleasure to use that you'll look forward to showers and baths!

How Soap Is Made

Soap is made when the chemical reaction of lye plus water further reacts with oil and turns the oil into a salt. This process is called *saponification*. It can take as little as 24 to 48 hours for cold process soap to saponify; for hot process, the saponification is complete when it's finished cooking (more on cold and hot process soaps in Part 2). Bar soap cannot be made without *alkalis;* sodium hydroxide and liquid soap cannot be made without potassium hydroxide. Both are caustic and can be dangerous if used improperly.

Lather Lingo

Saponification refers to the reaction of an alkali with a fat or oil and water to form soap. An **alkali** is a compound that has a pH greater than 7 (a base). Sodium hydroxide and potassium hydroxide are both alkalis. **Bases** are the oils you use in your soap recipe to stabilize the bar. **pH** is a factor that deals with the alkaline (drying) and the acid (conditioning) of the substance. The higher the pH number, the more cleansing and drying it is to the skin or hair. pH 7 is neutral. Most bar soaps have a pH of 10, and liquid soaps have a pH of between 9 and 9.5.

The caustic aspect isn't something to be feared, but it does need to be respected. All safety equipment and all safety procedures should be utilized throughout the whole soap-making process. Negligence to take proper safety precautions can cause injuries. We recommend you wait until the kids are at school, your spouse is at work, and the pets are outside or closed in another portion of the house before you start making soap.

When our grandmothers made soap, it was just a guesstimate in how much lye was to be used. Now we have soap calculators that calculate how much lye is needed. This means no more guessing and no more worries. With the proper use of a soap calculator (we give you a great one, SoapCalc, in Chapter 4), you'll feel certain that your soap won't be lye-heavy. With SoapCalc, you learn how to formulate a bar of soap to be exactly what you want.

Basic Soap Ingredients

The beauty of soap is that you need very few ingredients for a simple bar of soap. Fragrance, color, and embedded pieces are nice add-ins, but here's all you really need to make a basic bar of soap:

Oils/butters. These are the bases of your soap. Each oil and butter has a different property and a different use. Base oils are lard, tallow, and palm oil. Cleansing oils are coconut, babassu, and palm kernel oil. Castor oil is used for added lather and moisturizing. Many other oils/butters can be used for adding more conditioning to the soap.

Lye. This includes sodium hydroxide for bar soap and potassium hydroxide for liquid soap. Soap cannot be made without it.

Distilled water. Distilled water eliminates any contaminants or high amounts of minerals your water might contain.

Borax. This is used to neutralize any leftover lye in liquid soap, boost its cleaning power, and lower the pH. It is natural and mined from the earth. Borax is also known to be a disinfectant and deodorizer. Often borax is added to cold process or hot process soap when making a mechanic's soap bar.

Safety First _____

When lye is added to water and stirred to dissolve, it will produce a visible vapor. *Do not inhale this vapor.* When mixing, be sure you open a window, turn on a vent, or turn on the down-draft to draw the vapors out of the house and away from you.

Adding In Some Fun: Additives

Of course, you can get creative and add to that basic bar of soap with additives like herbs, honey, milk, colors, fragrance, micas, salt, and sugar. Anything other than oil, water, and lye are additives.

When working with fragrance oils, be sure to use only skin-safe fragrance oils. You can use essential oils to fragrance soap, but use sparingly because they're very potent and can burn the skin if you use too much. The average use ratio is a maximum of 3 percent, but a maximum of 2.5 percent is better for many of the essential oils. Also, several essential oils should not be used on children, pregnant women, or cancer patients. Be sure to check our chapter on essential oils (Chapter 3) before using them in soap. Liquid colorants are available, but we've found they don't always keep their color in the soap-making process. We use mostly micas and oxides. Any color used in soap has to be skin safe, and don't use crayons. Micas lose their "sparkle" during the saponification process, but when the bar is wet, you can once again see their beautiful sparkles and iridescent colors. Most oxides remain the same throughout the soap-making process.

And One More—for Safety

Vinegar, you might be thinking. *In soap?* Not exactly. Although vinegar doesn't go *in* the soap, it is very important to have on hand because vinegar neutralizes lye. If you spill lye on your skin, flush thoroughly with water and follow with vinegar to neutralize and remove all traces of the lye.

If you only flush with water, your skin will have a slick feel. Only when you apply the vinegar will the slick feeling go away.

The Importance of Safety Equipment

Speaking of safety, it's the number-one concern when making soap, and with just a few basic, inexpensive pieces of equipment, you can fully protect yourself from harm:

Safety glasses or a face shield. Any kind of heat-resistant, wrap-around safety goggles will do fine. Stay away from the type of goggles that look similar to eyeglasses as they tend to heat up and fog over, making it impossible to see what you are doing. A full-face shield also works great and isn't all that expensive. If you wear glasses, the shields are your best choice because you can wear them right over your glasses.

Gloves. Latex gloves like the ones dentists or doctors use are the best. They're inexpensive and readily available. You can find 100-count boxes at any drugstore.

Long-sleeved shirt. The splatter from the lye or potassium hydroxide mixture can be irritating to the skin but it can also eat holes in clothing, so wear an old long-sleeved shirt to cover your arms and protect the front of your shirt from splatters. You can also wear an apron to protect your pants.

Shoes. Never, *ever* make soap in your bare feet or sandals. Any splatter will sear your skin and hurt like crazy. Get a sturdy pair of closed shoes, and be sure they're ones you won't mind getting splattered.

Other Soap-Making Equipment You'll Need

Here again, just a few inexpensive items are needed to make soap:

Stainless-steel stockpot with a lid. Most of us have pots already and won't need to buy any. They will wash clean and still be food-ready. A 3- to 12-quart pot should allow you to make any size batch of soap you will want.

Safety First _____

Only use stainless-steel pots, never aluminum or enamelware, when making soap. Aluminum reacts with lye, causing the lye to eat holes in it. The lye etches enamelware and, in time, eats away at the enamel.

Handheld immersion blender. An immersion blender is a handheld, sticklike blender that has one spinning blade on the end. Mainly used for whipping cream or drinks, they're also a soaper's best friend because they reduce the amount of stirring time (and save your arm!). But they're optional if you'd rather SIY—stir it yourself.

Spoon or whisk. Again, stainless steel is best, or you can use utensils made for nonstick pans. Don't use wooden spoons, however. Over time, the wood dries out and little splinters will end up in the soap batch.

Spatula. Stainless or nonstick is best.

Bowls. Stainless-steel or plastic bowls are the best to use to weigh oils, butters, water, or lye. Zonella uses food-saver bowls to mix her lye. These come with lids that cut down on the chance of spills if the bowl gets turned over or bumped. Sally uses a tall plastic pitcher with a lid and secures the handle so the pitcher cannot be tipped or knocked over.

Plastic pitcher with a lid. You'll be using this to mix lye. Don't use a glass pitcher because it'll etch the glass. Lye heats up so much it could cause the glass to break—a very dangerous situation.

Scale. In soap-making, everything has to be weighed. You'll need a good electronic kitchen scale with a flat platform big enough to rest bowls and pitchers on and that measures to $\frac{1}{10}$ an ounce. It should also measure in grams.

 From the Soap Pot

Always use a scale to weigh your soap ingredients. Never use measuring cups, tablespoons, etc., because they measure *volume*. The weight of oils varies a lot; some are lighter than water, and some are heavier than water. The only way you'll get an exact amount is to use a scale.

Stainless-steel thermometer. A thermometer tells you the temperature of the oils and the lye/water so you know when to mix the oils and lye/water. The hotter the oils, the faster the soap will set up. If you don't have a thermometer, you can feel the outside of the pot or pitcher with your fingers. When it's ready to have the lye mixture added, it'll be comfortable to the touch.

Molds. We devote an entire chapter to molds (Chapter 5), so we won't go into detail here.

The Shelf Life of Soap

How long a soap will stay good varies. Sally once found some soap she'd put away, and it smelled and looked great. It was pushing five years old. Zonella, on the other hand, had some that didn't fare that long, but she had used sweet orange essential oil, which doesn't often stay well in soap.

WATERFORD TOWNSHIP
PUBLIC LIBRARY

110001

From the Soap Pot

Antioxidants prevent or retard oxygen reacting on a substance. Rosemary oleo resin added to short-life soaping oils extends their shelf life.

The shelf life of any soap is based on the iodine value. If the iodine is too high, it's going to produce DOS—dreaded orange spots—a sure sign the soap is going rancid.

So for soap with a long shelf life, pay close attention to the iodine value when you put your soap recipe in SoapCalc. The iodine value is part of the soap qualities.

Storing Your Soap

The main thing to remember when storing soap is that it will absorb scents very easily, so be careful where you store it. We like to store our soaps in lidded plastic containers, like plastic shoe boxes. With the lid on, the soap remains clean and the fragrance stays true and doesn't absorb any other fragrances.

Soap Stats

If your soap has lost its fragrance, place it in an airtight container along with either cloth or paper towels saturated with fragrance oil, and replace the lid. After a few weeks, you'll find that the soap once again has a fragrance.

These boxes also stack well in a small space. Be sure to label the boxes, including the name of the soap, fragrance, date, and the recipe if you like. It's so easy to forget what's in all those boxes!

If you smoke, don't allow the smoke to get close to your soap. There's nothing quite so bad as soap that smells like a dirty ashtray!

Frequently Asked Questions About Making Soap

What is meant by *trace*?   When you add the lye/water to the oils, a chemical reaction begins. The mixture begins to thicken just like pudding or gravy does when you're making it. The first stage of thickening is called *light trace*. If you dribbled some of the soap on top of the soap in the pot, it would leave a trace in the soap—hence the name. It will continue to thicken until it's a firm bar.

Does soap have to go through trace?   Yes. If it didn't, you wouldn't have soap.

What does it mean when you say the soap is "in the gel stage"?   The gel stage is when the soap has heated up so much it has the appearance of applesauce. It's liquid, hot, and almost finished in changing to soap. It's in full saponification.

WATERFORD TOWNSHIP
PUBLIC LIBRARY

Which way do you mix the lye and water together?   You always add the lye slowly to the water. *Never* pour water into the container with the lye.

Is it really necessary to wear safety glasses and gloves?   Yes. If lye gets on your skin it can burn you badly. You should immediately wash the area with lots of cold water. As mentioned earlier in this chapter, if you still can feel a slick feeling on your skin, follow with vinegar. The fumes can also burn your lungs, so don't put your face over the pitcher of lye solution. We recommend that you set your lye solution in a well-ventilated area while it's cooling.

How can I be sure my lye is good?   When you add the lye to the water, it will start a chemical reaction that will cause the water to become very hot. If the lye is bad or inactive, this heat-up won't happen.

What kind of lye do I use?   Many soap-makers use Red Devil lye, but that isn't always easy to get. You can order lye online from Boyer Corp. and from many online venders (find some in Appendix D). You have to use pure lye and one that says it's for soap-making.

I am afraid of using lye. Is there a safe way?   You can't make soap without lye. However, melt-and-pour (M&P) soap might be something you could try. It's already a finished soap product, so you don't add any lye. M&P soap base is easy, fast, and fun. But still, if you follow the directions and wear your safety gear, you should have no reason to fear using lye—just don't forget to respect lye and handle it properly.

Can I make soap in my kitchen when my children are home?   We never make soap when the kids are at home or when any of the pets are in the kitchen. Accidents can happen really fast when you turn your back for even a second.

Do I use the same lye to make hot process soap as I do to make cold process soap?   Yes, they both use sodium hydroxide. Both soaps become solid.

Do I use the same lye for making liquid soap as I do for making cold process or hot process soap?   No. For liquid soap, you use potassium hydroxide. This lye is in flakes or
diamond-shape pieces. With potassium hydroxide, the soap won't become solid. It stays a liquid.

Can I use Drano for my lye?   No. Although Drano has lye, it also has other chemicals that could be harmful when used in soap.

The Least You Need to Know

◆ You don't need a lot of expensive, hard-to-find ingredients to make soap. With some oil/butter, lye, water, and borax, you're on your way.

◆ Soap-making won't require a ton of new tools and equipment. It's likely you already have most of what you'll need in your kitchen.

◆ It's easy to get excited about all the wonderful and lovely soap combinations you can create, but never forget the importance of safety. Soap-making can be dangerous if you don't pay attention and respect your ingredients.

Chapter 2

Oils and Butters

In This Chapter

- ◆ Choosing oils and butters for your soap recipes
- ◆ Understanding how oils and butters work in your soap
- ◆ Grocery store oils—they're not just for cooking!

Without oil/butter, water, and lye, you can't make soap. The oils and butters you choose for your soap can do far more than just provide part of the chemical reaction needed for saponifying. They also have wonderful skin-loving properties. Many have healing properties for certain skin problems, while others have more specialized benefits.

Many oils and butters are still very expensive, but some you might *have* to try, no matter how expensive they are. You could spend a fortune buying all kinds of exotic oils and butters, but in reality, because soap is a wash-off product, unless you're making a specialty bar, stick with the basic, good oils.

If you can only buy one butter for soap making, make it shea butter. Shea brings wonderful skin-softening properties to the soap as well as increases the creamy lather. If you can only buy three oils to start your soap-making adventure, choose castor oil, coconut oil, and palm oil.

Soap-Making Oils and Butters

As you'll see, the list is quite long. With each oil, we've listed its shelf life, description, properties, and typical uses. We've also included the common name and the botanical name you'll use in labeling. (For more on labeling, see Appendixes B and C.)

Before we dig into the oils and butters you can use in your soaps, here are a few things to keep in mind. If unopened, peanut oil, corn oil, and other vegetable oils keep for at least a year. Once opened, they're good for 4 to 6 months.

Peanut oil, like olive oil, which is high in monounsaturates, is better stored in the refrigerator. Olive oil keeps for about 6 months in the cool, dark pantry, but stays up to a year in the refrigerator. It may become cloudy and thicken in the cold. Letting it warm to room temperature by sitting on your kitchen counter will restore its pouring capacity.

If you don't use an oil very often, you can store it in your freezer. Most oils don't actually freeze, but they will become very thick, and the cold temperature will extend their shelf life. Butters will actually freeze.

Adding rosemary oleo resin extract (ROE) to oils gives them a longer shelf life. Use 1 percent of the weight of the oils. So if you have 32 ounces (907.2 grams) oil, you would use 0.3 ounce (8.5 grams) ROE.

Now, on with the show!

Almond (Sweet) Oil (*Prunus amygdalus*)

Shelf life: 6 months to 1 year.

Properties and benefits: This oil is great for flaky, itching, or rough skin. It contains vitamins A, B_1, B_6, and E as well as fatty acids. In soap, it adds conditioning and is often used for mature skin or in facial bars. Almond oil isn't expensive, so it's widely used in many soaps, lotions, and other bath and body products for its skin-loving benefits as well as its low cost. When using this oil in soap-making, keep the percentage low because it will increase the iodine. Sweet almond oil is a very light gold color and produces a white bar of soap. This oil has a hardness of 7.

Apricot Kernel Oil (*Prunus armeniaca*)

Shelf life: 6 months to 1 year.

Properties and benefits: Apricot kernel oil is good for damaged or irritated skin. It contains vitamins A, C, E, and unsaturated fatty acid. More often it's used in lotions and body butters for its exceptional skin-healing properties. This oil isn't expensive and can be a wonderful addition to facial bars or for a gentle soap for mature or sensitive skin. It has a golden color and no fragrance. This oil has a hardness of 6.

Avocado Oil (*Persea gratissima*)

Shelf life: 1 year.

Properties and benefits: Contains vitamins A, B$_1$, B$_2$, D, and E; pantothenic acid; protein; lecithin; and fatty acids. Avocado hydrates and nourishes the skin. It is said to lighten age spots and increase the amount of collagen in the skin cells. This oil penetrates the skin quickly and easily, making it ideal for use in lotions and other leave-on products. In soaps, it's a favorite for shampoo bars, shampoo gel, and shower gel. Avocado oil is often used in facial bars because of its high vitamin content. The color varies from a light green to a clear oil, depending on the refining. This oil has a hardness of 22.

Babassu Oil (*Orbignya oleifera*)

Shelf life: 1 to 2 years.

Properties and benefits: There are three oils that are cleansing. Babassu is one of those oils. (The other two are coconut oil and palm kernel oil.) You increase the cleansing value of your soap bar by using a higher percentage of one of these three oils. This oil will also increase the lather and hardness in a bar of soap. Babassu is higher in lauric, myristic, palmitic, and stearic than coconut or palm kernel oil. It does not contain any linoleic acid. It offers very little moisturizing, so in soap-making, we use this oil only for its cleansing and bar-hardening values. Babassu is a hard oil that is semi-solid at room temperature. It has a hardness of 85.

Canola Oil (*Brassica campestris*)

Shelf life: Up to 1 year.

Properties and benefits: Canola oil is inexpensive, and you can buy it at your local grocery store so it is often used in place of the more pricey base oils, such as olive oil. It contributes moisturizing qualities to the soap and produces a creamy, stable lather, but it takes longer to saponify. Canola oil is made from genetically altered rapeseed. The name *canola* stands for "Canadian Oil Company." This oil is high in protein and fatty acids. It has a hardness of 6.

Castor Oil (*Ricinus communis*)

Shelf life: 2 years.

Soap Stats

Castor oil has many uses, from medicinal to cosmetics. It adds moisturizing properties to lipsticks and lip gloss, and it's used in other types of cosmetics because it doesn't contribute or cause acne. In soap-making it helps create lather without having to use the chemical SLS.

Properties and benefits: Using castor oil in soap increases the bubbly and creamy lather as well as the conditioning. If your bar of soap doesn't have a lot of lather, you can increase this oil to boost the lather your soap will produce. Note, however, that it also makes the soap bar softer. Using 10 to 15 percent castor in your soap batch gives a nice lather and increases the skin-conditioning qualities. We've experimented with using as much as 25 percent in bar soaps. For shower gels and shampoos, using 20 to 35 percent helps create a really nice lather. Castor oil is the only oil in this group that contains ricinoleic acid. It's a thick, clear oil with a hardness of 0.

Cocoa Butter (*Theobroma cacao*)

Shelf life: Up to 5 years.

Properties and benefits: Cocoa butter comes in three forms: natural, deodorized, and ultra-refined. Cocoa butter adds hardness to soaps and helps seal in moisture by forming a barrier on the skin. The average use in soaps is 3 to 5 percent, but in winter, some soap-makers increase that amount to 8 to 10 percent. Cocoa butter is the second-most-used butter in soaps, and it's widely used in many bath and body products. It's not recommended for oily skin, however. Natural cocoa butter has a rich, golden-yellow color and a delicate chocolate fragrance. That fragrance goes away within a few days after the soap is made. Deodorized cocoa butter is a light yellow and usually doesn't have any chocolate scent. Ultra-refined cocoa butter is white and has no scent. Cocoa butter has a hardness of 61.

Coconut Oil (*Cocos nucifera*)

Shelf life: 2 plus years.

Properties and benefits: Coconut oil is one of the three cleansing oils. It's inexpensive, at about 10¢ per ounce or less, depending on where and how much you buy. You can find this oil at your local grocery store on the isle with all the other cooking oils. Look for the oil with the brand name LouAna. It's in a white plastic jar with a green lid.

Soap-makers use coconut oil in all types of soap for its cleansing and cost factors. This oil is refined, bleached, and deodorized. It's high in lauric and myristic fatty acids, and has a high cleansing quality along with hardness and high bubbly lather. There are three types of coconut oil used in soap making: coconut 76 degree hardness is 79, coconut 92 degree hardness is 79, fractionated coconut hardness is 93. Coconut 76 degree is the type we most often use.

Corn Oil (*Zea mays*)

Shelf life: 1 year unopened; 4 to 6 months opened.

Properties and benefits: Corn oil creates a stable, creamy lather and is high in conditioning. Refrigeration helps extend corn oil's shelf life, or you can add 1 percent rosemary oleo resin extract. Corn oil contains the fatty acids palmitic, stearic, oleic, linoleic, and linolenic. You can easily find it in your local grocery store. It has a hardness of 14.

Emu Oil

Shelf life: Short. Refrigerate after opening.

Properties and benefits: Used in soap at 10 to 20 percent, emu oil makes a hard bar with a stable, moisturizing lather. This is another oil we often use in facial bars. It is known to sink deep into the tissues, bringing the other oils and essential oils with it. For those who want that type of benefit but who prefer not to use an animal by-product, Meadowfoam Seed oil is the vegan alternative. Emu oil contains palmetic and oleic fatty acids. It is an excellent choice to use when making a bar of soap for people with skin problems such as eczema or psoriasis. It has a hardness of 32.

From the Soap Pot

Use emu oil in massage or sports blends to help relieve soreness and inflammation.

Flaxseed Oil (Linseed)

Shelf life: 1 year. Refrigerate after opening.

Properties and benefits: Flaxseed oil must be blended with stable oils or an antioxidant such as rosemary oil extract (ROE). Use 1 percent per the weight of oil. If you have a 32-ounce (907.6-gram) bottle, use 0.3 ounce (8.5 grams) ROE. Flaxseed oil contains palmetic and oleic fatty acids. It is helpful for those who suffer from eczema, psoriasis, rosacea, acne, and dry or aging skin. It has a hardness of 9.

Grape Seed Oil (*Vitis vinifera*)

Shelf life: 6 months.

Properties and benefits: Grape seed oil is rich in flavonoids called procyanidolic oligomers (PCOs). These phytochemicals have antioxidant properties. (Antioxidants safeguard the cells against damage by unstable oxidant molecules called free radicals.) In addition, PCOs are thought to improve blood circulation and help strengthen blood vessels. Flavonoids also inhibit allergic reactions. These factors help fight against uncomfortable skin problems encountered with eczema. It is great for use in soap for those who suffer from skin problems such as eczema or psoriasis. It's also known to rebuild cellular tissue. This oil quickly and easily penetrates the skin, and it has almost no odor. Grapeseed oil is not an expensive oil, and it's a favorite for use in lotions and other leave-on products. Plus, it has a slight astringent property, which helps tighten pores and tones the skin. Grapeseed has a hardness of 12.

From the Soap Pot

To help prevent head lice in young children, add 1 ounce (28.4 grams) light oil such as almond or grapeseed oil mixed with ½ teaspoon (2.5 milliliters) tea tree essential oil and 7 ounces (198.5 grams) distilled water. Bottle the mixture in a fine mist spray bottle. After shampooing, spray the child's hair lightly while it is still wet. Tea tree essential oil repels the lice, and the oil helps detangle the hair. Be sure to shake the bottle before each use.

Hemp Seed Oil (*Cannabis sativa*)

Shelf life: 6 months to 1 year.

Properties and benefits: This oil is rich in vitamins A and E, is good for dry and/or irritated skin, and reduces inflammation. Hemp seed oil is used in similar ways as flaxseed oil. It's an excellent choice for use in shampoo bars for its hair-conditioning benefits, adding shine and silkiness to the hair. In soap, it adds conditioning and is an excellent choice for soap for mature skin. Use a small percent because it increases the iodine. Hempseed oil has a hardness of 8.

Illipe Butter (*Shorea stenoptera*)

Shelf life: 2 years.

Properties and benefits: Illipe butter is very hard and similar to cocoa butter. It can be used in soap-making to create firm and highly moisturizing bars with a creamy lather. Illipe butter is often substituted for cocoa butter in bath and body products. It has a hardness of 62.

Jojoba Oil (*Simmondsia chinensis*)

Shelf life: Infinite.

Properties and benefits: Jojoba oil is actually a liquid wax. In soap, it's often used in shampoo bars because it adds shine and gloss to the hair. It's very close to the natural oil, sebum, which the body produces for protecting the skin. Because of this, jojoba oil can be used in facial and other soaps for those who have acne. It can help control acne by tricking the glands into slowing down their sebum production. Jojoba oil can be used on all skin types. It's more often used in bath and body products. We use jojoba in our mineral makeup to help the powders adhere better to the skin. It's also an excellent makeup remover. Jojoba oil is a stable oil and often is used to extend the shelf life of other oils. When jojoba oil gets cold it becomes solid. It has a hardness of 0.

Soap Stats

During the 1930s, scientists analyzed the composition and properties of jojoba. They were surprised to find that jojoba is not based on triglycerides like most liquid oils and solid fats. It's actually liquid esters, making it a liquid wax.

Karanja Oil (*Pongammia glabra*)

Shelf life: 2 years.

Properties and benefits: Karanja oil is cold pressed from seeds. The oil is reddish-brown in color, rather viscous, and inedible. It has antiseptic properties, plus it's known for its natural insecticide qualities. To treat head lice without chemicals, add karanja oil to a small amount of shampoo, and wash the child's hair. We use karanja oil at the rate of 12 percent in soap. Most of the time it's combined with 10 percent neem oil for those who have eczema or psoriasis. This combination is also used in soaps for our pets because it repels fleas and ticks. Karanja oil has a hardness of 12.

Kokum Butter (*Garcinia indica*)

Shelf life: 2 years.

Properties and benefits: Kokum butter is a hard and brittle butter that's cream in color. It's the hardest butter with the highest melting point. Like cocoa butter, kokum butter melts quickly when it comes in contact with the skin. In soap, kokum butter can be used to

From the Soap Pot

When remelting kokum butter, be sure to leave empty space in your container in case the butter expands or "climbs" as it cools.

produce a hard, creamy bar of soap with high moisturizing properties. It has a hardness of 60.

Lanolin

Shelf life: 3 years.

Lanolin, known as wool oil or wool grease, has no useful benefits for making soap. It's a smelly, sticky substance that's actually a wax and not a fat or oil. Often lanolin is used in cosmetics. Its hardness is 0.

Lard

Shelf life: 12 to 18 months.

Properties and benefits: Lard, or pig fat, produces a moisturizing bar of soap but does not produce a lot of lather. To increase the lather and add cleansing in soap, you need to also use coconut oil and castor oil. Lard tends to make a soft soap and is often used in conjunction with tallow or vegetable oils like coconut or palm to increase the hardness. Lard is very inexpensive, and you can find it at your local grocery store. It makes a gentle white bar of soap. Lard has a hardness of 42.

Mango Butter (*Limnanthes alba*)

Shelf life: 2 to 3 years.

Properties and benefits: This white butter is hard and high in stearic acid. It's also a great source of essential fatty acids and antioxidants. Mango is one of our favorite butters, and we love to use it in our soap because it adds creamy lather and hardness to the bar. Mango butter has a similar conditioning value as shea butter. It's great for using in products such as lip balms and lotion bars because it adds firmness as well as moisturizing properties. Mango has a hardness of 53.

Mowrah Butter (*Madhuca latifolia*)

Shelf life: 1 year.

Properties and benefits: Mowrah butter is hard and solid at room temperature but melts quickly when it comes in contact with the skin. It has moisturizing properties and is known to help prevent wrinkles. In soap, it adds conditioning and a creamy lather. The ultra-refined mowrah butter is wonderful in lip balms and lipsticks, and gives them a rich and smooth texture while it helps keep the lips soft. Mowrah butter is a great addition to your lotions and creams. It's also excellent to put on a burn because it stops the pain and even stops blistering if it's used soon enough. This butter is one of the softer butters with a hardness of only 46.

Soap Stats _____

Mowrah butter is imported from India. Since 2009, this butter has become harder to buy. About all we can find is the gently refined version, which is a dark yellow color and has a strong nutty fragrance. For our products, we prefer the ultra-refined mowrah butter.

Neem Seed Oil (*Azadirachta indica*)

Shelf life: 2 years.

Properties and benefits: Neem seed oil gets rid of head lice and won't poison your child. Add 1 tablespoon (15 milliliters) neem seed oil to 8 ounces (226.8 grams) of your regular shampoo. It also gets rid of fleas and won't harm your pet with pesticides that are in commercial products. Neem seed oil is great to use in soap that's for eczema, psoriasis, and acne. It's considered safe and can be used in skin products. The only problem with this oil is that it doesn't have a pleasant smell. Bars of soap made with neem seed oil don't have an unpleasant smell after they've cured, and with the use of an essential oil like juniper, they can have a very nice smell. We've used neem seed oil at 10 percent in soap, up to 5 percent in hand- and foot-care products, and at 1 or 2 percent as an insect repellent. Neem seed oil has a hardness of 33.

Olive Oil (*Olea europaea*)

Shelf life: 1 year.

Properties and benefits: Olive oil is the oldest-known oil used for soap. It's the ideal soap for a newborn or anyone who has a problem with their skin. Soap containing at least 50 percent olive oil is called castile. It's not a high-lathering soap, so if you want, you can add coconut, babassu, or palm kernel oil to add cleansing. For more lather, add castor oil. 100 percent olive oil soap has a cleansing number of 0, but it's very high in conditioning. In soap-making, the bars made

Soap Stats _____

Because olive oil is naturally high in oleic acid, it is very stable and has a long shelf life. Several other oils we use are termed *high oleic*. These other oils have been bred to have less polyunsaturated fat and more monounsaturated (oleic acid) fat. The outcome gives these oils a longer shelf life and stability, similar to that of olive oil.

with high olive oil are very soft when you first remove them from the soap mold but in time, they become very hard. To help speed this curing and hardening time, use a water discount. Many soap-makers regularly use olive oil in their soap recipes. In liquid soap, a high amount of olive oil seems to help thicken the soap. It has a hardness of 17.

Olive Oil Pomace

Shelf life: 1 year.

Properties and benefits: This very stable oil does not go rancid easily and can be stored without refrigeration for a year. Olive oil pomace creates a long-lasting, nondrying, mild soap with a creamy lather. It's very gentle. This oil makes a great soap to use for babies and the elderly who have dry skin. The downside is that the oil often discolors the soap to a slight olive color. Some people may find certain grades unpleasantly strong-smelling. It has a hardness of 17.

Ostrich Oil

Shelf life: 1 year. Keep refrigerated.

Properties and benefits: Ostrich oil contains essential fatty acids known for their skin-conditioning properties, making it ideal for lotions, shampoos, creams, and soaps. Just like emu oil, ostrich oil is an excellent oil to use in your facial bars. Ostrich oil sinks deep into the skin's tissues and acts like a carrier, delivering all the other ingredients to the deep tissues at the same time. It has a hardness of 36.

Palm Oil (*Elaesis guineensis*)

Shelf life: 2 years.

Properties and benefits: Palm oil makes a nice, hard bar when used in combination with other oils such as coconut and olive oil. Soap-makers use this oil as a base and stabilizer. The difference between palm kernel oil (nut inside the fruit) and palm oil is that palm kernel is white and has a higher melting point. Palm kernel oil is also one of the three cleansing oils, whereas palm oil has no cleansing values. It is also solid at room temperature. Palm oil is beige-colored and has a lower melting point close to room temperature—unless it's homogenized, and then it will be the last to melt in your pot. Palm oil is like milk in that it separates when left sitting. Before you can use palm oil to make soap, you have to completely melt all the oil and stir it very well. If you don't, you may find white, chalky veins running through your soap. The chalky vein is the stearic acid that's separated. It doesn't hurt the oil to melt and then later reuse it over and over. During the winter months, you can buy homogenized palm oil, which does not need to be melted and stirred before use. Palm oil has a hardness of 50.

Soap Stats

Oils with higher melting points are hard and make harder soaps that take longer to melt in the bath or shower.

Palm Oil (Red Unrefined, Unbleached, Nondeodorized)

Shelf life: 2 years.

Properties and benefits: Unrefined, not bleached or deodorized, this oil contains vitamins K and E. In Africa, it's used mainly for cooking. We love this oil for all its skin benefits. Red palm oil is like whole milk; it separates. Before you can use the oil, you have to melt the entire container and stir the oil very well before it's ready to use. It doesn't hurt the oil to remelt it over and over again. If you fail to melt and stir the oil, your soap will have a waxy vain running through it. When the bar gets wet, the waxy vain washes away, leaving a gap in the soap bar. In soap and lotions, it produces a lovely apricot yellow color. It has a hardness of 50.

Soap Stats

Red palm oil contains very high levels of the two most important types of vitamin E and carotenoid, which our bodies changes to vitamin A. The vitamin A is what gives the red palm its deep-orange/red color.

Palm Kernel Oil (*Elaesis guineensis*)

Shelf life: 2 years.

Properties and benefits: Also known as palm nut, palm kernel oil is pressed from the kernels of the palm tree fruit. It has a high percentage of lauric acid, which is why palm kernel oil produces a hard soap and a rich lather. Soap made with this oil is white with a smooth texture. Palm kernel oil is often substituted in place of coconut oil because it's very stable. Palm kernel oil is one of the three oils you can use for adding cleansing to your soap. (The other two are coconut and babassu.) We don't recommend using two of the cleansing oils together in a batch of soap. Palm kernel oil comes in a flake form or solid in a container. It has a hardness of 70.

Peanut Oil (*Arachis hypogaea*)

Shelf life: 1 year.

Properties and benefits: Peanut oil has a high content of vitamin E. It's a thick conditioning oil that has a slight fragrance and is slow to penetrate so it leaves your skin with an oily feeling. It is good for all skin types. In soap-making, this oil is best when used in a small amount. It adds conditioning and has a long-lasting creamy lather. Many people have severe allergies to peanuts, so if you use this oil in your soap, you have to clearly mark it on the label. Peanut oil is easy to find in your local grocery store. It has a hardness of 11.

Safety First

Peanut oil should not be used by anyone allergic to peanuts.

Rice Bran Oil (*Oryza sativa*)

Shelf life: 1 year.

Properties and benefits: Rice bran oil is high in vitamin E. The oil comes from the husk part of rice. Many use this oil in place of the more expensive olive oil in soap-making. Blending rice bran oil in equal parts with sunflower oil, high oleic, gives you a less-expensive oil that's comparable to olive oil. It isn't a heavy oil, and it doesn't leave a greasy feel on the skin. It's an excellent moisturizer that's often used in massage oils, lotions, eye creams, and baby products. It's also good for liquid soaps. Rice bran oil has a hardness of 26.

Safflower Oil, High Oleic (*Carthamus tinctorius*)

Shelf life: Less than 3 months without refrigeration or 2 years mixed with 1 percent rosemary oleic resin extract. Keep refrigerated.

Properties and benefits: Safflower oil is very light and moisturizing; however, it's used more in leave-on products and not very often in soap-making. Because it doesn't stain sheets, it's often used with other oils in massage oils. You can find this oil at your local grocery store. It has a hardness of 7.

Sal Butter (*Shorea robusta*)

Shelf life: 1 year.

Properties and benefits: Sal butter, imported from India, is produced from the seeds of the sal tree. This hard, light-yellow butter is recommended for use in soap to add hardness and conditioning. It also has nice skin-softening qualities. It's more often used in body products such as lotions and creams because of its uniform triglyceride composition, which gives it high oxidative and emulsion stability. It's an ideal choice to use in balms and lotion bars. Like cocoa butter, sal butter melts easily on the skin. It has a hardness of 50.

Shea Butter (*Butyrospermum parkii*)

Shelf life: 1 to 2 years; longer if refrigerated.

Properties and benefits: Shea butter, a hard butter rich in vitamins A, E, and F, along with other vitamins and minerals, adds wonderful conditioning properties to soap. We have used from 5 percent up to 40 percent shea butter in soap and found that the magic number is around 10 percent for soap you want to use or sell now. A bar of soap made with 20 to 40 percent shea butter gets better with age. Letting it age for over a year, even 2 years, gives the soap time to fully come into its own and becomes an incredibly moisturizing bar of soap. Shea butter is also helpful for those who have eczema and psoriasis. It has a hardness of 45.

Soybean Oil (*Glycine soja*)

Shelf life: 1 year.

Properties and benefits: This high-protein oil contains lecithin; unsaturated fatty acid; sterols; and vitamins A, E, and K. It's easy to obtain from the grocery store, but it isn't an oil that has any special benefits for the skin. When you use it in a soap, you have to watch the iodine value because it is so high. When we used it in liquid soap the first time and weren't watching the iodine level, the soap went rancid in less than a month. It has a hardness of 16.

Soap Stats

The soybean oil we use is a European Union, non-GMO (genetically modified organism) type, which means the soybeans haven't been genetically modified through any biotechnology procedures to add a specific trait. These soybeans are stored untreated and without any chemical pesticides.

Sunflower Oil, High Oleic (*Helianthus annuus*)

Shelf life: 2 years.

Properties and benefits: Sunflower oil has a high vitamin E content and contains lecithin, tocopherols, carotenoids, and waxes. It resists infection by forming a protective barrier, and it's very moisturizing for the skin. This oil is the oil we most often use for infusing with herbs we want to use in our soaps or bath and body products. You can buy this oil at your local grocery store. There are two types of sunflower oil. We use the high oleic type. It has a hardness of 7.

Tallow, Beef

Shelf life: 1 year from manufacture.

Properties and benefits: Rendered from beef fat, tallow is high in oleic, palmitic, and stearic acids and is an inexpensive addition to soap. It adds some conditioning, cleansing, and creamy lather as well as hardens the bar of soap. It is also inexpensive, making your soap batch more cost-effective. Beef tallow, when combined with other oils, produces a hard, long-lasting, white soap bar that has a rich and silky lather. It has a hardness of 58.

Frequently Asked Questions About Oils and Butters

What kinds of oils do most soap-makers use?   There seem to be four favorites among soap-makers: castor oil, which adds lather and is moisturizing; coconut oil for cleansing; olive oil for moisturizing; and palm oil for hardness and stability.

Can I use motor oil for my soap?   No. It has no values that will interact with the lye.

Can I use LouAna Coconut Oil I see at the grocery store?   Yes, that is 76 degree coconut oil. That means the oil is solid if the temperature is cooler than 76 degrees Fahrenheit.

Is regular shortening from the grocery store okay to use?   Yes, you can use it. But other than the Spectrum brand, which is 100 percent palm oil that's been homogenized, regular shortening doesn't add much to your soap.

The Least You Need to Know

◆ The oils and butters available to use in your soaps is long and should inspire your creativity.

◆ Each oil and butter have specific properties and qualities, so you can more easily choose the best oil or butter for your soap.

◆ You can buy many of your soap-making oils in your local grocery store.

Fragrance and Essential Oils

In This Chapter

- ◆ Using fragrance oils in your soap
- ◆ Tips on blending fragrance oils
- ◆ A look at essential oils
- ◆ Tips for using essential oils in soap

Nearly every soap-maker becomes addicted to and excited about scents and scent blends. We joke with each other about our passion, that the family doesn't need groceries this week because there's a fragrance oil prebuy starting, and that's more important than food.

It's all in fun, but deep down, there's a grain of truth. We soap-makers love our fragrance and essential oils. Soon, you will, too.

Fun with Fragrance Oils

You've had a rough day. Traffic was terrible. Your boss scolded you for your co-worker's error. Your kids and their friends had made a mess of the kitchen by the time you got home from work. And to top it off, you've had a headache all day. You want to escape from it all in a bath filled with the scents of lavender and vanilla in a soap you made yourself. That's where fragrance oils come in.

Fragrance oils are soothing and relaxing. You can lie in your tub, surrounded by scents, and just let the world go by. Light a scented candle while you're at it, and relax even more. Before you know it, your headache is gone and you're rejuvenated, ready to face that huge mess in the kitchen!

Choose Your Scent

Fragrance oils are synthetic blends made from chemicals that mimic scents and essential oils that are then added to bases. Fragrance oils are formulated in different ways for specific products—candles, bath and body products, and soap. You can find any number of fragrance oils. Here's a list of a few of the most popular fragrances:

◆ Spellbound Woods is a seductive blend of top notes of amber, middle notes of cedar and sandalwood, and faint bottom notes hinting a touch of floral.

◆ Black Tea and Berries is a fresh and deliciously fruity blend of berries with a touch of red clover.

◆ Cool Mountain Lake is a fresh, crisp, and clean water fragrance.

◆ Lavender Rose is a lovely blend of French lavender with rose top notes complimented by musk, moss, and muget. Add a little powdery note, and you have a very romantic, soft, and sexy scent.

◆ Cucumber Mint is a rejuvenating blend of fresh mint and cold, crisp cucumbers.

◆ Hardwood Musk blooms with notes of sandalwood, cedarwood, oak, and myrtle woods with earthy base notes. This a very sexy male fragrance women love to smell on their fellas.

◆ Fresh Pomegranate is, just like the name implies, a sweet fruity-cranberry scent.

That's just a sampling of the more than 7,500 fragrances on the market today. Many are duplicates of popular colognes and commercial home fragrance lines. No matter what type of fragrance you love, you will certainly find plenty to choose from.

Safety First

It's important that you only use fragrances safe for skin in your soaps. Choose your vendor carefully, and know what you're buying.

You'll hear a lot about *phthalates* in fragrance oils and how harmful these are. There are several different types of phthalates, and some are more harmful than others. Phthalates are usually found in some of the bases manufacturers use, but you can find many phthalate-free fragrances.

Fragrance oils have what are called *flash points*. A flash point is the temperature at which the fragrance oil gives off just enough vapor that will ignite when an open flame is applied. Every fragrance oil is given a flash point number.

Lather Lingo

Phthalates are chemicals used to soften plastics and make them flexible. They're also in cosmetics, plastic toys, beverage bottles, flooring, furniture, wallpaper, and thousands of other everyday things. There are seven types of phthalate compounds. The one used in premade fragrance oil base is diethyl phthalate (DEP). It's considered safe and is used as a fragrance stabilizer. Many fragrance oil manufacturers are starting to offer phthalate-free fragrances.

Flash point is important when you're using a fragrance oil in candles. A too-low flash point could cause the candle to catch fire. If your wick burns at 160°F, you wouldn't want to use a fragrance oil with a flash point of 140°F. Flash point isn't as important in soap-making because we don't use open flames when making soap. That said, there are restrictions on how low a flash point can be and still be shipped by the postal service or allowed to be brought into other countries. Fragrance oils with flash points of 200°F and greater can be shipped through regular mail. All others have to be shipped by the other carriers.

How Much Do I Use in Soap?

You want your soap to smell nice, but you don't want it so strong you get a headache from the scent, so it's important to know how much fragrance oil to use. As a general rule of thumb, for stronger fragrance oils, use only .5 to .7 ounce per pound of oil. If it's a light fragrance, use 1 ounce per pound of oil. Bath and body products generally contain 1 to 3 percent fragrance oil.

Serious soap-makers have a lot of money invested in fragrances. The more concentrated the fragrance is, the higher the cost. You actually save money buying the higher-priced oil because you use less fragrance oil per pound of soap. With the cheaper and

Safety First

When it comes to fragrance oils, you get what you pay for.

weaker fragrances, you have to use 1 ounce or more per pound of soap and even then, the fragrance may fade within a month or two. As you learn more about soap-making, you'll see that $25-a-pound fragrance formulated for soap is usually more cost-effective than one of the much cheaper fragrances.

Blending Fragrance Oils

Many soap-makers enjoy blending their fragrance oils to create new scents. You can blend fragrances, even those from different manufacturers, or add an essential oil to a fragrance oil to make a new scent. As you saw in the list of fragrance oils earlier in this chapter, you have many options when it comes to fragrance oil scents. Be creative and have some fun. For example, to make a man's cologne fragrance oil into one suitable for a female fragrance, all you have to do is add a little floral fragrance oil. It's that easy!

Some soap-makers add the fragrance oil to the warm oils before adding the lye mixture. Some wait until light trace. We prefer waiting until light trace.

Frequently Asked Questions About Fragrance Oils

Are any fragrance oils made to be used only in soap? Yes, but you can also use them in all your other bath and body products, too. They are more expensive, but you use a lot less per pound of oil, so in the long run you save money.

Can I use any fragrance oil in soap? No. It has to be skin-safe. Don't use fragrance oil that's not labeled skin-safe.

Can I use my favorite perfume to scent my soap? No. You have to use fragrance oils or essential oils formulated to be used in soap-making. And remember, they have to be skin-safe.

Can I blend fragrances together to create my own scent even if they're from different vendors? Yes, as long as they're all skin-safe and formulated for the product you intend to make.

Enhancing Soaps with Essential Oils

You might be wondering why we've included *essential oils* in a book on making soap. Here's our line of thought: essential oils were our first "medicine," so why not add them to soap to help with different skin or hair problems? Not only can you use them for medicinal reasons, but some of them are also great for adding fragrance to the soap. (Be sure to write down all the combinations you like so you can remember them!)

Do not use essential oils as if they were fragrance oils. Because essential oils are distilled from the roots, bark, flower, stems, and leaves of plants, they contain the true essence of the plant they were derived from. Therefore, they're very potent and can be irritating if too strong. You are told in the recipes later in the book what percentage of essential oils to use.

Lather Lingo

Essential oils are volatile oils extracted from plant matter by distillation, expression, or solvents that can be blended together and with other natural essences to make scents for use in perfumes and colognes. Essential oils aren't just for scenting; they also have medicinal properties and are widely used in aromatherapy.

The Usefulness of Essential Oils in Soap

With more and more antibiotic-resistant bacteria, mutating viruses, disease-causing parasites, and infectious fungi in the news each day, it can be comforting to know we have essential oils to rely on because, although the mutating bacteria in viruses can become resistant to Western medicines, they never become resistant to essential oils. When essential oils were tested by diffusing, the report was that the essential oils killed 100 percent of bacteria and viruses in the room. A study in France showed the antiseptic qualities of 34 essential oils. Among them, thyme, origanum, sweet orange, lemongrass, Chinese cinnamon, and rose were so antiseptic that one part of these rendered 1,000 parts of raw sewage free of all living organisms.

Although this knowledge has been known and applied with great success for ages, it's just now being rediscovered. An inquisitive doctor put some of the microbe-laden air from a hospital into a flask containing just a few drops of essential oils, and after 20 minutes, 40 percent of the microbes were destroyed; 80 percent in an hour, and 100 percent in 9 hours!

Essential oils should be called germ-killing oils! They're so good to add to soaps for acne and other conditions where germs are a problem.

Adding Essential Oils to Soap

Peppermint, cinnamon, and clove all smell great in soap but can cause a great deal of pain and burning if you use too much. If you want the smell of cinnamon and clove in your soap, use the cooking herbs you have in the spice rack in the kitchen rather than essential oils. Or you can buy a skin-safe fragrance oil that's been formulated for use in making soap.

When adding essential oils to soap, never use them as if they were fragrance oils. They are too potent and could cause a skin problem. Most essential oils should only be used at .5 percent and never higher than .7 percent.

When using essential oils in creams or lotions, we suggest you buy a book that tells the percentages that have been tested for each and every essential oil. A great one is *Plant Aromatics* by Martin Watt (Martin Watt, 1992).

Common Essential Oils You Can Use

Now let's take a look at some of the essential oils you might use in your soaps.

Note: This information isn't meant to take the place of professional medical help. It's only a guideline of known uses for essential oils.

Balsam peru (*Myroxylon pereirae*)   Known uses: helps hold fragrance in products; good for chapped hands and feet; and relieves itching caused by scabies, eczema, and ringworm. Use a small amount at a time.

Basil, sweet (*Ocimum basilicum*)   Antibacterial, antispasmodic, and anti-inflammatory. Known uses: for pain relief, virus and chest infections, mouth ulcers, muscle aches, and infected gums; serves as a digestive aid; helps rheumatoid arthritis; and aids in circulation and urinary tract infections.

Bay laurel (*Laurus nobilis*)   Antiseptic and *expectorant.* Known uses: for colds, virus infections, muscle aches and pains, sprains, bruises, hair loss, greasy hair, and flaky scalp; can act as a scalp and hair tonic, respiratory system inhalant, and liver and kidney tonic. Try it in shampoo bars!

Lather Lingo

An **expectorant** thins and loosens mucus congestion in the lungs and bronchial tubes.

Bay rum (*Pimento racemosa*)   Known uses: for general aches and pains, scalp conditions, acne, dandruff, and greasy hair; acts as an appetite stimulant; and settles stomach pains. Try using it in a shampoo bar or gel.

Benzoin (*Styrax benzoin*)   Antiseptic and expectorant. Known uses: as a pulmonary antiseptic; for acne, eczema, and psoriasis; acts as a preservative in foods; and helps hold fragrance in soap.

Bergamot (*Citrus bergamia*)   Antiseptic, expectorant. Known uses: relaxes the nervous system; acts as a digestive aid and a gargle for sore throats; helps anxiety, depression, mild respiratory and urinary tract infections, wounds, herps, acne, and oily skin. Bergamot can be a photosensitizer (a substance that absorbs light), so use the bergaptene-free version. *Should not be used when pregnant.*

Cajeput (*Melaleuca leucadendron*)   Antiseptic, analgesic, and expectorant. Known uses: acts as an insect repellant; helps with skin care, wound cleansing; acts as a stimulant; soothes colic and vomiting; and helps respiratory tract infections, nasal and sinus congestion, headaches, gout, muscle stiffness, pain, fire ant bites, menstrual cramps, acne, genital herpes, hemorrhoids, and varicose veins. From the same family as tea tree and manuka.

Carrot seed (*Daucus carota*)   Stimulant. Known uses: acts as a tonic for liver regeneration and cholesterol control; helps mature wrinkled skin; tones the skin, stimulates blood cells; adds elasticity to the skin; helps burns, weeping sores, ulcers, boils, eczema, psoriasis, carbuncles, and scars; and can be used as a massage oil and blood purifier.

Cedarwood, atlas (*Cedrus atlantica*)   Antibacterial. Known uses: acts as an insecticide; helps remove body fat, cellulite, fluid retention, respiratory ailment discomfort, dandruff, oily skin and scalp, alopecia, acne, eczema, bladder and kidney functions, and psoriasis; reduces oily secretions; acts as a hair tonic for seborrhea of the scalp; can be used in chest rubs; helps hold fragrances. Can also be used in men's fragrances, in facial washes and shampoos, in tonics, and in chest rubs. This is a true cedar, also known as Atlantic cedar or Moroccan cedarwood.

Safety First _____

Do not confuse atlas cedarwood with Texas or Virginia cedarwood. And do not use on children or pregnant women.

Cinnamon bark (*Cinnamomum zeylanicum*)   Antibacterial, antispasmodic, antiseptic, aphrodisiac, and antifungal. Known uses: acts as an insecticide and room spray; can be inhaled for a respiratory and circulatory stimulant; helps exhaustion and depression. The bark oil is a dermal toxin, so don't use it on the skin. If you want a cinnamon-smelling soap, use the cinnamon you cook with instead.

Clary sage (*Salvia sclaria*)   Antispasmotic and analgesic. Known uses: helps nervous tension, fear, paranoia, depression; relaxes; inhibits prolactin; helps during menopause; sooths digestion; accelerates labor; helps throat and respiratory infections; cools inflammation; and helps hold fragrances in soaps, perfumes, and cosmetics. *Do not use while pregnant or nursing.*

Combava petitgrain (*Citrus hystrix*)   Antiseptic and anti-inflammatory. Known uses: acts as a liver decongestant and sedative; calms; and relieves stress, agitation, insomnia, skin inflammation, and acne. Do not use on sensitive skin. You can use it in soap for acne.

Coriander (*Coriandrum sativum*)   Anti-inflammatory. Known uses: for stress, anxiety, insomnia, to stimulate the mind, arthritis pain, migraines, clears black heads and tames oily skin.

Cypress (*Cupressus sempervirens*)   Antiseptic and antispasmodic. Known uses: acts as a deodorant, diuretic, haemostatic, hepatic, stryptic, vasoconstrictor, respiratory tonic, and sedative; can be inhaled for strength and comfort, or diluted in a carrier oil and used to massage varicose veins every day. Try it in a deodorant soap!

Elemi (*Canarium luzonicum*)   Antifungal, antiseptic, analgesic, and expectorant. It's nontoxic, nonirritating, and nonsensitizing. Known uses: helps nervous exhaustion and stress, skin and acne, cell regeneration, dry and mature skin, wounds, sores, inflamed skin, eczema, and dermatitis; balances sebum secretions; and controls heavy perspiration.

Eucalyptus (*Eucalyptus globulus*)   Also called blue gum. Antiseptic, antirheumatic, expectorant, analgesic, and insecticide. Known uses: acts as a decongestant, inhibits cold viruses, repels insects, lowers fevers, eases breathing, clears sinus congestion, loosens phlegm, and can be used in room sprays. Should never be taken internally.

Eucalyptus (*Eucalyptus radiate*)   Antiviral and expectorant. Known uses: same as eucalyptus globules. This one is gentler and a more pleasant oil to use. For a scent blend, try blending it with spearmint.

Eucalyptus, lemon (*Eucalyptus citriodora*)   Antiviral, antibacterial, antifungal, and analgesic. Known uses: helps viral, bacterial, and fungal skin infections; colds and flu; is calming; acts as a sedative and an antihypertensive. Useful in soap.

Fir needle (*Abies alba*)   Analgesic, antiseptic, expectorant, deodorant. Known uses: inhaled for anxiety, stress, and respiratory issues; is warming; good for massages; and relieves muscle aches, pain, and rheumatic or arthritic conditions.

Soap Stats _____

You can use essential oils to make room sprays to kill bacteria. Mix 1 teaspoon (5 milliliters) vodka or perfumer's alcohol with 7 ounces (198.5 grams) distilled water in a spray bottle. Add 1 teaspoon (5 milliliters) essential oil or essential oil blend. To help the oil blend with the water, you might want to add 1 teaspoon (5 milliliter) of an emulsifier such as polysorbate 20. Shake the bottle before each use.

Fir needle, Canada (*Abies canadensis*)   Canadian balsum and Siberian fir are favored for their wonderful fragrance. Known uses: good for respiratory problems, warming, massages, and deodorant and room sprays.

Frankincense (*Boswellia carteri*)   Also known as olibanum. Antiseptic and astringent. Known uses: for anxiety and stress, dry and mature skin, wrinkles, scars, and wounds; acts as a diuretic; helps digestion; and can be used as a sedative. Mix with myrrh for soap.

Geranium (*Pelargonium graveolens*)   A.k.a. rose geranium. Antidepressant, antiseptic, and analgesic. Known uses: helps depression, anxiety, and PMS; acts as a diuretic, detoxifier; helps stimulate the lymphatic system; balances sebum; helps oily skin, wounds, ulcers, and burns; and repels mosquitoes.

Grapefruit, pink (*Citrus paradise*)   Stimulant, antidepressant, antiseptic, disinfectant. Known uses: helps depression; acts as a detoxifier and diuretic; helps cellulite, digestion, congestion, oily skin, and acne; and can be used as a room spray.

Jasmine (*Jasminum grandiflorum*)   Antidepressant, aphrodisiac, antiseptic, and antispasmodic. Known uses: helps depression, headaches, nervous exhaustion, stress, skin care, dermatitis, and eczema.

Juniper berry (*Juniperus communis*)   Antiseptic, antispasmodic, astringent, and expectorant. Known uses: acts as a diuretic; helps the urinary tract, cystitis, kidney stones, gout, acne, blocked pores, weeping eczema, psoriasis, and inflammations; and eliminates uric acid. The berries and extracts are used in diuretics, laxatives, gout treatment, wart treatments, flea and tick repellants, spicy fragrances, and aftershaves.

Lavender (*lavandula officinalis*)   Known uses: helps burns, headaches, sleep, athlete's foot, and herpes and acts as an insect repellant. Great in scent for soap.

Lavender, Bulgarian (*lavender augustifolia*)   Antidepressant, analgesic, antirheumatic, antiseptic, antispasmodic, antiviral, antibacterial, antifungal, and decongestant. Known uses: acts as a diuretic, deodorant, sedative, fungicide, and bactericide; calms; lowers high blood pressure; helps insomnia, sunburns, and scars; promotes new skin cells; and can be used in room sprays. It's also great in soap!

Lavender, super (*Lavandula* hybrid var. super French)   Antispasmatic. Known uses: helps headaches, relaxation, inflammation, acne, scabies, skin infections, and respiratory disorders. It's great in soap!

Lavendin, grosso (*Lavandula* hybrid var. grosso French)   Anti-inflammatory and antiseptic. Known uses: acts as a stimulant; helps acne, scabies, skin infections, and respiratory disorders. This is wonderful in soap.

Lemongrass (*cymbopogon citratus*)   Anti-inflammatory. Known uses: helps high blood pressure, gastrointestinal problems, and fever; can be used in deodorants, skin care, fragrances, and insect repellants; also good for aromatherapy.

Lemongrass, East Indian (*cymbopogon flexuosus*)   Anti-inflammatory. This genus has 200 species. Known uses: acts as a stimulant; helps aching muscles, headaches, nervous exhaustion, and stress; aids the flow of milk; stimulates hair; helps acne, athlete's foot, and open pores; and prevents the spread of contagious diseases. It also smells divine in soap.

Lather Lingo

When discussing ingredients, such as an essential oil, **neat** means to use it as it is, not diluted.

Litsea cubeba (*Litsea cubeba*)   A.k.a. may chang. Antidepressant, antiseptic, astringent, insecticide. Known uses: helps depression; calms; promotes sleep; acts as a sedative; and helps indigestion, flatulence, lower back pain, chills, travel sickness, headaches, excessive perspiration, acne, and oily skin. Also helps hold sweet orange essential oil in soap. Do not use *neat*.

Manuka (*Leptospermum scoparium*)   Antibacterial, antifungal, and antiviral. Known uses: proven effective against both strep and staph infections. It's very similar to tea tree but smells better. It can be used in place of tea tree, and it's great to use in soap for acne.

Myrrh (*Commiphora myrrha*)   Antiseptic, astringent, disinfectant, and deodorant. Known uses: acts as a diuretic; stimulates the immune system; helps gum disorders, sore throat, excessive mucus, colds, coughs, flatulence, hemorrhoids, wounds, weepy eczema, athlete's foot, jock itch, mouth ulcers, gingivitis, and bleeding or spongy gums. Do not use during pregnancy.

Myrtle (*Myrtus communis*)   Antiseptic, astringent, antibacterial, and expectorant. Nonirritating and nonsensitizing. Similar to eucalyptus. Known uses: helps pulmonary and urinary infections, hemorrhoids, insomnia, and nervous conditions and acts as a sedative. It's revitalizing and balancing.

Neroli (*Citrus aurantium*)   Antispasmatic, antidepressant, antiseptic, stimulant, and deodorant. Known uses: helps digestion, anxiety, depression, stress, insomnia, broken capillaries, and oily or dry skin. Balances sebum.

Niaouli (*Melaleuca quinquenervia*)   Antiseptic, antibacterial, insecticide, decongestant, and vermifuge. This is another melaleuca, and you can use it instead of tea tree oil. Known uses: stimulating and for head and chest colds. Does not smell as bad as tea tree oil.

Oak moss absolute (*Evernia prunastri*)   Characterized by its earthy, mossy, musky odor, oak moss's properties are more emotional and spiritual than physical. It's soluble in alcohol and is used as an anchor in all types of perfume. Known uses: in fragrances and respiratory oils and relieves congested sinuses. It also smells wonderful in soap.

Orange, bitter (*Citrus sinensis*)   Antiseptic; comes from the peel of the orange. Known uses: aids in calming, helps nervousness, is disinfecting, and is used in men's fragrances. Must be diluted before use.

Oregano (*Oreganum vulgare*)   Antibiotic, anti-inflammatory, antioxidant, and expectorant. Known uses: helps infections; relieves pain, coughing, fever, and digestion; counters effects of poison; soothes muscle spasms; and aids wounds.

Patchouli (*Pogostemon patchouli*)   Antidepressant, antiseptic, astringent, antifungal, and insecticide. Known uses: helps depression, wounds, acne, eczema, scars, cracked skin, fungal infections, scalp disorders, wrinkles, and cellulite; tightens skin; and aids in tissue regeneration. Try mixing with lemon, lime, or lavender essential oils for a wonderful scent.

Soap Stats

If you could only get one essential oil for the medicine cabinet, it should be oregano. With the super bugs that have reared their ugly heads, this is one that can take them all on and win.

Peppermint (*Menthe piperita*)   Decongestant, expectorant, and *emmenagogue*. Known uses: for cooling, pain relief, muscle aches, cramps, diarrhea, colic, nausea, bruises, joint pain, insect bites; acts as a stimulant; and helps itching or irritation and travel sickness. Avoid during pregnancy. When using in soap, be careful not to use too much because it can cause a burning sensation in sensitive areas.

Lather Lingo

An **emmenagogue** helps stimulate the blood flow in the pelvic area. It can help stimulate menstrual flow or help with menstrual problems.

Rosalina (*Melaleuca ericifolia*)   A.k.a. lavender tea tree. Antiseptic, antispasmodic, expectorant, and anticonvulsant. Known uses: helps respiratory congestion, infections, stress, and insomnia; calms. This is a twin to rosewood essential oil, and it's wonderful in soaps.

Rosemary (*Rosemarinus officinalis*)   Antidepressant, antirheumatic, antispasmodic, astringent, antimicrobial, and antiseptic. Known uses: helps depression, digestion, hypertension, blood circulation, gout, and tired muscles; acts as a diuretic; lowers high blood sugar; enhances the color in dark hair; and reduces static charge. Do not use if epileptic, have high blood pressure, or are pregnant. Rosemary is great to use in a shampoo bar or gel.

Rosewood (*Aniba roseaodora*)   A.k.a. *bois de rose*. Antiseptic, antidepressant, aphrodisiac, deodorant, and insecticide. Known uses: helps depression, infections, and odors.

Sage, dalmatian (*Salvia officinalis*)   Anti-inflammatory, antibacterial, and antiseptic. Known uses: helps digestion, inflamed or oily skin, alopecia, baldness, joint pain, muscle pain, and arthritis; acts as a diuretic; and stimulates hair growth. Can be toxic if overused. Do not use if you're pregnant or have high blood pressure.

Sage, Spanish (*Salvia lavandulifolia*)   Anti-inflammatory, antibacterial, and antiseptic. Has all the uses of *Salvia officinalis* without the dangers. *Avoid while pregnant.*

Soap Stats

Rosewood is native to the Amazon and is being overharvested. We suggest using rosalina instead.

Sandalwood-mysore (*Santalum album*)   Antiseptic, antispasmodic, aphrodisiac, expectorant, and astringent. Known uses: calms; soothes mucous membranes; acts as a diuretic and sedative; helps acne, infections, insomnia, sore throats, dry cough, dry eczema, aging and dehydrated skin, arthritis, muscle injuries, premenstrual pain, insect bites and stings, and inflammation.

Spearmint (*Menthe spicata*)   Antispasmodic, insecticide, and stimulant. Has the properties of peppermint essential oil, but it's not as potent. This can be used on children, too, and it mixes great with other fragrances for use in soap-making.

Spikenard (*Nardostachys jatamansi*)   Antifungal. Known uses: calms; helps serious skin conditions, athlete's foot, and dandruff. This is one of the oldest of the sacred oils.

Spruce (*Tsuga canadensi*)   Known uses: helps stress, anxiety, muscle aches and pains, joint pain, poor circulation, muscle spasms, and respiratory conditions.

Spruce, black (*Picea mariana*)   Has the same benefits as the *Tsuga canadensi*. Wonderful evergreen scent.

Styrax resin (*Liquidambar styraciflua*)   American styrax or red gum. Known uses: helps with wounds, ringworm, and scabies.

Tangerine (*Citrus reticulate*)   Antiseptic and antispasmodic. Known uses: acts as a sedative; helps with the stomach, stretch marks, and acne; and stimulates circulation. Can be a photosensitizer.

Tea tree (*Melaleuca alternifolia*)   Antibacterial, antiseptic, expectorant, antiviral, and insecticide. Known uses: helps infections, fungus, scars, and acne. Do not use this oil neat; always dilute it with a carrier oil. It's good to use in soap for acne.

Tea tree, lemon scented (*Leptospermum petersonii*)   Antibacterial, antifungal, and expectorant. This is a cousin of Manuka. Known uses: helps oily skin and acne; kills mold, fungus, and bacteria; and repels insects. Use in candles or a room spray to kill mold, fungus, and bacteria in the air.

Thyme (*Thymus vulgaris*)   Antirheumatic, antiseptic, antispasmodic, aphrodisiac, expectorant, and insecticide. Known uses: acts as a diuretic; and helps the heart, cicatrizant, gout, scalp, hair loss, and dandruff. This is a great choice for a shampoo bar or gel.

Thyme, linalol (*Thymus vulgaris linalool*)   Antibacterial, anti-infectious, and antifungal. This is the mildest of the thymes.

Verbena (*Lippia citriodora*)   Antidepressant and antispasmodic. Known uses: helps depression, insomnia, nervous fatigue, stress, digestion, nausea, fever, and flatulence.

Vetiver, El Salvador (*Vetiveria zizanoides*)   Known uses: relaxing, mild sedative, balances sebum production. Used in making fragrances.

Violet leaf (*Viola odorata*)   Decongestant and stimulant. Known uses: helps the liver, aging and problem skin, enlarged pores, and blackheads; acts as a circulatory stimulant. Used in making fragrances.

Yarrow (*Achillea milleflorum*)   Anti-inflammatory and stimulant. Deep blue in color. Known uses: for acne, oily skin or scalp, hair growth, rheumatoid arthritis; acts as a circulatory stimulant; and repels ticks. *Do not use for pregnant women, small children, or babies.*

Ylang ylang (*Canangium odoratum*)   Antidepressant. Known uses: for depression, insomnia, constipation, dermatitis, diabetes, emotional exhaustion, epilepsy, blood pressure, indigestion, stomachaches, muscle spasms, nervous tension, temporomandibular joint disorder (TMJ), sexual difficulties, acne, and hair loss.

Frequently Asked Questions About Essential Oils

Is it safe to use essential oils for babies and young children?   Yes, but with one warning: do not use essential oils on a baby younger than 3 months. Along the same lines, there are some essential oils that pregnant women shouldn't use or come in contact with. We make a lavender bath oil with essential oil that helps calm children and ease them to sleep right after their bath. Now that's heaven!

My father is a diabetic. Can I use peppermint essential oil to scent soap for him? No. Everything we've read about diabetics and peppermint essential oil says not to mix the two.

Can you mix fragrance oils and essential oil to make a blend for soap? Yes, as long as the fragrance oil is rated as soap- and skin-safe. One of our favorite blends is made with equal parts patchouli essential oil, sandalwood fragrance oil, and ½ part English garden fragrance oil. We call that blend Peach on Earth!

The Least You Need to Know

- Essential oils can help with a multitude of aches and pains and other bothersome aspects of your everyday life.

- You can really get creative when you use essential oils.

- Certain essential oils are antibacterial and are great to use for a natural antibacterial soap.

Chapter 4

Say Hello to SoapCalc

In This Chapter

- Using SoapCalc
- What numbers do I want my soap to have?
- Formulating the type of soap you want

As you read in earlier chapters, you don't need a lot of different kinds of ingredients to make soap. Some oil/butter, some lye, some water, and you've got your basic recipe. But there's more to it than that, and that's where SoapCalc (soapcalc.net) comes in.

SoapCalc does all the work for you. For whatever type of soap you want to make, you enter the ingredients, choose some of the qualities you want your soap to have, click a button, and SoapCalc produces the recipe, adding the correct amount of water and lye you need in your recipe. But it doesn't stop there. It also tells you the properties your soap will have, including cleansing, hardness, lather, conditioning, and the iodine. All these things are very important when you're formulating a certain type of soap.

How to Use SoapCalc

First, go to soapcalc.net and click on the **SoapCalc** tab. This brings up the fill-in form you'll use over and over as you make different kinds of soaps. (You might want to bookmark this page for quick reference later.)

As you read through this chapter's tutorial, follow along on the SoapCalc website. This will help make everything easier to understand as you fill in numbers later.

Starting at the top left on the homepage, you'll notice that the topic boxes are numbered 1 through 8. If you click on the number in the box, you'll get an overview of what you're calculating in that box and why. We'll also use these numbers to identify what area of SoapCalc we're talking about. Let's take a look at each box.

Box 1: Type of Lye Used

In this box, you have two choices:

- **NaOH,** or sodium hydroxide, for making bar soap

- **KOH,** or potassium hydroxide, for making liquid soap

Click on the circle next to either NaOH or KOH, depending on the type of soap you're making. The default for bar soap is NaOH.

Box 2: Weight of Oils

This box is for the total weight of all the oils or butters you use in a recipe. You have three choices for which unit of measure you want to use:

- **Pounds**

- **Ounces**

- **Grams**

When you change the filled-in circle here, you'll notice that the green box underneath changes according to your choice, as does the far-right column in box 6 (unit measurement).

From the Soap Pot _____

When you choose **pounds** in box 2, it doesn't mean your calculations will make 1 pound of soap. Lye + oils + water = total weight of soap. "Pounds" in this box means 1 pound of *oils*, which will make 24.86 ounces (704.8 grams) of soap at full water of 38 percent. For an easy way to remember how much oil you need for a pound of soap, just think "11" (11 ounces oil plus 5 ounces water/lye equal 1 pound soap): 11 ounces of oils make 1 pound of soap; 22 ounces of oils makes 2 pounds of soap, and for 3 pounds of soap—you guessed it! You need 33 ounces of oils.

Box 3: Water

As you'll see, this box contains three calculations. Let's go through them one at a time.

Water as % of Oils   The default value for water is 38 percent. That means water weighs 38 percent of the weight of the oil used. This is the best percentage for soap, and the best one for beginners to use. We use the 38 percent of water when we make a batch of soap that will have a fragrance or essential oil in it we've not used before. This is because some fragrances, mainly florals, and some essential oils will accelerate trace (the thickening of the soap) so fast you won't have enough time to get the soap out of the pot. Using the full amount of water cuts down the chances of this happening. As you make more soap and becoming familiar with the process, you can start reducing the amount of water (called discounting water).

The soap may be softer than you like with the full amount of water, but it will harden in time. Sometimes it may take up to 2 weeks to fully harden.

If your finished soap is "soft," meaning you leave an indentation when you press on it with your finger, you can reduce the amount of water the next time you make it and it'll be harder. If in doubt as to how the fragrance is going to react, reduce the water to 34 percent on the second go-round with the recipe and fragrance. If the second batch of soap is still too soft, reduce the water to 30 percent. This usually makes a hard bar of soap.

Don't worry about making mistakes with the water calculation—a built-in warning box in SoapCalc will pop up if you try to reduce the water by too much, telling you it's not a safe thing to do.

From the Soap Pot _____

Keep notes on each batch of soap you make. If the soap turned out exactly like you expected, note that on the recipe. If it was too soft, write that down, too, so you'll know what you need to do the next time.

Lye Concentration   Another option to reducing the water in your soap recipe is using the lye concentration. This box is for advanced soap-making; if you're using the 38 percent water calculation, you don't need to do anything with this box.

Water : Lye Ratio   This box is for changing the water-to-lye ratio in your recipe. Again, this is advanced soap-making and you don't actually need to use this box at all, ever.

Box 4: Super Fat %

In this box, we are dealing with two topics:

- **Super Fat %**
- **Fragrance**

Super Fat % means there's been a reduction in the amount of lye, so a portion of the oils won't be turned to soap; instead, they serve to soothe the skin. The higher the super fat percentage, the more oils/butters are left to soothe the skin. The highest number we've super fatted with is 15 percent. Most soap-makers prefer to super fat at 5 to 8 percent for most bars of soap. During the summer months, 5 percent is good to use, and during the winter months, 8 percent is used more often. Still, it's a matter of which works best for your skin or purpose.

The default here is 5 percent because the super fat should never be below 5 percent or your soap would be lye-heavy. The scale we use isn't that accurate, and saponification numbers are averages that can change with each shipment to the United States. So with 5 percent as a buffer zone, you're safe. If you're making laundry soap, however, the rules change. You want 0 percent super fat for laundry soap and all liquid soaps. The super fat is set at a –13 for liquid soaps. (We explain why in Chapter 10.)

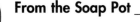

From the Soap Pot

Some soap-makers think that by super fatting to a higher number, the soap will go rancid and produce DOS (dreaded orange spots). This isn't so. DOS is caused by a high amount of iodine. This is why we advise to keep your iodine number under or as close as possible to 70.

The Fragrance field enables you to determine the amount of fragrance or essential oils for the recipe. The standard is from .5 to 1.0 ounces (14.7 to 28.4 grams) per 1 pound (453.6 grams) of oils. This is not the same thing as 1 pound of soap, remember. It's a pound of oil.

If your essential oil is a strong fragrance, use .5 ounce (14.7 grams) percent per 1 pound (453.6 grams) of oils. If your essential oil is a weaker fragrance, use .7 ounces (19.8 grams) per 1 pound (453.6 grams) of oils. This is the maximum amount of an essential oil you'll want to use because essential oils are *potent*.

For fragrance oils, you can use higher percentages. If it's a light fragrance, use 1.0 ounce (28.35 grams) per 1 pound (453.6 grams) of oils. If it's a very strong-smelling one, reduce the amount and use .5 ounce (14.3 grams) or even less. Some fragrances are so strong we use as little as .25 ounce (7.1 grams) per pound of oil.

Safety First _____

Be careful with hot essential oils, such as cinnamon and clove. They're not recommended for use on the skin because they can burn sensitive skin. You can use peppermint, but don't overdo it.

In box 4, type the amount you're going to use in the green box in line with **Oz per lb** or **Gm per Kg.** The amount to use will be displayed after you click **Calculate Recipe** and **View or Print Recipe.**

To figure how much fragrance oil to use in box 4, here's an ounces-to-grams conversion chart for fragrance:

   .5 per pound of oil = 31.25 per gram/kilogram

   .6 per pound of oil = 37.50 per gram/kilogram

   .7 per pound of oil = 43.75 per gram/kilogram

   .8 per pound of oil = 49.99 per gram/kilogram

   .9 per pound of oil = 56.25 per gram/kilogram

   1.0 per pound of oil = 62.50 per gram/kilogram

If you use pounds or ounces in the Weight of Oils, you would use .5 to 1.0 ounces (14.7 to 28.4 grams) per pound of oils in box 4 for the fragrance ratio. If you use grams, you'll use the per gram/kilogram numbers to fill in box 4 for the fragrance ratio. With these numbers, SoapCalc can calculate the amount of the fragrance oil or essential oil you need for your soap recipe.

Box 5: Soap Qualities and Fatty Acids

The soap quality numbers are the sum of all the fatty acids in all vegetable oils and butters. This section has two columns:

- ◆ **One,** on the left, represents the qualities for an individual oil/butter. If you click on an oil or butter in the scroll-down list on the right, you can see how the numbers change in this column.

- ◆ **All,** on the right, gives the combined weighted average of all the oils/butters in a recipe.

If you hover your cursor over each attribute on the left—Hardness, Cleansing, Conditioning (abbreviated as *Condition* here), Bubbly, Creamy, Iodine, and INS—a box will pop up showing the optimal value range. Each attribute represents a different aspect of the soap.

Here's a list of the attributes and what they do (their optimal value range is noted in parentheses):

Hardness (29 to 54)   This denotes the softness of a soap. The lower the number, the softer the soap will be. You want a hardness of 45 and up; otherwise you'll need to reduce the water to get a hard bar of soap without waiting for the cure to finish. We make a bar of soap for acne that is 100 percent coconut oil, and the hardness is 79. There's always an exception to every rule. Our facial bars will be very soft. Many times their number is 34 or below.

Cleansing (12 to 22)   This rates the harshness of the cleansing properties of a soap. The lower the number, the better it is for sensitive skin. We've found that people who have very sensitive skin need to reduce the cleansing to between 2 and 7. (2 is also a good level for those who are in chemotherapy.) For very oily skin or for those with acne, a range of 20 to 22 is optimal. During winter months, we like to lower the cleansing number and up the super fat to help combat winter skin dryness. Try super fat at 8 percent and the cleansing between 8 to 10.

Conditioning (44 to 69)   This notes a soap's ability to soften and soothe the skin. The higher the number of the conditioning, the greater the softening and soothing ability of the oils in your soap. If your soap recipe has 44 conditioning, you can raise the super fat number from 5 to 8 percent. This lowers the amount of lye used in the recipe so more oils are left to soothe the skin. Changing the super fat percentage won't show in the soap qualities. The only thing you'll notice is less lye. The iodine value will be the limiting factor to how much conditioning. Don't let the iodine go over 70.

Bubbly (14 to 46)   This refers to the soap's ability to lather up and get bubbly. The higher the number, the greater amount of lather your soap will produce. This lather is fluffier and is the first to go when left alone and the water isn't agitated.

Creamy (16 to 48)   This is the stable form of lather and is the last to dissipate. The higher the number, the more lather your soap will produce.

Iodine (41 to 70)   The iodine value represents the softness of the oil. The softer the oil, the higher the iodine value. The iodine value is the indicator if soap will go rancid in time. There are no optimum numbers here. If you keep the iodine value at 70 or below, you won't have a problem with rancidity. (We are still testing this to find the highest number we can use and *not* get rancidity.)

INS (136 to 165)   The INS, or iodine in SAP, indicates the moisturizing quality of the soap. The more moisturizing the soap is, the lower the INS number. A balanced bar of soap will have an INS number of 160. In bath bars, we try to get close to this number. Specialty soap, such as a facial bar, will be much lower. We have recipes that call for 121 and another one for 136.

Soap Stats _____

It may take a little practice to choose the right cleansing for your type of skin. You'll know it's right when you don't have itchy skin after you take a bath or shower. If the soap is right for your skin, you won't have to use lotion after your bath.

The rest of the list—Lauric, Myristic, Palmitic, Stearic, Ricinoleic, Oleic, Linoleic, and Linolenic—are the fatty acids. When you place your cursor on the individual fatty acid, a brief description pops up, and if you click on the name, a new window opens with a Wikipedia page definition. Lauric and myristic contribute to the hardness, cleansing, and bubbly lather. Palmitic and stearic contribute to hardness and creamy lather. Ricinoleic, which comes from castor oil, contributes to both creamy and bubbly lather and conditioning properties. Oleic, linoleic, and linolenic all contribute conditioning properties.

So when you're choosing oils and butters, keep an eye on these numbers to be sure they stay within the range you want for your particular soap recipe.

From the Soap Pot _____

The most commonly used coconut oil for soap-making is coconut 76 degree. The 76 degree means the oil is solid when room temperature is under 76 degrees and it's a liquid over 76 degrees. Another type of coconut oil is called coconut oil 92 degree, which is solid when room temperature is less than 92 degrees and a liquid when over 92 degrees. Both types are cleansing, but the 92 degree is a much harder oil when in its solid state, and therefore harder to dig out of the container. Both 76 and 92 degree have a long shelf life. The 76 degree type is more easily found at your local grocery store.

Box 6: Soap Recipe

Now, here's where the real fun really starts! This box is where you add your oils and butters. To the left is a scroll-down menu with all the oils and butters listed. To add an oil or butter to your recipe, just double-click the name in the scroll-down list and you will see it appear under Soap Recipe. (Notice that as you do this, the numbers in box 5 change.)

If you want to replace one oil/butter with another, simply single-click on the ingredient you want in the scroll-down list and then click the red **+** next to the ingredient you want to replace in your recipe. Voilà! The ingredient has been replaced. To remove an oil/butter, just click on the red **−** next to its name.

Each oil has another set of boxes next to it. The first box next to the oil is where you start playing with the percentages of the oils for the recipes. All recipe percentages will total 100 percent. You can raise or lower the percentage of an oil to change the qualities of the soap you're formulating. Keep a close eye on the iodine number, and keep it close to or under 70. To add more conditioning and lather, increase the percentage of castor oil. Note that the higher percentage the castor oil, the lower the hardness number is. To increase or decrease the cleansing, simply change the percentage for the cleansing oils. These oils are coconut, palm kernel, or babassu oil. Continue adding oils and playing with the percentages until you're satisfied with the recipe and the qualities of the soap you're formulating. SoapCalc completes the second box after you click on the Calculate Recipe button. That box will have the amount of each oil to be used in the type of weight measurement you chose—pounds, ounces, grams, or kilograms.

Box 7: Save Recipe

This is a button you may not feel a need to use. It's mainly here if you want to save your recipe instead of print it. But if you want to use this, after you click **Calculate Recipe** (box 8) you can save your recipe by clicking on this button. Then just choose a recipe name in the drop-down menu and click **Save Recipe.** You can choose to save your recipe in percentages, pounds, ounces, or grams by clicking on the button beside the type you want.

After you've done all this, you can't go back and change the name of the recipe.

Box 8: Calculate Recipe and View or Print Recipe

After you have your recipe completed, click **Calculate Recipe.** Look at the numbers for the iodine, hardness, lather, conditioning, and cleansing. If you're happy with the qualities, continue to the next step, which is to view or print your recipe. If you want to make any changes, now is the time to do so. When you've made your changes, then click **Calculate Recipe.** Continue doing making changes until you're satisfied with your soap recipe. Then, click the **View or Print Recipe** button. It's not unusual for soap-makers to spend hours playing around with the oils and amounts.

After you've clicked the View or Print Recipe button, a page will pop up with your recipe, including all the soap qualities and the amounts. This is the page you print out. Type or write the name of the soap at the top in the space provided. At the bottom you'll see buttons that say Show Graph and Hide Graph. You can either print the graph or just view it before you print out the recipe.

Space is provided at the bottom of the printed page for you to make your notes. Be sure to note all additives, including colorant, and all results in this space. Include the name of the fragrance oil you used here, too.

The **Reset Recipe** button clears all the oils/butters from the Soap Recipe in box 6. Before making another recipe, be sure the fields in boxes 1 through 4 are back to their default numbers.

Formulating Soap Using SoapCalc

Some of this may seem confusing, so let's look at some simple recipes. You'll learn a lot faster with some practice runs while you read these instructions than if you just read the instructions and tried to remember them.

Basic Soap

We are going to use a basic soap recipe—Palm 70%, coconut 20%, and castor oil 10%.

First, in box 2, click **Ounces** and type in **11.** Notice that the right column in box 6 has changed to **oz.**

Next, in box 3, change **Water as % of Oils** from the default (38%) to **30.**

In box 4, change the **Super Fat %** to **10**, and for fragrance, type in **.5.**

In the oil list, double-click on **Palm,** and you'll see it appear on the first line of the

From the Soap Pot _____

It's important to learn how to use percentages because everyone uses different-size molds. All you have to do is change the amount of oils in the Weight of Oils and SoapCalc does the rest. You can size up or down to fit any mold as long as you have your recipes in percentages.

recipe. Click the circle above the % symbol and the column will go green. Next to Palm, type in **70.**

Next, double-click **Coconut (76 deg, solid)** and type in **20** in the green field under %. Then double-click **Castor Oil** and type in **10** in the green field.

Click **Calculate Recipe** in box 8.

If your percentage isn't 100, you'll get a pop-up box telling you how much to add or subtract to get 100 percent.

Here are the soap qualities (box 5) of this recipe:

Hardness	51
Cleansing	14
Conditioning	46
Bubbly	23
Creamy	46
Iodine	48
INS	163

In box 8, click **View or Print Recipe.** A new window will open. This is your soap recipe.

 Lather Lingo

When we refer to the **hardness** with a number for a butter or oil, it has to do with the number in SoapCalc. All oils and butters have a hardness number. SoapCalc computes the numbers for hardness in your soap recipe and determines the total hardness number. Because of all the soft oils used in a facial bar, its hardness number may be in the low 30s. A bath bar will be in the 40s or 50s.

Olive Oil Soap

The oldest soap is olive oil soap, also called Castile soap. This soap is mild enough for using on a newborn baby. We're going to make a pound of soap with olive oil. You can use any of the olive oils. The highest grade will make a green-tinted soap; the golden olive doesn't.

Starting in box 2, click on the circle in front of **Ounces,** and type **11** in the green field below.

In box 3, change the 38 water to **25.** This is a soft oil and will take forever to harden.

Everything in box 4 is fine as is, so no changes here.

In box 6, double-click **Olive** and type in 100 under **%.** Click **Calculate Recipe** and then click **View or Print Recipe.**

Here are the soap qualities:

Hardness	15
Cleansing	0
Conditioning	83
Bubbly	0
Creamy	15

Let's take a look at these numbers. A 15 for Hardness means this soap is very soft. And with Cleansing at 0, the soap will clean you, but it won't do well against oil and grease. The 83 for Conditioning is very good. The 15 for Creamy means there will be some lather, just not a lot.

So let's change this a bit. In box 6, change the **Olive** to 80, and add **Coconut (76 deg, solid)** at 20%. Now click **Calculate Recipe.** The revised soap qualities are as follows:

Hardness	28
Cleansing	13
Conditioning	68
Bubbly	13
Creamy	14

As you can see, the cleansing and bubbly lather are much higher.

Now, let's say you wanted more cleansing and more lather. Add **Castor Oil** to the recipe and type in **10.** Then, change Olive to **70** and Coconut to **20** and click **Calculate Recipe.** Now the soap qualities are as follows:

Hardness	26
Cleansing	13
Conditioning	70

Bubbly	22
Creamy	22

Lard Soap

Lard is another old standby that can be found at any grocery store. The lard makes a slightly soft soap, so you can reduce the water to **30** instead of 38. With **100** percent lard, the soap qualities are as follows:

Hardness	42
Cleansing	1
Conditioning	52
Bubbly	1
Creamy	41

Now, change Lard to **80.** Add **Coconut (76 deg, solid),** and set it to **20.** The qualities of this soap are as follows:

Hardness	49
Cleansing	14
Conditioning	44
Bubbly	14
Creamy	35

With the addition of the coconut, cleansing is up 13 percent, and the combined bubbly and creamy lather is up from 42 to 49.

Now let's try it with Lard at **70** and **Coconut (76 deg, solid)** at **20.** Add **Castor Oil,** and set at **10.** The soap qualities are these:

Hardness	45
Cleansing	14
Conditioning	48
Bubbly	23
Creamy	40

Now the conditioning is up and the combined lather is up from 49 to 63! If you want soap for very sensitive skin, you can cut down on the amount of coconut oil or not use it at all.

Beef Tallow Soap

Beef tallow is another old-time soap ingredient. When used at **100** percent, beef tallow (listed as **Tallow Beef** on SoapCalc) makes a very nice bar of soap. Change the water to **38** because beef tallow makes a hard bar of soap. Here are the soap qualities:

Hardness	58
Cleansing	8
Conditioning	40
Bubbly	8
Creamy	50

Now, change the beef tallow to **92** and add **Coconut (76 deg, solid)** at **8.** The soap qualities are as follows:

Hardness	60
Cleansing	13
Conditioning	38
Bubbly	13
Creamy	47

Soap Stats _____

Beef tallow makes a hard, white bar of soap, but it offers very little conditioning or lather. You can increase both the conditioning and the lather by adding castor oil. Beef tallow is also inexpensive. It also comes in a cube, so all you have to do is use a knife to slice off the amount you need. Very easy!

Change the beef tallow to **82** and the **Coconut (76 deg, solid)** to **8.** Add **Castor Oil** and set to **10.** Here are the soap qualities:

Hardness	54
Cleansing	12

Conditioning	43
Bubbly	21
Creamy	51

When working with beef tallow, change the super fat to 10%, because the conditioning is in the low 40s. During the summer months, that's fine, but in the winter, when your skin gets so dry, the added conditioning is a great benefit.

The Least You Need to Know

♦ Formulating your own batch of soap can be fun and so rewarding!

♦ Not only are these oils great for making soap, but you can actually see what qualities the oils add up to in your soap batch.

♦ The math part of soap-making won't be scary because SoapCalc does all the work for you.

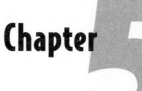

Chapter

Soap Molds

In This Chapter

- Finding—or making—a soap mold
- Determining how much soap a mold holds
- Instructions for lining a soap mold
- A look at M&P molds
- Tips for removing soap from molds

So far we've learned about the basics of soap-making and what oils, butters, and other ingredients you need, plus some of the fragrances and essential oils you can add in to create one-of-a-kind soaps at home. But there's one more very important piece of equipment you need if you're making bar soap, and that's a soap mold. It's what holds everything together—literally!

In this chapter, we look at everything mold-related, from finding a mold—or even making your own—to lining your mold, to unmolding your finished soap.

What Can I Use for a Soap Mold?

The better question is, what *can't* you use! Just about any container works as a soap mold—except anything metal, which would react with the lye and ruin your soap. If you're a first-time soap-maker, we suggest you start with a box or tray as your mold. You could even use a food storage container or buy the small, 2-pound plastic tray mold that makes pretty designs on the top of your soap bar. Some soap-makers use Pringle potato chip cans or PVC pipe to make round soap bars. Shoeboxes can also be used if you line them with freezer paper first. As long as it's at least 5×6 inches, it'll hold a 1.5-pound (24-ounce; 680.4-gram) batch of soap. That should make four bars each measuring 3×2.5 inches and weighing 6 ounces. As you make more and more soap, you'll find yourself looking at different types of containers and thinking *That might make a really cool soap mold!*

You can find many types of wooden, plastic, and acrylic molds in soap-making supply shops and online, in all sizes, from a 1-pound mold up to a 25-pound mold for the professional soap-makers. There are log molds, slab molds, upright molds, and trays, and while you're shopping, you're sure to come across log soap molds that have a soap bar cutter, divided molds that make perfect bars, and even molds with slits in the sides so you can cut perfect bars with your soap knife. You'll find no-liner molds and others that come with premade liners you just place up against the sides and bottom of the mold. Let's not forget about the individual plastic soap molds that make one bar at a time with a pretty design on the bar. Or a soap bar stamp! You can have them custom made, for a reasonable cost, so you can stamp your name or logo on the top of each soap bar.

From the Soap Pot

We've found that the premade liners often leave a weird texture on the outside of the soap bars.

Making Your Own Soap Mold

Yes, you can make your own soap mold, and we bet you'll find it easy and fun. The final product might not be all that pretty, but if it works, that's what counts!

To start, you'll need some wood. The easiest thing to do, if you don't have wood handy at home, is to go to your local lumber store and buy either the precut .5-inch-thick wood pieces close to the necessary sizes and then finish them at home, or have a store employee cut the pieces the exact sizes you need. Here's your wood list:

- 2 pieces, each .5 inch thick, 13 inches long, and 2.5 inches wide

- 2 pieces, each .5 inch thick, 11 inches long, and 2.5 inches wide

- 1 piece 12 inches long and 10 inches wide

You'll also need these:

- Wood glue

- 1 small package of 1-inch nails

- At least 2 C clamps

- Hammer

- Sandpaper

- Varnish (optional)

Safety First _____

Before you start putting together your mold, please put on your safety glasses to protect your eyes from flying nails or bits of wood.

This mold measures 10×12×2 inches inside, holds 6.5 pounds (2,948.4 grams), and makes 16 bars of soap each weighing about 6.5 ounces (184.3 grams). This shape mold is called a slab mold and is the easiest mold to use for doing swirls, embeds, and other fun and fancy designs.

Here's how to assemble your slab mold:

1. Starting with one 11×2.5-inch piece and one 13×2.5-inch piece, apply wood glue to the end edge of the 11-inch piece. Butt that piece flush against the inside edge of the 13-inch piece, lining up the edges so they're even. The pieces will make a right angle and look sort of like an L.

2. While holding everything tightly in place, nail the pieces together from the outside with three evenly spaced nails.

3. Do the same with the other two 11×2.5-inch and 13×2.5-inch pieces. You should now have one 12×10 piece, which is the bottom of the mold, and two L-shape pieces, which are the sides.

4. Apply wood glue to the two edges of the first L piece and on the lower $\frac{1}{4}$ of the bottom edge, where it will butt up to the edge of the mold bottom. Line those pieces up against the mold bottom, and nail into place. Space the nails 2 inches apart.

5. Do the same with the second L piece, and let the glue thoroughly dry overnight.

6. Sand the inside and outside of your mold, and apply a coat or two of wood varnish (if desired).

Soap Stats

Using a wood varnish on your wood soap mold isn't absolutely required. The molds do absorb some oil during the soap-making process, and spills do happen. But a coat or two of wood varnish protects the mold and makes cleaning up spills easier. At the very least, you should use a sealant.

How Much Soap Will My Mold Hold?

How much soap you'll use in a mold varies greatly depending on the type of oils and butters you use in the recipe. Butters weigh more than oils. Get out your calculator, because we're going to run some numbers.

First, you have to decide how much you want each bar to weigh. Many soap-makers like their bars to weigh 6 ounces after they have cured. To end up with 6-ounce bars, they have to start out weighing 6.5 ounces. (They lose the water weight during the curing.) Multiply that number by how many bars your mold makes. For example, in our 10×12 molds, we make 16 bars, so we multiply 6.5×16 to get 104 ounces. We then divide 104 by 16 ounces to get 6.5 pounds. So 6.5 pounds is the total weight of oils, water, and lye this size of mold will hold.

Now let's use the dimensions of the mold to determine the approximate weight the mold will hold. To do this, multiply the width (10) by the height of the bars (1.5 inches). Multiply that number by the length (12) and then again by .58 for a total of 104.4 ounces (2,948.4 grams). Then divide that by 16 ounces (453.6 grams) for a total of 6.5 pounds (104 ounces; 2,948.4 grams). This mold will hold 6.5 pounds (104 ounces; 2,948.4 grams) without coming to the very top and possibly spilling over the edge during gel stage. (That would make a *huge* mess!)

You can calculate the weight of a log mold the same way you do the slab molds. If the inside measurements of your log mold are (like ours) 3.5 inches wide by 2.5 inches tall by 15 inches long, and you cut your bars 1.25 inches thick, you'll get 12 bars. So multiply 3.5 (the width) by 2.5 (the height) by 15 inches (the length) by .58, and you'll get 76.13 ounces, which, rounded down, is 76 ounces (2,154.6 grams). Now divide 76 ounces (2,154.6 grams) by 16 ounces (453.6 grams), and you have 4.75 pounds.

Now to check the math, multiply 6.5 (1,842.75 grams; the weight of bars) by 12. That's 78 ounces (2,211.3 grams), and that's pretty darn close. Our bars come out weighing between 6.3 ounces (1,786.05 grams) and 6.5 ounces (1,842.75 grams), depending on the recipe.

Okay, if you're still with us after all that math, now we need to figure out how many ounces of oil per pound of soap the mold will hold. Remember, it takes 11 ounces (311.85 grams) of oil plus the water and lye to make 1 pound (16 ounces; 453.6 grams) of soap. In SoapCalc, you need to know how many ounces to put in the box for total weight of oils.

The math for this part is a little different from the math formula we just used. Once again, we multiply the width (3.5 inches) by the height (2.5 inches) by the length (15 inches) by .38 for a total of 49.88 ounces (2,494.8 grams). Round that up to 50 ounces (1,417.5 grams). That's the number you'll use for your total weight of oils, depending on your recipe. You may have to add or subtract 1 or 2 ounces (28.35 or 56.7 grams), but this formula gives you a starting place for determining your total weight of oils.

Lining Your Mold

When I first started making soap, I bought a plastic no-line mold (that in reality needed to be lined!) … and I thought I'd *never* get the soap out! I finally stuck the mold in the freezer and left it overnight. The cold shrank the soap enough that it released from the mold and the soap came out. What a relief! From then on, I've always used white freezer paper to line my molds … and I haven't had any more problems.

Soap-makers talk about using everything from cling film to trash bags to line their molds, followed by the lament that they're always having to fight to have a smooth lining for a smooth bar. And we've tried just about every way there is to line our soap molds, from making complicated measurements and cutting out parts for the corners to the simple and easy method we now use— white freezer paper.

From the Soap Pot

The easiest and best thing to use for lining your soap mold is freezer paper. Yep, this is the same thing you can buy at your local grocery store. Turn the shiny side up so it's next to the soap, and when you're unmolding, the paper will peel right off the soap. No wrinkles or dents from crumpled liners!

We use freezer paper, shiny side up, so it won't stick to the soap. Using one large sheet and making folds and a slit in each corner, you, too, can line your mold in just a couple minutes. There are no leaks because there are no cutouts and very little if any waste. Freezer paper is readily available, even in your grocery store. It's on the aisle with the foil and waxed paper.

Here's how to line your soap mold with freezer paper:

1. Measure the length of your mold, and add 13 inches. The lining has to completely cover the inside of your mold, up the sides and ends with a little extra for folding over each top edge of the mold. Roll out your freezer paper, measure the length, and mark and cut it.

2. Lay the paper, shiny side up, lengthwise next to your mold. Fold up one edge 3 or 4 inches the whole length of the paper. Line the folded edge of the paper against the inside edge of the mold. With your thumb, make a crease in the paper along the other inside edge of the mold. That will be your next fold line. After you've folded the second side, place the folded paper in your mold to be sure it fits smoothly and evenly. If not, make the proper adjustments.

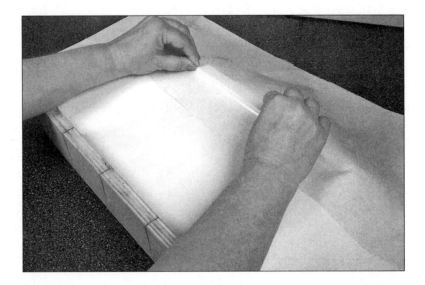

3. Using the point of your scissors, crease the paper where it butts up smoothly on each end. Crease and fold down each end, as you did with the sides.

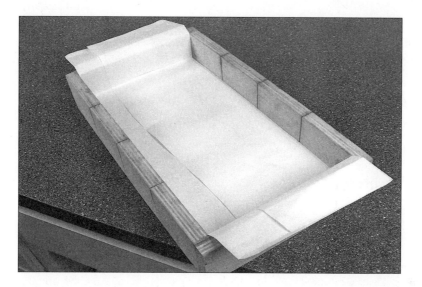

4. Next, pull up the long sides and smooth them into place. Working with one corner at a time, pull up the end piece while holding down the side piece, and crease the triangle fold so it lies flat and smooth against the mold. Make a slit in the corner edge of the paper. Repeat this in the other corner on that same end. Now fold the paper over the edge on the end and tape it securely. Repeat for the other end.

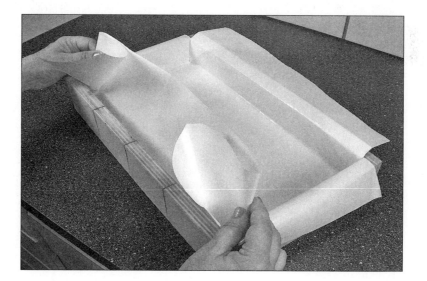

5. Fold the paper over the edges of the mold and tape securely. Check to be sure the lining is still smooth and flat. Now you have a perfectly lined mold that won't hold on to your soap for dear life!

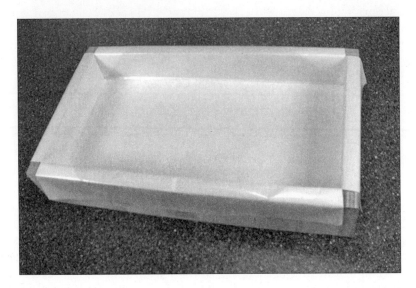

See how easy that was? You'll be even more surprised how easily your finished soap comes out of your freezer paper–lined mold!

Melt-and-Pour Soap Molds

There are many high-quality plastic and silicone soap molds on the market designed for melt-and-pour (M&P) soap base. These molds don't have to be lined, but you might want to spray a cooking spray in the mold before you pour in the M&P soap. This will help you remove your soap after it has hardened. You can also buy a silicone spray mold release if you want—many are available online. These molds range in price from $2 or $3 and up. (The silicone molds cost more but they have a longer use life.)

You can also make your own silicone mold using a silicone product designed for this purpose. There are two kinds of silicone. With one kind, you paint the silicone over the object you want to make a mold of. With the other type, you fill a container with the appropriate amount of silicone and insert the object upside down in the container. Both of these silicone products are easy to use. The painted-on type will not last through very many uses, but the other type will.

Unmolding Your Soap

Depending on what type of mold you're using, and whether or not you lined it, removing soap from the mold can be a frustrating ordeal. It doesn't matter if you've used M&P or made cold process soap; the best way to get a stubborn soap out of the mold, especially an unlined plastic tray or PVC pipe mold, is to put the filled mold in the freezer. Some will only need to be in the freezer for a few minutes while others will need to be kept there overnight.

Depending on what type of mold you're using, you have some options for removing the soap.

First, let's look at removing soap from a plastic tray mold. When the soap is ready to come out of the freezer, you'll see that it has retracted from the edges of the mold. Let the mold sit on the counter for about 5 minutes. Place a piece of waxed paper on your counter, and turn the soap tray upside down onto the paper. Gently press on the center of the back of the tray. You should be able to see the soap releasing from the mold. Continue to press until the soap pops completely out of the mold. If the tray is a slab type with bars, allow the soap to thaw to room temperature before cutting into bars.

Next up, let's look at plastic PVC pipe molds. I made soap in a round PVC pipe once—and only once. I froze it. I banged it. But no matter what I did, I couldn't get the soap out of the pipe. Two months later, I saw a big, hairy spider in my workshop so I grabbed the closest thing to me to whack it with, the PVC pipe still full of soap. When I slung the pipe to hit the spider, the soap shot out and went flying across the room. It had finally dried enough to let go of the sides of the PVC pipe. Imagine the look of shock and amazement on my daughter's face as she watched the soap roll fly out of the mold, across the room, and make a loud thud as it hit the floor. The spider ran off, safe to taunt me another day. The soap and the PVC mold went directly in the trash.

Although plastic no-line CP soap molds are very convenient molds to use, they can be hard to remove the soap from. But if you use the freezer method explained earlier in this section, you should be okay. I had problems with mine, so now I line my no-line mold whenever I use it.

Lined molds are the easiest type of mold to remove your soap from. Start by placing a piece of waxed paper on the counter. Loosen the taped sides, turn the mold upside down on the waxed paper, and pull the mold straight up. Gently pull the freezer paper off the soap, and then let the soap sit out in the open air for a few hours or a day, depending on how soft the soap is, before cutting.

If you're using a lined mold with knife slits, loosen the taped sides and, using your large soap knife, place the knife where it will fit into both slits, one on each side of the mold. Gently guide the knife down through the soap. Do this both across and length-wise to cut your perfectly shaped bars. Lay a piece of waxed paper on the counter, and turn the soap mold upside down. Pull the mold up, and place to the side. Very gently remove the freezer paper from the cut bars of soap, careful not to nick or bump the bars. Set bars on a wire rack or in an open box to dry. Wire cookie racks work really well for drying soap!

You are now ready to choose the type of soap mold you want to try first. Be sure to gather all the things you will need to use with your mold before you start making your soap batch. Lining your mold first is the best way to get started. Don't wait until your soap is ready to be poured to line the mold. Have it ready and waiting.

The Least You Need to Know

◆ Choosing or making your own soap mold can be a little fun-filled adventure!

◆ Don't be afraid to try different sizes and shapes of soap molds! You might love the results, but if you don't, move on to the next experiment.

◆ If you are math challenged, don't worry—store-bought soap molds come with specific instructions on how much the mold will hold so you don't have to do any number-crunching.

Part 2

Making Cold and Hot Process Soap

Now you really start your soap-making adventure! In Part 2, you learn how to make soap in the oven, on the stove, and even in a slow cooker. In the following chapters, we also give you recipes for everything from goat milk bar soap to liquid laundry detergent.

But watch out—soap-making can become an addiction! You might soon find yourself wanting to make soap instead of doing ... well, anything else! It happens to us all, new soap-makers as well as long-time soap-makers. And a heads-up: you'll likely also become very fond of fragrance oils, often finding yourself pacing past your front door waiting for the UPS man, who you've been on a first-name basis with for some months now, to deliver those lovely bottles of oils and potions. That's all part of the fun!

Chapter 6

Cold Process Soap

In This Chapter

- ◆ All about cold process soap
- ◆ Understanding super fatting
- ◆ A quick look at cold process oven process soap
- ◆ How to make cold process soap

I was so nervous the first time I made soap. I had read and reread everything I could find about making cold process soap, but still, I couldn't find enough information to explain many of the steps or equipment. For example, I had no idea what an immersion blender was, or what trace looked like. It took several months for me to muster the courage to jump right in and make my first batch of cold process soap.

That first batch took *5 hours* to come to trace. Why? Because I didn't have an immersion blender and was using a stainless-steel spoon to stir the soap batch. (At least I had the right kind of spoon!) The soap was also slow to trace because the recipe I used contained a lot of peanut oil. (Peanut oil is very slow to trace and is sometimes used to slow down a recipe when a touchy floral fragrance oil is being used.) In addition, the soap took several days to harden enough that I could remove it from the soap mold—a mold I'd made myself, by the way.

Needless to say, this wasn't the ideal soap-making experience, and I began to think that if all soap took that long, then my soap-making career was going to come to an end right then and there. Before throwing in the towel, however, I went online, found a soap-makers group at Yahoo! Groups, and joined. I posted a question as to why my soap took 5 hours to trace. Zonella answered that post, and together we began our soap-making adventure.

I do have to tell you that the peanut oil soap I first made turned out to be one of my favorite bars of soap. I have since fixed the recipe and have several immersion blenders. Trace no longer takes 5 hours.

The Basics of Cold Process Soap

Cold process (CP) soap is one method of soap-making where the saponification takes place in the mold. As you learned in Chapter 1, saponification is the chemical reaction of the lye attaching to the oils. This method takes longer to *cure*.

During this process, the soap batch goes through a very hot gel stage. After you've mixed your oils and lye and brought the batch to trace, you pour the soap into the mold, cover it with waxed paper, and walk away. Saponification begins once the soap becomes solid in the mold.

Lather Lingo

Curing is when the water is evaporating and the bar of soap hardens.

This is the hardest part for me because I want to peek and see what my swirls look like. I have to force myself not to touch it—which is important because it's hot and you can get lye burns on your fingers if you touch it.

Cold process soap has a creamier texture than hot process soap. As you become more experienced with making soap, you might want to try discounting the water phase to help speed up the curing. This isn't something for a beginner to try, though, so only try this method after you've gotten the knack of soap-making. I prefer not to discount the water phase. When you do, often *trace* will come faster, and I like to have the time to swirl several colors or make layers with my soap.

Lather Lingo _____

Trace is when the soap batch becomes thick. There are three stages of trace: light, medium, and thick. When trace starts, you'll start seeing a little ripple behind your spoon or immersion blender as you move it through the soap. Light trace looks like a thin sauce. Medium trace looks like gravy. Thick trace looks like pudding. All soap has to go through trace for it to properly saponify.

In all the soap-making classes I teach, I tell every student to save their exotic and more expensive oils for the leave-on products so the user will get the most benefits from these oils. Soap is a wash-off product, and even though you'll get some of the benefits by taking a bath rather than a shower, it all still just goes down the drain. Unless you're making a certain type of bar designed for a certain reason, stick with the basic oils:

- Babassu oil
- Castor oil
- Coconut oil
- Olive oil
- Palm oil

- Palm kernel oil
- Peanut oil
- Cocoa butter
- Shea butter

These will get the job done well and also keep the cost per bar reasonable. If you want a little more conditioning, you can increase the super fat (oil that's not attached to lye—more on super fatting coming right up), but don't go over 8 percent.

Keep it simple. You don't need to put 1 ounce of this and 2 ounces of that in your batch to have a great bar of soap. Stick to the basics, and your soap will be wonderful as well as cost-effective.

One final tip: remember, always weigh your ingredients instead of using volume measures such as cups and tablespoons. Many of the oils weigh more than others, so if you use volume, you may have not enough or too much lye. Be very accurate when weighing your ingredients.

Soap Stats _____

Facial bars are one of the exceptions to the rule for the more exotic and expensive oils. Rosehip oil added to the formula for a facial bar helps lighten age spots. Flaxseeds or flaxseed oil added to a bath bar helps with certain skin disorders.

The Skinny on Super Fatting

Many times we've heard new soap-makers—and sometimes even those more experienced—say "My soap is super fatted with shea butter" or that their soap is super fatted with shea butter because they added it at trace.

This is scientifically impossible when you're making cold process soap. If you're making hot process soap, however, you can super fat after the cook phase and just before the soap goes into the mold.

We mentioned *super fatting* briefly in earlier chapters, but just what is super fatting? Basic chemistry tells you that in cold process soap, the lye doesn't know the difference between the oils or when the oil/butter was added. All the oils and butters are in the pot together. All the oil molecules mingle with all the lye molecules. When all the lye molecules have attached to the oil molecules, what's left is the oil that's called the super fat. These unsaponified oil molecules provide extra conditioning for the skin. Adding the oil or butter at trace does not keep that oil/butter from being saponified when making cold process because saponification takes place over a period of 48 hours.

Lather Lingo

Super fatting is the process of reducing the amount of lye in a soap recipe so more oils are left un-saponified and can then soothe the skin.

Most soap-makers super fat at 5 percent. In winter, you can raise it to 8 percent to help combat winter dryness.

Cold Process, Only Faster: Cold Process Oven Process

The cold process oven process (CPOP) method is perfect for those who are in a hurry to use or sell their soaps because it forces the gel stage and dries out the soap faster—sometimes in as little as 2 or 3 days, your soaps are hard and ready for use. To make CPOP soap, simply follow the directions for making regular cold process soap, except put the soap-filled mold in the oven.

Here's how: just before you're ready to start mixing together the lye and oils, preheat the oven to 170°F. Follow the directions for making CP soap, and pour your soap into the mold. Cover the top with waxed paper. Now turn *off* your oven, turn the oven light on, and put your mold in the oven on the middle rack. Shut the door and leave it until tomorrow. The next day, remove the mold from the oven, let it stand a few hours to cool before you remove the soap from the mold, and cut it into bars. Then let the bars sit for another couple days.

Unmolding and Cutting Your Soap

Many people choose to unmold their soap batch after 24 hours, but we think this is too soon. The soap will still be too soft, and the lye will still be active. It's best to wait 48 hours before you take your soap out of the mold and set it on a drying rack.

When your soap is ready, cover a section of your workspace with a piece of waxed paper. Loosen the tape that held the freezer paper lining in place. Slowly turn the soap out onto the waxed paper. Let the soap dry for a day or two before you try to cut it into bars.

Sally uses a ruler to first measure and mark the bars. Most soap-makers cut their bars 3.25 inches long and 2.25 inches wide.

Stand with the soap directly in front of you so you can push the cutter or knife straight down into the soap, making a clean, straight cut. To cut your soap, you can use a handheld soap cutter or a knife. Once you've cut the bars, set them up on their sides to dry. Many people use cardboard as soap-drying trays, and some use professionally made drying racks, but whatever you have will be fine as long as the soap is open to the air. Avoid drying your soap in a humid area; instead of drying, they'll absorb the moisture in the air and become mushy.

Making Cold Process Soap

Are you ready? Let's make a batch of cold process soap! First, gather all your equipment. Here's what you'll need (turn back to Chapter 1 if you need a refresher on these items):

- Stainless-steel stock pot
- Several paper cups or measuring cups
- Scale
- Stainless-steel thermometer
- Long-handled stainless-steel spoon
- Thin latex gloves
- Safety glasses
- Freezer paper
- Waxed paper
- Soap mold
- Paper towels
- Skin-safe fragrance or essential oil
- Soap-safe colorant
- Oil(s)
- Sodium hydroxide lye
- Distilled water
- Stove

Always run your recipe through a lye calculator before you start to be sure your lye and water phase are correct. This is a good habit to get into right from the start.

For every pound of soap, you'll need 11 ounces of oils. The rest of the pound comes from the lye and water. So if you have a 3-pound mold, you'll need 33 ounces of oils. For the following Basic Recipe for Cold Process Soap, we'll be making a 3-pound batch. So in SoapCalc's Weight of Oils section, choose **ounces** and type **33** in the green box.

Basic Cold Process Soap

Here's what to put in SoapCalc:

Weight of Oils	33 ounces
Water as % of Oils	38
Super Fat %	5
Fragrance Oz per Lb	1
Distilled water	12.5 ounces (355.5 grams)
Lye—sodium hydroxide	4.6 ounces (131.0 grams)
Castor oil	6.6 ounces (187.1 grams) (20%)
Coconut oil (76 degree)	6.6 ounces (187.1 grams) (20%)
Palm oil	19.8 ounces (561.3 grams) (60%)

Here are the soap qualities:

Hardness	46
Cleansing	14
Conditioning	51
Bubbly	32
Creamy	50
Iodine	51
INS	156

Always put on your gloves and safety glasses before you begin.

1. Line your mold with freezer paper (shiny side up), following the directions in Chapter 5. If you're using a plastic tray mold, you don't need to line it.

2. Set your scale to ounces (or grams if you're an international reader). Place your empty plastic pitcher on the scale, and push the tare button to zero out the weight of the pitcher, and wait for the scale to read 0. Start pouring the water into the pitcher until it weighs 12.5 ounces (355.5 grams). Remove the pitcher from the scale, and set it aside for now.

3. Put a bowl on the scale, push the tare button, and wait for the scale to read 0. Using a spoon or scoop, add the lye to the bowl until your scale reads 4.6 ounces (131.0 grams). Remove the bowl from the scale.

4. Have the pitcher of water sitting in the sink or on a counter several inches away from you. Open a near window or turn on an extracting fan. Slowly add the lye to the water and stir until the lye is totally dissolved. You'll know your lye is good because the water will become hot.

5. Put the pitcher of lye/water in a safe place to cool. This takes about 1 hour.

> **Safety First** _____
>
> Follow all the safety instructions while working with lye. Wear your safety glasses and latex gloves, and have the area well ventilated. When mixing the lye and water, slowly add the lye to the water, and never put your face over the pitcher of lye.

6. Before you can weigh all your oils, the palm oil has to be completely melted and stirred because, like milk, palm oil separates. If you don't melt and stir the oil, you'll have chalky white veins running throughout your soap batch. You can return this unused palm oil to the container and use it at another time.

7. Once your palm oil has melted, and you've stirred it well, weigh 19.8 ounces (561.3 grams) on your scale and place the oil in a stainless-steel pot. Do the same with the castor oil for 6.6 ounces (187.1 grams) and coconut oil for 6.6 ounces (187.1 grams).

8. Put on your safety glasses and latex gloves again.

9. When the lye and oils have cooled to less than 90°F, it's time to make soap! Slowly pour your lye/water solution into your oils.

10. Once your oils are well blended with the lye water, it's time to add your fragrance.

11. Continue stirring until you start to see trace. This is like the beginning of gravy or pudding where you can see a little thickening as your spoon treads through the soap.

When poured from the spoon, the soap at light trace makes a thin stream. It should look similar to buttermilk or a thin sauce.

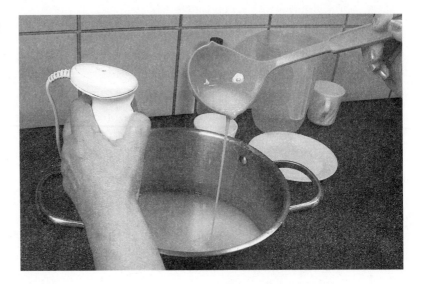

12. At this point, if I've used a fast-moving or floral fragrance oil I pour the batch into the mold. Otherwise, continue to stir until you reach a medium trace and then pour the soap into the prepared mold. Don't overstir, or you'll end up with hard trace and it'll be very hard to pour it smoothly into the mold.

Medium trace soap is thicker than light trace when you pour it, but it still flows freely. It looks more like a medium gravy.

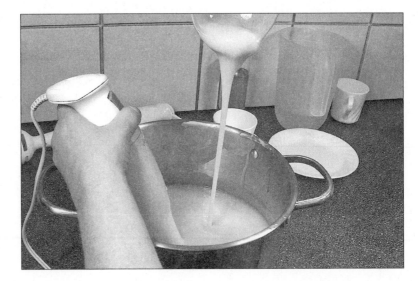

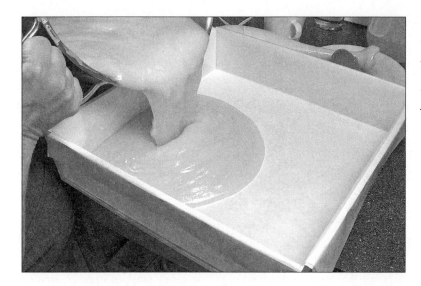

Thick trace is the "pudding" stage. The soap no longer pours freely but globs out of the pot and into the mold. Any thicker than this, and you'll have to push and shove the soap into the mold!

13. Cover the top of the soap with a piece of waxed paper. If you have a lid for your mold, put that on. Leave the soap for 48 hours. During this time your soap will go through the gel stage, which is when it saponifies. The oils and lye/water are going through chemical changes, too, and these changes are what make it soap as the lye molecules attach to the oil molecules. It takes 48 hours for your lye to complete its work and become neutralized.

Congratulations! You've just made your first batch of soap. If you're not addicted yet, you soon will be!

Forty-eight hours later, your soap should be ready to come out of the mold. Place a piece of waxed paper on your counter, and gently turn the soap mold upside down and place your soap on the paper. Let the soap air for several hours before you cut it into bars. Be sure you're wearing latex gloves while doing this so you don't get any *lye bites*.

Lather Lingo

While the lye is still active, it can burn your skin. Such **lye bites** occur when little bits of soap that contain still-active lye touch your skin and give you a little shock or burn.

Your soap will need time to cure so the water can evaporate and the bars harden. If you use your soap without it properly curing, it will melt faster in the shower or bath.

From the Soap Pot

When using your soap in the shower, keep it away from the spray of the water or move it where it doesn't sit in water because the water exposure will melt it very quickly. For longest life, set the soap on a slated soap dish out of the path of the water.

The Zap Test

Before you use or give a fresh bar of soap, it's a good idea to be sure the lye has completely neutralized. This is where the zap test—or the lick, *yuck*, and spit test—comes in handy.

The test is easy: simply touch the tip of your tongue to the bar of soap. If you get nothing but the yucky taste of soap, then that soap is safe to use. However, if you get a little tingle or zap, the lye is still active and the soap needs more time to cure before it can be safely used.

You've now made your first batch of soap! Congratulations! But waiting to use it will be a killer! If you don't mind it melting in the water quicker, you could sneak just one bar out of the batch to use after the soap has been sitting 3 or 4 days—do the zap test first!—just so you can see how nice it is! Nothing feels as nice on your skin as hand-made soap. And if you think you'll get to keep your soap batch all to yourself, think again! Once your family and friends find out you're making soap, they'll all want to try a bar! By that time, you'll love your new craft so much you won't mind making soap to share. Plus, it will give you a great excuse to buy more fragrances! There's one more addiction to add to the pot!

The Least You Need to Know

◆ Following the easy instructions makes working with lye safe and not so scary!

◆ Making a batch of soap is very fun and addicting. But the best part is using it!

◆ You will have so much fun experimenting with fragrance and essential oils, colorants, and embeds! A batch of soap can be an artist's canvas.

Chapter 7

Hot Process Soap

In This Chapter

- All about hot process soap
- How to make stovetop hot process soap
- How to make slow cooker hot process soap
- How to make oven hot process soap

Need some soap quickly but don't want to wait 2 to 4 weeks for the soap to cure? Then let me introduce you to hot process soap! Hot process soap needs little to no cure time! You still need the same oils, type of lye, and equipment, but the difference is: cold process soap goes through saponification in the mold, and hot process goes through saponification over heat in the pot. Both methods produce lovely soap. Let's get started!

The Basics of Hot Process Soap

Hot process soap-making is a method of cooking the soap mixture on the stove until it has completely finished saponifying (made into soap). When the soap has finished cooking and has cooled, it's ready to use. With this process, you can add oils after the cooking stage to super fat because the saponification process has already used up all the lye. Hot process soap-making does not make as pretty a bar of soap as cold process soap, but it does offer instant gratification!

There's a new way to make hot process soap. You start out with cold process soap, and after pouring the soap into the mold, place it in an oven preheated to 170°F. Allow the soap to cook at this temperature for 4 hours, turn off the heat, and leave the mold in the oven until it has cooled. When you get it out of the oven, it's ready to cut and use. The heat of the oven forces the soap into saponification and holds it there for a few hours. With this method, you have the beauty of cold process soap and the no-wait of the hot process soap—the best of both worlds!

The one downside to hot process soap is that it's hard to get out of the mold. But there's a simple fix for that: line your mold with freezer paper, with the shiny side against the soap. Then your soap will slip out of the mold with ease.

Soap Stats _____

Unsaponifiables are the part of oils and butters that don't react with the lye—the sodium hydroxide or potassium hydroxide—and are left in the soap in their original state. These later help moisturize the user's skin.

Making Hot Process Soap

Before we begin, be sure you have everything you need at hand. When things get going, you won't have time to go looking for things you've forgotten. Trust us—we know this for a fact! Here's what you'll need (turn back to Chapter 1 if you need a refresher on these items):

- Safety glasses or face shield
- Thin latex gloves
- Plastic pitcher
- Scale
- Plastic or glass cereal bowl and 1 small glass or stainless-steel cup
- 1 stainless-steel or glass bowl or 2-cup measuring cup
- Long-handled stainless-steel spoon or plastic spoon
- Immersion blender
- Large stainless-steel (stock) pot
- Mold lined with freezer paper
- Stove with an oven

We give you a basic recipe in this section, but any recipe will do if you want to try something different. Just remember to run it through SoapCalc to be sure the lye amount is right and see if the recipe has the qualities you want. Don't do a water discount.

Basic Hot Process Soap

This is a hard bar of soap. The cleansing is mild, and the conditioning is a little low, but putting 8 percent in the super fat instead of 5 percent improves the conditioning (although it won't change the 48 conditioning in the soap qualities on SoapCalc). And with a combined bubbly and creamy lather amounts, at 67, this soap produces loads of lather. This recipe makes a total of 17.11 ounces (485.1 grams) of soap.

Here's what to put in SoapCalc:

Weight of Oils	11 ounces
Water as % of Oils	38
Super Fat %	8
Fragrance Oz per Lb	.7
Distilled water	4.18 ounces (118.503 grams)
Lye—sodium hydroxide	1.454 ounces (41.232 grams)
Beef tallow	7.92 ounces (224.532 grams) (72%)
Coconut oil	.88 ounce (24.948 grams) (8%)
Olive oil	1.10 ounces (31.185 grams) (10%)
Castor oil	1.10 ounces (31.185 grams) (10%)
Fragrance oil	.481 ounce (13.640 grams)

If you want to add a colorant to your soap, now is the time to get it ready. Measure the manufacturer's recommended use amount for the size of soap batch you're making, and put it in the 2-cup measuring cup or stainless-steel bowl. If you're using a powder colorant, you need to add a little oil to wet the colorant so it will be ready when it's time to color. (See Chapter 11 for more information on using colorants.)

Here are the soap qualities:

Hardness	50
Cleansing	11
Conditioning	48
Bubbly	20

Creamy	47
Iodine	50
INS	146

Before we go any further, let's discuss recipes a little more, especially the percentages used in them. Don't freak out if you get a recipe that only lists percentages for the oils. Using percentages for a recipe makes it very easy to size up or size down the soap batch to fit the mold you want to use. For every pound of soap it takes 11 ounces oil and 5 ounces water/lye solution. If your mold is a 3-pound mold, you'll multiply 3×11 and get 33—that's the number to add into SoapCalc for total weight of oil. After that, you put in the oils from the recipe and the percentages. Click **Calculate Recipe,** and SoapCalc converts the recipe to fit your soap mold. It's as easy as that! All the recipes in this book list the percentages as well as the ounces to be used for a specified batch size, but you can make it any size you want by using the percentages.

You can also multiply the percentage of the oil by the amount of the total weight of oils for the size batch you want. Let's say for a 1-pound batch you need 11 ounces oils. If the palm is 72, multiply by 11 (the amount of oils you're going to use), and you get 7.92 ounces (224.5 grams). Easy! If you want to make 2 pounds of soap, multiply all the percentages in the recipe by 22, the ounces of oils it takes to make 2 pounds of soap. To check if your math is right, add all the ounces, and you should have either 11 ounces (for 1 pound of soap) or 22 ounces (for 2 pounds of soap). How can 11 ounces of oils be 1 pound of soap? Remember, you add the water and lye to the oils to get the weight of the soap.

Now, back to the recipe. Always put on your gloves and safety glasses before you begin.

1. Line your mold with freezer paper (shiny side up), following the directions in Chapter 5. If you're using a plastic tray mold, you don't need to line it.

2. Set your scale to ounces (or grams if you're an international reader). Place the ceramic bowl on the scale, and push the tare button to zero out the weight of the cup, and wait for the scale to read 0. Start pouring the fragrance oil into the bowl until it weighs .481 ounce (13.640 grams). Remove the bowl from the scale, and set it aside for now.

3. Do the same for the colorant, and set aside.

4. Place a cereal bowl–size bowl on the scale, and push the tare button to zero out the weight of the bowl. Weigh each oil individually and add to the stockpot.

5. Place the stockpot of oils over medium-low heat. Let the oils completely melt.

6. Put on your safety glasses and latex gloves again.

7. While the oils are heating, place a plastic bowl on the scale, and push the tare button to zero out the weight of the bowl. Weigh the sodium hydroxide (lye) in the bowl. Remove the bowl from the scale, and set it aside.

8. Place a pitcher on the scale, and push the tare button to zero out the weight of the pitcher. Weigh the distilled water. Remove the pitcher from the scale, and set it aside.

9. When the oils have completely melted, it's time to mix your lye into the water. Put on your safety glasses and latex gloves again. Now slowly sprinkle the lye into the water, stirring while you do this and keeping your face away from the pitcher until all the lye has dissolved. Remember, the fumes from the lye can burn your eyes and lungs, so don't get your face too close to that pitcher!

Safety First _____

Always slowly add the lye to the water—*never* the other way around. Doing it the other way around can cause a volcanic reaction.

10. With the pot still over medium-low heat, slowly pour the lye/water mixture into the oils. Using an immersion blender, blend until the oils and water come together.

From the Soap Pot _____

A fellow soap-maker shared this tip: add 1 ounce of a soft oil, such as sweet almond oil, to the hot process soap batch when it reaches the mashed potato stage, stir it well, and add your fragrance oil and colorant. That's actually adding a little more super fat to the soap, which gives it more conditioning. The results are fantastic.

11. Continue stirring, with the pot on the heat, as the soap starts coming to trace.

12. Don't stop cooking yet! The soap will now go through the next stage. This is when the soap looks like it is falling apart, but it's supposed to do this. You will see the oils coming to the top. This is the "applesauce" stage. The soap is going through gel and is saponifying.

With your oils and lye in the pot on the stove, stir or use an immersion blender to bring it to trace.

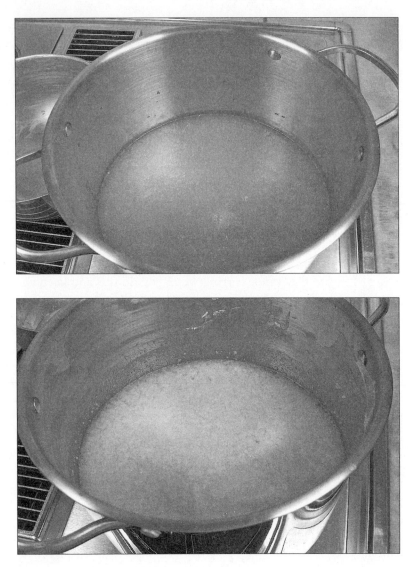

The soap will thicken and come to a full trace.

13. Continue cooking through the applesauce stage. It will saponify and then start to smooth out. This is the "mashed potato" stage, and now is the time to add the fragrance and color. Add your fragrance first and stir until it's well incorporated. How much coloring you use depends on how dark or light you want the finished soap to be. Using your long-handled spoon, scoop out about 1 cup (8 ounces) of the soap and add it to the bowl with the colorant. Stir well until the mixture is one uniform color. Add the colored soap back into the pot, and stir in the color until you have the desired effect—less stirring gives you a two-colored, swirled bar; the more you stir, the more you get one color. If the color is too light,

remove another cup of soap and add more colorant. Stir it well and return it to the soap pot. You do have to work quickly before the soap batch starts setting up.

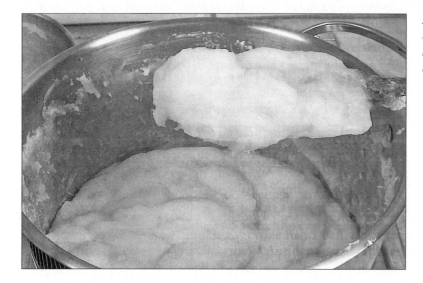

After trace and during the cook stage, the soap batch falls apart. Don't worry! It has to do this.

14. Pour the soap into the freezer paper–lined mold. Smooth down the top as best you can. Bang the mold on the counter a few times to get the air bubbles out. Now let the soap cool. You can leave your soap to cool on your counter or put it in a cold oven, with the oven door slightly cracked open, so the soap is out of the way. After it has completely cooled, the only thing left to do is to cut it into bars, and your soap is ready to use.

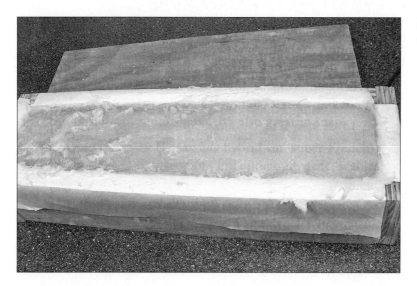

Let the cooked soap cool in the mold.

15. You'll need a soap cutter or a long knife. Use a ruler to measure and mark the cutting line. Then, place your cutter over the first cutting line and push firmly straight down all the way through the soap. If you stand directly over the soap, you'll increase your chances of cutting straight.

Making Slow Cooker Hot Process Soap

Soap? In a slow cooker? You bet! It's just as fast and just as easy as making soap on the stove. The only difference is your stove and stockpot are free for simmering a pot of stew while you make soap in your slower cooker. After dinner you could relax in a nice hot bath using a bar of your freshly made soap! That's a perfect ending to a busy day if you ask me.

In addition to most of the equipment listed earlier in the "Making Hot Process Soap" section, you will obviously need a good-quality slow cooker. Some have two temperature settings (low and high), and some have three (low, medium, and high). We recommend using a slow cooker with three settings, as the one with two settings gets a bit too hot when set on low.

Safety First

Once you use a slow cooker for soap, it is no longer safe to use for food. Over time, the lye will destroy the surface of the slow cooker bowl. Even with one use, you'll see that the bowl's surface isn't as shiny as it was.

Slow Cooker Hot Process Soap

This easy, hands-off recipe will yield 17.2 ounces (487.6 grams) of soap.

Here's what to put in SoapCalc:

Weight of Oils	11 ounces
Water as % of Oils	38
Super Fat %	8
Fragrance Oz per Lb	.07
Distilled water	4.18 ounces (118.501 grams)
Lye—sodium hydroxide	1.498 ounces (42.455 grams)
Palm oil	7.92 ounces (224.528 grams) (72%)
Coconut oil	1.98 ounces (56.132 grams) (18%)

| Castor oil | 1.10 ounces (31.184 grams) (10%) |
| Fragrance oil | .481 ounce (13.64 grams) (.7%) |

Here are the soap qualities:

Hardness	50
Cleansing	13
Conditioning	47
Bubbly	22
Creamy	46
Iodine	49
INS	160

Always put on your gloves and safety glasses before you begin.

1. Line your mold with freezer paper (shiny side up), following the directions in Chapter 5. If you're using a plastic tray mold, you don't need to line it, but it does help if you spray the mold with a cooking oil spray.

2. Put a ceramic bowl on the scale, and push the tare button to zero out the weight of the cup. Weigh the fragrance oil, and set it aside.

3. Do the same for the colorant, and set aside.

4. Heat the slow cooker to high.

5. Place a cereal bowl–size bowl on the scale, and push the tare button to zero out the weight of the bowl. Weigh each oil individually and add to the slow cooker.

6. Put on your safety glasses and latex gloves again.

7. While the oils are heating, put a plastic bowl on the scale, and push the tare button to zero out the weight of the bowl. Weigh the sodium hydroxide in the bowl. Remove the bowl from the scale, and set it aside.

8. Place a pitcher on the scale, and push the tare button to zero out the weight of the pitcher. Weigh the distilled water. Remove the pitcher from the scale, and set aside.

9. When all the oils have melted, it's time to mix the lye and water. Slowly add the lye to the pitcher of water and stir with a long-handled spoon. Stir the mixture until all the lye has dissolved. Do not put your face close to the pitcher. The vapor from the lye can burn your eyes and lungs.

10. Slowly pour the lye/water mixture into the slow cooker. Using an immersion blender, blend until the soap comes to trace/starts to thicken. This may take 10 to 15 minutes. Once it has come to trace, stop blending, turn the heat to low, and put on the lid. Let it rest as you do the next step.

11. Pour some of the oxides/glycerin mix into a bowl. Dry oxides also work—just mix your dry oxides with the glycerin. I can't tell you how much to start with; this is a trial-and-error thing. Set the colors and fragrance aside.

12. This is the stage when your soap will start to separate, and oil will start coming to the top. Don't worry—this is part of the gel stage, and it's supposed to do this. Keep stirring! The soap may try to climb out of the pot or boil over if you don't keep stirring. Once you reach the mashed potato stage, you can turn off the heat. Stir the soap while it cools down some. If your slow cooker is the type that can be removed from the base, remove it to help the soap cool a little faster.

From the Soap Pot

We use mostly mica or oxides mixed with glycerin to color our soap. We've used liquid colorants but find some of them don't hold their color as well as the oxides.

From the Soap Pot

Sometimes you'll have a hard time getting the soap out of the molds. When using the Milky Way brand molds, we've found that by placing them in the freezer for a few hours (the longer the better), the soap comes out with ease.

13. When the soap has cooled, add the fragrance oil and mix well. Using your long-handled spoon, scoop out about 1 cup soap and add it to the bowl with the colorant. Stir well until the colorant is incorporated. Add the colored soap back to the bowl, and stir in the color until you have the desired effect—less stirring gives you a two-colored, swirled bar; the more you stir, the more you get one color.

14. Pour the soap into the freezer paper–lined mold. Smooth down the top as best you can. Bang the mold on the counter a few times to get the air bubbles out. Let the soap completely cool. You can leave the soap mold on your kitchen counter while it cools or put it in a cold oven to get it out of the way. Cut into bars, and your soap is ready to use.

Making Cold Process Oven Process Soap

Cold process oven process (CPOP), hot process oven process (HPOP), in the mold oven process (ITMOP)—whatever you call it, you're talking about the same thing:

hot process soap that was poured into the mold and then placed in the oven to finish cooking. It's cold process soap put in the oven to force the gel stage and speed up saponification. This is a good way to make a 48-hour process happen in 4 hours! It's the best of both worlds—the smoothness of cold process soap without the cure time.

In addition to most of the equipment listed earlier in the "Making Hot Process Soap" section, you also need an acrylic mold if you opt to only use the oven light for heat. Be sure to line your mold. You can use a wooden mold for the light-on method.

The recipes in this section make approximately 1 pound of soap. The first one has a cleansing of 13, the second one has a cleansing of 11, and the third has a cleansing of 8. The 13 is best suited for normal skin, and the 8 works well for dry skin.

Cold Process Oven Process Soap for Normal Skin

This recipe yields 17.2 ounces (487.6 grams) of soap.

Here's what to put in SoapCalc:

Weight of Oils	11 ounces
Water as % of Oils	38
Super Fat %	8
Fragrance Oz per Lb	.07
Distilled water	4.180 ounces (118.501 grams)
Lye—sodium hydroxide	1.498 ounces (42.455 grams)
Palm oil	7.92 ounces (224.528 grams) (72%)
Coconut oil	1.98 ounces (56.132 grams) (18%)
Castor oil	1.10 ounces (31.184 grams) (10%)
Fragrance oil	.481 ounce (13.64 grams) (.7%)

Here are the soap qualities:

Hardness	50
Cleansing	13
Conditioning	47
Bubbly	22
Creamy	46

Iodine	49
INS	160

The conditioning is low for this soap, but we fixed that by changing the super fat to 8 percent. Even though this number doesn't change on SoapCalc, we know we've added conditioning by raising the super fat. This lowers the amount of lye and leaves more of the oils free to moisturize and condition the skin.

You'll start this soap on the stove and finish it in the oven. You have two choices for the heat: you can either turn on the light in the oven before you start measuring out the oils or preheat the oven to 170°F.

Always put on your gloves and safety glasses before you begin.

1. Line your mold with freezer paper (shiny side up), following the directions in Chapter 5. If you're using a plastic tray mold, you don't need to line it.

2. Place the plastic pitcher on the scale, and push the tare button to zero out the weight of the pitcher. Pour the exact amount of water called for in the recipe into the pitcher, and set it aside.

3. Place the plastic bowl on the scale, and weigh out the exact amount of lye called for in the recipe.

4. Pour the lye into the water in the pitcher and stir until completely dissolved. Put the lid on the pitcher so the lye/water won't make a crust on top. Place at the back of the counter so no one can accidentally turn it over. You won't use this until it's cool.

5. Weigh all oils on the scale and add them to the stockpot. You can stir them at this point if you want, but you don't have to. Set over low heat, and allow the oils to melt. Don't let them get too hot, though. We usually leave some of the coconut or palm unmelted. (The oils will be warm enough to continue melting the little bit that hasn't melted after you remove the pot from the heat. And this way, you don't have to wait as long.) You want the oils to cool down to between 95° and 100°F. The lye should be close to that, too. Don't worry if both of them get cooler than this. It will still make soap.

6. Weigh the fragrance oil in the cup, and set it aside. If you're going to color your soap, have that measured, ready, and waiting nearby.

7. When the oils and lye/water have cooled down, pour the fragrance oil into the other oils. (Or you may wait and add the fragrance at trace if you want to.) Pour

the lye/water into the oils, and stir with spoon or whisk. When you see light trace, pour the soap into the mold and use a spatula to get all the soap out of the pot.

 From the Soap Pot

> When working with floral or fast-moving fragrance oils, a few tricks might help. First, you can add an extra 1 or 2 ounces water to slow the trace. Or you could add the extra water and let the oils and lye cool way down, almost cold. After you've mixed your lye/water into the soap and it's starting to trace, remove the immersion blender, add the fragrance, and use a spoon to hand-stir. Move quickly, because you won't have much time to get the soap into the mold. Pour as soon as all the fragrances are well incorporated. It will take some practice to master the temperamental fragrance oils, but you can do it!

8. If you're using a wooden mold, place it on the top shelf of the oven, and close the door. Leave the oven on for 2 hours and then turn it off, leaving the soap alone, inside the closed oven, until the next morning. Don't open the oven!

   If you're using just the light (and an acrylic mold), leave the light on for 6 hours and then turn it off and leave the soap in the oven until the next morning. Again, don't open the oven door. The soap will still be a little warm the next day.

9. Remove the mold from the oven, and let cool. Remove the soap from the mold, cut it, and it's ready to use.

Soap Stats

> If you see any wrinkles on the top of the soap, that means it got too hot. We've found that when we put two molds in the oven at once, we have to turn off the light or the soap gets too hot and has wrinkles or waves on the top. (This is an easy fix; just plane, or shave, off some of the wrinkles until the soap is smooth.)

Cold Process Oven Process Soap for Mild Skin

This is one of our favorite recipes. You can make the recipe to fit your soap mold using the percentages listed next to each oil. This recipe yields 17.3 ounces (490.5 grams) of soap.

Here's what to put in SoapCalc:

Weight of Oils	11 ounces
Water as % of Oils	38

Super Fat %	8
Fragrance Oz per Lb	.7
Distilled water	4.180 ounces (118.501 grams)
Lye—sodium hydroxide	1.485 ounces (42.099 grams)
Palm oil	8.25 ounces (233.883 grams) (75%)
Coconut oil	1.65 ounces (46.777 grams) (15%)
Castor oil	1.10 ounces (31.184 grams) (10%)
Fragrance	.481 ounce (13.64 grams)

Here are the soap qualities:

Hardness	49
Cleansing	11
Conditioning	48
Bubbly lather	20
Creamy lather	48
Iodine	50
INS	157

You probably noticed that with a cleansing of 11, this soap is a little milder than the preceding recipe, which has a cleansing of 13.

Prepare as instructed for the preceding Cold Process Oven Process Soap for Normal Skin recipe.

Cold Process Oven Process Soap for Sensitive Skin

This mild soap is perfect for those of you who have sensitive skin. This recipe yields 17.2 ounces (487.6 grams) of soap.

Here's what to put in SoapCalc:

Weight of Oils	11 ounces
Water as % of Oils	38
Super Fat %	8
Fragrance Oz per Lb	.7

Distilled water	4.180 ounces (118.501 grams)
Lye—sodium hydroxide	1.464 ounces (41.505 grams)
Palm oil	8.8 ounces (249.476 grams) (80%)
Coconut oil	1.1 ounces (31.184 grams) (10%)
Castor oil	1.1 ounces (31.184 grams) (10%)
Fragrance oil	.481 ounce (13.640 grams) (.7%)

Here are the soap qualities:

Hardness	48
Cleansing	8
Conditioning	50
Bubbly	17
Creamy	49
Iodine	52
INS	151

As you can see, this recipe is even a little milder than the preceding two. The more sensitive the skin, the lower the cleansing needs to be.

Prepare as instructed for the previous Cold Process Oven Process Soap for Normal Skin recipe.

Cold Process Oven Process Soap for Difficult Skin

This soap is great for eczema or for dogs who get hot spots in the summer. This recipe yields 17 ounces (482 grams) soap.

Here's what to put in SoapCalc:

Weight of Oils	11 ounces
Water as % of Oils	38
Super Fat %	5
Fragrance Oz per Lb	.5 (This is an essential oil so use less.)
Distilled water	4.18 ounces (118.501 grams)

Lye—sodium hydroxide	1.45 ounces (41.102 grams)
Palm oil	6.6 ounces (187.107 grams) (60%)
Coconut oil	1.1 ounces (31.184 grams) (10%)
Karanja oil	1.1 ounces (31.184 grams) (10%)
Neem oil	1.1 ounces (31.184 grams) (10%)
Castor oil	1.1 ounces (31.184 grams) (10%)
Juniper essential oil	.34 ounce (9.750 grams)

Here are the soap qualities:

Hardness	42
Cleansing	7
Conditioning	54
Bubbly	16
Creamy	44
Iodine	59
INS	149

This soap will be a little soft, but it'll harden up in a few days.

Prepare as instructed for the previous Cold Process Oven Process Soap for Normal Skin recipe.

The Least You Need to Know

◆ With the methods in this chapter, you can make soap faster and use it the same day!

◆ Your oven isn't only for baking—it's also perfect for making soap!

◆ Drag out your slow cooker from the closet! It has a new use—making soap!

Chapter 8

Cold and Hot Process Soap Recipes

In This Chapter

- ◆ Recipes for cold and hot process soap
- ◆ Tips for coloring your soap
- ◆ Ideas for decorating your bars
- ◆ Finishing and packaging your soap

Now that we've covered the basics of cold and hot process soap-making in the preceding two chapters, it's time to get down to business and start making some super soaps.

In this chapter, we give you a few recipes to get started. These recipes, which work for either cold or hot process soap, are relatively easy to do, but the soaps they produce are absolutely wonderful.

We start with a very simple recipe, and each subsequent recipe takes you another step forward in your soap-making education. By the time you've made all the recipes in this chapter, you'll be well on your way to being a good soap-maker. Enjoy, remember to be creative, and above all else, have fun!

A Few Notes Before We Begin

As mentioned, these recipes all work for either cold or hot process method. Simply follow the appropriate directions from either Chapter 6 for cold process soap or Chapter 7 for hot process soap.

Use SoapCalc to check the recipes and print out the recipe you want to make so you'll have it in front of you while you make the soap batch. Also, by using SoapCalc and the percentages next to each of the oils in the recipes, you can increase or decrease the size of the soap batch to fit your needs and the size of your mold.

From the Soap Pot

Please read all directions before you start. Hindsight is 20/20, and a little foresight/reading can save the soap—and lots of time and frustration!

If you plan on coloring your soap, before you start making any, be sure to read the section on coloring your soap in Chapter 11. We suggest you do a solid color the first time. Choose your colorant and have it ready. If you plan on using oxide for your colorant, you need to wet it first. You do this by putting about 1 teaspoon (5 milliliters) oxide in a glass container and wet it with one of the oils in the recipe or with glycerin. When the oils have melted, add the color-ant directly to the oils and use your immersion blender to mix the colorant before you add the lye solution to the oils. If you're using a liquid colorant, when the oils are melted, just add the recommended amount and use your immersion blender to mix them well before you add the lye solution. But more on that in Chapter 11.

Beginner Batch 1 (2-Pound Mold)

This is a small recipe for you to start with. We suggest using a 2-pound (32-ounce; 907.2-gram), 8-bar plastic tray mold for this soap (find one online or at your local candle and soap supply store). It makes eight 4-ounce (113.4-gram) bars. We are start-ing with this very simple recipe, with no color, so you can concentrate on the steps of making the soap first. When you've completed this recipe without making any mistakes, you can move on to the next recipe. This recipe yields 2 pounds (32 ounces; 907.2 grams).

Here's what to put in SoapCalc:

Weight of Oils	22 ounces
Water as % of Oils	38
Super Fat %	5

Fragrance Oz per Lb	.7 ounces (19.8 grams)
Distilled water	8.4 ounces (237.0 grams)
Lye—sodium hydroxide	3.1 ounces (87.4 grams)
Castor oil	4.4 ounces (124.7 grams) (20%)
Coconut oil	4.4 ounces (124.7 grams) (20%)
Olive oil	4.4 ounces (124.7 grams) (20%)
Palm oil	13.2 ounces (374.2 grams) (60%)
Fragrance oil	1.4 ounces (39.7 grams) (.7 ounce per pound of oils [ppo])

Here are the soap qualities:

Hardness	46
Cleansing	14
Conditioning	51
Bubbly	32
Creamy	49
Iodine	51
INS	158

Beginner Batch 2 (5×6 Mold)

This is the same recipe as Beginner Batch 1, only it's been cut down to fit a 5×6 box mold. You may also want to cut the sides of the box down to 3 inches (7.62 cm). This will make it easier to line the mold. This recipe yields 1.5 pounds (24 ounces; 680.4 grams).

Here's what to put in SoapCalc:

Weight of Oils	16 ounces
Water as % of Oils	38
Super Fat %	5
Fragrance Oz per Lb	.7 ppo
Distilled water	6.1 ounces (172.4 grams)

Lye—sodium hydroxide	2.2 ounces (63 grams)
Castor oil	3.2 ounces (90.7 grams) (20%)
Coconut oil (76 degree)	3.2 ounces (90.7 grams) (20%)
Olive oil	3.2 ounces (90.7 grams) (20%)
Palm oil	6.4 ounces (181.4 grams) (40%)
Fragrance oil	1 ounce (28.4 grams) (.7 ppo)

Here are the soap qualities:

Hardness	39
Cleansing	14
Conditioning	58
Bubbly	32
Creamy	43
Iodine	57
INS	150

Baby Your Baby Soap

We formulated this recipe especially for babies and young children. Babies 3 months old and younger shouldn't have essential oils used on them. You might want to use fragrance oil, such as the Baby Magic Type, for this soap instead. This recipe is also great for more mature skin because it's very gentle and has a lot of moisturizing properties. We usually don't add any colorants to our baby soap, but you can if you want to. A skin-safe colorant won't harm babies or young children. This recipe yields 2 pounds (32 ounces; 907.2 grams).

Here's what to put in SoapCalc:

Weight of Oils	22 ounces
Water as % of Oils	38
Super Fat %	5
Fragrance Oz per Lb	.7 ppo
Distilled water	8.4 ounces (237 grams)
Lye—sodium hydroxide	2.9 ounces (82.2 grams)

Coconut oil (76 degree)	.7 ounces (18.7 grams) (3%)
Cocoa butter	1.1 ounces (31.2 grams) (5%)
Sunflower oil	1.1 ounces (31.2 grams) (5%)
Castor oil	3.7 ounces (106 grams) (17%)
Olive oil	5.5 ounces (156 grams) (25%)
Palm oil	9.9 ounces (280.7 grams) (45%)
Fragrance oil	1 ounce (28.4 grams) (.7 ppo)

Here are the soap qualities:

Hardness	33
Cleansing	2
Conditioning	66
Bubbly	18
Creamy	45
Iodine	56
INS	128

Safety First

This soap is not tear-free. Keep it out of little ones' eyes because it will burn.

Sweetheart Soap for Dry Skin

For this gentle soap that has extra conditioning for dry skin, let's try using a soap-safe strong pink colorant. You'll add the colorant to the soap before you add the lye to the oils. Because floral fragrances can be touchy to work with, hand-stir the fragrance into the soap. Trace will come quickly, so have your mold lined and already close at hand. If you'd prefer to use another fragrance or essential oil, feel free to do so. This recipe yields 3 pounds (48 ounces; 1,360.8 grams).

Here's what to put in SoapCalc:

Weight of Oils	33 ounces
Water as % of Oils	38
Super Fat %	5
Fragrance Oz per Lb	.7 ppo
Distilled water	12.6 ounces (355.5 grams)
Lye—sodium hydroxide	4.5 ounces (126.6 grams)

Cocoa butter	1.7 ounces (46.8 grams) (5%)
Olive oil	3.3 ounces (93.6 grams) (10%)
Coconut oil (76 degree)	3.3 ounces (93.6 grams) (10%)
Castor oil	6.6 ounces (187.1 grams) (20%)
Palm oil	18.15 ounces (514.6 grams) (55%)
Fragrance oil	2 ounces (56.7 grams) (.7 ppo)

Here are the soap qualities:

Hardness	40
Cleansing	7
Conditioning	58
Bubbly	25
Creamy	51
Iodine	58
INS	143

If you make this recipe using the hot process method and want to add a little pizzazz to the finished soap, you can cover the top of the soap with pink or red dried rose petals after you've poured the soap into the mold. It makes a striking bar of soap! (You cannot put the dried rose petals on top of a cold process batch because the active lye will turn the petals brown during the gel stage.)

For this soap, we use White Roses fragrance oil. It's soft and spicier than the regular full-bodied rose fragrances.

From the Soap Pot _____

Many of our fragrance oils can speed trace so fast that you end up with a glob of soap on a stick. There are several ways to help slow these fast fragrance oils. You can add the fragrance oil directly to the pot of soap oils before you add the lye solution. Or you can add a little extra water to the lye. Cool temperature for lye and oils helps. Using soft oils such as olive oil helps slow the trace, too. Always hand-stir the soap after you've added a floral or touchy fragrance oil.

Lavender Bar Soap

This is a completely decadent soap. Once your lavender soap has cured, run to your bathroom, lock the door, light a candle, fill your tub with warm water, and enjoy this soap! Don't forget to hang a "Do Not Disturb" sign outside your bathroom door. This recipe yields 3 pounds (48 ounces; 1,360.8 grams).

Here's what to put in SoapCalc:

Weight of Oils	33 ounces
Water as % of Oils	38
Super Fat %	5
Fragrance Oz per Lb	.7 ppo
Distilled water	12.6 ounces (357.2 grams)
Lye—sodium hydroxide	4.5 ounces (127.6 grams)
Shea butter	1.7 ounces (46.8 grams) (5%)
Olive oil	3.3 ounces (93.6 grams) (10%)
Coconut oil (76 degree)	4.6 ounces (131 grams) (14%)
Castor oil	6.6 ounces (187.1 grams) (20%)
Palm oil	16.8 ounces (477.1 grams) (51%)
Fragrance oil	2 ounces (56.7 grams) (56.7%)

Here are the soap qualities:

Hardness	41
Cleansing	10
Conditioning	57
Bubbly	28
Creamy	49
Iodine	57
INS	145

When we color this soap, we remove about 2 or 3 cups (453.6 to 680.4 grams) of the soap base and, using a large measuring cup, mix in a soft purple (or a purple and a lavender!) soap-safe colorant. Follow the instructions for swirling your soap in Chapter 11. After you've colored your soap and removed the part to be colored, add the fragrance.

Safety First _____

The strength of fragrances can vary greatly between manufacturers and vendors, so adjust the amount of fragrance you use in these recipes according to the manufacturer's recommended use. Even if it is a weak fragrance oil, please don't use more than 3 percent of the total weight of your recipe.

Choose a nice lavender fragrance oil or lavender essential oil, but know that lavender is a floral and can speed trace. Use a stainless-steel spoon, and hand-stir the fragrance into the batch. Pour the base soap into the mold and start swirling your color into the soap base. Follow the rest of the directions for swirling your soap batch.

If you don't want to swirl, you can color the batch solid with a soap-safe lavender colorant. If you used the hot process method, try sprinkling lavender buds on the top after you pour it into your mold. Be creative!

Manly Man's Soap

Soaps for men should have a nice outdoorsy or cologne fragrance, and there are many on the market today for you to choose from. Try Irish Green Tweed or Cool Water. Sandalwood is also good. This recipe yields 3 pounds (48 ounces; 1,360.8 grams).

Here's what to put in SoapCalc:

Weight of Oils	33 ounces
Water as % of Oils	38
Super Fat %	5
Fragrance Oz per Lb	.7 ppo
Distilled water	12.6 ounces (357.2 grams)
Lye—sodium hydroxide	4.6 ounces (129.9 grams)
Olive oil	3.3 ounces (93.6 grams) (10%)
Coconut oil	6.6 ounces (187.1 grams) (20%)
Castor oil	8.3 ounces (233.9 grams) (25%)

Palm oil	14.6 ounces (421 grams) (45%)
Fragrance oil	2 ounces (56.7 grams) (.7 ppo)

Here are the soap qualities:

Hardness	40
Cleansing	14
Conditioning	57
Bubbly lather	36
Creamy lather	49
Iodine	56
INS	151

Men need a higher cleansing number than most women. This bar has a higher castor oil percentage so it will be a softer bar in the beginning and will need a little extra time to cure. Thanks to the increased castor oil, this soap has lots of lather.

You can leave this bar plain and uncolored, or you can swirl it with more masculine colors. When we use the Irish Green Tweed fragrance, we swirl in green, black, and brown.

Buttery and Nice Soap

During the winter, your skin needs extra oils and conditioning, so we formulated this recipe just for winter skin. The super fat is 8 percent, the shea butter is used for its moisturizing properties, and the cocoa butter helps protect the skin and seals in moisture. This recipe yields 3 pounds (48 ounces; 1,360.8 grams).

Here's what to put in SoapCalc:

Weight of Oils	33 ounces
Water as % of Oils	38
Super Fat %	8
Fragrance Oz per Lb	.7 ppo

Distilled water	12.5 ounces (355.5 grams)
Lye—sodium hydroxide	4.4 ounces (124.2 grams)
Peanut oil	1 ounce (28.4 grams) (3%)
Cocoa butter	1.7 ounces (46.8 grams) (5%)
Shea butter	1.7 ounces (46.8 grams) (5%)
Olive oil	1.7 ounces (46.8 grams) (5%)
Coconut oil (76 degree)	4.6 ounces (131 grams) (14%)
Castor oil	5 ounces (140.3 grams) (15%)
Palm oil	17.5 ounces (495.8 grams) (53%)
Fragrance oil	2 ounces (56.7 grams) (.7 ppo)

Here are the soap qualities:

Hardness	44
Cleansing	10
Conditioning	53
Bubbly lather	23
Creamy lather	48
Iodine	54
INS	149

Safety First _____

Be sure anyone who might use this bar of soap is aware that it contains peanut oil.

We sometimes play around with using natural spices, herbs, and clays to color our soaps. In this soap, we usually use cocoa powder to color a part of the soap batch for swirling. We like the "in the pot" method for this so there are different shades of brown and cream as part of the swirl. Looks good enough to eat!—but don't because, after all, it's soap!

Cool, Fresh Cucumber Soap

This is a refreshing soap, perfect for hot summer days. To this soap base you add 2 ounces of fresh puréed cucumber just before you add the fragrance. What better fragrance to use than a crisp cucumber fragrance oil? We love making a green swirl in this soap, too. This recipe yields 3 pounds (48 ounces; 1,360.8 grams).

Here's what to put in SoapCalc:

Weight of Oils	33 ounces
Water as % of Oils	388
Super Fat %	5
Fragrance Oz per Lb	.7 ppo
Distilled water	12.5 ounces (355.5 grams)
Lye—sodium hydroxide	4.6 ounces (129.3 grams)
Avocado oil	1.7 ounces (45.8 grams) (5%)
Castor oil	5 ounces (140.3 grams) (15%)
Olive oil	5 ounces (140.3 grams) (15%)
Coconut oil	5.6 ounces (159.0 grams) (17%)
Palm oil	15.8 ounces (449.0 grams) (48%)
Fragrance oil	2 ounces (56.7 grams) (.7 ppo)
Puréed fresh cucumber (added to soap at trace)	2 ounces (56.7 grams)

Here are the soap qualities:

Hardness	41
Cleansing	12
Conditioning	56
Bubbly lather	25
Creamy lather	43
Iodine	57
INS	148

From the Soap Pot

When making shampoo bars, you might want to add some proteins and vitamins. Panthenol B5, honeyquat, and silk amino acid are very conditioning. Some essential oils also help correct scalp or hair problems. Check out Chapter 3 for which essential oils would be helpful for your needs. You would add these additives when you add the fragrance or essential oil.

Shampoo Bar Soap

For this shampoo bar, the super fat is higher to give the hair a little extra conditioning. And the hempseed and avocado oils used are also wonderful for the hair. This recipe yields 2 pounds (32 ounces; 907.2 grams).

Here's what to put in SoapCalc:

Weight of Oils	22 ounces
Water as % of Oils	38
Super Fat %	8
Fragrance Oz per Lb	.7 ppo
Distilled water	6.1 ounces (172.4 grams)
Lye—sodium hydroxide	2 ounces (57.9 grams)
Hempseed oil	.67 ounce (18.7 grams) (3%)
Coconut oil	1 ounce (28.4 grams) (6%)
Avocado oil	1.1 ounces (31.8 grams) (7%)
Castor oil	5.6 ounces (158.8 grams) (35%)
Palm oil	7.8 ounces (222.2 grams) (49%)
Fragrance oil	1 ounce (28.4 grams) (.7 ppo)

Here are the soap qualities:

Hardness	31
Cleansing	5
Conditioning	67
Bubbly lather	36
Creamy lather	58
Iodine	68
INS	128

Safety First _____

Avoid getting this soap in your eyes; it will burn.

This bar will be soft at first and may need extra time in the mold before removing it. Castor oil takes longer to saponify, and because this bar has a high castor oil percentage, the cure time will be up to 4 to 6 weeks. Letting the soap stay in the mold an extra couple days will also be helpful when trying to remove it. It's definitely worth the wait! The castor oil is what gives this bar such an abundance of lather.

As with all fresh soap batches, this one will be soft at first, and removing it from an unlined plastic mold can be difficult. We recommend that you put the plastic mold in your freezer overnight before trying to unmold your soap. The next morning, turn the mold upside down on a piece of waxed paper. Press in the center of the mold, and the soap should release. If not, wait a few minutes and try again. Once soap has been removed from the plastic tray mold, let the soap warm up to room temperature before cutting it into bars. If the soap is frozen, it'll shatter when you cut it.

Facial Bar for Normal Skin

This chapter wouldn't be complete if we didn't include a facial bar. You can choose a single fragrance oil or blend a few together for their skin benefits. A blend we like contains .3 ounce (8.5 grams) each of Bulgarian lavender, lemongrass, and geranium essential oils. If you can find red palm oil (natural unrefined), that addition would make the bar perfect! Red palm oil is very high in 2 types of vitamin E and A and will make your soap a lovely apricot-yellow color. Super fat this bar at 8 percent. This recipe yields 2 pounds (32 ounces; 907.2 grams.)

Here's what to put in SoapCalc:

Weight of Oils	22 ounces
Water as % of Oils	38
Super Fat %	8
Fragrance Oz per Lb	.7 ppo (1 ounce; 28.4 grams) (or the essential oil blend)
Distilled water	8.4 ounces (237.0 grams)
Lye—sodium hydroxide	2.8 ounces (80.3 grams)
Evening primrose oil	.67 ounce (18.7 grams) (3%)
Rosehip oil	1 ounce (28.4 grams) (6%)
Shea butter	.67 ounce (18.7 grams) (3%)
Cupuacu butter	.67 ounce (18.7 grams) (3%)
Coconut oil	1.1 ounces (31.8 grams) (5%)
Castor oil	4.4 ounces (124.7 grams) (20%)

| Palm oil | 13.2 ounces (374.2 grams) (60%) |
| Fragrance oil | .9 ounce (25.5 grams) for essential oil and 1 ounce for fragrance oil (28.4 grams) (.7 ppo) (You will always use less essential oil or essential oil blend than fragrance oil.) |

Here are the soap qualities:

Hardness	31
Cleansing	5
Conditioning	67
Combined lather	94
Iodine	68
INS	128

Finishing Your Soap Bars

Once your soap has had a day or two to harden, it will be time to give it a finished and professional look, no matter if you're keeping it for yourself, giving it as a gift, or selling it.

To even out any uneven edges and sides, we use a soap planer. If you don't have a planer, you can use something like a cheese cutter. Some soap-makers even use a potato peeler. You may also want to bevel the edges of your soap to take off the sharp edge. It's completely up to you how you want to finish the bars.

Using a soft cloth removes any little bits that may be on the surface of the soap, and the cloth also gives the soap bar a nice shine. After you've cleaned and polished your soap, place the bars back on the drying rack or box and let them continue to cure.

If you've decided to use the hot process method and added rose petals or lavender buds to the top of your soap bar, you won't be able to use a planer to even up the edges. So instead, cut the soap using a wavy soap cutter. As a bonus, this can hide uneven cuts!

To prevent our soap from getting nicks and dents, we use shrink-wrap tubing to protect it. All you have to do is cut the shrink-wrap .5 inch longer than the soap on each end. You want the edges of the wrap to only cup over the ends of the soap bar. Slide the soap into the shrink-wrap tube, center it, and, using a hairdryer on high or a heat gun, shrink the wrap over the soap. Don't hold the dryer or heat gun too close to the soap bar, or you'll burn a hole in the wrap. Leave the ends open so the soap can continue to evaporate the excess water.

After you've shrink-wrapped your soap, you could package it in soap boxes. These are very handy for putting the labels on and offer a nice space on the back of the box for the ingredient label. These boxes can be expensive, so you might want to buy them in bulk for discount. If you don't want to go the box route, there are hundreds of other cute and eye-catching ways to package your soap.

 Soap Stats

The shrink-wrapping also prevents the soap from absorbing all the smells in the air such as cigarette smoke. If you're a smoker, you may not be able to smell the cigarette smoke, but nonsmokers will. The same is true for pet odors and hairs.

A Little Soap Humor

We are both part of several Yahoo! soap-makers lists, and those groups like to have fun making soapy songs or soapy raps. One afternoon we got to talking about the warning labels we put on our soap. You know the kind—"if irritation occurs, discontinue use." These are no-brainers, but we still have to have them on the labels.

One of the members started being very creative with her warnings. She came up with, "If soap gets in mouth, stop cussing." This had everyone laughing. Before we knew it, others were joining in with other funny warnings, like "If gets in eyes, shut your eyes next time!" or "Of course it tastes bad—it's soap!"

Soap-making is fun, and we soap-makers have fun talking with each other about all types of soap projects, including humorous labeling and funny stories of mishaps.

The Least You Need to Know

◆ For soap-making success, have everything you need ready and waiting before you start.

◆ You can blend together essential oils and fragrance oils to create unique and personal scents.

◆ Be creative and add extra goodies to your soap using additives such as seeds or jojoba beads to exfoliate the skin. Just add them at trace!

Chapter 9

Goat Milk Soap

In This Chapter

- The benefits of goat milk soap
- Preventing your goat milk soap from discoloring
- Two great recipes for goat milk soap

Milk has long been reputed to be a rejuvenator and moisturizer for the human skin. Even Cleopatra bathed in full tubs of milk to keep her skin soft and youthful!

Soap made with milk is one thing, but soap made with goat milk is quite something else. It's ultra gentle and perfectly suited for delicate and sensitive skin.

The Basics of Goat Milk Soap

When making 100 percent goat milk soap, any recipe you have will do. You'll simply substitute goat milk for the water called for in the recipe. Beyond that, making soap with goat milk is a little different from making soap with water—but it's so worth the extra trouble!

Not everyone will have the luxury of having fresh goat milk, so if this is the case with you, you'll have to use either canned or powdered milk. Before Zonella found her local goat farm, she used canned and powdered milk. You can use the canned milk straight, or you can dilute it. The powdered milk will have directions on the package, or you can mix 1 ounce (28.35 grams) milk to 8 ounces (803.7 grams) water.

From the Soap Pot

Look for goat milk in the canned-milk section of your grocery store. For fresh goat milk, look for a local goat farm in your area. You might also find a health food store in your area that carries fresh goat milk.

Goat milk soap will turn wheat-colored if it isn't put in a refrigerator or freezer. The hotter it gets, the darker it will go. If you prefer your soap to be white, put it in the refrigerator as soon as you pour it in the mold.

Also, soap made with canned and powdered milk won't be as white as soap made with fresh milk.

Making Goat Milk Soap

As with any other kind of soap, you need to assemble the equipment you'll need ahead of time. After you start, you won't have time to go look for something! Here's what you'll need (turn back to Chapter 1 if you need a refresher on these items):

- Safety glasses
- Thin latex gloves
- Scale
- Plastic pitcher
- Cereal bowl–size glass or plastic bowls (for oils and butters)
- Long-handled stainless-steel or plastic spoon

- Meat or candy thermometer
- Immersion blender
- Freezer paper
- Mold
- Stove

100 Percent Goat Milk Soap

The goat milk in this recipe is used frozen. That helps the milk/lye solution cool faster and prevents the milk from getting as hot from the heat of the lye. When the milk gets hot, the sugars in it turn dark, making the soap brown. That's also why the soap goes through gel in the refrigerator. This recipe yields 15.64 ounces (443.4 grams).

Here's what to put in SoapCalc:

Weight of Oils	11 ounces
Water as % of Oils	34
Super Fat %	10
Fragrance Oz per Lb	.7
Goat milk	2.74 ounces (77.691 grams)
Lye—sodium hydroxide	1.412 ounces (40.023 grams)
Palm oil	6.6 ounces (187.107 grams) (60%)
Coconut oil	1.1 ounces (31.184 grams) (10%)
Castor oil	2.2 ounces (62.369 grams) (20%)
Sunflower (High Oleic)	1.1 ounces (31.184 grams) (10%)
Cucumber-mint fragrance oil	.481 ounces (13.640 grams) (.7 ppo)

Here are the soap qualities:

Hardness	39
Cleansing	7
Conditioning	59
Bubbly	25
Creamy	49
Iodine	58
INS	142

Soap Stats

There's a big difference between high-oleic and regular sunflower oil, so when putting this recipe in SoapCalc, be sure to click the right one.

Freeze the goat milk before you begin making this soap. Do this with whichever type you use—canned, powdered, or fresh. You want it frozen solid. Measure the 2.74 ounces (77.691 grams) of goat milk into a zipper-lock bag, and lay it flat in the freezer. Right before you add it to the recipe, drop the bag on the counter or the floor a few times to break the frozen milk into pieces. (This works better than hitting it with a hammer, which might break the bag and cause a big mess.)

Always put on your gloves and safety glasses before you begin.

1. Line your mold with freezer paper (shiny side up), following the directions in Chapter 5. If you're using a plastic tray mold, you don't need to line it, but using a cooking or silicone mold spray will help the soap release from the mold easier. Check your refrigerator, and clean out a spot to put it when the time comes.

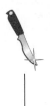

Safety First _____

Remember to use and wear the appropriate safety equipment when you're making soap.

2. Weigh the fragrance oil, and set it aside.

3. Weigh the lye, and set it aside. Be sure it has a lid on it so it won't spill.

4. Weigh all the oils, and place in the stockpot. Set the pot over low heat, and heat until all the oils are melted. Remove from heat, and set aside to cool to 95°F.

5. When the oils reach 95°F, remove the milk from the freezer, and drop it on the counter to break into pieces.

6. Place the frozen pieces of milk into the container you've set aside to hold the lye/milk mixture. Pour the lye over the frozen pieces of milk, and stir slowly until all the milk and lye are dissolved. Don't rush this step; it's very important that all of the lye and milk dissolve.

7. When the lye/milk are dissolved, slowly add them to the cooled oil mixture, and blend with a spoon.

8. Add the fragrance oil, and stir to combine. The cucumber mint doesn't accelerate the soap to trace, so you can use the immersion blender if you like. If you're going to use a fragrance that accelerates the trace, stir with a spoon.

9. As soon as the soap begins to thicken, pour it into the prepared mold. Because of the high sugar in the milk, the soap will turn dark if you allow it to go into gel mode. (The soap gets very hot when it starts to saponify.)

10. If you don't want your soap to darken, place it in the refrigerator as soon as you pour it into the mold. (Don't have any cut onions or anything else that has a strong odor in the refrigerator, or your soap will absorb the odor!) The cooler the soap, the lighter it will be. Leave the mold in the refrigerator for 24 to 36 hours. Thirty-six hours is better because it's less likely to be lye-active after that long, and the additional cooling time takes some of the moisture out of the soap.

From the Soap Pot _____

If you don't have a refrigerator handy to put the soap in, you can place a fan to blow on the soap to help keep it cooler. But do not insulate. It even helps to elevate the mold by putting a support under each corner so the air from the fan can get under the mold, too, and help keep the soap cooler.

11. Remove the soap from the mold, cut into bars, and allow to dry. You may have lye activity up to 48 hours after pouring into the mold. That's okay, and it'll eventually settle down.

Because this soap has 20 percent castor oil, it needs to cure for 4 to 6 weeks before using. The soap won't hurt you if you use it right away; it just won't be as moisturizing. It just takes the added time for the lye to make the castor oil let go of its wonderful moisturizing qualities. But it's well worth the wait.

50 Percent Goat Milk/50 Percent Water Soap

This recipe is a bit easier and less time-consuming than the 100 Percent Goat Milk Soap recipe earlier in this chapter because you don't have to freeze the milk first. This recipe yields 15.7 ounces (445.1 grams) of soap.

Here's what to put in SoapCalc:

Weight of Oils	11 ounces
Water as % of Oils	38
Super Fat %	8
Fragrance Oz per Lb	.7 ppo
Distilled water	1.37 ounces (38.840 grams)
Lye—sodium hydroxide	1.41 ounces (40.023 grams)
Goat milk	1.37 ounces (38.840 grams)
Palm oil	6.6 ounces (187.107 grams) (60%)
Coconut oil	1.1 ounces (31.184 grams) (10%)
Castor oil	2.2 ounces (62.369 grams) (20%)
Sunflower (high oleic)	1.1 ounces (31.184 grams) (10%)
Cucumber-mint fragrance oil	.48 ounce (13.640 grams) (.7 ppo)

Here are the soap qualities:

Hardness	39
Cleansing	7
Conditioning	59
Bubbly	25

Creamy	49
Iodine	58
INS	142

Always put on your gloves and safety glasses before you begin.

1. Line your mold with freezer paper (shiny side up), following the directions in Chapter 5. If you're using a plastic tray mold, you don't need to line it.

2. Weigh the fragrance oil and set aside.

3. Weigh the water, and add the lye. Stir until dissolved.

4. Weigh the milk, and set it aside in its own container.

5. Weigh each oil and add to the pot. Set over low heat, and heat to 95°F. If you get the oils too hot, let them cool to the proper temperature.

6. When the oils are cooled to 95°F, pour in the fragrance oils and blend with the immersion blender. Or if you like, you can wait until the soap traces to add the fragrance.

7. Add the milk to the lye/water mixture, stir, and immediately pour into the oils. Don't allow the lye/water/milk to set for any time, or it will begin to turn orange and smell. As soon as you add the milk to the lye/water mixture, add it to the oils.

8. Blend with the immersion blender until the soap reaches light trace (just a slight thickening). Change to a spoon or spatula, so you can feel the soap get thicker. You want the soap just a little past light trace. If you're going to use another fragrance oil, use a spoon to stir, not an immersion blender. The immersion blender brings the soap to trace faster, and the fragrance oil accelerates it, too. The soap will zoom right on past light trace and be too firm to pour into the mold.

9. Pour the soap into the lined mold, and place into the refrigerator for 24 to 36 hours.

10. Remove the soap from the mold, cut into bars, and allow to dry. Let at least 4 weeks go by before you use the soap. If you wait, it will be so much more moisturizing than when first made.

Castor oil is the hardest oil to saponify, and it will take up to 4 weeks for the lye to make the castor oil give up its good qualities to the soap.

In the past I have added castor oil to the lye/water mix instead of adding to the oils in the pot. This has proven to make the soap bars even harder. If you decide to try this, heat all your oils except for the castor oil. Save it, and add it to the lye/water solution, stirring well, just before you add the solution to the cooled oils.

The Least You Need to Know

- There's an easy way to keep your goat milk soap from turning brown. The secret is to keep the milk cold. Very cold. Frozen, even.

- We have recipes for you using 100 percent and 50 percent goat milk. Which do you want to use?

- It's important to read all instructions, lay out all your equipment, and get all your safety gear in place when making soap.

Liquid Soap

In This Chapter

- Formulating liquid soap using SoapCalc
- Easy instructions for making liquid soap
- Recipes for household and laundry soap
- Shower gel and shampoo recipes
- Recipes for facial and hand soaps

Liquid soap is so much fun to make. Although it does take a lot of time to cook and dilute, don't be afraid to try this type of soap. It's very easy once you get the hang of it.

In this chapter, you learn an easy way to make a basic liquid soap you can use for many purposes, as well as some terrific shower gels and shampoos for every type of skin and hair.

Using SoapCalc to Formulate Your Soap

Before you start making your soap, always check your recipe in SoapCalc. This is a very important habit to get into, and one we always advise new soap-makers to do. Anyone can make a mistake or enter an incorrect number, and checking the recipe makes good soap sense, no matter who wrote it.

All liquid soap is made basically the same way, so this formula works for any kind of liquid soap. Here's what to put in SoapCalc:

Type of Lye used	KOH
Weight of Oils	ounces
Water as % of Oils	80
Super Fat %	–13

The rest of the settings for the laundry soap and shower gels are different, so you'll enter the specifics when you get to those recipes, but this is the basic setup for liquid soaps.

When you've put in all the information, you'll be ready to formulate or check your recipe. It's as easy as that!

Increasing and Decreasing Batches

It's easy to increase or decrease the size of a batch of liquid soap once you know the percentage of each oil. Just remember that the weight of your paste (the oils and lye) is half of the total weight of your batch. So to find out how much paste you need, you divide the total weight of your desired finished batch by 2. Let's say you want 32 ounces (907.2 grams) of shower gel. 32 ÷ 2 = 16. So for 32 ounces of shower gel, you'll need 16 ounces (453.6 grams) of paste.

Soap Stats _____

Household detergent was introduced and produced in the United States in the 1930s. It became popular after World War II.

Now, to figure out the total weight of oils you need, divide your number by 2 again: 16 ounces (453.6 grams) ÷ 2 = 8. The total weight of oils for your 32-ounce batch is 8 ounces (226.8 grams). This is the number you enter for Total Weight of Oils on SoapCalc. Then you can add in the individual oils and their percentages in the oil columns. Click the Calculate Recipe button, and you're done!

Let's try another one. Say the recipe is written for a 64-ounce (1,814.4-gram) batch of liquid soap, and you want 256 ounces (7,257.6 grams). 256 ÷ 2 = 128 ounces (3,628.8 grams). This is both the paste weight and the dilute water weight. Now, divide by

2 once again to get the total weight of oils. 128 ÷ 2 = 64 ounces (1,814.4 grams). Type 64 in the Total Weight of Oils box in SoapCalc. Then, again, add the oils and their percentages in the oil column and calculate the recipe.

Now that we have our basics, let's make some soap!

Making Liquid Soap and Shampoo

You'll need certain supplies for making any kind of liquid soap, shower gel, or shampoo. Here's what you'll need (turn back to Chapter 1 if you need a refresher on these items):

- Safety glasses
- Thin latex gloves
- Scale
- Immersion blender
- Meat or candy thermometer
- Stove
- Cereal bowl–size glass or plastic bowl

- Plastic pitcher
- Large stainless-steel stockpot with a solid stainless-steel lid (no plastic handles or knobs), or aluminum foil for cover
- Long-handled stainless-steel or plastic spoons
- Plastic funnel
- Plastic bottle to store the soap

You'll notice that liquid soap is made using potassium hydroxide lye instead of sodium hydroxide, the kind of lye used for bar soap. Potassium hydroxide comes in flake or diamond-shape pieces. With this type of lye, your oil won't become solid and hard, and the soap remains in a liquid form. Liquid soap also has a lower pH than bar soaps, which helps the liquid soap hold together. Borax is used to neutralize any leftover lye and lower the soap's pH.

Safety First _____

If the pH is too high, your soap will separate. Same is true if the pH is too low. It's best to keep the pH around 9.5. You'll know your soap has separated when the bottom is opaque and the top is clear. It can take a couple days or weeks for this to happen. There's no way to save a batch of liquid soap if it has separated. You have to toss it out and start over.

Although there are several products to choose from to thicken your shower gels, our favorite is HEC (hydroxyethyl cellulose). This natural product is made from polymer cellulose, is water soluble, and stays clear. You can also use citric acid, although it can make the end product cloudy. Boric acid is another choice, but HEC is still our favorite.

You'll need a 1-gallon (128-ounce; 3628.8-gram) container to store your Basic Household and Laundry Soap. An empty used laundry detergent bottle that's been cleaned also works. What won't work, however, is a plastic milk jug. The plastic is too thin, and the soap will soon leak out.

For shower gel storage, we recommend 8-ounce (226.8-gram) or 16-ounce (453.6-gram) PET-type plastic bottles. These bottles are made from recycled plastic. You can find them online at several of the venders we list on Appendix D.

Making Household and Laundry Soap

At less than $5 per batch (depending on where you get your ingredients), homemade liquid soap is not only a fantastic bargain, but it also does a great job cleaning everything from your clothes to your kitchen, bathroom, and walls. Your stovetop will shine like new when you clean it with this soap, and it's excellent for hand-washing dishes. Don't try it in your dishwasher, though—unless you're planning on mopping your floor that day!

Soap Stats

For some reason, spiders don't like coconut oil. After I'd been using this soap to clean my tile floors, I noticed I no longer saw spider webs in the corners of ceilings. We live in the country, so I used to find a lot of spiders who made their way into the house. Now I hardly ever see them or any evidence they've been around.

As a laundry detergent, there's nothing better. You'll get 64 loads of laundry out of this batch in hard water and 128 loads of clothes in soft water—and it's biodegradable, so it can be used in front-load washers. This soap also rinses completely out of your clothes and removes all the buildup that's been left by store-bought detergents. You'll also notice that your clothes are softer and no longer need fabric softeners or dryer sheets—another great way to save a few pennies!

Please be sure to read all the instructions before you start. And remember, some oils are thicker and therefore weigh more than others, so you must always weigh—not measure—all ingredients.

Basic Household and Laundry Soap

You'll love this all-around soap and find new uses for it all the time. This recipe yields 1 gallon (128 ounces; 3,628.8 grams; 3.78 liters).

Here's what to put in SoapCalc—remember to adjust the Type of Lye used, Weight of Oils, Water as % of Oils, and Super Fat % categories as instructed earlier in this chapter:

Weight of Oils	32 ounces (908.8 grams)
Water as % of Oils	80
Super Fat %	−13
Fragrance Oz per Lb	(See the later "Scenting Your Household and Laundry Soap" section.)
Coconut oil (76 degree)	8 ounces (226.7 grams) (25%)
Palm kernel oil	8 ounces (226.8 grams) (25%)
Lard	16 ounces (276 grams) (50%)
Distilled water (for lye)	25.6 ounces (725.7 grams)
Lye—potassium hydroxide	8.1 ounces (230.7 grams)
Distilled water (for dilution and borax)	64 ounces (1,814.4 grams)
Borax	2.5 ounces (70.9 grams)
Fragrance oil (if desired)	1.5 to 3 ounces (42.5 to 85.0 grams) (This is added after the cook and dilution.)

For more cleaning power, you can increase the borax. We've increased the borax to as much as 8 ounces. But a word of warning: if you plan to use the soap to mop your floors and you have pets, don't increase the borax to more than 3 ounces. It may cause irritation to your pet's feet. If your pet is chewing on its feet, decrease amount of borax. And always rinse the floors after mopping with this soap.

Always put on your gloves and safety glasses before you begin.

1. Place the plastic pitcher on the scale, and push the tare button to zero out the weight of the pitcher. Weigh the coconut oil in the pitcher and pour into the pot.

2. Weight the palm kernel oil and pour into the pot.

3. Set the pot of oils over medium-low heat. If you're using a candy thermometer, attach it to the side of the pan now.

4. While the oil is heating, put the plastic bowl on the scale and zero out the weight of the bowl. Weigh the potassium hydroxide in the bowl. Set aside.

5. Place a pitcher on the scale, zero out the weight of the pitcher, and weigh the distilled water. Set aside.

Safety First

Always slowly add the lye to the water, *never* the other way around. Doing it the other way around can cause a volcanic reaction.

6. Check the temperature of the oils. When the oil has reached 160°F (71°C), it's time to mix the lye and water. Slowly add the lye to the pitcher of water and stir. You will hear a "swoosh" as the lye dissolves in the water. Stir the mixture until all the lye has dissolved. Do not put your face close to the pitcher. The vapor from the lye can burn your eyes and lungs.

7. Keeping the pot on the burner still set on medium-low, slowly pour the lye/ water mixture into the batch of oils. Using an immersion blender, blend until the oils and water come together. Bring the mixture to a thick trace by blending for a few minutes and then stopping for a few minutes. Be patient; bringing the mixture to a thick trace takes some time—sometimes up to 45 minutes! When it reaches thick trace, it will look like very thick pudding.

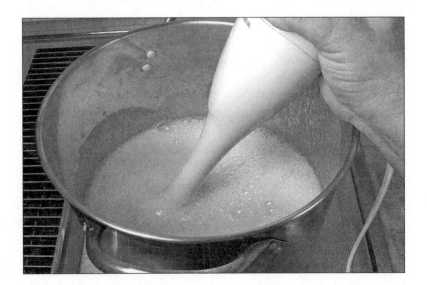

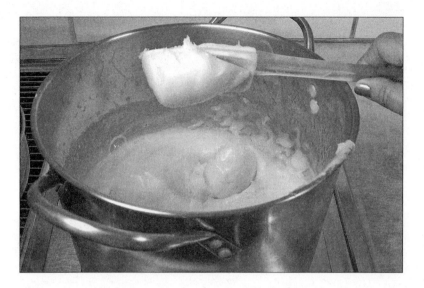

8. Remove the blender and set it aside when the soap has become too thick to stir. Remove the pot from the heat and let it sit on the counter while the soap continues to harden into a paste. This can take up to 30 minutes.

9. While you're waiting for the soap to form a hard paste, preheat the oven to 200°F (93°C). When the soap has reached the hard paste stage, cover the pot with the lid or aluminum foil, and put the pot in the oven for 4 hours or until the paste is transparent. (Remove a little bit of paste and spread it out over a piece of paper or a plate to test this. Not all paste will be completely transparent.)

From the Soap Pot _____

Just as your soap is starting to come to trace, you might notice a little thickening and foam around the edge of the pot. This is perfectly normal.

10. Place the plastic bowl on the scale, zero out the weight, and weigh the borax. Set aside.

11. Place the pitcher on the scale, zero out the weight, and weigh 4 ounces distilled water. Pour the water into a stainless-steel pan and add the borax. Stir, and place on the stove over medium heat. Bring to a boil and continue a simmering boil until the borax is completely dissolved.

12. Weigh the rest of your water in the pitcher on the scale, and pour it into another pan. Set over high heat, bring to a boil, and add it to the soap paste.

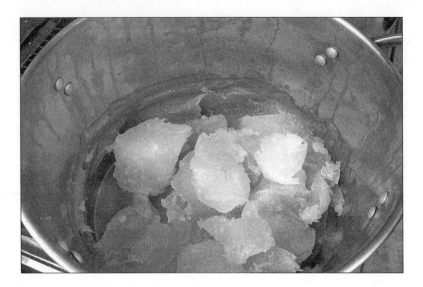

Soap Stats

You don't have to dilute the paste the same day you make it. You can leave it out overnight to dilute the next day. You can also put it in a baggie and freeze it until you're ready.

13. Slowly pour the borax mixture into the paste, put the lid back on, set the diluted mixture over medium heat, and let it all melt down. Keep a close watch on this because it might boil over, or you can put the burner on low and check on it every 30 minutes.

14. When the soap is completely melted, remove it from heat. Let it cool down in the pot for at least an hour. The sides of the pot should feel only slightly warm to the touch.

15. Add the fragrance, if desired, and stir to thoroughly combine. When the soap has completely cooled, pour it into your plastic bottles.

Another Easy Household and Laundry Soap

We love making this soap with 100 percent coconut oil (76°F). It costs a little bit more, but you may find it worth it because you won't have to buy palm kernel oil, too. You can use LouAna coconut oil from your local grocery store. This recipe yields 1 gallon (128 ounces; 3,627.2 grams).

Here's what to put in SoapCalc—remember to adjust the Type of Lye used, Weight of Oils, Water as % of Oils, and Super Fat % categories as instructed earlier in this chapter:

Weight of Oils	32 ounces (907.2 grams)
Water as % of Oils	80
Super Fat %	–13
Fragrance Oz per Lb	(See the "Scenting Your Household and Laundry Soap" section.)
Coconut oil (76 degree)	32 ounces (907.2 grams) (100%) (Don't forget to add the borax when you dilute the paste!)

Follow the same directions as you did for the Basic Household and Laundry Soap, using the amount of water and potassium hydroxide SoapCalc calls for in this recipe.

From the Soap Pot

You can also use the soap paste undiluted for cleaning hard surfaces. Just pinch off a little of the paste, and using a wet rag, clean that baked-on grease off your vent hood or the bottom of your pots and pans.

Scenting Your Household and Laundry Soap

Scenting this type of soap is done a little differently. You use less scent because fragrance and essential oils can leave oil spots on your clothes if you use too much. You also may not want the scent in your laundry soap so it won't overpower your perfume or cologne.

If you're using a fragrance oil whose recommended use is .5 ounce (14.2 grams) fragrance per 1 pound soap, then use 1 ounce (28.4 grams) for these recipes. If the fragrance oil is recommended at 1 ounce (28.4 grams) per 1 pound soap, use a total of 2 ounces (56.7 grams) for these recipes. If you like more scent, increase it another 1 ounce (28.4 grams); if you don't like it that strong, decrease the amount. We usually use 3 ounces (85.05 grams) fragrance oil in laundry soap, but you can make it as strong or mild as you like. You also might like orange essential oil for its cleaning properties, but know that it will make the soap very cloudy-looking.

Making Shower Gels

To make shower gel, you follow the basic step-by-step directions for the liquid soap. The only difference is the amount of distilled water, lye, borax, and additives you may want to add.

From the Soap Pot

Remember that the total weight of oils, lye, and water will make the paste that you'll dilute into the finished product at a ratio of 1:1. That means 1 ounce paste to 1 ounce water. If your paste weighs 32 ounces, you'd dilute with 32 ounces (907.2 grams) water and 1 ounce (28.35 grams) borax. This would make the total finished product 65 ounces.

For shower gels and shampoos, we've found that a low cleansing number is best so they don't dry out your skin or hair. We cannot super fat liquid soaps the way we do bar soap, so that number is changed by lowering the percentage of the three cleansing oils—coconut, palm kernel, or babussa oil.

When you're lowering the cleansing oil percentages on SoapCalc, the most important thing to remember is that you don't want to have your iodine number go over 70—that's the magic number. Let's say you lower the coconut oil from 14 to 8 percent. You will then need to increase one of the other oils in the recipe by 6 percent and recalculate the recipe. If, after you've recalculated the recipe and the cleansing is still too high, lower the percentage of the coconut oil again and raise the percentage of another one of the oils in the recipe.

For those in England and in Europe, where the use of borax isn't allowed for skin products, you can use citric acid instead to neutralize any leftover lye. Citric acid also lowers the pH. The ratio is the same as for borax.

Basic Shower Gel

This small, basic recipe is terrific for getting you started making shower gel. This recipe yields 32 ounces (907.2 grams; .945 liters).

Here's what to put in SoapCalc—remember to adjust the Type of Lye used, Weight of Oils, Water as % of Oils, and Super Fat % categories as instructed earlier in this chapter:

Weight of Oils	8 ounces (226.8 grams)
Water as % of Oils	80
Super Fat %	–13
Fragrance Oz per Lb	(See the "Scenting Your Household and Laundry Soap" section.)
Castor oil	2.6 ounces (72.6 grams) (32%)
Coconut oil (76 degree)	1.1 ounces (31.7 grams) (14%)
Olive oil	2.4 ounces (68.0 grams) (30%)
Palm oil	1.9 ounces (54.4 grams) (24%)
Distilled water (for lye)	6 ounces (170.1 grams)
Lye—potassium hydroxide	1.8 ounces (50.8 grams)
Distilled water (for borax)	2 ounces (56.7 grams) plus 1.6 ounces (45.4 grams) (for diluting paste)
Borax	.5 ounce (13.6 grams)
HEC (or other thickener)	.5 ounce (13.6 grams)

Here are the soap qualities:

Cleansing	10
Conditioning	69
Bubbly	38
Creamy	47
Iodine	66
INS	133

Always put on your gloves and safety glasses before you begin.

The basic instructions for shower gels are similar to the laundry soap—just the ingredients and measurement ratios are different. Please follow steps 1 through 9 of the Basic Household and Laundry Soap instructions and then come back here to finish your shower gel.

10. Put a small plastic or glass bowl on the scale, zero out the weight, and weigh out .48 ounce (13.6 grams) borax or citric acid. (This is to neutralize any lye that may be left in the gel.) Set it aside for now.

11. Put a plastic pitcher on the scale, zero out the weight, and weigh 30 ounces (850.5 grams) distilled water. Add the borax or citric acid to the water, and stir.

12. Put the pot with the paste back over medium heat, and add the distilled water solution to the paste.

13. When the paste has completely melted, remove it from the heat. Let it cool until the sides of the pot only feel warm, not hot, to the touch.

From the Soap Pot

To help speed the melting stage, boil the distilled water. Add a few extra ounces to compensate for evaporation while bringing it to boil. Weigh the amount of water your recipe calls for before you pour it into the soap pot.

14. Put a plastic bowl on the scale, zero out the weight, and weigh the HEC. Set aside.

15. Weigh 2 ounces (56.7 grams) very warm distilled water. Add to the thickener, and stir to completely dissolve. Add the thickener to the soap pot and, using an immersion blender, incorporate the mixture. If you're using HEC, the mixture will thicken on its own. (If you're using GuarCat as your thickener, you'll need to continue with the blender until the mixture thickens.)

16. Once the mixture has thickened, weigh any other additives you desire, including fragrance or essential oil. Add these to the soap, and stir to incorporate fully.

17. Let the gel cool completely. This will take several hours. Pour the finished soap into bottles.

After you've finished making soap, wipe any oils from your pots and spoons with a paper towel before you load them into your dishwasher. Then pour 1 ounce (28.4 grams) or more vinegar in the Jet-Dry reservoir. This will cut any bubbles caused by the oil residue.

Shower Gel for Normal Skin

This recipe is great for busy families who have normal skin and want a shower gel with a little more cleansing power. It lathers up a storm when used with a bath pouf or wash cloth. This recipe yields 65 ounces (1,842.8 grams; 1.92 liters).

Here's what to put in SoapCalc—remember to adjust the Type of Lye used, Weight of Oils, Water as % of Oils, and Super Fat % categories as instructed earlier in this chapter:

Weight of Oils	16 ounces
Water as % of Oils	80
Super Fat %	–13
Fragrance Oz per Lb	(See the "Scenting Your Household and Laundry Soap" section.)
Castor oil	5.6 ounces (158.8 grams) (30%)
Coconut oil (76 degree)	2.2 ounces (63.5 grams) (14%)
Cocoa butter	.5 ounce (13.6 grams) (3%)
Olive oil	4 ounces (113.4 grams) (25%)
Palm oil	3.7 ounces (104.3 grams) (28%)
Distilled water (for lye)	12.8 ounces (362.9 grams)
Lye—potassium hydroxide	3.6 ounces (102.1 grams)

After the soap has been cooked:

Distilled water (for borax)	32 ounces (907.2 grams) plus 2 ounces (56.7 grams)
Borax	1 ounce (28.35 grams) (1.5%)
HEC (or other thickener)	1 ounce (28.35 grams) (1.5%)
Fragrance or essential oil	1 ounce (28.35 grams) (1.5%)

Here are the soap qualities:

Cleansing	10
Conditioning	69
Bubbly	37
Creamy	48
Iodine	65
INS	136

Cooking time for hard paste: 5 or 6 hours

Shower Gel for Mature Skin

This is the recipe most popular with women who are still pretty active but who also have delicate skin. With the cleansing of 5, it gets you clean while it conditions. This recipe yields 64 ounces (1,814.4 grams; 1.9 liters).

Here's what to put in SoapCalc—remember to adjust the Type of Lye used, Weight of Oils, Water as % of Oils, and Super Fat % categories as instructed earlier in this chapter:

Weight of Oils	16 ounces
Water as % of Oils	80
Super Fat %	−13
Fragrance Oz per Lb	124
Castor oil	5.6 ounces (158.8 grams) (35%)
Coconut oil (76 degree)	1.3 ounces (36.3 grams) (8%)
Cocoa butter	1.3 ounces (36.3 grams) (8%)
Olive oil	5.6 ounces (158.8 grams) (35%)
Palm oil	2.25 ounces (63.5 grams) (14%)
Distilled water (for lye)	12.8 ounces (362.9 grams)
Lye—potassium hydroxide	3.5 ounces (99.1 grams)

After the soap has been cooked:

Distilled water (for borax)	32 ounces (907.2 grams) plus 2 ounces (56.7 grams)
Borax	1 ounce (28.35 grams) (1.5%)
HEC (or other thickener)	1 ounce (28.35 grams) (1.5%)
Fragrance or essential oil	1 ounce (28.35 grams) (1.5%)

Here are the soap qualities:

Cleansing	5
Conditioning	74
Bubbly	37
Creamy	50

Iodine	70
INS	123

Cooking time for hard paste: 5 to 6 hours.

Shower Gel for Sensitive Skin

This shower gel is excellent for toddlers, the elderly, cancer patients, or anyone who has very dry skin. To add extra skin healing, use sunflower oil that's been infused with the herb calendula. Calendula is also great for preventing and soothing diaper rash. This recipe yields 42 ounces (1,190.7 grams; 1.2 liters).

Here's what to put in SoapCalc—remember to adjust the Type of Lye used, Weight of Oils, Water as % of Oils, and Super Fat % categories as instructed earlier in this chapter:

Weight of Oils	10.5 ounces
Water as % of Oils	80
Super Fat %	–13
Fragrance Oz per Lb	(See the "Scenting Your Household and Laundry Soap" section.)
Castor oil	2.5 ounces (70.9 grams) (25%)
Coconut oil (76 degree)	.3 ounce (8.5 grams) (3%)
Cocoa butter	.5 ounce (14.2 grams) (5%)
Olive oil	3 ounces (85 grams) (30%)
Sunflower oil	.5 ounce (14.2 grams) (5%)
Palm oil	3.2 ounces (90.7 grams) (32%)
Distilled water (for lye)	8 ounces (226.8 grams)
Lye—potassium hydroxide	2.2 ounces (61.7 grams)

After the soap has been cooked:

Distilled water (for borax and diluting)	20.2 ounces (572.7 grams) plus 2 ounces (56.7 grams)
Borax	.6 ounce (17 grams) (1.5%)

| HEC (or other thickener) | .6 ounce (17 grams) (1.5%) |
| Fragrance or essential oil | .6 ounce (17 grams) (1.5%) |

Here are the soap qualities:

Cleansing	2
Conditioning	72
Bubbly	25
Creamy	47
Iodine	72
INS	120

Cooking time for hard paste: 5 or 6 hours.

This recipe has a high percentage of olive oil, so it thickens nicely with less HEC. The olive oil reacts with the borax and thickens the soap.

Even though we have it listed here, you can omit the HEC in this recipe if you like. If you decide later that you want it thicker, reheat the soap to 110°F and add the HEC dissolved in 2 ounces (56.7 grams) almost-hot distilled water and add to the soap. Incorporate it well using an immersion blender, and let cool.

Safety First _____

Do not use essential oils in products for babies 3 months old or younger because they can't tolerate the essential oils. Essential or fragrance oils also shouldn't be used on cancer patients while they're going through chemotherapy.

Making Shampoos

Shampoos are made just like the shower gels, but they also include a few other conditioning ingredients, namely vitamin B_5 (liquid form; also called DL Panthenol B5), silk amino acid, and honeyquat. These are basic conditioning ingredients. As you get more shampoo-making experience, you might want to add others as well or adjust these to fit your hair type better. You will also need a much lower cleansing number. Through trial and error, we finally worked out the best cleansing numbers for each hair type.

From the Soap Pot _____

It's important to use the liquid type of DL Panthenol B5 for the shampoo recipes. We've found the powdered form too tricky to work with and can cause the shampoo to separate.

These homemade shampoos aren't super fatted, so you'll need to follow with a good conditioning rinse. Don't worry—we give you a recipe later in this chapter!

Shampoo for Normal Hair

This shampoo has a cleansing of 2, which you might think is too low. It really isn't—remember, you can't super fat liquid soap. This recipe works very well cleansing normal hair and removing any buildup and pollution. This recipe yields 32 ounces (907.2 grams; .945 liters).

Here's what to put in SoapCalc—remember to adjust the Type of Lye used, Weight of Oils, Water as % of Oils, and Super Fat % categories as instructed earlier in this chapter:

Weight of Oils	8 ounces (226.8 grams)
Water as % of Oils	80
Super Fat %	−13
Castor oil	2 ounces (56.7 grams) (25%)
Coconut oil (76 degree)	.24 ounce (6.8 grams) (3%)
Avocado oil	.4 ounce (11.34 grams) (5%)
Olive oil	1.6 ounces (45.4 grams) (20%)
Hemp oil	.2 ounce (4.5 grams) (2%)
Palm oil	3.6 ounces (102.1 grams) (45%)
Distilled water (for lye)	6 ounces (170.1 grams)
Lye—potassium hydroxide	1.8 ounces (49.6 grams)

After the soap has been cooked:

Distilled water (for borax and dilution)	16 ounces (453.6 grams)
Borax	.5 ounce (14.7 grams) (1.5%)
HEC	.5 ounce (14.7 grams) (1.5%)
Vitamin B_5	.3 ounce (8.5 grams) (1%)
Silk amino acid	.64 ounce (18.2 grams) (2%)
Honeyquat	1 ounce (28.4 grams) (3%)
Fragrance oil	.5 ounce (14.7 grams) (1.5%)

Here are the shampoo qualities:

Cleansing	2
Conditioning	69
Bubbly	25
Creamy	50
Iodine	70
INS	123

Always put on your gloves and safety glasses before you begin.

Follow the Basic Household and Laundry Soap instructions 1 through 9. Then follow the Basic Shower Gel instructions 1 through 8. You will add the conditioning ingredients just before you add the thickener.

Shampoo for Dry, Limp Hair

This recipe has a cleansing of 1 and increased additives to add more conditioning, and after using it, your hair will be more manageable and shiny. For extra shine and control, you could increase the honeyquat. You can also substitute shea butter for the cupuacu butter. This recipe yields 32 ounces (907.2 grams; .945 liters).

Here's what to put in SoapCalc—remember to adjust the Type of Lye used, Weight of Oils, Water as % of Oils, and Super Fat % categories as instructed earlier in this chapter:

Weight of Oils	8 ounces
Water as % of Oils	80
Super Fat %	–13
Castor oil	2 ounces (56.7 grams) (25%)
Coconut oil (76 degree)	.08 ounce (2.3 grams) (1%)
Avocado oil	.4 ounce (11.34 grams) (5%)
Olive oil	1.4 ounces (38.6 grams) (17%)
Hemp oil	.2 ounce (4.5 grams) (2%)
Cocoa butter	.24 ounce (6.8 grams) (3%)
Peach kernel oil	.2 ounce (4.5 grams) (2%)
Cupuacu butter	.24 ounce (6.8 grams) (3%)

Palm oil	3.4 ounces (95.3 grams) (42%)
Distilled water (for lye)	6 ounces (170.1 grams)
Lye—potassium hydroxide	1.7 ounces (49.2 grams)

After the soap has been cooked:

Distilled water (for borax and dilution)	16 ounces (453.6 grams)
Borax	.5 ounce (14.7 grams) (1.5%)
HEC	.5 ounce (14.7 grams) (1.5%)
Vitamin B$_5$	.5 ounce (14.7 grams) (1.5%)
Silk amino acid	.64 ounce (18.2 grams) (2%)
Honeyquat	.64 ounces (18.2 grams) (2%)
Fragrance oil	.5 ounce (14.7 grams) (1.5%)

Here are the shampoo qualities:

Cleansing	1
Conditioning	69
Bubbly	24
Creamy	51
Iodine	70
INS	122

Follow the Basic Household and Laundry Soap instructions 1 through 9. Then follow the Basic Shower Gel instructions 1 through 8. You will add the conditioning ingredients just before you add the thickener.

Shampoo for Slightly Oily Hair

If your hair is only slightly oily, this is the perfect recipe for your type of hair. It has a little more cleansing than the normal hair shampoo but a lot lower cleansing than the oily hair shampoo. This recipe yields 32 ounces (907.2 grams; .945 liters).

Here's what to put in SoapCalc—remember to adjust the Type of Lye used, Weight of Oils, Water as % of Oils, and Super Fat % categories as instructed earlier in this chapter:

Weight of Oils	8 ounces (226.8 grams)
Water as % of Oils	80
Super Fat %	−13
Castor oil	2 ounces (56.7 grams) (25%)
Coconut oil (76 degree)	.4 ounce (11.34 grams) (5%)
Avocado oil	.4 ounce (11.34 grams) (5%)
Olive oil	1.6 ounces (45.4 grams) (20%)
Hemp oil	.2 ounce (4.5 grams) (2%)
Cocoa butter	.24 ounce (6.8 grams) (3%)
Palm oil	3.2 ounces (90.7 grams) (40%)
Distilled water (for lye)	6 ounces (170.1 grams)
Lye—potassium hydroxide	1.8 ounces (49.8 grams)

After the soap has been cooked:

Distilled water (for borax and dilution)	16 ounces (453.6 grams)
Borax	.5 ounce (14.7 grams) (1.5%)
HEC	.5 ounce (14.7 grams) (1.5%)
Vitamin B_5	.3 ounce (8.5 grams) (1%)
Silk amino acid	.64 ounce (18.2 grams) (2%)
Honeyquat	.64 ounce (18.2 grams) (2%)
Fragrance oil	.5 ounce (14.7 grams) (1.5%)

Here are the shampoo qualities:

Cleansing	4
Conditioning	67
Bubbly	26
Creamy	49
Iodine	69
INS	126

Follow the Basic Household and Laundry Soap instructions 1 through 9. Then follow the Basic Shower Gel instructions 1 through 8. You will add the conditioning ingredients just before you add the thickener.

Shampoo for Oily Hair

This shampoo removes the excess oil, buildup, and pollution from your hair. Be sure to follow it with a light conditioner. This recipe yields 32 ounces (907.2 grams; .945 liters).

Here's what to put in SoapCalc—remember to adjust the Type of Lye used, Weight of Oils, Water as % of Oils, and Super Fat % categories as instructed earlier in this chapter:

Weight of Oils	8 ounces (226.8 grams)
Water as % of Oils	80
Super Fat %	−13
Castor oil	2 ounces (56.7 grams) (25%)
Coconut oil (76 degree)	.7 ounce (20.4 grams) (9%)
Cocoa butter	.4 ounce (11.3 grams) (5%)
Olive oil	1.6 ounces (45.4 grams) (20%)
Palm Oil	3.3 ounces (92.9 grams) (41%)
Distilled water (for lye)	6.4 ounces (181.4 grams)
Lye—potassium hydroxide	1.8 ounces (50.6 grams)

After the soap has been cooked:

Distilled water (for borax and dilution)	16 ounces (453.6 grams)
Borax	.5 ounce (14.7 grams) (1.5%)
HEC	.5 ounce (14.7 grams) (1.5%)
Vitamin B_5	.3 ounce (8.5 grams) (1%)
Silk amino acid	.64 ounce (18.2 grams) (2%)
Honeyquat	.64 ounce (18.2 grams) (2%)
Fragrance oil	.5 ounce (14.7 grams) (1.5%)

Here are the shampoo qualities:

Cleansing	6
Conditioning	64
Bubbly	29

Creamy	50
Iodine	63
INS	135

Follow the Basic Household and Laundry Soap instructions 1 through 9. Then follow the Basic Shower Gel instructions 1 through 8. You will add the conditioning ingredients just before you add the thickener.

Conditioning Rinse

This is a very simple conditioner you can use on your hair after shampooing. It's easy to make and leaves your hair soft, easy to comb, and manageable. This recipe yields 32 ounces (907.2 grams; .945 liters).

Distilled water	28.8 ounces (816.5 grams) (90%)
BTMS Conditioning Emulsifier	1.6 ounces (45.4 grams) (5%)
Meadowfoam seed oil (or oil of choice)	1 ounce (28.4 grams) (3%)
Optiphen Plus preservative	.3 ounce (8.5 grams) (1%)
Fragrance oil	.3 ounce (8.5 grams) (1%)

1. Put a pitcher on the scale, zero out the weight of the pitcher, and weigh out 28.8 ounces (816.5 grams) distilled water.

2. In a medium stockpot set over medium-low heat, add the distilled water.

3. In separate small containers, weigh out the other ingredients. Set them aside for now.

4. When water reaches 180°F, add the BTMS Conditioning Emulsifier. When most of the BTMS has melted, use your immersion blender to bring about a good emulsion. This may take a minute or two.

5. Remove the pot from the heat, and add the oil. Again use your immersion blender to incorporate the oil.

6. Let soap cool to 110°F. Now add the preservative and fragrance oil. Use your immersion blender to incorporate the ingredients.

7. Let cool overnight. Bottle and use.

Making Other Useful Liquid Soaps

Now that you know how to make shower gel and shampoo, how about a few recipes for liquid hand and facial soaps? Your liquid hand soap will be antibacterial because you add an across-the-board preservative that preserves the soap and kills mold, fungus, and bacteria. We recommend Optiphen ND, but read about these preservative systems and make you own choice.

Liquid Hand Soap

The cleansing in this soap is high, making it suitable to use in the kitchen before and after you handle food. If you handle a lot of garlic or onions, try adding a coffee fragrance oil to help remove their odors from your hands. This recipe yields 32.5 ounces (921.4 grams; .945 liters).

Here's what to put in SoapCalc—remember to adjust the Type of Lye used, Weight of Oils, Water as % of Oils, and Super Fat % categories as instructed earlier in this chapter:

Weight of Oils	8 ounces (226.8 grams)
Water as % of Oils	75
Super Fat %	−13
Castor oil	2 ounces (56.7 grams) (25%)
Coconut oil (76 degree)	1.6 ounces (45.4 grams) (20%)
Olive oil	1.6 ounces (45.4 grams) (20%)
Palm oil	2.8 ounces (79.4 grams) (35%)
Distilled water	6 ounces (170.1 grams)
Lye—potassium hydroxide	1.8 ounces (52.3 grams)

After the soap has been cooked:

Distilled water (for borax and dilution)	16 ounces (453.6 grams)
Borax	.5 ounce (14.7 grams) (1.5%)
HEC	.5 ounce (14.7 grams) (1.5%)
Optiphen ND Preservative	.3 ounce (8.5 grams) (1%)
Fragrance oil	.3 ounce (8.5 grams) (1%)

Here are the shampoo qualities:

Safety First _____

This soap will burn if it gets in the eyes, so be careful to avoid the eye area. If soap does get in eyes, flush with lots of cool water.

Cleansing	14
Conditioning	60
Bubbly	36
Creamy	45
Iodine	59
INS	147

Follow the instructions just like you did for making shower gels.

Liquid Facial Soap for Normal Skin

Handcrafted soaps, both bar and liquid, will completely dissolve all makeup, leaving your skin totally clean. Be sure to follow with by splashing your face with cool water to close your pores and add a light moisturizer. To add even more skin-loving benefits, use an essential oil blend that will best suit your skin needs. This recipe yields 32.5 ounces (921.4 grams; .945 liters).

Here's what to put in SoapCalc—remember to adjust the Type of Lye used, Weight of Oils, Water as % of Oils, and Super Fat % categories as instructed earlier in this chapter:

Weight of Oils	8 ounces (226.8 grams)
Water as % of Oils	75
Super Fat %	−13
Castor oil	2.8 ounces (79.4 grams) (35%)
Coconut oil (76 degree)	.4 ounce (11.3 grams) (5%)
Olive oil	2 ounces (56.7 grams) (25%)
Cocoa butter	.4 ounce (11.3 grams) (3%)
Palm oil	2.6 ounces (72.6 grams) (32%)
Distilled water	6 ounces (170.1 grams)
Lye—potassium hydroxide	1.8 ounces (52.3 grams)

After the soap has been cooked:

Distilled water (for borax and dilution)	16 ounces (453.6 grams)
Borax	.5 ounce (14.7 grams) (1.5%)
HEC	.5 ounce (14.7 grams) (1.5%)
Optiphen ND preservative	.3 ounce (8.5 grams) (1%)
Fragrance oil	.3 ounce (8.5 grams) (1%)

Here are the shampoo qualities:

Cleansing	4
Conditioning	72
Bubbly	35
Creamy	54
Iodine	54
INS	124

Follow the instructions just like you did for making shower gels.

Liquid Facial Soap for Teenagers

For better results and clearer skin, use a single essential oil or make a blend from these oils: elemi, bay rum, bergamot, cedarwood, sandalwood, coriander, geranium, pink grapefruit, tangerine, yarrow, tea tree, patchouli, litsea, and juniper. You only need .3 ounce essential oil or blend. This recipe yields 32.5 ounces (921.4 grams; .945 liters).

Here's what to put in SoapCalc—remember to adjust the Type of Lye used, Weight of Oils, Water as % of Oils, and Super Fat % categories as instructed earlier in this chapter:

Weight of Oils	8 ounces (226.8 grams)
Water as % of Oils	75
Super Fat %	−13
Castor oil	2.0 ounces (56.7 grams) (25%)
Palm kernel oil	2.7 ounces (63.5 grams) (28%)

Olive oil	2.0 ounces (45.35 grams) (25%)
Sunflower oil (high oleic)	1.1 ounces (31.8 grams) (14%)
Shea butter	.64 ounce (18.1 grams) (8%)
Distilled water	6.4 ounces (181.4 grams)
Lye—potassium hydroxide	1.3 ounces (37.0 grams)

After the soap has been cooked:

Distilled water (for borax and dilution)	16 ounces (453.6 grams)
Borax	.5 ounce (14.7 grams) (1.5%)
HEC	.5 ounce (14.7 grams) (1.5%)
Optiphen ND preservative	.3 ounce (8.5 grams) (1%)
Essential oil	.3 ounce (8.5 grams) (1%)

Here are the shampoo qualities:

Cleansing	6
Conditioning	64
Combined lather	79
Iodine	63
INS	135

Follow the instructions just like you did for making shower gels.

The Least You Need to Know

- Even though making liquid soap is advanced soap-making, we've made it simple and easy!

- Throw out the store-bought laundry soap and make your own all-natural version—it's easier than you think!

- You will find so many uses for these homemade liquid soaps!

- Weigh twice, pour once: precise measurements are the key to perfect liquid soap.

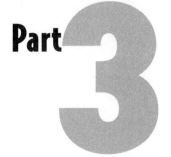

Part 3

Getting Creative with Your Soap

Soap-making is so much more than just throwing together a bunch of oil, water, and lye. Soap-makers like to be very artistic and creative, making beautiful bars of soap. And why not, when you consider what amazing things you can do with a batch of soap! Don't limit yourself to plain white or one-color soap. Shakespeare said, "If music be the food of life, then play on." And we say, "Being creative in our craft brings so much color to the world."

Adding color, making swirls, and embedding objects are just some of the ways you can make your soap bars art and uniquely yours. In Part 3, we hope to inspire you and jump-start your creative side. Start with adding a colorant. Then try swirling color into the soap. Once you've mastered those steps, you can add embeds. Let your imagination run wild—and have fun!

Chapter

11

Coloring Your Soap

In This Chapter

- ◆ Types of colorants for your soap
- ◆ All about swirling
- ◆ Tips for marbleizing your soap
- ◆ Colorant cautions

When I (Sally) first met Zonella, she hardly used colorant in her soap. When she did, it was either one solid color in the bar or a tiny thin little vein of swirl. I, on the other hand, jumped right in and began swirls with two, three, or even four or more colors at a time. (Needless to say, I love color!) Slowly, as I rubbed off on her, Zonella has become a little more adventurous and is now making bolder swirls—even using *two* colors at a time!

When adding color to your soap, try to match the color to the fragrance. Or if you're in a creative mood, throw in a wild group of colors. Somehow it always works out as long as you don't overstir. You just have to take the bull by the horns and get in there and swirl. Don't be shy. This is where you can really be creative and show off a little.

In this chapter, you learn about the different colorants you can use and how to use them to do one or more color swirls. This is the fun part of soap-making—well, *one* of the many fun parts!

Types of Colorants

Many types of colorants on the market today are made for coloring soaps. Before you buy a soap colorant, be sure it's right for the type of soap you're making. Most liquid soap colorants tend to stay true to color in melt-and-pour soap but mutate in cold process or hot process soap. Some liquid colorants are specially made for the high-pH types of soap. Oxides stay true in any type of soap, and you can blend them together to make more colors.

In this chapter, we dig into all the different types of colorants, including spices and clays. Look around your kitchen, and you're sure to find some spices you can use to color your soap.

I blend my own oxides and soap-safe dyes to create many pastel, bright, and neon colors I call "Berry-Liscious." In addition, I also like Select Shades. You will have to try different ones until you find your favorite.

Liquid Colors

Liquid soap colorants are very convenient to use and less messy than some of the other types of colorants. You can find these colorants online or at many of your local supply stores.

One of my favorite brands, Select Shades, offers eight basic shades. Using their online color chart, you can easily create many colors. Some of their colors will mutate in cold and hot process soap. I found that out recently when I thought I was making a beautiful blue swirl through a white soap base with Cool Water for men as the fragrance. Within minutes of finishing my swirl, the beautiful blue swirl started turning pink! In the end, it had turned a pinkish-purple and no longer looked like a man's soap. It is the high pH of cold and hot process that causes this sort of color change. Still, these are really nice colorants and I use them for many projects.

Other liquid colors are just that—greens, yellows, blues, etc.—and you have to buy each color. From this type of colorants I've used the Peacock colors and enjoyed working with them. They are vivid and stay true to color. However, they can be expensive. Even though they are very concentrated, it takes more than a few drops to have the vivid colors once the soap has saponified. It's also impossible to buy only one or two colors. They're so pretty, you'll want to buy every color available!

You can also use Peacock colorants in liquid soaps, lotions, and creams as well as in bar soaps.

Oxides for Colorants

Oxides are powder colorants, now made in a lab for sanitary reasons, but they are exactly duplicated from the natural oxides that were once mined from the earth. Micas and oxides are the only colorants approved by the FDA. Even though the oxides are messy, they're what I use most of the time. I can blend them with white titanium dioxide (TD) to lighten the color to a pastel or add a touch of black to make the color darker. You can even mix together colors to make even more colors. The possibilities are endless.

Oxides stay pretty true to color no matter what type of product they're used in. Mineral makeup is made with the very same oxides and micas you'll use in soap. The use rate for oxide colorants is about 1 teaspoon (5 ml) per pound of soap.

You can also find soap-safe neon colorants. Like oxides, these neon colors don't change and are also in a powder form.

Once you've chosen or blended the color you want, you have to "wet" the oxide with glycerin or some of the oil from your soap batch so the oxide dissolves before you add it to your soap batch or add the soap for coloring to the oxide. If you skip that step, you'll have little clumps of color in your soap instead of even color throughout. The colors in the final soap stay pretty true to what you see while you're making the soap.

You can use oxides in liquid soap, bar soap, lotions, creams, and types of makeup.

Micas

Micas are also a powder, now being made in labs for sanitary reasons, and are exact duplicates from the natural mica that was once mined from the earth. They come in beautiful colors, but they don't do well in cold process, hot process, or liquid soap because the high pH causes the mica to morph in color and lose its sparkle.

From the Soap Pot

For more information on making your own makeup, check out our companion book, *The Complete Idiot's Guide to Making Natural Beauty Products* (Alpha Books, 2010).

Micas do work well in most melt-and-pour soaps as well as in lotions, creams, and other bath and body products. Micas are also used in mineral makeup for lipsticks, blush, and eye shadows among many other products.

Natural Colorants

Many natural cosmetic-grade clays can be used for coloring your soaps while adding extra benefits for the skin. Clays are available in yellow, green, red, rose, white, pink, and coral, just to mention a few. But did you know you can also go to your spice cabinet and find many useful colorants?

Color	Colorants
White	Titanium dioxide, kaolin clay
Yellow	Ground calendula petals, curry powder, safflower, turmeric (gold), saffron
Yellow-orange	Annatto seed (steep in oil first), carrots (shredded or ground), pumpkin (puréed)
Green	Alfalfa (medium), chlorophyll, cucumber, henna (ground), kelp/seaweed, sage, spinach
Blue-green	Spirulina
Blue	Indigo root (can stain), poppy seeds (blue-gray to dark specks)
Red	Moroccan red clay, rose pink clay, cochineal powder, madder root (rosy red-purple)
Purple	Alkanet (steep in oil first), rattan jot (lavender to purple)
Tan to brown	Coffee/coffee grinds, cocoa powder, cinnamon (can irritate), cloves, comfrey root, milk, rosehip seeds

Safety First

Do not use crayons to color your soap. Use only colorants approved for use in soap, or use natural ingredients such as cocoa powder.

For a solid-colored batch of soap, you can add the colorant to the oils after you've removed them from the heat. There's no real rule to follow for how much to use. It all depends on the size of your batch, the colorant you're using, and how intense or light you want the finial color to be. For most colorants, it's 1 teaspoon per 1 pound of soap. You'll have to add it to the oils and see if that's enough color for what you want.

Keep in mind, too, that the color will be lighter after you've added the lye/water to the oils.

The Basics of Swirling

This is the fun part. You can be very colorful and swirl four or five colors or be more conservative and swirl only one or maybe two. Be creative and have fun, no matter how many colors you choose.

To create beautiful swirls, you must be quick and light-handed. Overdoing it will only make a mess.

Once you've chosen your colorant, you'll want to have it ready for when the soap comes to light trace. You won't have time at that point to measure out the colorant or anything else, so do it ahead of time. The soap continues to set up even though you've stopped stirring or blending it.

The next thing you'll have to decide is how you're going to swirl—in the pot or in the mold. I like both ways, but if I'm using more than one color, I use the in-the-mold method. Swirling in the mold gives you time to drag the color into designs.

If you're going to swirl in the mold, you'll need a "swirling tool." I use a dowel rod about the size of a pencil, cut to 12 to 18 inches long. Some people use a small spatula, while others use stainless-steel forks. Use what works best for you and gives you the effect you're looking for.

Safety First _____

As always, before you begin, be sure to put on your safety glasses and latex gloves.

The Blind Swirl

Even a soap that will turn dark because of the fragrance oil can be swirled. We call this a *blind swirl*. To do this type of swirl, you use titanium dioxide (TD) or kaolin clay.

When you reach light trace, before you add the fragrance, remove about a third of the soap base and pour it into a big measuring cup that already has the dissolved TD or clay in it. Stir the colorant into the soap.

You'll need to use around 2 teaspoons TD or clay per 1 cup soap base, depending on how dark the fragrance will turn the soap. The more vanilla there is in a fragrance, the darker the soap will be.

The In-the-Pot Swirl

For this method, remove the amount of soap to be colored and stir in the colorant well. Next, add the fragrance to the base soap in the pot and stir until the fragrance is well incorporated into the soap base.

Next, pour the soap into the pot and give it a light, quick stir. Don't overdo it! Then slowly pour your soap into your mold.

As the soap cures, the uncolored part will start to darken, and your white soap swirls will become more visible. This method works beautifully with any color, not just with a blind swirl.

The In-the-Mold Swirl

For this method, you pour the soap base into the mold. Holding your hand above the mold and raising it higher and lower as you pour, dribble and trickle the soap using a grid pattern or any sort of pattern you choose. Then, drag your swirling tool through the soap, making whatever design you like.

Again, don't overdo this. The less you mess with it, the better your swirl will turn out.

The White-on-White Swirl

You can also swirl your white-colored soap into the base to create a beautiful white-on-white soap bar. Bars of soap are never really white (unless you use TD to make it so); they're more of a whitish-cream color, so doing this swirl makes a really pretty bar of soap.

You can also do this same type of swirl with soap that doesn't discolor or only slightly discolors.

Swirling Your Soap

Now let's get down to business—and have some fun!

Before you even start your soap batch, decide on your color (or colors). I usually try to match the colors with the name of the fragrance. Then you can prepare the colorant and have it ready and waiting in a container (I like to use a 4-cup measuring cup for this) to add to the soap later. Have your mold already lined and close by. You'll have to work quickly before the soap sets up and becomes hard.

Here's what to do:

1. In a large measuring cup, add about 1 or 2 teaspoons of colorant. If your colorant is a powder, you'll need to wet it, either with glycerin or the oil from your soap batch. You don't need a lot, just enough to cover the powder well. Let it sit a minute and then stir it well, making sure it has all dissolved.

2. Add the lye/water to the oils and, using an immersion blender, blend until the soap base reaches light trace.

3. Remove a quarter to a third of the soap base, and add it to the prepared colorant. Stir well, making sure all the soap is evenly colored.

4. Now add the fragrance oil and hand-stir until it's blended.

5. You have to work quickly now. Pour the colored soap into the pot, and give it a quick stir. Don't overdo it!

6. Gently pour the soap into the mold. Cover with wax paper, and leave for 48 hours.

Some people like to use a wooden lid for their mold. That's fine, but you'll still need to cover the soap with waxed paper before you place the lid on top.

Swirling in the Mold

Prepare your mold and colorant just like you would do if you were going to swirl in the pot. (See steps 1 through 3 from the "Swirling Your Soap" section.) Then continue:

4. Add the fragrance to the soap base still in the pot. Hand-stir, and when it's totally incorporated, pour the base soap into the mold.

5. Holding your hand at different heights above the base, pour or drizzle the colored soap into the base soap, making a design or a grid.

6. Using your swirling tool or a stainless-steel fork, drag the colored soap through the soap base, making a nice design as you go. Once again, don't overdo this or you may end up with a mess. Keep it light and feathery.

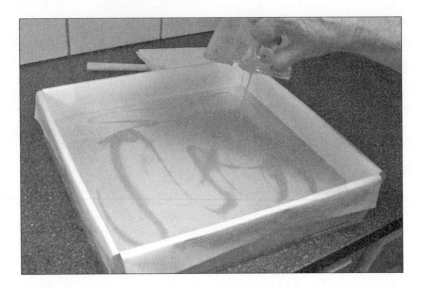

7. Cover with waxed paper, and leave for 48 hours.

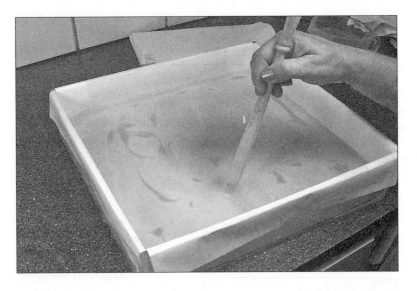

This is the hardest part, but no peeking! The finished product will be worth the wait.

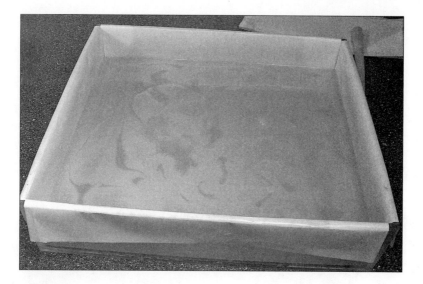

Swirling Two Colors

To be able to swirl two or more colors, the soap batch has to be at least a 3-pound (1020.6-gram) batch. The larger the soap batch, the prettier a two- or more-color swirl will be. Color combinations can be as simple as two soft pastels or two bright neon colorants.

To swirl, follow the same directions as for a single-color swirl. But instead of removing 1½ to 2 cups (340.2 to 453.6 grams) of soap from the base, remove 3 or 4 cups (680.4 to 907.2 grams) and divide it between two measuring cups that already contain the colorants. You don't have to pour the colored soap into the mold with one cup in each hand, although it is fun to do it that way. You could also use a ladle to scoop.

Remember, for swirling in the mold, to hold the measuring cup at different heights while pouring, so the colored soap will go all the way through the base soap in the mold.

Marbleizing

Marbleizing is an in-the-mold swirl. You can use one color or two, but we don't recommend doing more than that, or you could easily end up with an ugly mess.

To marbleize your soap, you'll pour the base into the mold. With your colored soap ready, start pouring in even lines lengthwise with 1 or 2 inches of space between the lines. Next, pour even lines going across your mold, perpendicular to your first lines. Sometimes you can use a second color for these lines.

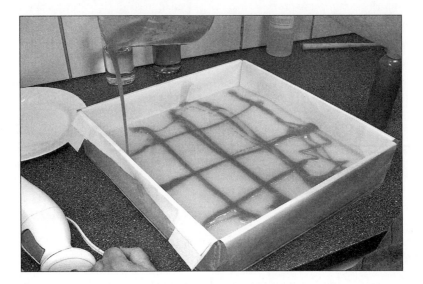

After you've poured your grid of color, start dragging your swirling tool down the lines lengthwise. Do the same with the lines going horizontally. Now make a few circles, dragging both colors.

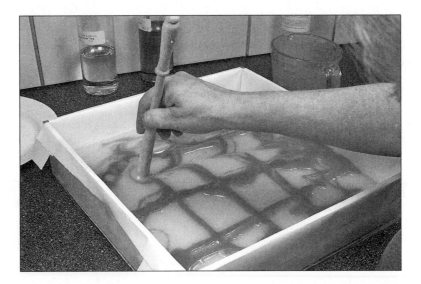

When you're satisfied with your design, cover with waxed paper and leave it 48 hours.

Pitfalls to Avoid

Now that we've learned what to do when coloring soap, let's look at what *not* to do. Working with oxides can create beautiful swirls and colors for your soaps. However, using too much oxide can cause a few problems.

For example, black can stain washcloths if you use too much, so don't use it heavily. Black oxide would be better to use as an accent color instead of as the main color swirl, unless you do the swirl as a thin line.

The next potential troublemaker is red oxide. Red is one of my favorite colors, but I learned a valuable lesson about using too much of it when I made a special batch of soap for my husband. He grew up in London during the 1960s, so for his birthday one year, I decided to make a batch of soap and color it with a paisley design in his favorite fragrance oil, sandalwood. Sandalwood turns the soap medium-dark brown, which makes a perfect background color for English paisleys. The fragrance was not one that speeds trace, but to be sure I'd have enough time to create my her design, I added 2 ounces (56.7 grams) extra water and increased the olive oil in the recipe.

For the design I used red oxide, blue ultramarine, yellow oxide, green oxide, orange oxide, and black oxide. I wanted the red to stand out and help make the paisley design more visible, so I used a little extra red oxide. That was my mistake. After I had completed the swirl, I was very pleased with how it looked. You could actually see the paisleys!

When the time came to cut the soap, I couldn't wait any longer to show it to my husband. He was very impressed with my artistic talent, and grabbed one of the paisley soap bars and headed to the shower. And that's when I learned a valuable lesson: too much red oxide can be a problem.

When the bar of soap got really wet in the shower, the red oxide turned loose and turned the water a bright red, just like blood. At first he thought he'd cut himself. But it was just the red oxide. Let this be a lesson, and make a note not to overdo the red oxide. It can cause a panic!

A few months later, I gave a bar of that same soap to our friend KC, but this time, I warned him the water might turn red due to the red oxide. Sure enough, even after months of curing, the shower water turned bright red when it hit the soap.

No matter how long you let the bar cure, if you have used too much red oxide, you'll have a "bloody" mess! So use about half of the red oxide you'd normally use to color the soap. Or don't, and watch the panic ensue!

The Least You Need to Know

◆ Making pretty swirled designs in your soap is easy once you know the basics.

◆ There's no magic involved in coloring soap. But there are things to keep in mind.

◆ By using colorants and a little imagination, you can turn your bars of soap into small works of art!

Taking Your Soap to the Next Level

In This Chapter

◆ Making layers in your soap

◆ Having fun with cutouts, curls, and confetti

◆ Adding pizzazz with plaids

We've said it before, but it bears repeating: experiment with soap-making. Try different colors. Play with new techniques. Go online and visit soap-maker groups and websites. All the things being done with soap these days are pretty amazing. Soap-makers have been pushing the creative envelope and the results are stunning.

In this chapter, we give you a few ideas and techniques so you can begin to think creatively and really see what you can do with your soaps.

Making Layered Soap

When I pour my cold process soap in layers, I usually make three different layers using three colors and three scents. I also use a log mold to show off the layers.

To make the three different batches of soap, you have to adjust the original recipe. First, divide the amount of total oils by 3. Then, use SoapCalc to formulate the ⅓ recipe you'll use to make all three layers.

My log mold's total weight of oils is 54 ounces (1,530.9 grams). So dividing 54 by 3, that means each of the three layers' total weight of oils is 18 ounces (510.3 grams).

After you've lined your mold, you make each layer one right after the other. You want the soap you just poured into the mold to become hard before you pour in the next layer, but you don't want it to go into gel stage before you've finished pouring all three layers.

From the Soap Pot

The usual use amount of oxides is 1 teaspoon (5 milliliters) per pound of soap but when you are doing a blind swirl you increase the amount of titanium dioxide so that the swirled (white) soap stays very white.

Let's see how this all works with our Coffee Mocha Delight cold process soap.

Coffee Mocha Delight

You'll make three batches of soap for this recipe, each one a different color and fragrance. We start out with a blind swirl, a white/creamy color layer with a vanilla fragrance. To this layer you'll add 2 teaspoons (10 milliliters) to 1 tablespoon (15 milliliters) titanium dioxide (TD) and remove 1 cup (237 milliliters) soap before you mix in the fragrance oil to keep the soap from going dark. The second layer will be a dark chocolate-brown color with chocolate fragrance oil. The third layer will be white/cream with a chocolate color swirl and a coffee fragrance.

Here's what to put in SoapCalc:

Weight of Oils	18 ounces
Water as % of Oils	38
Super Fat %	5
Fragrance Oz per Lb	.7 ounce
Distilled water	6.8 ounces (193.9 grams)
Lye—sodium hydroxide	2.4 ounces (66.7 grams)

Cocoa butter	1.3 ounces (35.2 grams) (7%)
Peach kernel oil	1.8 ounces (51 grams) (10%)
Coconut oil	2 ounces (56.1 grams) (11%)
Olive oil	2.7 ounces (76.5 grams) (15%)
Castor oil	3.6 ounces (102.1 grams) (20%)
Palm oil	6.7 ounces (188.8 grams) (37%)
Fragrance oil	1.1 ounces (31.2 grams) (.7 ppo)

Here are the soap qualities:

Hardness	35
Cleansing	8
Conditioning	63
Bubbly	26
Creamy	45
Iodine	64
INS	136

From the Soap Pot

To keep cocoa butter from becoming grainy when you're melting it, don't melt it all the way. When the butter is just about totally melted, remove it from the stove or microwave and hand-stir it until it has finished melting. You can also save cool-down time for your batch of oils by melting the cocoa butter before you add it to the pot of oils. You won't have to get your oils as hot over the burner because it takes longer to melt cocoa butter than most of the other hard oils.

Always put on your gloves and safety glasses before you begin.

1. Weigh all three amounts of water, and have each amount in its own pitcher.

2. Do the same with the sodium hydroxide.

3. Slowly add the lye to the water for each batch. Stir each one until the lye has dissolved. Set them aside to cool.

4. Next, weigh the oils, each in its own pot.

5. Weigh the cocoa butter, and melt it in the microwave set on low power so it doesn't burn. Do this with each batch of butter, and pour into the pots with the oils. Or you can melt it on your stove top over low heat. Don't let the cocoa butter totally melt over the heat. Remove it from either the microwave or stove top before it has totally melted. It will continue melting while you stir it.

6. Weigh the rest of your oils and pour them into the pots. Give each pot a stir, and set them aside for now.

7. In a small measuring cup or other glass container, weigh the three fragrance oils. You'll need 1.1 ounces (31.2 grams) each of vanilla, chocolate or mocha, and coffee fragrance oils.

8. Line your mold with freezer paper (shiny side up), following the directions in Chapter 5. If you're using a plastic tray mold, you don't need to line it.

When the lye has cooled down to about 90°F, it's time to put together the soap.

Here's how to make the first layer:

1. In a measuring cup, add 1 tablespoon (15 milliliters) TD and about 3 tablespoons (45 milliliters) oil from your soap pot or glycerin. Stir and let the oxide dissolve.

2. Slowly pour one pitcher of lye/water solution into one pot of soap oils. Use an immersion blender to incorporate the lye and the oils. Just as you see the soap base is starting to thicken, remove about 1½ cups of the base and add it to the TD in the measuring cup. Using a small stainless-steel or plastic spoon, stir the soap until the colorant is spread evenly.

3. Working quickly, add the fragrance oil to the soap base in the pot. Hand-stir until all the fragrance is incorporated.

4. Pour the colored soap back into the pot. Give it a quick stir—don't overdo it— and pour the first layer of your soap into the mold. Don't worry that you can't see the color right now. Over the next week or two, the vanilla fragrance will darken the soap that doesn't have the TD and create a strikingly beautiful layer. Leave the mold to stand and let this first layer harden enough for the next layer. By the time you're ready to pour the next layer, this layer should be firm enough to support it.

Soap Stats

Fragrance oil with vanilla in the formula always turns the soap from tan to a dark brown, depending on the vanilla content.

5. Again using a measuring cup, add 1 heaping teaspoon dark-brown oxide mixed with a pinch of black oxide or cocoa powder and 3 tablespoons soap oil or glycerin. Stir until it dissolves.

6. As in step 2, slowly pour the lye into the oils. Blend with the immersion blender until the soap base begins to thicken. Remove about $1\frac{1}{2}$ cups soap and add it to the oxide or cocoa powder. Stir well until the soap base is evenly colored.

7. Repeat steps 3 and 4. This time, stir in the colorant to color all the base soap and use the chocolate or mocha fragrance oil.

8. Gently touch the top of the first layer to be sure it's hard enough to support the second layer. If it is, pour in the second layer.

9. For the third layer, repeat steps 1 through 4. Use 1 teaspoon dark-brown oxide or cocoa powder to color about $1\frac{1}{2}$ cups soap base. The fragrance for this layer is coffee. Before you pour the colored soap back into the pot, add 2 teaspoons TD, already dissolved in oil, into the soap base so it stays white/cream color. Then add your coffee fragrance and stir well. After you've stirred the color evenly into the soap base in the measuring, pour it back into the pot. Quickly stir and then pour it on top of the second layer.

10. Cover top of soap with waxed paper, and leave it for 48 hours.

There's no end to the layers and colorants you can do. Be creative and try different methods. The base soap recipe can work with any colorants or fragrance oils you want to use. And you're not limited to always making three layers. Do however many you want!

From the Soap Pot

Even coffee fragrance oil may contain some vanilla. When making the Coffee Mocha Delight soap, add some titanium dioxide to the soap base to keep it white/creamy in color. If you don't want to swirl the top layer, you could use a little ground coffee, already brewed and removed from the filter, in the layer for a speckled effect.

Making Cold Process Embeds

Embeds are shapes and pieces of cold process soap and other items you can insert into a larger soap batch. You can arrange them so you have one in each bar of soap or many scattered throughout the mold. With melt-and-pour (M&P) soap, you can embed cutout shapes made with M&P soap or even embed small toys to amuse your children. You can use hot process soap to make embeds, but it becomes brittle and hard, and that makes it difficult to cut shapes out of. Cold process soap is still soft enough when it comes out of the mold for you to easily cut shapes. You can cut shapes with a knife and cut the shapes freehand or use small cookie cutters. It's fun to do and adds art and interest to the soap bars.

To make cold process embeds, you need either a box or a log mold. Line the mold, and make a small 1- or 2-pound batch of soap. Don't use a water discount for the soap batch. Instead, use full water so you can cut the soap easily. Color it or not—it's up to you and what you want to create. Using a log mold for this project will show off the soap layers better when it's cut into bars.

Sometimes I cut the soap into strips or shapes using a cheese slicer and then a knife to cut the strips. Other times I use small cookie cutters to cut hearts, doves, or trees. The possibilities are endless. Be creative and let your imagination go! For Valentine's Day, for example, you could make X's and O's for hugs and kisses and embed them in a soap fragranced with a duplication of your favorite perfume.

 From the Soap Pot

Once cold process soap has already been through saponification, it won't be effected when it's used as an embed in a freshly poured batch of cold process soap going through its saponification. It will not melt or change. On the other hand, I've used M&P soap for embeds in cold process soap and had mixed results. Some worked well when the mold was simply left on the counter to saponify, but when I used the oven to speed up the saponification, the heat melted the M&P embeds. Lesson learned.

Making Cutouts

If you're going to go the cookie cutter route, you won't want to pour the soap thicker than the height of the cookie cutter.

Once you've made, colored, and poured your soap, let it go through saponification. Then remove the soap from the mold.

For the next part you'll want to have on latex gloves in case the lye is still active.

While the soap is still soft, cut out the shapes and gently move them to a cookie sheet for drying and hardening. Give them a day or two before you insert them in a batch of soap.

Making Curls

Curls are made the same as cutouts, but you'll use a long box or a log mold and pour the soap only about ¼ or ½ inch thick. After the soap has gone through the gel stage and has cooled down enough to handle—but is still warm—you'll make your curls.

With gloves on, cut strips the height of the soap or soap layer you're going to use the curls in. Gently bend the strips of soap around a pencil to help curl it. Set the soap curl on a cookie sheet to dry and harden. Continue to do this until you have as many curls as you need. Let them harden for a couple days before use.

Making Plaids

For plaids, you'll follow the same directions as for cutouts and curls, but instead of cutting the strips the height of the soap bars, cut them in thinner strips so you can lay out a plaid or checked pattern. The strips should be as thin as you can make them. Try for about ⅛ inch thick. Repeat the layer at least three or four times so you achieve a nice plaid pattern in the soap.

The first layer will be short pieces the width of the mold. Lay these pieces all the way down the mold. The second layer will be the long pieces going the length of the mold. Repeat this until the mold is full. Then gently pour in your soap base. Cover and wait 48 hours before removing from the mold.

You can also make plaid melt-and-pour (M&P) embeds this same way.

Making Confetti

Soap confetti is very simple to make. Just cut up a few bars of different-color soap into tiny pieces, and throw them into the soap batch just before you pour the soap into the mold.

Making Stained-Glass M&P Pieces

The addition of stained-glass M&P pieces makes a striking bar of soap. And they're easy to do.

Melt a couple ounces of clear M&P soap base, coloring each one with a bright liquid colorant. Pour a thin layer of one color into one container. Wait about 5 to 10 minutes for the soap to set up and then remove it and cut it into pieces—squares, diamonds, or whatever shape you want. Repeat this until you have all the colors you want to use.

After you've made your CP soap and are ready to pour it into the mold, add your stained-glass pieces and stir. Pour the soap into the mold, cover, and let set for 48 hours.

One of my favorite soap batches contained stained-glass pieces. I made bright green, red, bright blue, and orange M&P pieces, all fragranced with lemon fragrance oil. I then made CP soap and colored it a light sun yellow, also using lemon fragrance oil. I threw all the different-colored M&P pieces into the soap, stirred them around, and poured the batch into the mold. When the bars were cut, the stained-glass pieces made a very colorful and lovely bar of soap. (See Chapter 13 for lots more on M&P soap.)

Tips for Laying Embeds in the Mold

For certain effects, you may have to choose between using a flat slab mold or a log mold.

With the slab mold, you need to mark where the cut lines for the bars will be so you can center the embeds properly. Having a slab mold that already has slits in the wood for the knife makes it a lot easier to see where the cuts will be. Otherwise, you can use a ruler and mark the cut lines on the sides of the mold. Then use string and make the grid, taping the string to each side of the mold exactly where the soap will be cut. When it comes time to pour your soap into the mold, be very careful not to pour it on the strings. It's best to pour at light traces. From that point on, you have to work quickly to get all your embeds placed in the mold before the soap sets up and becomes too hard.

With log molds, you cut the soap bars from the end and make slices—like cutting butter into patties. You start by pouring the soap at medium trace so it can support the weight of the embeds. If you pour at light trace, most of, if not all, the embeds will sink to the bottom of the mold. So to avoid this, pour some of the soap base and then sprinkle or layer the embed pieces, depending on the effect you're going for. Then continue pouring, sprinkling, and pouring again until the mold is full.

The Least You Need to Know

- Love striped soap? It's easier to make than you might think. You can even make plaid soap.

- Adding embeds enables you to personalize your soaps to fit whatever décor you have.

- You can make beautiful soaps with special occasion or holiday embeds. These are great to give as gifts!

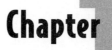

Chapter 13

-and-Pour

n cold pro-
get too hot
tor and let

supervision
when they

It sets up
out of the

bases have
milk M&P.
nd called

base, includ-
ver to
the base has
ent power.
ntil the base is
the soap base
to become

the lid cover-
p base come

tir the soap,

he commer-
ge containers,
ontainers

p

ng melt-and-pour soap

our soap

vith melt-and-pour (M&P) soap yet,
re many things you can do with M&P
&P soap on top of hot process soap for a
pretty bar of soap that had, as the bottom
vith a layer of hot process soap, and on
tP soap. You can add colored pieces of
n interesting stained-glass look, as we did
ap.

eate embeds, or add-in pieces, for their
use M&P soap is already a finished soap,
hen added as embeds to cold or hot

process soap. The only thing you can't do when you have M&P embeds cess soap is to place the mold in an oven for the gel stage. The soap will and melt the embeds. Just leave the mold on a counter or in the refriger the soap go through gel stage normally.

M&P is also kid-friendly. Because there's no lye involved, under parental children can enjoy making fun soapy projects. Bath time is a lot more fu get to use a soap they helped to make!

The Basics of M&P Soap

M&P soap is what it sounds like: you *melt* it and then *pour* it into a mole quickly, doesn't need a cure time, and is ready to use as soon as it comes mold. Easy, fast, and artsy!

Many types of bases are sold for M&P soap, from clear to opaque. Some shea butter, and others contain olive oil and aloe. You can even buy goat Read the label ingredients and decide which type you'd like to use. A br SFI(c) seems to be the favorite among serious M&P soap-makers.

Soap Stats

Many M&P soap bases aren't soap at all but made with detergent. Some don't even have real glycerin in the base.

There are several ways to melt the soap ing in your microwave oven. Set the pc medium, and use short cook times unti melted—try 30-second bursts at 50 per You might have to heat it a few times u completely melted. Be careful not to le boil, though. Boiling can cause the soap brittle and prone to cracking.

The favored method for melting the soap base is in a double boiler with ing the pot with the soap over medium-low heat. Again, don't let the so to a boil.

Either method you use for melting your base is fine. You won't need to but you might want to push the clumps around to help them melt.

M&P Soap Molds

You can use many different containers as a mold for your M&P soap— cial plastic or silicone molds work fine, too, of course. Plastic food store PVC pipe, plastic candy molds, tart molds, and even empty, clean food work. There are also sprays that help the soap release more easily from the molds, or you can use a vegetable spray like PAM.

Plastic molds are cheap and easy to work with. But don't grab any old plastic mold. Be sure you have a thick plastic mold made for soap. Many use plastic candy molds, but after a few uses, these molds start cracking and leaking. Some tray molds make eight 4-ounce (113.4-gram) or single soap molds.

Another option is a 3-D mold. Go online and look at all the beautiful 3-D silicone molds available. (We've listed a few websites for these molds in Appendix D.)

Soap Stats _____

I once used a 3-D silicone mold of an angel on a soap bar. I poured the angel with white M&P. Once that part had set up, I melted more of the white M&P base, added pink colorant, and then poured the "bar" part of the mold. Once it was set, I carefully removed the soap. Using a silvery white mica called Sparks and an eye shadow brush, I dusted the angel with the mica. This enhanced all the details of the angel and made a beautiful bar of soap.

M&P Colorants, Additives, and Scents

You can use any colorant designed for soap in M&P soaps. Cosmetic-grade oxide and micas are also safe for coloring M&P soap.

You can use liquid soap colorants, but be sure they're soap-safe before adding to the M&P base. It only takes a drop or two to color the soap. Because M&P soap base is already a completed soap, what you see is what you get.

Many beautiful oxides and micas are available to color M&P soap. They come as a dry powder, so you'll need to wet the oxide or mica with a little oil or glycerin before you add it to the M&P soap base. It only takes a little colorant to color this type of soap.

Safety First _____

Please do not use crayons for coloring M&P soap. They are not intended for this purpose.

You can also use the oxides and/or micas dry and rub them on the soap after it has come out of the soap mold. Use your finger or a makeup brush to rub the micas onto the soap, or for more detailed work, try a thin paintbrush or an eyeliner brush.

You can also use natural herbs, ground spices, and cosmetic clays listed in Chapter 11 to add color to your M&P soap. Additives such as shea or cocoa butter are wonderful additions, too. Oatmeal ground to a very fine powder is a nice additive for a facial bar. It will help to gently exfoliate the skin.

Chamomile and calendula are the only dried flowers that will retain their color when added to the M&P soap. All other dried flowers will turn brown and yucky.

Start by using 1 teaspoon of your chosen additive per 1 pound of soap. If that's not enough, you can increase the amount, but don't use more than 1 tablespoon per pound.

With all skin- and soap-safe fragrance and essential oils, the recommended amount to use is 1 to 3 percent per pound. We've found that you use less with M&P than you do with cold or hot process soap. Add the scent just before you pour the soap into the mold. If you're only making one bar of soap at a time, use ¼ teaspoon (1.25 milliliters) of fragrance. Any more than that will be too strong.

Fun M&P Projects

You can make many fun projects with M&P soap base. Let your imagination run wild! Following are a few fun projects to get you started.

Making Soap Paints

For fun soap projects, you may want to make your own soap paints. This is very easy to do using micas, and the colors look beautiful and bright.

Here's what you need:

- Clear or light liquid dish soap
- Clear M&P soap base
- Mica or oxide colors

- Glycerin
- Alcohol (This helps the paint dry after you've painted with it.)

Make very small amounts of paint at a time so it doesn't dry out.

Start with 1 tablespoon (15 milliliters) liquid dish soap (or our Basic Household and Laundry Soap from Chapter 10!). Add 1 teaspoon (1.25 milliliters) glycerin and ½ to 1 teaspoon (2.5 to 5 milliliters) alcohol, and stir until well blended. Add a very small amount of the mica or oxide at a time, and stir until the colorant has evenly colored the base. If that's not enough color, add a little more until you reach the desired shade.

Use a paint brush to apply the paint to your soap. And for a little more pizzazz in your soap paint, add a little very fine glitter to the paint.

Making Soap Bar Embeds

Making embeds is fun and easy. You can make strips or even cut out shapes to put in soap you make later. Small cookie cutters are great to use for making embeds. Let your creative side loose and have some fun!

Choose your design and decide what color you want it to be. Melt and color your M&P soap base. Pour the soap into a small container until it's ¼ inch to ½ inch deep. Let the soap sit for about 5 minutes. Remove and, using the cookie cutters or a knife and template, cut out your shapes. You can now start making your soap bars.

To make a geometric design with M&P soap base, pour the cutouts as thick as the bar of soap will be so your design will be all the way through the soap bar. Most bars of soap are 1 to 1¼ inch thick, so pour the soap base for your cutout shapes accordingly. It will take more time for the thicker soap to set.

When it's time to add the M&P shapes to your soap, line a 5×6-inch mold. This mold will make four bars of soap, each 3 inches long, 2½ inches wide, and 1 to 1¼ inches thick.

Safety First

Don't let the soap become so hard that it's too brittle to cut into the geometric shapes. As soon as it feels firm to the touch, you can begin cutting your shapes.

Using a ruler, make marks on the box showing the bar's width and length. On the outside of the box, mark your pour-to line of 1 or 1½ inches. This will help you when you place your cutouts and tell you how full to fill the box with your remaining soap.

So you'll know how much base soap you need, weigh your cutouts. The 5×6-inch mold holds 26 ounces (737.1 grams) of soap and makes four 6.5-ounce (104.3-gram) bars. Subtract the weight of your cutouts from 26 ounces (737.1 grams) to determine how much soap base you need to fill the rest of the mold.

Carefully place your embed shapes in the mold and create your design. Then melt, color, and scent the remaining soap. Pour the base soap slowly and carefully around the cutout shapes, being careful not to disturb them. Set the mold aside and allow the soap to harden.

When the soap has hardened, remove it from the mold. Using a ruler, mark the cut lines and cut the bars.

Making Soapy Bath-Time Crayons

Children love to draw, and what could be more fun at bath time than to wash and draw in the tub with their own soapy crayons? Your kids (or grandkids) can use the soapy crayons to draw on the tile and tub. But never fear!—it washes right off with just a wipe of a rag.

You can buy premade crayon molds online or simply buy trays for making the long, thin ice cubes for sports-drink bottles. They are about 4 inches long and .5 inch around, and each tray makes 8 cubes—or in this case, soapy crayons.

Liquid colorants work best for this project. Sally uses red, blue, yellow, pink, green, and purple. You'll need about $\frac{1}{8}$ teaspoon (0.625 milliliter) of colorant per soapy crayon.

Using a paper towel, lightly coat the inside of the molds with Vaseline. Mix the colorant in the M&P soap base, and pour it into one cylinder of the ice tray. Do this with each color and then let the soap set.

When it's time to remove the soap, you may need to put it in the freezer for 15 minutes so it will retract from the sides of the ice cube tray. When you've removed all the soapy crayons from the mold, use a large pencil sharpener to sharpen one end.

Making Dipping Petals

These one-time-use soaps for hand-washing are a fun and popular item at weddings and parties—and they're very simple to make.

Start with silk rose or other flower petals. Some people also buy silk leaves for festive fall fun. You'll also need to find something to dry the dipped petals on. Or you can hang the petals, lay them out one at a time on a wire screen, or lay them out on waxed paper. Whichever you chose will be fine.

For this project you will need these:

- Clear M&P soap base
- Silk petals or leaves
- Fragrance oil
- Tweezers (to hold petal when dipping)
- Drying rack or waxed paper

Melt the soap base either on the stove in a double boiler or in the microwave set on 50 percent power. When the soap is melted, add the fragrance.

Using your tweezers, hold a petal by the tip and gently dip it into the soap base. Hold it over the soap container for a second so any extra soap can drip off the petal. Lay the petal out on the rack or paper and allow to dry. This only takes a few minutes. You can reheat the soap base whenever needed.

Keep these petals in a small, pretty dish beside the bathroom sink. Use one petal to wash your hands and then throw away the petal.

Final Thoughts

You can color and mold M&P soap to look like just about anything you can think of. It's easy to work with and can be used as soon as the soap comes out of the mold, with no wait time like with the lye methods. This chapter offered just a few of the many things you can do with M&P soap. The rest is up to you.

If you've read this book chapter by chapter, you should have a good foundation for becoming a great soap-maker. We've given you the main methods to make soap, many of our favorite recipes, as well as information we've learned from experience and experimenting. Don't be afraid to experiment and see what happens. Sometimes it's great, and sometimes it's not. We still have failures, even with all our experience, but that's just life and we make our notes and go on to make the next batch. Don't let a failed soap batch discourage you from trying again. The mistakes teach us the most and make the successes that much sweeter.

As we close this book, we'd like to say that it's been a pleasure and a privilege to share our combined knowledge of soap-making with you. We hope you'll enjoy making and using your own handcrafted soap for many years to come.

The Least You Need to Know

- Just about anything can be a mold for M&P soap. Use your imagination and see what you can come up with!

- M&P soap is kid-friendly, so let them join in the fun.

- Another bonus of M&P soap: there's no waiting or cure time—you can use it right away.

Glossary

additive A substance that's added to soap, such as herbs, honey, milk, colorants, fragrance, salt, or sugar. Anything other than oils, butter, water, and lye is an additive.

alkali An alkali is any sort of base that dissolves in water and also neutralizes acids. In soap-making, sodium hydroxide or potassium hydroxide are the alkalis.

aloe vera A plant whose juice or gel obtained from the leaves. It has soothing and healing properties.

antioxidant A substance that's synthetic or natural material that extends a product's shelf life.

ash A white, powderlike covering that forms on the surface of soap. It doesn't harm the soap and can be washed or wiped off.

base In soap-making, a base is your basic oils used in the soap recipe or the type of melt-and-pour soap you use. For cold and hot process soap, the base most soap-makers start with is olive, coconut, or palm oil.

beeswax Wax obtained from processing the honeycomb. It's used in candles, soaps, and lip balms. Beeswax reduces the lather in a soap.

bleaching A process used to remove the color of an oil or fat. Palm oil is a bright orange until it's bleached, when it lightens to a beige color.

borax Sodium borate, a white powdery mineral generally used as an emulsifier, water softener, pH buffer, viscosity modifier, foam booster, and stabilizer in liquid soap. Look for 20 Mule Team Borax, Natural Laundry Booster in stores. It's usually found close to the laundry soap.

Castile   A region in Spain known for producing olive oil–based soaps in the thirteenth century. Soap having a large percentage of olive oil is called Castile soap.

castor oil   Oil derived from the beans of the castor plant. It's used in soap for added creaminess, bubbly lather, and conditioning. It's also used in many cosmetic and body products.

caustic potash   *See* potassium hydroxide.

caustic soda   *See* sodium hydroxide.

coconut milk (CM)   The milk that comes from the fruit (nut) of the coconut tree. Like all milk, it contains sugars and will turn your soap dark if it's allowed to get hot during the gel stage.

coconut oil (CO)   An oil that's expeller-pressed from the fruit (nut) of the coconut tree. It's one of top cleansing oils used in soap-making.

cold process (CP)   A method of soap-making that relies on saponification for the heat to produce soap. The only heat that's applied is to melt the oils and butters.

colorants   Dyes, pigments, oxides, micas, neons, herbs, spices, and tea used to color soap. Never use children's crayons for colorants.

copra   The dried flesh or meat from a coconut, which coconut oil is obtained from.

cucumber   Puréed and added to soap at trace, cucumber can be used in facial creams, lotions, cleansers, and soaps. It's known for its astringent and soothing properties, as well as an anti-inflammatory agent.

cure   The time after a soap is made (about 4 to 6 weeks) during which the water evaporates out of the soap, making the bar harder. This is also the time needed for a soap that is 100 percent coconut to become mild and more user-friendly. This is the time needed for a high percentage of castor oil to let go of all its benefits of lather and moisturizing and make your soap bar luscious.

deodorized   The process during which some ingredients that have strong scents are removed from an oil or fat. Cocoa butter is a good example.

direct heat hot process (DHHP)   Hot process soap saponifying over direct heat from a stove burner, oven, or slow cooker.

double boiler hot process (DBHP)   The process of making hot process soap using a double boiler on a stove.

dreaded orange spots (DOS)   Spots that appear on soap that's going rancid from having a too-high iodine value.

embeds   Items placed inside a bar of soap. For example, if you see a blue bar of soap with a white dove in the middle of the bar, the dove is the embed.

emollient   Something that softens and lubricates the skin; it's moisturizing and soothing, and also stops itching and scaling of the skin.

essential oil (EO)   A liquid from a plant. It is distilled, highly concentrated, and very aromatic.

exothermic   The reaction between lye, fat, and water that results in soap.

felting   The process during which a soap bar is encased with wool to make a washcloth and soap in one.

fixative   An additive used to retain a scent in a soap.

fixed oil   Oil that can be raised to a high temperature without evaporating. Vegetable oil is a fixed oil. Fragrance and essential oils can evaporate.

fragrance oil (FO)   Synthetic oils that mimic natural fragrances and are used in soap, cosmetics, and candles. Only skin-safe fragrance oils can be used in soap.

gel stage   The final stage that soap goes through before it becomes soap. This is the stage some refer to as "applesauce." Most soap-makers want to have their soap go into this gel stage, but if you're making goat milk soap, you don't want this to happen. The extreme heat causes the soap to darken.

glycerin   Glycerin comes from the saponifying of oils and fats. It's a thick and clear by-product of soap-making and is used in cosmetics and many other products. It adds lather in soaps and helps prevent ash on the soap.

goat milk powder (GMP)   This is goat milk that's been dehydrated into a powder. Simply mix it with water to make it liquid again. It contains natural sugars that will turn your soap dark if it's allowed to get hot during the gel stage.

goat milk soap   Cold processed soap made with fresh, frozen, or powdered goat milk.

hard oils   Any oils that are solid at room temperature.

hot process (HP)   A soap-making method where the oils, water, and lye are cooked for a period of time using an external heat source such as a burner, slow cooker, double boiler, or oven to accelerate the saponification process. You can use hot process soap as soon as it comes out of the mold.

humectant   Absorbs and holds water or moisture from the air. Glycerin and honey are natural humectants.

hygroscopic   An ingredient such as lye that absorbs moisture from the air. If you put a few grains of lye on a saucer, soon little drops of water will appear where each grain of lye was. This is why it's so important to have the lye packaged in a plastic bag inside a lidded bucket. You can twist down the plastic bag onto the lye as you use it, and the bucket with lid keeps it safe from kids and animals.

immersion blender   A long, skinny, handheld blender used to blend milk shakes, smoothies—and soap!

infusion   A mixture made by steeping herbs in oil or water. It's then used in soap to get the benefit from the herbs.

International Nomenclature of Cosmetic Ingredients (INCI)   When labeling soaps marketed in the United States, the INCI name is required if you make any claims on the soap, such as "moisturizing." If you don't make any claims, you don't *have* to list anything on your soap. But it's wise to list all ingredients on the soap so people with allergies can decide if the soap is safe for them to use.

iodine in sap (INS)   A number derived from the iodine and saponification numbers found in SoapCalc that indicates a balanced bar.

KOH   *See* potassium hydroxide.

lanolin   Wool fat. This fatty, waxy substance is obtained from wool and used in soaps as a moisturizer.

lard   The semi-solid or solid fat rendered from a hog.

layering   The process of pouring different colors of soap into one mold, one layer at a time. Cold process soap works well for layering.

loofah   A tropical and subtropical vine in the Luffa family. They look a lot like deeply ridged rough-coated cucumbers. Before maturity it's edible as a vegetable, but after maturity, the inside material can be dried and used as an exfoliating sponge.

lye   The common name of sodium hydroxide (caustic soda) and potassium hydroxide (caustic potash).

melt-and-pour (M&P) soap   Soap that's basically a ready-made base you can melt, add fragrance and additives like shea to, and pour into a mold. If you're concerned about the dangers of using lye, try this lye-free soap.

melting point   The temperature that has to be attained before something becomes a liquid.

milling   The process of grating an already-made cold or hot processed soap batch or bars, remelting them on the stove top, and pouring the milled soap into molds. When the soap has melted, you can add butters, colorants, and scents to the soap before molding it into bars. Also called rebatching.

NaOH   *See* sodium hydroxide.

natural soap   Homemade soap made of natural ingredients, free of petroleum and chemicals.

natural source   Essential oils are derived from a natural source, plants.

oatmeal (OM)   Common oatmeal that, when ground to a fine powder, can be added to soap for sensitive skin.

oatmeal, milk, and honey (OMH)   The name of a fragrance oil often used by soap-makers.

oven hot process soap (OHP)   Cold process soap that's finished in the oven.

per pound of oil (PPO)   The ratio used to determine how much fragrance oil to use in a soap recipe.

pH   A scale used to measure the acidity or alkalinity of a substance. The scale goes from 0 (very acidic) to 14 (very alkaline), with 7 being neutral. Soap should have a pH between 9 and 10.5.

phthalates   A chemical compound used by fragrance manufacturers in the ready-made bases for stabilizing fragrance oils. Some of the ready-made bases used have higher or lower amounts of phthalates. Some types of phthalates are also used to make hard plastics soft and flexible, but those aren't the same type used in fragrance oil manufacturing.

potassium hydroxide (KOH)   A caustic, white granular powder used to make liquid soap.

pumice   A porous lava rock used in solid forms as a smoothing stone for dry heels. In powdered form, it acts as an abrasive and is good in mechanic's soap.

rebatching   The process of shredding soap; adding a small amount of liquid; and then melting over low heat, in a double boiler, or in the oven to save a ruined batch of soap.

refined   The process of removing all impurities from oil or butter.

refined, bleached, deodorized (RBD)   Oils such as coconut and palm that are refined, bleached, and deodorized.

rendering   The process of heating fat from a hog, cow, sheep, or deer to release the liquid oil. The liquid oil from hogs becomes lard. Tallow is from cows, sheep, and deer.

SAP   The value number of an oil that relates to the amount of potassium hydroxide or sodium hydroxide in milligrams required to saponify 1 gram oil.

saponification   The reaction of an alkali (base) with a fat or oil and water to form soap.

seize   A term used to describe soap that's changed from a lovely pourable mixture to a hard mass in the pot.

soap   The result of a combination of oils and fats reacting with an alkali.

soap on a stick   The term used to describe a batch of soap that's seized with the immersion blender still in it.

soda ash   A powdery white residue that can form on soap. It isn't harmful and can be removed by wiping it off. Glycerin added to your soap seems to stop this from happening.

sodium hydroxide   An alkali used to make bar soap, commonly called lye or caustic soda.

sodium lactate (SL)   This is the sodium salt that comes from lactic acid. It's used in soap to make the bar harder.

stainless steel (SS)   A type of metal that's nonreactive with lye so it's safe to use for soap-making.

stearic acid   An acid obtained from animal and vegetable fats used in soaps to make the bar harder.

super fatting   The process of reducing the amount of lye in the soap recipe so more oils are left unsaponified and can then soothe the skin.

synthetic   Something that's artificially produced. Fragrance oils, for example, are synthetic fragrances. Essential oils are natural and distilled from the actual plant and plant matter.

tallow   Hard fat obtained from around the organs of cattle, sheep, hogs, and deer. It was once used to make candles, leather dressing, and lubricants. The term now seems to refer to any fat rendered from cattle, sheep, hogs, and deer. Rendered hog fat oil is called lard.

titanium dioxide (TD)   An opaque white pigment in powder form that's used in many products such as cosmetics and soap. In soap, it's used to make the bar really white. It can also be mixed with other oxides to create pastel colors that are then added to or swirled into the soap.

tongue test   A test to see if any lye is still active in your soap. You can either touch the very end of your tongue to the soap or wet your finger and then touch your finger to your tongue. Either way, if you get a zap, burning sensation, or tingling, the lye is still active. Wait a day or so, and the lye will no longer be active.

trace   The term used when the soap is beginning to thicken like gravy. The term came about because when you drop a bit of the soap back on itself, it will leave a "trace" and remain visible for a little while on the surface.

turkey red oil (TRO)   An oil, also known as sulfated castor oil, you can use in liquid soap to add moisturizing. It's the only oil that's completely dispersed in water.

unrefined   A natural, unaltered state of an oil or butter that still has all the original color.

unsaponifiables   Components of the fat/oil that don't combine with the lye to form soap. Instead, these components contribute to the soap's moisturizing qualities.

vegetable shortening   A solid fat made from vegetable oils. Crisco is one example.

INCI Labeling Names

When making labels for your soap, you need to use the International Nomenclature of Cosmetic Ingredients (INCI) names of the oils you use in your soap. The following table lists both the botanical name and the label name for many different types of soap ingredients.

Botanical Name	Label Name
Almond (sweet) oil (*Prunus amygdalus*)	Prunus amygdalus (sweet almond) oil
Apricot kernel (*Prunus armeniaca*)	Prunus armeniaca (apricot kernel) oil
Avocado (*Persea gratissima*)	Persea gratissima (avocado) oil
Babassu (*Orbignya oleifera*)	Orbignya oleifera (babassu) oil
Canola (*Brassica campestris*)	Brassica campestris (canola) oil
Castor (*Ricinus communis*)	Ricinus communis (castor) seed oil
Cocoa butter (*Theobroma cacao*)	Theobroma cacao (cocoa) butter
Coconut oil (*Cocos nucifera*)	Cocos nucifera (coconut) oil
Corn oil (*Zea mays*)	Zea mays (corn) oil
Emu oil	Emu oil

Botanical Name	Label Name
Flaxseed oil (Linseed)	Linum usitatissimum (linseed) seed oil
Grapeseed (*Vitis vinifera*)	Vitis vinifera (grape) seed oil
Hemp seed oil (*Cannabis sativa*)	Cannabis sativa (hemp) seed oil
Illipe butter (*Shorea stenoptera*)	Shorea stenoptera (illipe) butter
Karanja (*Pongammia glabra*)	Pongammia glabra (karanja) oil
Kokum butter (*Garcinia indica*)	Garcinia indica (kokum) butter
Lanolin	Lanolin
Lard	Lard
Macadamia (*Macadamia integrifolia*)	Macadamia integrifolia (macadamia) oil
Mango butter (*Mangifera indica*)	Mangifera indica (mango) butter
Milk fat (Bovine)	Bovine (milk) fat
Neem seed oil (*Azadirachta indica*)	Azadirachta indica (neem) seed oil
Olive (*Olea europaea*)	Olea europaea (olive) oil
Olive oil pomace	Olea europaea (olive) oil pomace
Ostrich oil	Ostrich oil
Palm (*Elaesis guineensis*)	Elaesis guineensis (palm) fruit oil
Palm—red unrefined, bleach, or deodorized	Elaesis guineensis (palm) fruit oil
Palm kernel (*Elaesis guineensis*)	Elaesis guineensis (palm) kernel oil)
Peanut oil (*Arachis hypogaea*)	Arachis hypogaea (peanut) oil
Rice bran (*Oryza sativa*)	Oryza sativa (rice) bran oil
Sal butter (*Shorea robusta*)	Shorea robusta (sal) butter
Shea (*Butyrospermum parkii*)	Butyrospermum parkii (shea) butter
Soybean (*Glycine soja*)	Glycine soja (soybean) oil
Sunflower—high oleic (*Helianthus annuus*)	Helianthus annuus (sunflower) oil
Tallow, beef	Tallow (beef)

Appendix **C**

FDA Labeling Rules

When it comes to labeling, the FDA holds soap in a special category that needs a little extra explanation. The regulatory definition of soap is different from the way most people use the word. Products that meet the definition of soap are exempt from the provisions of the FD&C Act because—even though Section 201(i)(1) of the act includes "articles … for cleansing" in the definition of a cosmetic—Section 201(i)(2) excludes soap from the definition of a cosmetic.

How the FDA Defines Soap

Not every product marketed as soap meets the FDA's definition of the term. The FDA interprets the term *soap* to apply only when the following conditions are met:

♦ The bulk of the nonvolatile matter in the product consists of an alkali salt of fatty acids, and the product's detergent properties are due to the alkali-fatty acid compounds.

♦ The product is labeled, sold, and represented solely as soap (21 CFR 701.20).

Further, the FDA states that if a product intended to cleanse the human body does not meet all the criteria for soap, it's either a cosmetic or a drug. For example …

♦ If a product consists of detergents or primarily of alkali salts of fatty acids and is intended not only for cleansing but also for other cosmetic uses, such as beautifying or moisturizing, it's regulated as a cosmetic.

◆ If a product consists of detergents or primarily of alkali salts of fatty acids and is intended not only for cleansing but also to cure, treat, or prevent disease or to affect the structure or any function of the human body, it's regulated as a drug.

◆ If a product is intended solely for cleansing the human body and has the characteristics consumers generally associate with soap, but doesn't consist primarily of alkali salts of fatty acids, it may be identified in labeling as soap, but it's regulated as a cosmetic.

Defining "True" Soaps

"Ordinary" soap is made solely of fats and an alkali. In the past, homemade soap was made from animal fats and wood ashes. Today you'll find very few true soaps, in the traditional sense, on the market. There are a few; look for them marketed with terms such as *pure*. "True" soaps are regulated by the Consumer Product Safety Commission, not the FDA, and they don't require ingredient labeling.

Most commercial body cleansers are actually synthetic detergent products and come under the jurisdiction of the FDA. These detergent cleansers are popular because they produce suds easily and don't form gummy deposits. Some of these detergent products are actually marketed as soap, but they're not true soap in the common and legal definition of the word.

If a cosmetic claim, such as moisturizing or deodorizing, is made on the label of a true soap or cleanser, the product must meet all FDA requirements for a cosmetic, and the label must list all ingredients. An ingredient listing is not required on soaps that make no cosmetic claims.

If a drug claim, such as antibacterial, antiperspirant, or anti-acne, is made on a cleanser or soap, the product is considered a drug, and the label must list all active ingredients, as is required for all drug products.

Frequently Asked Questions About Labeling

Do I have to put the weight on my soap? Yes, you have to include the exact weight, and it cannot be "approximately 5 ounces" or "not less than 5 ounces" To get an accurate weight, weigh the same bar of soap, freshly made, at 6 months old, and again at 1 year old. The last weight, at 1 year, is what you should put on the package.

We're guessing your soap will lose between .6 to .9 ounces over the year. Our soap loses .6 ounces in a year's time. If you use full water to make your soap, yours will lose even more.

When we plane our soap, we make sure it's 5.7 ounces. With the soap cut at that size, it will be 5 ounces when it's old. So if we put "5 ounces" on the package, that will be acceptable by the rules and regulations of soap.

Do I have to put my name and address on my soap if I sell it? Yes, you do. You don't have to put your phone number, but you can if you want to.

Appendix D

Resources

Now that you've got the soap-making bug, we're sure you'll want to expand your skills and learn even more. Here are some of our favorite venders to help you find the supplies and ingredients you'll need.

Lye and Oils

Boyer Corporation
PO Box 10
La Grange, IL 60525
1-800-323-3040
www.boyercorporation.com

Oils by Nature
30300 Solon Industrial Parkway,
Suite E
Solon, OH 44139
440-498-1180
info@oilsbynature.com
www.oilsbynature.com

Soaper's Choice
A division of Columbus Foods
Company
30 E Oakton Avenue
Des Plaines, IL 60018
Contact: Mike Lawson
773-265-6500 or 1-800-322-6457
www.soaperschoice.com

Soap Colorants

Apples, Woods and Berries
www.awbsupplies.com/berry-liscious_
colors.htm

Ellen's Essentials
Houston, Texas 77072
www.ellensessentials.com

Select Shades
PO Box 1220
Bath, SC 29842
803-593-0675 (for orders)
www.selectshades.com/chart/clear.html

TKB Trading, LLC
1101 9th Avenue
Oakland, CA 94606
510-451-9011
tkbtrading@sbcglobal.net
www.tkbtrading.com

Soap Molds

Anhoki's Place
www.bunniesworkshop.com/soap_molds.
html

Kelsei's Creations
3193 W FM 2002
Lamesa, TX 79331
806-462-7370
www.kelseiscreations.com

Milky Way Molds
www.milkywaymolds.com

Upland Soap Factory
213 Flynn Branch Road
Marshall, NC 28753
828-649-0303
www.uplandsoapfactory.com

Essential and Fragrance Oils

Camden-Grey
3579 NW 82 Avenue
Doral, FL 33122
305-500-9630 or 1-866-503-8615
www.camdengrey.com

Stony Mountain Botanicals
www.wildroots.com

Wholesale Supplies Plus, Inc.
www.wholesalesuppliesplus.com

General Soap-Making Supplies

Apples, Woods and Berries
www.awbsupplies.com
(This is Sally's shop. She carries highly concentrated fragrance oils for soap and all bath and body products. You can also find soap colorants and cosmetic-grade oxides for making mineral makeup here.)

Bramble Berry, Inc.
2138 Humboldt Street
Bellingham, WA 98225
(not open to the public; online orders only)
360-734-8278 or 1-877-627-7883
www.brambleberry.com

Kangaroo Blue
PO Box 9021
Naperville, IL 60567-9021
630-999-8132
www.kangarooblue.com

Oregon Trail Soap Supplies and More
PO Box 669
Rogue River, OR 97537
541-582-3393
www.oregontrailsoaps.com

Taylored Concepts, Inc.
12021 Plano Road, Suite #190
Dallas, TX 75243
972-671-5661 or 1-866-322-9944
www.tayloredconcepts.com

Wholesale Supplies Plus, Inc.
10035 Broadview Road
Broadview Heights, OH 44147
440-526-6556 or 1-800-359-0944
www.wholesalesuppliesplus.com

Packaging Supplies

Shrink Wrap Store
www.shrinkwrapstore.com

Wholesale Supply Plus, Inc.
www.wholesalesuppliesplus.com

Yahoo! Soap-Makers Groups

AplesNBerries@yahoo.com
This is Sally's group. You can find us here just about any day of the week. We answer all questions and teach soap-making as well as other bath and body products on this group.

SoapMaker_Haven@yahoo.com
This is a wonderful list co-owned by two of our very good friends. San, the leader, is one of Sally's very closest and trusted friends. These ladies are always willing to help if a list-member is in need.

TheRedBarn@yahoo.com
Suz, of Oregon Trail Soap, Supplies, and More Soap owns this soap-maker's group. She covers lots of activities as well as specials and sales announcements for Oregon Trail.

Index